PA...
QUIC... ...S

Textbook of Pathology
7th Edition

PATHOLOGY
QUICK REVIEW AND MCQs
FOURTH EDITION

Based on
Textbook of Pathology
7th Edition

Harsh Mohan
MD, FAMS, FICPath, FUICC
Professor & Head
Department of Pathology
Government Medical College
Sector-32A, Chandigarh-160 031
INDIA

E-mail: *drharshmohan@gmail.com*

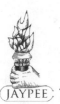 JAYPEE The Health Sciences Publishers

New Delhi | London | Philadelphia | Panama

Jaypee Brothers Medical Publishers (P) Ltd.

Headquarters
Jaypee Brothers Medical Publishers (P) Ltd.
4838/24, Ansari Road, Daryaganj
New Delhi 110 002, India
Phone: +91-11-43574357
Fax: +91-11-43574314
Email: jaypee@jaypeebrothers.com

Overseas Offices

J.P. Medical Ltd.
83, Victoria Street, London
SW1H 0HW (UK)
Phone: +44-20 3170 8910
Fax: +044(0)20 3008 6180
Email: info@jpmedpub.com

Jaypee Medical Inc.
The Bourse
111, South Independence Mall East
Suite 835, Philadelphia, PA 19106, USA
Phone: +1 267-519-9789
Email: jpmed.us@jaypeebrothers.com

Jaypee Brothers Medical Publishers (P) Ltd.
Bhotahity, Kathmandu, Nepal
Phone: +977-9741283608
Email: kathmandu@jaypeebrothers.com

Jaypee-Highlights Medical Publishers Inc.
City of Knowledge, Bld. 237, Clayton
Panama City, Panama
Phone: +1 507-301-0496
Fax: +1 507-301-0499
Email: cservice@jphmedical.com

Jaypee Brothers Medical Publishers (P) Ltd.
17/1-B, Babar Road, Block-B, Shaymali
Mohammadpur, Dhaka-1207
Bangladesh
Mobile: +08801912003485
Email: jaypeedhaka@gmail.com

Website: www.jaypeebrothers.com
Website: www.jaypeedigital.com

© 2015, Harsh Mohan

Pathology Quick Review and MCQs

First Edition : 2000
Second Edition : 2005
Third Edition : 2010
Reprint : 2013
Fourth Edition : 2015

Assistant Editors: Praveen Mohan, Tanya Mohan, Sugandha Mohan

ISBN: 978-93-5152-370-3

Printed at Replika Press Pvt. Ltd.

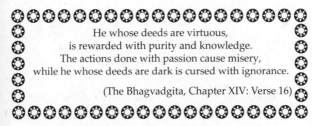

He whose deeds are virtuous,
is rewarded with purity and knowledge.
The actions done with passion cause misery,
while he whose deeds are dark is cursed with ignorance.

(The Bhagvadgita, Chapter XIV: Verse 16)

To my family, friends, colleagues and students,
All of you matter so much to me ......
Life would truly be so incomplete without you!

Preface

I am pleased to present 4th revised Edition of *Pathology Quick Review and MCQs* for users of my 7th Edition of *Textbook of Pathology* as a package. Based on feedback from users of previous edition who found this condensed material very useful and attractive, the past practice of this combination of new edition of companion-book with revised edition of the mainbook started 15 years back has been continued this time too. Thus, the revised editions of both the books have been prepared and released simultaneously.

This pocket-sized, handy and user-friendly book is the abridged version of 7th revised edition of my textbook, yet containing adequate learning material, and is aimed to serve the following purposes:

❖ For beginner students of Pathology who have undertaken an in-depth study of the mainbook earlier may like to revise the subject in a relatively short time from this book and may also undertake self-test on the MCQs given at the end of each chapter.

❖ For senior students, interns and those preparing for their postgraduate and other entrance examinations or interview who are confronted with revision of vast medical subjects in a limited time, this book is expected to act as the main source material for quick revision and also expose them to MCQs based on applied pathology.

❖ The material contained in the book may be considered adequate for students of some courses such as those pursuing paramedical courses.

Pathology Quick Review book has the same 28 chapters divided into three sections as in the main textbook—*Section I:* Chapters 1-9 (General Pathology), *Section II:* Chapters 10-12 (Haematology and Lymphoreticular Tissues), *Section III:* Chapters 13-28 (Systemic Pathology) and three *Appendices (A-I:* Basic Diagnostic Cytology, *A-II:* Clinical Cases and *A-III:* Normal Values). Each major heading in the small book has cross-references of page numbers of the 7th edition of my textbook so that an avid and inquisitive reader interested in simultaneous consultation of the topic or for clarification of a doubt, may refer to it conveniently. Self-Assessment by MCQs given at the end of every chapter which sets this book apart from other pocket-books, has over 50 new questions, mostly on clinical focus, raising their number to over 750 MCQs in the revised edition, besides modifying many old ones. While much more knowledge has been condensed in the baby-book from the added material in the main textbook, effort has been made to keep its volume reasonable. It is hoped that the book with enhanced and updated contents continues to be user-friendly in learning the essential aspects of pathology, while at the same time, retaining the ease with which it can be conveniently carried by the users in the pocket of their white coats.

Preparation of this little book necessitated selection from enhanced information contained in the revised edition of my textbook and therefore, required application of my discretion. In this regards, generous suggestions and comments from colleagues and users of earlier edition have been quite helpful and are gratefully acknowledged.

I thank profusely the entire staff of M/s Jaypee Brothers Medical Publishers (P) Ltd, New Delhi, India, for their ever-smiling support and coope-ration in completion of the book in a relatively short time, just after we had completed the mammoth task of revision work of 7th edition of the main textbook.

Finally, although sincere effort has been made to be as accurate as possible, element of human error is still likely; I shall humbly request the users to continue giving their valuable suggestions directed at further improvements of its contents.

Government Medical College
Sector-32A
Chandigarh-160 031
INDIA
E-mail: *drharshmohan@gmail.com*

Harsh Mohan
MD, FAMS, FICPath, FUICC
Professor & Head
Department of Pathology

Contents

Abbreviations Used

Throughout the book following abbreviations have been used:

G/A   for Gross Appearance.

M/E   for Microscopic Examination.

EM   for Electron Microscopy.

IF   for Immunofluorescence Microscopy.

1 Introduction to Pathology

STUDY OF PATHOLOGY *(p. 1)*

The word *'Pathology'* is derived from two Greek words—*pathos* (meaning suffering) and *logos* (meaning study). Pathology is, thus, scientific study of changes in the structure and function of the body in disease.

For the student of any system of medicine, the discipline of pathology forms a vital bridge between initial learning phase of preclinical sciences and the final phase of clinical subjects.

HEALTH AND DISEASE *(p. 1)*

In simple language, disease is opposite of health i.e. what is not healthy is disease. *Health* may be defined as a condition when the individual is in complete accord with the surroundings, while *disease* is loss of ease (or comfort) to the body (i.e. dis+ease).

COMMON TERMS IN PATHOLOGY *(p. 1)*

It is important for a beginner in pathology to be familiar with the language used in pathology:

◆ *Patient* is the person affected by disease.

◆ *Lesions* are the characteristic changes in tissues and cells produced by disease in an individual or experimental animal.

◆ *Pathologic changes* or *morphology* consist of examination of diseased tissues. These can be recognised with the naked eye *(gross or macroscopic changes)* or are studied by *microscopic examination* of tissues.

◆ Causal factors responsible for the lesions are included in *etiology* of disease (i.e. 'why' of disease).

◆ Mechanism by which the lesions are produced is termed *pathogenesis* of disease (i.e. 'how' of disease).

◆ Functional implications of the lesion felt by the patient are *symptoms* and those discovered by the clinician are the *physical signs*.

◆ Clinical significance of the morphologic and functional changes together with results of other investigations which help to arrive at an answer to what is wrong *(diagnosis)*, what is going to happen *(prognosis)*, what can be done about it *(treatment)*, and finally what should be done to avoid complications and spread *(prevention)* (i.e. 'what' of disease).

EVOLUTION OF PATHOLOGY *(p. 2)*

Pathology as the scientific study of disease processes has its deep roots in medical history. Pathology has evolved over the years as a distinct discipline from anatomy, medicine and surgery, in that sequence.

PREHISTORIC TIMES TO MEDIEVAL PERIOD *(p. 2)*

Present-day knowledge of primitive culture which was prevalent in the world in prehistoric times reveals that religion, magic and medical treatment were quite linked to each other in those times. The link between medicine and religion became so firmly established throughout the world that different societies had their gods and goddesses of healing; for example:

mythological Greeks had *Aesculapius* and *Apollo* as the principal gods of healing, *Dhanvantri* as the deity of medicine in India.

The insignia of healing, the Caduceus, having snake and staff, is believed to represent the god Hermes or Mercury, which according to Greek mythology has power of healing since snake has regenerative powers expressed by its periodic sloughing of its skin.

But the real practice of medicine began with *Hippocrates* (460–370 BC), the great Greek clinical genius of all times and regarded as 'the father of medicine'. Hippocrates dissociated medicine from religion and magic. Instead, he firmly believed in study of patient's symptoms and described methods of diagnosis. Hippocrates followed rational and ethical attitudes in practice and teaching of medicine and is revered by the medical profession by taking *'Hippocratic oath'* at the time of entry into practice of medicine.

Galen postulated humoral theory, later called Galenic theory. This theory suggested that the illness resulted from imbalance between *four humors* (or body fluids): blood, lymph, black bile (believed at that time to be from the spleen), and biliary secretion from the liver. The hypothesis of disequilibrium of four elements constituting the body *(Dhatus)* similar to Hippocratic doctrine finds mention in ancient Indian medicine books compiled about 200 AD—*Charaka Samhita*, a finest document by *Charaka* on medicine and *Sushruta Samhita,* similar book of surgical sciences by *Sushruta*.

HUMAN ANATOMY AND ERA OF GROSS PATHOLOGY (p. 3)

Dissection of human body was started by *Vesalius* (1514–1564) on freshly executed criminals. His pupils, *Gabriel Fallopius* (1523–1562) who described human oviducts (Fallopian tubes) and *Fabricius* who discovered lymphoid tissue around the intestine of birds (bursa of Fabricius) further popularised the practice of human anatomic dissection for which special postmortem amphitheatres came in to existence in various parts of ancient Europe.

Antony van Leeuwenhoek (1632–1723), a cloth merchant by profession in Holland, during his spare time invented the first ever microscope by grinding the lenses himself. *Marcello Malpighi* (1624–1694) used microscope extensively and observed the presence of capillaries and described the malpighian layer of the skin, and lymphoid tissue in the spleen (malpighian corpuscles). Malpighi is known as 'the father of histology.' The credit for beginning of the study of morbid anatomy (pathologic anatomy), however, goes to Italian anatomist-pathologist, *Giovanni B. Morgagni* (1682–1771). He, laid the foundations of clinicopathologic methodology in the study of disease and introduced the concept of clinicopathologic correlation (CPC), establishing a coherent sequence of cause, lesions, symptoms, and outcome of disease.

The era of gross pathology had three more illustrious and brilliant physician-pathologists in England who were colleagues at Guy's Hospital in London:

❖ *Richard Bright* (1789–1858) who described non-suppurative nephritis, later termed glomerulonephritis or Bright's disease;

❖ *Thomas Addison* (1793–1860) who gave an account of chronic adrenocortical insufficiency termed Addison's disease; and

❖ *Thomas Hodgkin* (1798–1866), who observed the complex of chronic enlargement of lymph nodes, often with enlargement of the liver and spleen, later called Hodgkin's disease.

R.T.H. Laennec (1781–1826), another French physician, dominated the early part of 19th century by his numerous discoveries. He described several lung diseases (tubercles, caseous lesions, miliary lesions, pleural effusion, and bronchiectasis), chronic sclerotic liver disease (later called Laennec's cirrhosis) and invented stethoscope. Morbid anatomy attained its zenith with appearance of *Carl F. von Rokitansky* (1804–1878), self-taught German pathologist who performed nearly 30,000 autopsies himself.

ERA OF TECHNOLOGY DEVELOPMENT AND CELLULAR PATHOLOGY *(p. 4)*

Pathology started developing as a diagnostic discipline in later half of the 19th century with the evolution of cellular pathology which was closely linked to technology advancements in machinery manufacture for cutting thin sections of tissue, improvement in microscope, and development of chemical industry and dyes for staining. The discovery of existence of disease-causing micro-organisms was made by French chemist *Louis Pasteur* (1822–1895), thus demolishing the prevailing theory of spontaneous generation of disease and firmly established germ theory of disease. Subsequently, *G.H.A. Hansen* (1841–1912) in Germany identified Hansen's bacillus in 1873 as the first microbe causative for leprosy (Hansen's disease).

Developments in chemical industry helped in switch over from earlier dyes of plant and animal origin to synthetic dyes. Simultaneous technological advances in machinery manufacture led to development and upgrading of microtomes for obtaining thin sections of organs and tissues for staining by dyes for enhancing detailed study of sections.

Until the end of the 19th century, the study of morbid anatomy had remained largely autopsy-based and thus had remained a retrospective science. *Rudolf Virchow* (1821–1905) in Germany is credited with the beginning of microscopic examination of diseased tissue at cellular level and thus began histopathology as a method of investigation. Virchow hypothesised cellular theory having following two components:

◈ All cells come from other cells.

◈ Disease is an alteration of normal structure and function of these cells.

Virchow was revered as Pope in pathology in Europe and is aptly known as the 'father of cellular pathology'.

Karl Landsteiner (1863–1943) described the existence of major human blood groups in 1900 and is considered "father of blood transfusion"; he was awarded Nobel prize in 1930.

The development of exfoliative cytology for early detection of cervical cancer began with *George N. Papanicolaou* (1883–1962), a Greek-born, American pathologist, in 1930s and is known as 'father of exfoliative cytology'.

MODERN PATHOLOGY *(p. 6)*

Following strides made in the latter half of 20th century until recent times in 21st century have made it possible to study diseases at genetic and molecular level, and provide an evidence-based and objective diagnosis that may enable the physician to institute targeted therapy:

◈ Description of *the structure of DNA* of the cell by Watson and Crick in 1953.

◈ Identification of *chromosomes and their correct number* in humans (46) by *Tijo* and *Levan* in 1956.

◈ The era of *stem cell research* started in 2000s by harvesting these primitive cells isolated from embryos and maintaining their growth in the laboratory. There are 2 types of sources of stem cells in humans: embryonic stem cells and adult stem cells, the former being more numerous. Stem cells are seen by many researchers as having virtually unlimited applications in the treatment of many human diseases such as Alzheimer's disease, diabetes, cancer, strokes, etc.

◈ *Human Genome Project (HGP)* consisting of a consortium of countries was completed in April 2003 coinciding with 50 years of description of DNA double helix by Watson and Crick in April 1953. The sequencing of human genome reveals that it contains approximately 3 billion base pairs of amino acids, which are located in the 23 pairs of chromosomes within the nucleus of each human cell. Each chromosome contains an estimated 30,000 genes in the human genome which carry the instructions for making proteins. The

HGP has given us the ability to read nature's complete genetic blueprint used in making of each human being (i.e. gene mapping).

TELEPATHOLOGY AND VIRTUAL MICROSCOPY (p. 7)

Telepathology is defined as the practice of diagnostic pathology by a remote pathologist utilising images of tissue specimens transmitted over a telecommunication network. The main *components* of a telepathology system are as under:

◈ Conventional light microscope.
◈ Method of image capture, commonly a camera mounted on light microscope.
◈ Telecommunications link between sending and receiving side.
◈ Workstation at receiving end with a high quality monitor.

Depending upon need and budget, telepathology system is of two *types*:
1. Static (store-and-forward, passive telepathology).
2. Dynamic (Robotic interactive telepathology).

SUBDIVISIONS OF PATHOLOGY (p. 7)

Human pathology is conventionally studied under two broad divisions: *General Pathology* dealing with general principles of disease, and *Systemic Pathology* that includes study of diseases pertaining to the specific organs and body systems. In general, the study of pathology includes morphological and non-morphological disciplines as follows:

MORPHOLOGICAL BRANCHES (p. 7)

These branches essentially involve application of microscope as an essential tool for the study and include histopathology, cytopathology and haematology.

A. HISTOPATHOLOGY Histopathology, used synonymously with anatomic pathology, pathologic anatomy, morbid anatomy, or tissue pathology, is the classic method of study and still the most useful one which has stood the test of time. Anatomic pathology includes the following subdivisions:

1. **Surgical pathology** It deals with the study of tissues removed from the living body by biopsy or surgical resection.

2. **Experimental pathology** This is defined as production of disease in the experimental animal and study of morphological changes in organs after sacrificing the animal.

3. **Forensic pathology and autopsy work** This includes the study of organs and tissues removed at postmortem for medicolegal work and for determining the underlying sequence and cause of death. The significance of a careful postmortem examination is appropriately summed up in the old saying 'the dead teach the living'.

B. CYTOPATHOLOGY It includes study of cells shed off from the lesions (exfoliative cytology) and fine-needle aspiration cytology (FNAC) of superficial and deep-seated lesions for diagnosis (Appendix I).

C. HAEMATOLOGY Haematology deals with the diseases of blood. It includes laboratory haematology and clinical haematology.

NON-MORPHOLOGICAL BRANCHES (p. 8)

These diagnostic branches of pathology include clinical pathology, clinical biochemistry, microbiology, immunology, genetics and molecular pathology. In these diagnostic branches, qualitative, semi-quantitative or quantitative determinations are carried out in the laboratory. Microscope may also be required for at least some of these lab tests.

1. The concept of clinicopathologic correlation (CPC) by study of morbid anatomy was introduced by:
   A. Hippocrates
   B. Virchow
   C. John Hunter
   D. Morgagni

2. ABO human blood group system was first described by:
   A. Edward Jenner
   B. Karl Landsteiner
   C. Hippocrates
   D. Laennec

3. Structure of DNA of the cell was described by:
   A. Watson and Crick
   B. Tijo and Levan
   C. Ruska and Lorries
   D. Barbara McClintock

4. Exact number of human chromosomes was first described in the year:
   A. 1947
   B. 1950
   C. 1953
   D. 1956

5. Which of the following was discovered first in human beings:
   A. Number of chromosomes
   B. Structure of DNA
   C. In situ hybridisation
   D. Polymerase chain reaction

6. Father of cellular pathology is:
   A. Carl Rokitansky
   B. Rudolf Virchow
   C. G. Morgagni
   D. FT Schwann

7. Humans genome consists of following approximate number of genes:
   A. 20,000
   B. 30,000
   C. 50,000
   D. 100,000

8. Stem cell research consists of:
   A. Human cells grown in vitro
   B. Plant cells grown in vitro
   C. Cadaver cells grown in vitro
   D. Synonymous with PCR

9. Human genome project was completed in:
   A. 2001
   B. 2002
   C. 2003
   D. 2004

10. Frozen section is employed for the following purposes except:
    A. Fat demonstration
    B. Amyloid
    C. Rapid diagnosis
    D. Enzymes

11. For frozen section, the tissue should be sent to the laboratory as under:
    A. In 10% formalin
    B. In Carnoy's fixative
    C. In saline
    D. Fresh unfixed

12. Usual chromogens used in immunohistochemical staining techniques impart the following colour to indicate positivity:
    A. Pink
    B. Blue
    C. Brown
    D. Red

13. Immunohistochemistry is employed for the following purpose:
    A. To distinguish neoplastic from non-neoplastic lesion
    B. To distinguish benign and malignant lesion
    C. To localise the cell of origin of tumour
    D. To detect autoantibodies in the serum

KEY

1 = D	2 = B	3 = A	4 = D	5 = B
6 = B	7 = B	8 = A	9 = C	10 = B
11 = D	12 = C	13 = C		

2

Cell Injury, Cellular Adaptations and Cellular Ageing

CELL INJURY (p. 9)

Cell injury is defined as the effect of a variety of stresses due to etiologic agents a cell encounters, resulting in changes in its internal and external environment. The cellular response to stress may vary and depends upon following two variables:

i)   Host factors i.e. the type of cell and tissue involved.
ii) Factors pertaining to injurious agent i.e. extent and type of cell injury.
     Various forms of cellular responses to cell injury may be as follows:

1.   When there is increased functional demand, the cell may adapt to the changes which are expressed morphologically, which then revert back to normal after the stress is removed (*cellular adaptations*).

2.   When the stress is mild to moderate, the injured cell may recover (*reversible cell injury*), while persistent and severe form of cell injury may cause cell death (*irreversible cell injury*).

3.   The residual effects of reversible cell injury may persist in the cell as evidence of cell injury at subcellular level (*subcellular changes*), or metabolites may accumulate within the cell (*intracellular accumulations*).

ETIOLOGY OF CELL INJURY (p. 9)

The cells may be broadly injured by two major ways:
A.   Genetic causes
B.   Acquired causes
     The acquired causes of disease comprise vast majority of common diseases afflicting mankind. Based on underlying agent, the acquired causes of cell injury can be further categorised as under:

1.   Hypoxia and ischaemia
2.   Physical agents
3.   Chemical agents and drugs
4.   Microbial agents
5.   Immunologic agents
6.   Nutritional derangements
7.   Ageing
8.   Psychogenic diseases
9.   Iatrogenic factors
10. Idiopathic diseases.

HYPOXIA AND ISCHAEMIA   Cells of different tissues essentially require oxygen to generate energy and perform metabolic functions. Deficiency of oxygen or hypoxia results in failure to carry out these activities by the cells. Hypoxia is the most common cause of cell injury. Hypoxia may result from the following 2 ways:

◈   The most common mechanism of hypoxic cell injury is by reduced supply of blood to cells due to interruption i.e. ischaemia.

◈   Hypoxia may also result from impaired blood supply from causes other than interruption e.g. disorders of oxygen-carrying RBCs (e.g. anaemia, carbon monoxide poisoning), heart diseases, lung diseases and increased demand of tissues.

PHYSICAL AGENTS   (i) mechanical trauma (e.g. road accidents); (ii) thermal trauma (e.g. by heat and cold); (iii) electricity; (iv) radiation (e.g. ultraviolet and ionising); and (v) rapid changes in atmospheric pressure.

CHEMICALS AND DRUGS (i) chemical poisons such as cyanide, arsenic, mercury; (ii) strong acids and alkalis; (iii) environmental pollutants; (iv) insecticides and pesticides; (v) oxygen at high concentrations; (vi) hypertonic glucose and salt; (vii) social agents such as alcohol and narcotic drugs; and (viii) therapeutic administration of drugs.

MICROBIAL AGENTS Injuries by microbes include infections caused by bacteria, rickettsiae, viruses, fungi, protozoa, metazoa, and other parasites.

IMMUNOLOGIC AGENTS Immunity is a 'double-edged sword'—it protects the host against various injurious agents but it may also turn lethal and cause cell injury e.g.
i) immunodeficiency diseases;
ii) hypersensitivity reactions;
iii) anaphylactic reactions; and
iv) autoimmune diseases.

NUTRITIONAL DERANGEMENTS A deficiency or an excess of nutrients may result in nutritional imbalances.
◈ Nutritional deficiency diseases may be due to overall deficiency of nutrients (e.g. starvation), of protein calorie (e.g. marasmus, kwashiorkor), of minerals (e.g. anaemia), or of trace elements.
◈ Nutritional excess is a problem of affluent societies resulting in obesity, atherosclerosis, heart disease and hypertension.

AGEING Cellular ageing or senescence leads to impaired ability of the cells to undergo replication and repair, and ultimately lead to cell death culminating in death of the individual.

PSYCHOGENIC DISEASES There are no specific biochemical or morpho-logic changes in common acquired mental diseases due to mental stress, strain, anxiety, overwork and frustration e.g. depression, schizophrenia. However, problems of drug addiction, alcoholism, and smoking result in various organic diseases such as liver damage, chronic bronchitis, lung cancer, peptic ulcer, hypertension, ischaemic heart disease etc.

IATROGENIC CAUSES Although as per Hippocratic oath, every physician is bound not to do or administer anything that causes harm to the patient, there are some diseases as well as deaths attributed to iatrogenic causes (owing to physician).

IDIOPATHIC DISEASES Idiopathic means "of unknown cause". Finally, although so much is known about the etiology of diseases, there still remain many diseases for which exact cause is undetermined. For example, most common form of hypertension (90%) is idiopathic (or essential) hypertension.

PATHOGENESIS OF CELL INJURY *(p. 10)*

The underlying alterations in biochemical systems of cells for reversible and irreversible cell injury by various agents are complex and varied. However, in general, irrespective of the type, following common scheme applies to most forms of cell injury by various agents:

1.   Factors pertaining to etiologic agent and host (i) Type, duration and severity of injurious agent; (ii) Type, status and adaptability of target cell.

2.   Common underlying mechanisms Irrespective of other factors, following essential intracellular biochemical phenomena underlie all forms of cell injury:
i) Mitochondrial damage causing ATP depletion.
ii) Cell membrane damage disturbing the metabolic and trans-membrane exchanges.
iii) Release of toxic free radicals.

3.   Usual morphologic changes The morphologic changes of rever-sible cell injury (e.g. hydropic swelling) appear earlier while later morphologic alterations of cell death are seen (e.g. in myocardial infarction).

4.   Functional implications and disease outcome Eventually, cell injury affects cellular function adversely which has bearing on the body.

Consequently, clinical features in the form of symptoms and signs would appear.

PATHOGENESIS OF ISCHAEMIC AND HYPOXIC INJURY

Ischaemia and hypoxia are the most common forms of cell injury. Although underlying intracellular mechanisms and ultrastructural changes seen in reversible and irreversible cell injury by hypoxia-ischaemia (depending upon extent of hypoxia and type of cells involved) are a continuation of the process, these mechanisms are discussed separately below.

REVERSIBLE CELL INJURY If the ischaemia or hypoxia is of short duration, the effects may be reversible on rapid restoration of circulation e.g. in coronary artery occlusion, myocardial contractility, metabolism and ultrastructure are reversed if the circulation is quickly restored. The sequential biochemical and ultrastructural changes in reversible cell injury are as under.

1.   Decreased generation of cellular ATP: Damage by ischaemia from interruption *versus* hypoxia from other causes All living cells require continuous supply of oxygen to produce ATP which is essentially required for a variety of cellular functions (e.g. membrane transport, protein synthesis, lipid synthesis and phospholipid metabolism). ATP in human cell is derived from 2 sources:
◈   *Firstly,* by aerobic respiration or oxidative phosphorylation (which requires oxygen) in the mitochondria.
◈   *Secondly,* cells may subsequently switch over to anaerobic glycolytic oxidation to maintain constant supply of ATP (in which ATP is generated from glucose/glycogen in the absence of oxygen).
    Ischaemia due to interruption in blood supply as well as hypoxia from other causes limit the supply of oxygen to the cells, thus causing decreased ATP generation from ADP:
◈   In *ischaemia* from interruption of blood supply, aerobic respiration as well as glucose availability are both compromised resulting in more severe and faster effects of cell injury. Ischaemic cell injury also causes accumulation of metabolic waste products in the cells.
◈   On the other hand, in *hypoxia from other causes* (RBC disorders, heart disease, lung disease), anaerobic glycolytic ATP generation continues, and thus cell injury is less severe.
    However, highly specialised cells such as myocardium, proximal tubular cells of the kidney, and neurons of the CNS are dependent solely on aerobic respiration for ATP generation and thus these tissues suffer from ill-effects of ischaemia more severely and rapidly.

2.   Intracellular lactic acidosis: Nuclear clumping Due to low oxygen supply to the cell, aerobic respiration by mitochondria fails first. This is followed by switch to anaerobic glycolytic pathway for the requirement of energy (i.e. ATP). This results in rapid depletion of glycogen and accumulation of lactic acid lowering the intracellular pH.

3.   Damage to plasma membrane pumps: Hydropic swelling and other membrane changes Lack of ATP interferes in generation of phospholipids from the cellular fatty acids which are required for continuous repair of membranes. This results in damage to membrane pumps operating for regulation of sodium-potassium and calcium.

4.   Reduced protein synthesis: Dispersed ribosomes As a result of continued hypoxia, membranes of endoplasmic reticulum and Golgi apparatus swell up. Ribosomes are detached from granular (rough) endoplasmic reticulum and polysomes are degraded to monosomes, thus dispersing ribosomes in the cytoplasm and inactivating their function. Similar reduced protein synthesis occurs in Golgi apparatus.
    Ultrastructural evidence of reversible cell membrane damage is seen in the form of loss of microvilli, intramembranous particles and focal projections of the cytoplasm (blebs). *Myelin figures* may be seen lying in the cytoplasm or present outside the cell.

Up to this point, withdrawal of acute stress that resulted in reversible cell injury can restore the cell to normal state.

IRREVERSIBLE CELL INJURY Persistence of ischaemia or hypoxia results in irreversible damage to the structure and function of the cell (cell death). Two essential phenomena always distinguish irreversible from reversible cell injury.

◈ Inability of the cell to reverse *mitochondrial dysfunction* on reperfusion or reoxygenation.

◈ *Disturbance in cell membrane function* in general, and in plasma membrane in particular.

In addition, there is further reduction in ATP, continued depletion of proteins, reduced intracellular pH, and leakage of lysosomal enzymes into the plasma. These biochemical changes have effects on the ultrastructural components of the cell.

1. **Calcium influx: Mitochondrial damage** As a result of continued hypoxia, a large cytosolic influx of calcium ions occurs, especially after reperfusion of irreversibly injured cell.

2. **Activated phospholipases: Membrane damage** Damage to membrane function in general, and plasma membrane in particular, is the most important event in irreversible cell injury. Increased cytosolic influx of calcium in the cell activates endogenous *phospholipases*. These, in turn, degrade membrane phospholipids progressively which are the main constituent of the lipid bilayer membrane.

3. **Intracellular proteases: Cytoskeletal damage** The normal cytoskeleton of the cell (microfilaments, microtubules and intermediate filaments) which anchors the cell membrane is damaged due to degradation by activated intracellular proteases or by physical effect of cell swelling producing irreversible cell membrane injury.

4. **Activated endonucleases: Nuclear damage** DNA or nucleoproteins are damaged by the activated lysosomal enzymes such as proteases and endonucleases. Irreversible damage to the nucleus can be in three forms:
i) Pyknosis: Condensation and clumping
ii) Karyorrhexis: Fragmentation
iii) Karyolysis: Dissolution.

5. **Lysosomal hydrolytic enzymes: Lysosomal damage, cell death and phagocytosis** The lysosomal membranes are damaged and result in escape of lysosomal hydrolytic enzymes. The dead cell is eventually replaced by masses of phospholipids called *myelin figures* which are either phagocytosed by macrophages or there may be formation of calcium soaps.

Liberated enzymes leak across the abnormally permeable cell membrane into the serum, the estimation of which may be used as clinical parameters of cell death.

ISCHAEMIA-REPERFUSION INJURY AND FREE RADICAL-MEDIATED CELL INJURY

Depending upon the duration of ischaemia/hypoxia, restoration of blood flow may result in the following 3 different consequences:

1. **From ischaemia to reversible injury** *When the period of ischaemia is of short duration,* reperfusion with resupply of oxygen restores the structural and functional state of the injured cell i.e. reversible cell injury.

2. **From ischaemia to irreversible injury** *Another extreme is when much longer period of ischaemia* has resulted in irreversible cell injury *during ischaemia itself* i.e. when so much time has elapsed that neither blood flow restoration is helpful nor reperfusion injury can develop.

3. **From ischaemia to reperfusion injury** *When ischaemia is for somewhat longer duration,* then restoration of blood supply to injured but viable cells (i.e. reperfusion), rather than restoring structure and function of the cell, paradoxically deteriorates the already injured cell and leads it to cell death. This is termed ischaemia-reperfusion injury.

Ischaemia-reperfusion injury occurs due to excessive accumulation of free radicals or reactive oxygen species. The mechanism of reperfusion injury by free radicals is complex but following three aspects are involved:

1. CALCIUM OVERLOAD Upon restoration of blood supply, the ischaemic cell is further bathed by the blood fluid that has more calcium ions at a time when the ATP stores of the cell are low.

2. EXCESSIVE GENERATION OF FREE RADICALS Although oxygen is the lifeline of all cells and tissues, its molecular forms as reactive oxygen radicals or reactive oxygen species can be most devastating for the cells.

Oxygen free radical generation The normal reaction of O_2 to H_2O involves 'four electron donation' in four steps involving transfer of one electron at each step. Free radicals are intermediate chemical species having a single unpaired electron in its outer orbit. Three intermediate molecules of partially reduced species of oxygen are generated depending upon the number of electrons transferred:

i) Superoxide oxygen (O'_2): one electron
ii) Hydrogen peroxide (H_2O_2): two electrons
iii) Hydroxyl radical (OH^-): three electrons

Other free radicals In addition to superoxide, H_2O_2 and hydroxyl radicals generated during conversion of O_2 to H_2O reaction, a few other free radicals active in the body are: (i) Nitric oxide (NO) and peroxynitrite (ONOO); (ii) Halide reagent (chlorine or chloride) and (iii) Exogenous sources of free radicals include some environmental agents such as tobacco and industrial pollutants.

Cytotoxicity of free radicals Free radicals are formed in physiologic as well as pathologic processes. The rate of spontaneous destruction is determined by catalytic action of certain enzymes such as superoxide dismutase (SOD), catalase and glutathione peroxidase (GSH). The net effect of free radical injury in physiologic and disease states, therefore, depends upon the rate of their formation and rate of their elimination.

However, if not degraded, then free radicals are highly destructive to the cell since they have electron-free residue and thus bind to all molecules of the cell; this is termed *oxidative stress*. Out of various free radicals, hydroxyl radical is the most reactive species. Free radicals may produce membrane damage by the following mechanisms: (i) Lipid peroxidation; (ii) Oxidation of proteins; (iii) DNA damage; and (iv) Cytoskeletal damage.

Conditions with free radical injury (i) Ischaemic reperfusion injury; (ii) Ionising radiation by causing radiolysis of water; (iii) Chemical toxicity; (iv) Chemical carcinogenesis; (v) Hyperoxia (toxicity due to oxygen therapy); (vi) Cellular ageing; (vii) Killing of microbial agents; (viii) Inflammatory damage; (ix) Destruction of tumour cells; (x) Atherosclerosis.

Antioxidants Antioxidants are endogenous or exogenous substances which inactivate the free radicals e.g.
i) Vitamins E, A and C (ascorbic acid)
ii) Sulfhydryl-containing compounds e.g. cysteine and glutathione.
iii) Serum proteins e.g. ceruloplasmin and transferrin.

3. SUBSEQUENT INFLAMMATORY REACTION Ischaemia-reperfusion event is followed by inflammatory reaction. Incoming activated neutrophils utilise oxygen quickly (*oxygen burst*) and release large excess of oxygen free radicals.

STRESS PROTEINS IN CELL INJURY

When cells are exposed to stress of any type, a protective response by the cell is by release of proteins that move molecules within the cell cytoplasm; these are called stress protein. There are 2 types of stress-related proteins: *heat shock proteins (HSP)* and *ubiquitin* (so named due to its universal presence in the cells of the body).

PATHOGENESIS OF CHEMICAL INJURY

Chemicals induce cell injury by one of the two mechanisms:

Direct cytotoxic effects The cytotoxic damage is usually greatest to cells which are involved in the metabolism of such chemicals e.g. in mercuric chloride poisoning, the greatest damage occurs to cells of the alimentary tract where it is absorbed and the kidney where it is excreted. Cyanide kills the cell by poisoning mitochondrial cytochrome oxidase thus blocking oxidative phosphorylation.

Conversion to reactive toxic metabolites This mechanism involves metabolic activation to yield ultimate toxin that interacts with the target cells. The target cells in this group of chemicals may not be the same cell that metabolised the toxin. Example of cell injury by conversion of reactive metabolites is toxic liver necrosis caused by carbon tetrachloride (CCl_4), acetaminophen (commonly used analgesic and antipyretic) and bromobenzene.

PATHOGENESIS OF PHYSICAL INJURY

Injuries caused by mechanical force are of medicolegal significance. But they may lead to a state of shock. Injuries by changes in atmospheric pressure (e.g. decompression sickness). Radiation injury to human by accidental or therapeutic exposure is of importance in treatment of persons with malignant tumours as well as may have carcinogenic influences.

MORPHOLOGY OF REVERSIBLE CELL INJURY *(p. 17)*

HYDROPIC CHANGE

Hydropic change means accumulation of water within the cytoplasm of the cell. Other synonyms used are *cloudy swelling* (for gross appearance of the affected organ) and *vacuolar degeneration* (due to cytoplasmic vacuolation). Hydropic swelling is an entirely reversible change upon removal of the injurious agent.

ETIOLOGY The common causes include acute and subacute cell injury from various etiologic agents such as bacterial toxins, chemicals, poisons, burns, high fever, intravenous administration of hypertonic glucose or saline etc.

PATHOGENESIS Cloudy swelling results from impaired regulation of sodium and potassium at the level of cell membrane. This results in intra-cellular accumulation of sodium and escape of potassium. This, in turn, is accompanied with rapid flow of water into the cell to maintain iso-osmotic conditions and hence cellular swelling occurs. In addition, influx of calcium too occurs.

G/A The affected organ such as kidney, liver, pancreas, or heart muscle is enlarged due to swelling.

M/E The features are as under:
i)   The tubular epithelial cells are swollen and their cytoplasm contains small clear vacuoles.
ii) Small cytoplasmic blebs may be seen.
iii) The nucleus may appear pale.
iv) The microvasculature of the interstitium is compressed due to swollen tubular cells.

HYALINE CHANGE

The word 'hyaline' or 'hyalin' means glassy (*hyalos* = glass). Hyaline change is seen in heterogeneous pathologic conditions and may be intracellular or extracellular.

INTRACELLULAR HYALINE Intracellular hyaline is mainly seen in epithelial cells.

1.   *Hyaline droplets* in the proximal tubular epithelial cells due to excessive reabsorption of plasma proteins in proteinuria.

2.   *Hyaline degeneration* of rectus abdominalis muscle called Zenker's degeneration, occurring in typhoid fever.

3.   *Mallory's hyaline* represents aggregates of intermediate filaments in the hepatocytes in alcoholic liver cell injury.

4.   Nuclear or cytoplasmic *hyaline inclusions* seen in some viral infections.

5.   *Russell's bodies* representing excessive immunoglobulins in the rough endoplasmic reticulum of the plasma cells.

EXTRACELLULAR HYALINE Extracellular hyaline commonly termed hyalinisation is seen in connective tissues.

1.   Hyaline degeneration in *leiomyomas* of the uterus.

2.   Hyalinised *old scar* of fibrocollagenous tissues.

3.   *Hyaline arteriolosclerosis* in renal vessels in hypertension and diabetes mellitus.

4.   Hyalinised glomeruli in *chronic glomerulonephritis*.

5.   *Corpora amylacea* seen as rounded masses of concentric hyaline laminae in the enlarged prostate in the elderly, in the brain and in the spinal cord in old age, and in old infarcts of the lung.

MUCOID CHANGE

Mucoid means mucus-like. Mucus is the secretory product of mucous glands and is a combination of proteins complexed with mucopolysaccharides. Both epithelial and connective tissue mucin are stained by alcian blue. However, epithelial mucin stains positively with periodic acid-Schiff (PAS), while connective tissue mucin is PAS negative but is, instead, stained positively with colloidal iron.

EPITHELIAL MUCIN (1) Catarrhal inflammation of mucous membrane (e.g. of respiratory tract, alimentary tract, uterus); (2) Obstruction of duct leading to mucocele in the oral cavity and gallbladder; (3) Cystic fibrosis of the pancreas; and (4) Mucin-secreting tumours (e.g. of ovary, stomach, large bowel etc).

CONNECTIVE TISSUE MUCIN (1) Mucoid or myxoid change in some tumours e.g. myxomas, neurofibromas, fibroadenoma, soft tissue sarcomas etc.; (2) Dissecting aneurysm of the aorta due to Erdheim's medial degeneration and Marfan's syndrome; (3) Myxomatous change in the dermis in myxoedema; (4) Myxoid change in the synovium in ganglion on the wrist.

INTRACELLULAR ACCUMULATIONS *(p. 19)*

Intracellular accumulation of substances in abnormal amounts can occur within the cytoplasm (especially lysosomes) or nucleus of the cell.

Abnormal intracellular accumulations can be divided into 3 groups:

i)   *Accumulation of constituents of normal cell metabolism produced in excess* e.g. accumulations of lipids (fatty change, cholesterol deposits), proteins and carbohydrates.

ii)   *Accumulation of abnormal substances* produced as a result of abnormal metabolism due to lack of some enzymes e.g. storage diseases or inborn errors of metabolism. These are discussed in Chapter 9.

iii)   *Accumulation of pigments* e.g. endogenous pigments under special circumstances, and exogenous pigments due to lack of enzymatic mechanisms to degrade the substances or transport them to other sites.

FATTY CHANGE (STEATOSIS)

Fatty change, steatosis or fatty metamorphosis is the intracellular accumulation of neutral fat within parenchymal cells. Fatty change is particularly common in the liver but may occur in other non-fatty tissues as well e.g. in the heart, skeletal muscle, kidneys (lipoid nephrosis or minimum change disease) and other organs.

FATTY LIVER

Liver is the commonest site for accumulation of fat because it plays central role in fat metabolism.

ETIOLOGY Fatty change in the liver may result from one of the two types of causes:

1. Conditions with excess fat These are conditions in which the capacity of the liver to metabolise fat is exceeded e.g.
i) Obesity
ii) Diabetes mellitus
iii) Congenital hyperlipidaemia

2. Liver cell damage These are conditions in which fat cannot be metabolised due to liver cell injury e.g.
i) Alcoholic liver disease (most common)
ii) Starvation
iii) Protein calorie malnutrition
iv) Chronic illnesses (e.g. tuberculosis)
v) Acute fatty liver in late pregnancy
vi) Hypoxia (e.g. anaemia, cardiac failure)
vii) Hepatotoxins (e.g. carbon tetrachloride, chloroform, ether, aflatoxins and other poisons)
viii) Drug-induced liver cell injury (e.g. administration of methotrexate, steroids, CCl_4, halothane anaesthetic, tetracycline etc)
ix) Reye's syndrome

PATHOGENESIS Mechanism of fatty liver depends upon the stage at which the etiologic agent acts in the normal fat transport and metabolism.

Normally, most of free fatty acid is esterified to triglycerides by the action of α-glycerophosphate and only a small part is changed into cholesterol, phospholipids and ketone bodies. While cholesterol, phospholipids and ketones are used in the body, intracellular triglycerides are converted into lipoproteins, which require 'lipid acceptor protein'. Lipoproteins are released from the liver cells into circulation as plasma lipoproteins (LDL, VLDL).

In fatty liver, intracellular accumulation of triglycerides occurs due to defect at one or more of the following *6 steps* in the normal fat metabolism:
1. Increased entry of free fatty acids into the liver.
2. Increased synthesis of fatty acids by the liver.
3. Decreased conversion of fatty acids into ketone bodies resulting in increased esterification of fatty acids to triglycerides.
4. Increased α-glycerophosphate causing increased esterification of fatty acids to triglycerides.
5. Decreased synthesis of 'lipid acceptor protein' resulting in decreased formation of lipoprotein from triglycerides.
6. Block in the excretion of lipoprotein from the liver into plasma.
   In most cases of fatty liver, one of the above mechanisms is operating. But liver cell injury from chronic alcoholism is multifactorial as follows:
i) Increased lipolysis
ii) Increased free fatty acid synthesis
iii) Decreased triglyceride utilisation
iv) Decreased fatty acid oxidation to ketone bodies
v) Block in lipoprotein excretion
   Even a severe form of fatty liver may be reversible if the liver is given time to regenerate and progressive fibrosis has not developed. For example, intermittent drinking is less harmful because the liver cells get time to recover; similarly a chronic alcoholic who becomes teetotaler the enlarged fatty liver may return to normal if fibrosis has not developed.

G/A The liver in fatty change is enlarged with a tense, glistening capsule and rounded margins. The cut surface bulges slightly and is pale-yellow to yellow and is greasy to touch.

M/E Characteristic feature is the presence of numerous lipid vacuoles in the cytoplasm of hepatocytes.

i) The vacuoles are initially small and are present around the nucleus (*microvesicular*).

ii) With progression of the process, the vacuoles become larger pushing the nucleus to the periphery of the cells (*macrovesicular*).

iii) At times, the hepatocytes laden with large lipid vacuoles may rupture and lipid vacuoles coalesce to form fatty cysts.

iv) Fat can be demonstrated in fresh unfixed tissue by frozen section by *fat stains* e.g. Sudan dyes (Sudan III, IV, Sudan black) and oil red O.

STROMAL FATTY INFILTRATION

Stromal fatty infiltration is the deposition of mature adipose cells in the stromal connective tissue in contrast to intracellular deposition of fat in the parenchymal cells in fatty change. The condition occurs most often in patients with obesity. The two commonly affected organs are the heart and the pancreas.

INTRACELLULAR ACCUMULATION OF PROTEINS

1. In *proteinuria*, there is excessive renal tubular reabsorption of proteins by the proximal tubular epithelial cells which show pink hyaline droplets in their cytoplasm.

2. The cytoplasm of actively functioning plasma cells shows pink hyaline inclusions called *Russell's bodies* representing synthesised immuno-globulins.

3. In $\alpha 1$-*antitrypsin deficiency*, the cytoplasm of hepatocytes shows eosinophilic globular deposits of a mutant protein.

4. *Mallory's body* or alcoholic hyaline in the hepatocytes is intracellular accumulation of intermediate filaments of cytokeratin and appear as amorphous pink masses.

INTRACELLULAR ACCUMULATION OF GLYCOGEN

1. In *diabetes mellitus*, there is intracellular accumulation of glycogen in different tissues because normal cellular uptake of glucose is impaired. Best's carmine and periodic acid-Schiff (PAS) staining may be employed to confirm the presence of glycogen in the cells.

2. In *glycogen storage diseases or glycogenosis*, there is defective metabolism of glycogen due to genetic disorders.

PIGMENTS *(p. 22)*

There are 2 broad categories of pigments: endogenous and exogenous.

A. ENDOGENOUS PIGMENTS

Endogenous pigments are either normal constituents of cells or accumulate under special circumstances e.g. melanin, alkaptonuria, haemoprotein-derived pigments, and lipofuscin.

MELANIN

Melanin is the brown-black, non-haemoglobin-derived pigment normally present in the hair, skin, mucosa at some places, choroid of the eye, meninges and adrenal medulla. In skin, it is synthesised in the melanocytes and dendritic cells, both of which are present in the basal cells of the epidermis and is stored in the form of cytoplasmic granules in the phago-cytic cells called the melanophores, present in the underlying dermis. Melanocytes possess the enzyme tyrosinase necessary for synthesis of melanin from tyrosine.

Various disorders of melanin pigmentation cause generalised and localised hyperpigmentation and hypopigmentation:

i) Generalised hyperpigmentation (a) In Addison's disease; (b) Chloasma observed during pregnancy; and (c) In chronic arsenical poisoning.

ii) Focal hyperpigmentation:

a) *Cáfe-au-lait spots* are pigmented patches seen in neurofibromatosis and Albright's syndrome.

b) *Peutz-Jeghers syndrome* is characterised by focal peri-oral pigmentation.

c) *Melanosis coli* is pigmentation of the mucosa of the colon.

d) *Melanotic tumours*, both benign such as pigmented naevi, and malignant such as melanoma, are associated with increased melanogenesis.

iii) Generalised hypopigmentation   *Albinism* is an extreme degree of generalised hypopigmentation in which tyrosinase enzyme is genetically defective and no melanin is formed in the melanocytes. Oculocutaneous albinos have no pigment in the skin and have blond hair, poor vision and severe photophobia. They are highly sensitive to sunlight. Chronic sun exposure may lead to precancerous lesions and squamous and basal cell cancers of the skin in such individuals.

iv) Localised hypopigmentation (a) Leucoderma; (b) Vitiligo; and (c) Acquired focal hypopigmentation can result from various causes such as leprosy, healing of wounds, DLE, radiation dermatitis etc.

HAEMOPROTEIN-DERIVED PIGMENTS

These pigments are haemosiderin, acid haematin (haemozoin), bilirubin, and porphyrins.

1.   HAEMOSIDERIN   Iron is stored in the tissues in 2 forms:

◈   *Ferritin,* which is iron complexed to apoferritin and can be identified by electron microscopy.

◈   *Haemosiderin*, which is formed by aggregates of ferritin and is identifiable by light microscopy as golden-yellow to brown, granular pigment, especially within the mononuclear phagocytes of the bone marrow, spleen and liver where break-down of senescent red cells takes place. Haemosiderin is ferric iron that can be demonstrated by Perl's stain that produces Prussian blue reaction.

Excessive storage of haemosiderin occurs in conditions when there is increased break-down of red cells systemic overload of iron. This may occur due to primary (idiopathic, hereditary) haemochromatosis, and secondary (acquired) causes such as in chronic haemolytic anaemias (e.g. thalassae-mia), sideroblastic anaemia, alcoholic cirrhosis, multiple blood transfusions etc.

Accordingly, the effects of haemosiderin excess are as under:

a)   Localised haemosiderosis   This develops whenever there is haemorrhage into the tissues. With lysis of red cells, haemoglobin is liberated which is taken up by macrophages where it is degraded and stored as haemosiderin. A few examples are as under:

◈   Changing colours of a bruise or a black eye.

◈   Brown induration of the lungs.

b)   Generalised (Systemic or Diffuse) haemosiderosis   Systemic overload with iron may result in generalised haemosiderosis.

◈   *Parenchymatous deposition* occurs in the parenchymal cells of the liver, pancreas, kidney, and heart.

◈   *Reticuloendothelial (RE) deposition* occurs in the RE cells of the liver, spleen, and bone marrow.

Causes for generalised or systemic overload of iron may be as under:

i)   Increased erythropoietic activity: In various forms of chronic haemo-lytic anaemia, there is excessive break-down of haemoglobin and hence iron overload. The deposits of iron in these cases, termed as *acquired haemosiderosis,* are initially in reticuloendothelial tissues but may eventually affect the parenchymal cells of the organs.

ii) Excessive intestinal absorption of iron: A form of haemosiderosis in which there is excessive intestinal absorption of iron even when the intake is normal, is known as *idiopathic or hereditary haemochromatosis.* It is an autosomal dominant disease associated with much more deposits of iron than in cases of acquired haemosiderosis.

iii) ***Excessive dietary intake of iron:*** An example of excessive iron absorption is *African iron overload* (earlier called *Bantu siderosis*) seen in blacks in South Africa.

2. ACID HAEMATIN (HAEMOZOIN) Acid haematin or haemozoin, also called malarial pigment, is a haemoprotein-derived brown-black pigment containing haem iron in ferric form in acidic medium. But it differs from haemosiderin because it cannot be stained by Prussian blue (Perl's) reaction, probably because of formation of complex with a protein so that it is unable to react in the stain.

3. BILIRUBIN Bilirubin is the normal non-iron containing pigment present in the bile. Normal level of bilirubin in blood is less than 1 mg/dl. Excess of bilirubin or hyperbilirubinaemia causes an important clinical condition called jaundice. Jaundice may appear in one of the following 3 ways:

i) An increase in the rate of bilirubin production due to excessive destruction of red cells (predominantly unconjugated hyperbilirubinaemia).

ii) A defect in handling of bilirubin due to hepatocellular injury (biphasic jaundice).

iii) Some defect in bilirubin transport within intrahepatic or extrahepatic biliary system (predominantly conjugated hyperbilirubinaemia).

Skin and sclerae become distinctly yellow. In infants, rise in unconjugated bilirubin may produce toxic brain injury called *kernicterus*.

4. PORPHYRINS Porphyrins are normal pigment present in haemoglobin, myoglobin and cytochrome. Porphyria refers to an uncommon disorder of inborn abnormality of porphyrin metabolism. It results from genetic deficiency of one of the enzymes required for the synthesis of haem, resulting in excessive production of porphyrins. Its major types are:

(a) Erythropoietic porphyrias These have defective synthesis of haem in the red cell precursors in the bone marrow.

(b) Hepatic porphyrias These are more common and have a normal erythroid precursors but have a defect in synthesis of haem in the liver.

LIPOFUSCIN (WEAR AND TEAR PIGMENT)

Lipofuscin or lipochrome is yellowish-brown intracellular lipid pigment (*lipo* = fat, *fuscus* = brown). The pigment is often found in atrophied cells of old age and hence the name 'wear and tear pigment'. It is seen in the myocardial fibres, hepatocytes, Leydig cells of the testes and in neurons in senile dementia.

M/E The pigment is coarse, golden-brown granular and often accumulates in the central part of the cells around the nuclei. In the heart muscle, the change is associated with wasting of the muscle and is commonly referred to as 'brown atrophy'.

By electron microscopy, lipofuscin appears as intralysosomal electron-dense granules in perinuclear location. Lipofuscin is an example of residual bodies.

B. EXOGENOUS PIGMENTS

Exogenous pigments are the pigments introduced into the body from outside such as by inhalation, ingestion or inoculation.

INHALED PIGMENTS

The lungs of most individuals, especially of those living in urban areas due to atmospheric pollutants and of smokers, show a large number of inhaled pigmented materials. The most commonly inhaled substances are carbon or coal dust; others are silica or stone dust, iron or iron oxide, asbestos and various other organic substances. These substances may produce occupational lung diseases called pneumoconiosis.

INGESTED PIGMENTS

i) *Argyria* is chronic ingestion of silver compounds.
ii) *Chronic lead poisoning* may produce the characteristic blue lines on teeth at the gumline.
iii) *Melanosis coli* results from prolonged ingestion of certain cathartics.
iv) *Carotenaemia* is yellowish-red colouration of the skin caused by excessive ingestion of carrots which contain carotene.

INJECTED PIGMENTS (TATTOOING)

Pigments like India ink, cinnabar and carbon are introduced into the dermis in the process of tattooing where the pigment is taken up by macrophages and lies permanently in the connective tissue.

MORPHOLOGY OF IRREVERSIBLE CELL INJURY (CELL DEATH) *(p. 26)*

Cell death is a state of irreversible injury. It may occur in the living body as a local or focal change (i.e. autolysis, necrosis and apoptosis) and the changes that follow it (i.e. gangrene and pathologic calcification), or result in end of the life (somatic death).

AUTOLYSIS

Autolysis (i.e. *self-digestion*) is disintegration of the cell by its own hydrolytic enzymes liberated from lysosomes. Autolysis can occur in the living body when it is surrounded by inflammatory reaction *(vital reaction)*, but the term is generally used for postmortem change in which there is complete absence of surrounding inflammatory response. Autolysis is *rapid* in some tissues rich in hydrolytic enzymes such as in the pancreas, and gastric mucosa; *intermediate* in tissues like the heart, liver and kidney; and *slow* in fibrous tissue.

NECROSIS

Necrosis is defined as a localised area of death of tissue followed later by degradation of tissue by hydrolytic enzymes liberated from dead cells; it is invariably accompanied by inflammatory reaction.

Necrosis can be caused by various agents such as hypoxia, chemical and physical agents, microbial agents, immunological injury, etc.

Based on etiology and morphologic appearance, there are 5 types of necrosis: coagulative, liquefaction (colliquative), caseous, fat, and fibrinoid necrosis.

1. COAGULATIVE NECROSIS This is the most common type of necrosis caused by irreversible focal injury, mostly from sudden cessation of blood flow (ischaemic necrosis), and less often from bacterial and chemical agents. The organs commonly affected are the heart, kidney, and spleen.

G/A Focus of coagulative necrosis in the early stage is pale, firm, and slightly swollen and is called infarct. With progression, the affected area becomes more yellowish, softer, and shrunken.

M/E The hallmark of coagulative necrosis is the conversion of normal cells into their 'tombstones' i.e. outlines of the cells are retained and the cell type can still be recognised but their cytoplasmic and nuclear details are lost. The necrosed cells are swollen and have more eosinophilic cytoplasm than the normal. These cells show nuclear changes of pyknosis, karyorrhexis and karyolysis.

2. LIQUEFACTION (COLLIQUATIVE) NECROSIS Liquefaction or colliquative necrosis also occurs commonly due to ischaemic injury and bacterial or fungal infections but hydrolytic enzymes in tissue degradation have a dominant role in causing semi-fluid material. The common examples are infarct brain and abscess cavity.

G/A The affected area is soft with liquefied centre containing necrotic debris. Later, a cyst wall is formed.

M/E The cystic space contains necrotic cell debris and macrophages filled with phagocytosed material. The cyst wall is formed by proliferating capillaries, inflammatory cells, and gliosis (proliferating glial cells) in the case of brain and proliferating fibroblasts in the case of abscess cavity.

3. CASEOUS NECROSIS Caseous (caseous= cheese-like) necrosis is found in the centre of foci of tuberculous infections. It combines features of both coagulative and liquefactive necrosis.

G/A Foci of caseous necrosis resemble dry cheese and are soft, granular and yellowish. This appearance is partly attributed to the histotoxic effects of lipopolysaccharides present in the capsule of the tubercle bacilli, *Mycobacterium tuberculosis*.

M/E Centre of the necrosed focus contain structureless, eosinophilic material having scattered granular debris of disintegrated nuclei. The surrounding tissue shows characteristic granulomatous inflammatory reaction consisting of epithelioid cells (modified macrophages having slipper-shaped vesicular nuclei), interspersed giant cells of Langhans' and foreign body type and peripheral mantle of lymphocytes.

4. FAT NECROSIS Fat necrosis is a special form of cell death occurring at mainly fat-rich anatomic locations in the body. The examples are: traumatic fat necrosis of the breast, especially in heavy and pendulous breasts, and mesenteric fat necrosis due to acute pancreatitis.

G/A Fat necrosis appears as yellowish-white and firm deposits. Formation of calcium soaps imparts the necrosed foci firmer and chalky white appearance.

M/E The necrosed fat cells have cloudy appearance and are surrounded by an inflammatory reaction. Formation of calcium soaps is identified in the tissue sections as amorphous, granular and basophilic material.

5. FIBRINOID NECROSIS Fibrinoid necrosis is characterised by deposition of fibrin-like material which has the staining properties of fibrin such as phosphotungistic acid haematoxylin (PTAH) stain. It is encountered in various examples of immunologic tissue injury (e.g. in immune complex vasculitis, autoimmune diseases, Arthus reaction etc), arterioles in hypertension, peptic ulcer etc.

APOPTOSIS

Apoptosis is a form of 'coordinated and internally programmed cell death' having significance in a variety of physiologic and pathologic conditions (*apoptosis*=falling off or dropping off, as that of leaves or petals). Unlike necrosis, apoptosis is not accompanied by any inflammation and collateral tissue damage.

APOPTOSIS IN BIOLOGIC PROCESSES Apoptosis is responsible for mediating cell death in a wide variety of physiologic and pathologic processes as under:

Physiologic Processes:
1. Organised cell destruction in sculpting of tissues during *development of embryo*.
2. Physiologic involution of cells in *hormone-dependent tissues* e.g. endometrial shedding, regression of lactating breast after withdrawal of breast-feeding.
3. Normal cell destruction followed by *replacement proliferation* such as in intestinal epithelium.
4. *Involution of the thymus* in early age.

Pathologic Processes:
1. Cell death in tumours exposed to *chemotherapeutic agents*.
2. *Cell death by cytotoxic T cells* in immune mechanisms such as in graft-versus-host disease and rejection reactions.
3. . Progressive *depletion of CD4+T cells* in the pathogenesis of AIDS.
4. *Cell death in viral infections* e.g. formation of Councilman bodies in viral hepatitis.
5. *Pathologic atrophy* of organs and tissues on withdrawal of stimuli e.g. prostatic atrophy after orchiectomy, atrophy of kidney or salivary gland on obstruction of ureter or ducts, respectively.
6. Cell death in response to low dose of *injurious agents* involved in causation of necrosis e.g. radiation, hypoxia and mild thermal injury.
7. In *degenerative diseases of CNS* e.g. in Alzheimer's disease, Parkinson's disease, and chronic infective dementias.
8. *Heart diseases* e.g. in acute myocardial infarction (20% necrosis and 80% apoptosis).

M/E The major features are:
1. Involvement of *single cells or small clusters of cells* in the background of viable cells.
2. Apoptotic cells are round to oval *shrunken masses* of intensely eosinophilic cytoplasm (mummified cell) containing shrunken or almost-normal organelles.
3. Nuclear chromatin is condensed under the nuclear membrane i.e. *pyknosis*.
4. The cell membrane may show *blebs or projections* on the surface.
5. There may be formation of membrane-bound near-spherical bodies containing condensed organelles around the cell called *apoptotic bodies*.
6. Characteristically, unlike necrosis, there is *no acute inflammatory reaction* around apoptosis.

Techniques to identify and count apoptotic cells
1. Staining of chromatin condensation by haematoxylin, Feulgen stain.
2. Fluorescent stain with acridine orange dye.
3. Flow cytometry to visualise rapid cell shrinkage.
4. DNA changes detected by *in situ* techniques or by gel electrophoresis.
5. Immunohistochemical stain with annexin V for plasma membrane of apoptotic cell having phosphatidylserine on the cell exterior.

MOLECULAR MECHANISMS OF APOPTOSIS Several physiologic and pathologic processes activate apoptosis in a variety of ways. However, in general the following molecular events sum up the sequence involved in apoptosis:

1. Initiators of apoptosis All cells have inbuilt effector mechanisms for cell survival and signals of cell death; it is the loss of this balance that determines survival or death of a cell.
i) *Withdrawal of normal cell survival signals* e.g. absence of certain hormones, growth factors, cytokines.
ii) *Agents of cell injury* e.g. heat, radiation, hypoxia, toxins, free radicals.

2. Initial steps in apoptosis After the cell has been initiated into self-destruct mode, cell death signaling mechanisms gets activated from *intrinsic (mitochondrial)* and *extrinsic (cell death receptor initiated)* pathways as outlined below. However, finally mediators of cell death are activated caspases. Caspases are a series of proteolytic or protein-splitting enzymes which act on nuclear proteins and organelles containing protein components.

i) Intrinsic (mitochondrial) pathway: This pathway of cell death signaling is due to increased mitochondrial permeability and is a major mechanism. The major mechanism of regulation of this mitochondrial protein is by pro- and anti-apoptotic members of Bcl proteins. Bcl-2 oncogene was first detected on B-cell lymphoma and hence its name. Bcl-2 gene located on the mitochondrial inner membrane is a human counterpart of *CED-9 (cell death)* gene regulating cell growth and cell death. Among about 20 members of Bcl family of oncogenes, the growth promoter (anti-apoptotic) proteins are Bcl-2,

Bcl-x and Mcl-1, while pro-apoptotic proteins are Bim, Bid and Bad which contain single Bcl-2 homology domain (also called BH-only proteins). The net effect on the mitochondrial membrane is based on the pro-apoptotic and anti-apoptotic actions of Bcl-2 gene family. This, in turn, activates caspase cascade.

ii) Extrinsic (cell death receptor initiated) pathway: This signaling pathway of cell death is by activation of death receptors on the cell membrane. An important cell death receptor is type 1 tumour necrosis factor receptor (TNF-R1) and a related transmembrane protein called Fas (CD95) and its ligand (FasL).

3. Final phase of apoptosis The final culmination of either of the above two mechanisms is activation of caspases. Mitochondrial pathway activates caspase–9 and death receptor pathway activates caspases-8 and 10.

4. Phagocytosis The dead apoptotic cells develop membrane changes which promote their phagocytosis.

CHANGES AFTER CELL DEATH *(p. 32)*

Two types of pathologic changes may superimpose following cell injury: gangrene (after necrosis) and pathologic calcification (after degenerations as well as necrosis).

GANGRENE

Gangrene is necrosis of tissue associated with superadded putrefaction, most often following coagulative necrosis due to ischaemia (e.g. in gangrene of the bowel, gangrene of limb). On the other hand, *gangrenous or necrotising inflammation* is characterised primarily by inflammation provoked by virulent bacteria resulting in massive tissue necrosis.

There are 2 main types of gangrene—dry and wet, and a variant of wet gangrene called gas gangrene.

DRY GANGRENE

This form of gangrene begins in the distal part of a limb due to ischaemia. The typical example is the dry gangrene in the toes and feet of an old patient due to severe atherossclerosis. Other causes of dry gangrene foot include thromboangiitis obliterans (Buerger's disease), Raynaud's disease, trauma, ergot poisoning.

G/A The affected part is dry, shrunken and dark black, resembling the foot of a mummy. The line of separation usually brings about complete separation with eventual falling off of the gangrenous tissue if it is not removed surgically.

M/E There is necrosis with smudging of the tissue. The line of separation consists of inflammatory granulation tissue.

WET GANGRENE

Wet gangrene occurs in naturally moist tissues and organs such as the bowel, lung, mouth, cervix, vulva etc. Two other examples of wet gangrene having clinical significance are as follows:

◈ *Diabetic foot* which is due to high glucose content in the necrosed tissue which favours growth of bacteria.

◈ *Bed sores* occurring in a bed-ridden patient due to pressure on sites like the sacrum, buttocks and heel.

Wet gangrene usually develops due to blockage of both venous as well as arterial blood flow and is more rapid. The affected part is stuffed with blood which favours the rapid growth of putrefactive bacteria. The toxic products formed by bacteria are absorbed causing profound systemic manifestations of septicaemia, and finally death. The spreading wet gangrene generally lacks clear-cut line of demarcation and may spread to peritoneal cavity causing peritonitis.

G/A The affected part is soft, swollen, putrid, rotten and dark. The classic example is gangrene of the bowel, commonly due to strangulated hernia, volvulus or intussusception.

M/E There is coagulative necrosis with stuffing of affected part with blood. The mucosa is ulcerated and sloughed. Lumen of the bowel contains mucus and blood. There is intense acute inflammatory exudates and thrombosed vessels. The line of demarcation between gangrenous segment and viable bowel is generally not clear-cut.

GAS GANGRENE It is a special form of wet gangrene caused by gas-forming clostridia (gram-positive anaerobic bacteria) which gain entry into the tissues through open contaminated wounds, especially in the muscles, or as a complication of operation on colon which normally contains clostridia.

PATHOLOGIC CALCIFICATION

Deposition of calcium salts in tissues other than osteoid or enamel is called pathologic or heterotopic calcification. Two distinct types of pathologic calcification are recognised:
◈ *Dystrophic calcification* is characterised by deposition of calcium salts in dead or degenerated tissues with normal calcium metabolism and normal serum calcium level.
◈ *Metastatic calcification*, on the other hand, occurs in apparently normal tissues and is associated with deranged calcium metabolism and hypercalcaemia.

M/E Calcium salts appear as deeply basophilic, irregular and granular clumps. The deposits may be intracellular, extracellular, or at both locations. Calcium deposits can be confirmed by special stains like silver impregnation method of *von-Kossa* producing black colour, and *alizarin red S* that produces red staining.

ETIOPATHOGENESIS

DYSTROPHIC CALCIFICATION It occurs in degenerated or dead tissues. **Calcification in dead tissue** (1) Caseous necrosis in tuberculosis; (2) Liquefaction necrosis in chronic abscesses; (3) Fat necrosis following acute pancreatitis or traumatic fat necrosis; (4) Gamna-Gandy bodies in chronic venous congestion (CVC) of the spleen; (5) Infarcts; (6) Thrombi, especially in the veins; (7) Haematomas; (8) Dead parasites like in hydatid cyst, Schistosoma eggs, and cysticercosis; and (9) Microcalcification in breast cancer.

Calcification in degenerated tissues (1) Dense old scars; (2) Atheromas in the aorta and coronaries; (3) Mönckeberg's sclerosis shows calcification in the degenerated tunica media of muscular arteries; (4) Stroma of tumours such as uterine fibroids; (5) Goitre of the thyroid; (6) Psammoma bodies or calcospherites such as in meningioma, papillary serous cystadenocarcinoma of the ovary and papillary carcinoma of the thyroid; (7) Cysts which have been present for a long time e.g. epidermal and pilar cysts; (8) Calcinosis cutis is nodular deposit of calcium salts in the skin and subcutaneous tissue; and (9) Senile degenerative changes e.g. in costal cartilages, tracheal or bronchial cartilages, and pineal gland in the brain etc.

Pathogenesis of dystrophic calcification The process of dystrophic calcification has been likened to the formation of normal hydroxyapatite of bone i.e. binding of phosphate ions with calcium ions to form precipitates of calcium phosphate. It involves phases of initiation and propagation.

METASTATIC CALCIFICATION Since metastatic calcification occurs in normal tissues due to hypercalcaemia, its causes would include either of the following two groups of causes:

Excessive mobilisation of calcium from the bone For example:
1. *Hyperparathyroidism* which may be primary such as due to parathyroid adenoma, or secondary such as from parathyroid hyperplasia, chronic renal failure etc.

2. *Bony destructive lesions* such as multiple myeloma, metastatic carcinoma.
3. *Hypercalcaemia* as a part of paraneoplastic syndrome.
4. *Prolonged immobilisation* of a patient results in disuse atrophy of the bones.

Excessive absorption of calcium from the gut   For example:
1. *Hypervitaminosis D* from excessive intake or in sarcoidosis.
2. *Milk-alkali syndrome* caused by excessive oral intake of calcium in the form of milk.
3. *Idiopathic hypercalcaemia of infancy* (Williams syndrome).
4. *Renal causes* such as in renal tubular acidosis.

Sites of metastatic calcification   Metastatic calcification may occur in any normal tissue of the body but preferentially affects the following organs and tissues:
1. *Kidneys*, especially at the basement membrane of tubular epithelium and in the tubular lumina causing nephrocalcinosis.
2. *Lungs*, especially in the alveolar walls.
3. *Stomach*, on the acid-secreting fundal glands.
4. *Blood vessels*, especially on the internal elastic lamina.
5. *Cornea* is another site affected by metastatic calcification.
6. *Synovium* of the joint causing pain and dysfunction.

Pathogenesis of metastatic calcification   Metastatic calcification occurs due to excessive binding of inorganic phosphate ions with elevated calcium ions due to underlying metabolic derangement. This leads to precipitates of calcium phosphate at the preferential sites, due to presence of acid secretions or rapid changes in pH levels at these sites.

ADAPTIVE DISORDERS *(p. 37)*

Adaptive disorders are the adjustments which the cells make in response to stresses which may be for physiologic needs *(physiologic adaptation)* or a response to non-lethal pathologic injury *(pathologic adaptation)*. Broadly speaking, such physiologic and pathologic adaptations occur by following processes:
◈   Decreasing or increasing their size i.e. *atrophy* and *hypertrophy* respectively, or by increasing their number i.e. *hyperplasia* (postfix word -*trophy* means nourishment; -*plasia* means growth of new cells).
◈   Changing the pathway of phenotypic differentiation of cells i.e. *metaplasia* and *dysplasia* (prefix word *meta*- means transformation; *dys*- means bad development).
    In general, the adaptive responses are reversible on withdrawal of stimulus.

ATROPHY *(p. 37)*

Reduction of the number and size of parenchymal cells of an organ or its parts which was once normal is called atrophy.

CAUSES   Atrophy may occur from physiologic or pathologic causes:

A.   Physiologic atrophy (i) Atrophy of lymphoid tissue with age; (ii) Atrophy of thymus in adult life; (iii) Atrophy of gonads after menopause; (iv) Atrophy of brain with ageing; and (v) Osteoporosis with reduction in size of bony trabeculae due to ageing.

B.   Pathologic atrophy (1) *Starvation atrophy;* (2) *Ischaemic atrophy* Gradual diminution of blood supply due to atherosclerosis may result in shrinkage of the affected organ; (3) *Disuse atrophy* Prolonged diminished functional activity is associated with disuse atrophy of the organ; (4) *Neuropathic atrophy* Interruption in nerve supply leads to wasting of muscles e.g. poliomyelitis; (5) *Endocrine atrophy* Loss of endocrine regulatory mechanism results in reduced metabolic activity of tissues and hence atrophy; and (6) *Pressure atrophy* Prolonged pressure from benign tumours or cyst or aneurysm may cause compression and atrophy of the tissues.

G/A The organ is small, often shrunken. The cells become smaller in size but are not dead cells.

M/E Shrinkage in cell size is due to reduction in cell organelles, chiefly mitochondria, myofilaments and endoplasmic reticulum. There is often increase in the number of autophagic vacuoles containing cell debris.

HYPERTROPHY *(p. 38)*

Hypertrophy is an increase in the size of parenchymal cells resulting in enlargement of the organ or tissue, without any change in the number of cells.

CAUSES Hypertrophy may be physiologic or pathologic. In either case, it is caused by increased functional demand or by hormonal stimulation.

A. Physiologic hypertrophy Enlarged size of the uterus in pregnancy is an example of physiologic hypertrophy as well as hyperplasia.

B. Pathologic hypertrophy
1. *Hypertrophy of cardiac muscle* may occur in a number of cardiovascular diseases e.g. systemic hypertension
2. *Hypertrophy of smooth muscle* e.g. cardiac achalasia (in oesophagus)
3. *Hypertrophy of skeletal muscle* e.g. hypertrophied muscles in athletes and manual labourers.
4. *Compensatory hypertrophy* may occur in an organ when the contralateral organ is removed e.g. following nephrectomy on one side.

G/A The affected organ is enlarged and heavy. For example, a hyper-trophied heart of a patient with systemic hypertension may weigh 700-800 g as compared to average normal adult weight of 350 g.

M/E There is enlargement of muscle fibres as well as of nuclei.

HYPERPLASIA *(p. 39)*

Hyperplasia is an increase in the number of parenchymal cells resulting in enlargement of the organ or tissue. Quite often, both hyperplasia and hypertrophy occur together. Hyperplasia occurs due to increased recruitment of cells from G0 (resting) phase of the cell cycle to undergo mitosis, when stimulated.

CAUSES These may be physiologic or pathologic.

A. Physiologic hyperplasia Examples are:

1. *Hormonal hyperplasia* e.g.
i) Hyperplasia of female breast at puberty, during pregnancy and lactation.
ii) Hyperplasia of pregnant uterus.
iii) Proliferative activity of normal endometrium after a normal menstrual cycle.
iv) Prostatic hyperplasia in old age.

2. *Compensatory hyperplasia* e.g.
i) Regeneration of the liver following partial hepatectomy.
ii) Regeneration of epidermis after skin abrasion.
iii) Following nephrectomy on one side, there is hyperplasia of nephrons of the other kidney.

B. Pathologic hyperplasia Examples are:
i) Endometrial hyperplasia following oestrogen excess.
ii) In wound healing, there is formation of granulation tissue due to proliferation of fibroblasts and endothelial cells.
iii) Formation of skin warts from hyperplasia of epidermis due to human papilloma virus.
iv) Pseudocarcinomatous hyperplasia of the skin occurring at the margin of a non-healing ulcer.
v) Intraductal epithelial hyperplasia in fibrocystic change in the breast.

G/A & M/E There is enlargement of the affected organ or tissue and increase in the number of cells.

METAPLASIA *(p. 39)*

Metaplasia is defined as a *reversible change of one type of epithelial or mesenchymal adult cells to another type of adult epithelial or mesenchymal cells*, usually in response to abnormal stimuli, and often *reverts back to normal on removal of stimulus*.

Metaplasia is broadly divided into 2 types:

A. EPITHELIAL METAPLASIA Depending upon the type of epithelium transformed, two types of epithelial metaplasia are seen: squamous and columnar.

1. Squamous metaplasia This is more common. Various types of specialised epithelium are capable of undergoing squamous metaplastic change due to chronic irritation that may be mechanical, chemical or infective in origin e.g.
i)   In *bronchus* (normally lined by pseudostratified columnar ciliated epithelium) in chronic smokers.
ii)   In *uterine endocervix* (normally lined by simple columnar epithelium) in prolapse of the uterus and in old age.
iii) In *gallbladder* (normally lined by simple columnar epithelium) in chronic cholecystitis with cholelithiasis.

2. Columnar metaplasia There are some conditions in which there is transformation to columnar epithelium e.g.
i)   Intestinal metaplasia in healed chronic gastric ulcer.
ii)   Columnar metaplasia in Barrett's oesophagus, in which there is change of normal squamous epithelium to columnar epithelium.

B. MESENCHYMAL METAPLASIA Less often, there is transformation of one adult type of mesenchymal tissue to another.

1. Osseous metaplasia Osseous metaplasia is formation of bone in fibrous tissue, cartilage and myxoid tissue e.g.
i)   In arterial wall in old age (Mönckeberg's medial calcific sclerosis)
ii)   In soft tissues in myositis ossificans
iii) In cartilage of larynx and bronchi in elderly people.

2. Cartilaginous metaplasia In healing of fractures, cartilaginous metaplasia may occur where there is undue mobility.

DYSPLASIA *(p. 41)*

Dysplasia means 'disordered cellular development', often preceded or accompanied with metaplasia and hyperplasia; it is therefore also referred to as *atypical hyperplasia*. Dysplasia occurs most often in epithelial cells. Epithelial dysplasia is characterised by cellular proliferation and cytologic changes as under:
1.   Increased number of layers of epithelial cells
2.   Disorderly arrangement of cells from basal layer to the surface layer
3.   Loss of basal polarity i.e. nuclei lying away from basement membrane
4.   Cellular and nuclear pleomorphism
5.   Increased nucleocytoplasmic ratio
6.   Nuclear hyperchromatism
7.   Increased mitotic activity.

The two most common examples of dysplastic changes are the *uterine cervix* and *respiratory tract*.

Dysplastic changes often occur due to chronic irritation or prolonged inflammation. On removal of the inciting stimulus, the changes may disappear. In a proportion of cases, however, dysplasia may progress into carcinoma *in situ* (cancer confined to layers superficial to basement membrane) or invasive cancer.

Old age is a concept of longevity in human beings. The consequences of ageing appear after reproductive life when evolutionary role of the individual has been accomplished.

The average age of death of primitive man was barely 20-25 years. However, currently average life-expectancy in the west is about 80 years. In India, due to improved health care, it has gone up from an average of 26 years at the time of independence in 1947 to 64 years at present. In general, survival is longer in women than men (3: 2). In general, the life expectancy of an individual depends upon the following factors:

1. *Intrinsic genetic process* i.e. the genes controlling response to endogenous and exogenous factors initiating apoptosis in senility.

2. *Environmental factors* e.g. consumption and inhalation of harmful substances, type of diet, role of antioxidants etc.

3. *Lifestyle of the individual* such as diseases due to alcoholism (e.g. cirrhosis, hepatocellular carcinoma), smoking (e.g. bronchogenic carcinoma and other respiratory diseases), drug addiction.

4. *Age-related diseases* e.g. atherosclerosis and ischaemic heart disease, diabetes mellitus, hypertension, osteoporosis, Alzheimer's disease, Parkinson's disease etc.

THEORIES OF AGEING (p. 42)

Although no definitive biologic basis of ageing is established, most acceptable theory is the functional decline of non-dividing cells such as neurons and myocytes. The following hypotheses based on investigations mostly in other species explain the cellular basis of ageing:

1. **Experimental cellular senescence** It has been observed that with every cell division there is progressive shortening of *telomere* present at the tips of chromosomes, which in normal cell is repaired by the presence of RNA enzyme, *telomerase*. However, due to ageing there is inadequate presence of telomerase enzyme; therefore lost telomere is not repaired resulting in interference in viability of cell.

2. **Genetic control in invertebrates** Clock *(clk)* genes responsible for controlling the rate and time of ageing have been identified in lower invertebrates.

3. **Diseases of accelerated ageing** A heritable condition associated with signs of accelerated ageing process, *progeria,* seen in children is characterised by baldness, cataracts, and coronary artery disease.

4. **Oxidative stress hypothesis (free radical-mediated injury)** Ageing is partly caused by progressive and reversible molecular oxidative damage due to persistent oxidative stress on the human cells. The role of antioxidants in retarding the oxidant damage has been reported in some studies.

5. **Hormonal decline** With age, there is loss of secretion of some hormones resulting in their functional decline.

6. **Defective host defenses** Ageing causes impaired immune function and hence reduced ability to respond to microbes and environmental agents.

7. **Failure to renew** Ageing causes accumulation of senescent cells without corresponding renewal of lost cells.

ORGAN CHANGES IN AGEING (p. 43)

1. *Cardiovascular system:* Atherosclerosis, arteriosclerosis with calcification, Mönckeberg's medial calcification, brown atrophy of the heart, loss of elastic tissue from aorta and major arterial trunks causing their dilatation.

2. *Nervous system:* Atrophy of gyri and sulci, Alzheimer's disease, Parkinson's disease.

3. *Musculoskeletal system*: Degenerative bone diseases, frequent fractures due to loss of bone density, age-related muscular degeneration.
4. *Eyes:* Deterioration of vision due to cataract and vascular changes in retina.
5. *Hearing:* Disability in hearing due to senility is related to otosclerosis.
6. *Immune system:* Reduced IgG response to antigens, frequent and more severe infections.
7. *Skin:* Laxity of skin due to loss of elastic tissue.
8. *Cancers:* 80% of cancers occur in the age range of 50-80 years.

SELF ASSESSMENT

1. **Tissues for electron microscopy are fixed in:**
   A. Carnoy's fixative
   B. 10% buffered formalin
   C. Saline
   D. 4% glutaraldehyde

2. **The DNA molecule is a double helical strand having the following nucleotide bases:**
   A. Cytosine, thymine, alanine, guanine
   B. Adenine, guanine, valine, thymine
   C. Cytosine, lysine, adenine, guanine
   D. Adenine, guanine, cytosine, thymine

3. **Actin and myosin proteins are found in:**
   A. Microtubules
   B. Microfilaments
   C. Intermediate filaments
   D. Ribosomes

4. **In ischaemia-reperfusion cell injury, there are:**
   A. Increased Ca^{++} ions in the extracellular fluid
   B. Increased Ca^{++} ions in the cytosol
   C. Ca^{++} ions are equal in the cytosol and in extracellular fluid
   D. Ca^{++} ion equilibrium is unaffected

5. **The major mechanism of damage to plasma membrane in ischaemia is:**
   A. Reduced intracellular pH
   B. Increased intracellular accumulation of sodium
   C. Increased Ca^{++} ions in the cytosol
   D. Reduced aerobic respiration

6. **Out of various free radical species, the following radical is most reactive:**
   A. Superoxide ($O_2^{.}$)
   B. Hydrogen peroxide (H_2O_2)
   C. Hydroxyl (OH^-)
   D. Nitric oxide (NO)

7. **In fatty liver due to chronic alcoholism, the following mechanisms are involved <u>except</u>:**
   A. Increased free fatty acid synthesis
   B. Decreased triglyceride utilization
   C. Increased α-glycerophosphate
   D. Block in lipoprotein excretion

8. **The following pigments are stainable by Prussian blue reaction <u>except</u>:**
   A. Haemosiderin
   B. Ferritin
   C. Haematin
   D. Haemochromatosis

9. **Enzymatic digestion is the predominant event in the following type of necrosis:**
   A. Coagulative necrosis
   B. Liquefactive necrosis
   C. Caseous necrosis
   D. Fat necrosis

10. **Mechanism of mammalian apoptosis involves the most important role of the following protein:**
    A. Receptor for TNF
    B. *BCL-2*
    C. *TP53*
    D. *CED-9*

11. **Apoptosis has the following features <u>except</u>:**
    A. There is cell shrinkage in apoptosis
    B. There are no acute inflammatory cells surrounding apoptosis
    C. There may be single cell loss or affect clusters of cells
    D. Apoptosis is seen in pathologic processes only

12. **Diabetic foot is an example of:**
    A. Dry gangrene   B. Wet gangrene
    C. Gas gangrene   D. Necrotising inflammation

13. **Idiopathic calcinosis cutis is an example of:**
    A. Necrotising inflammation   B. Dystrophic calcification
    C. Metastatic calcification   D. Calcified thrombi in veins

14. **In atrophy, the cells are:**
    A. Dead cells   B. Shrunken cells
    C. Irreversibly injured cells   D. Reversibly injured cells

15. **For metaplasia the following holds true:**
    A. It is a disordered growth
    B. It affects only epithelial tissues
    C. It is a reversible change
    D. It is an irreversible and progressive change

16. **In cell cycle, signal transduction system is activated by:**
    A. G protein receptors   B. Selectins
    C. Cadherins   D. Integrins

17. **Immune system in the body is activated by:**
    A. Cell adhesion molecules   B. Cytokines
    C. G-protein receptors   D. Ion channels

18. **Which of the following genes is proapoptotic:**
    A. *p53*   B. *Bcl-2*
    C. *RB*   D. *Bax*

19. **Annexin V is used as a marker for:**
    A. Necrosis   B. Fatty change
    C. Apoptosis   D. Gangrene

20. **Enzyme which prevents ageing is:**
    A. Catalase   B. Superoxide dismutase
    C. Metalloproteinase   D. Telomerase

<u>KEY</u>

1 = D	2 = D	3 = B	4 = B	5 = C
6 = C	7 = C	8 = C	9 = B	10 = B
11 = D	12 = B	13 = B	14 = B	15 = C
16 = A	17 = B	18 = D	19 = C	20 = D

3 Immunopathology Including Amyloidosis

Broadly speaking, immunity or body defense mechanism is divided into 2 types, natural (innate) and specific (adaptive), which are interlinked to each other in their functions:

Natural or innate immunity is *non-specific* and is considered as the first line of defense without antigenic specificity. It has 2 major components:
a) *Humoral:* comprised by complement.
b) *Cellular:* consists of neutrophils, macrophages, and natural killer (NK) cells.

Specific or adaptive immunity is *specific* and is characterised by antigenic specificity. It too has 2 main components:
a) *Humoral:* consisting of antibodies formed by B cells.
b) *Cellular:* mediated by T cells.

    The **major functions of immune system** are as under:
i) Recognition of self from non-self
ii) Mounting a specific response against non-self
iii) Memory of what was earlier recognised as non-self
iv) Antibody formation
v) Cell-mediated reactions

ORGANS AND CELLS OF IMMUNE SYSTEM (p. 44)

Although functioning as a system, the organs of immune system are distributed at different places in the body. These are as under:

a) Primary lymphoid organs:
i) Thymus
ii) Bone marrow

b) Secondary lymphoid organs:
i) Lymph nodes
ii) Spleen
iii) MALT (Mucosa-Associated Lymphoid Tissue located in the respiratory tract and GIT).

CELLS OF IMMUNE SYSTEM

The cells comprising immune system are as follows:
i) Lymphocytes
ii) Monocytes and macrophages
iii) Mast cells and basophils
iv) Neutrophils
v) Eosinophils

LYMPHOCYTES

Lymphocyte is the master of human immune system. Morphologically, lymphocytes appear as a homogeneous group but functionally two major lymphocyte populations, *T and B lymphocytes*, are identified; while a third type, *NK (natural killer) cells*, comprises a small percentage of circulating lymphocytes having the distinct appearance of *large granular lymphocytes*.

    Just as other haematopoietic cells, all three subtypes of lymphocytes are formed from lymphoid precursor cells in the bone marrow. However, unlike other haematopoietic cells, lymphocytes undergo maturation and differentiation in the bone marrow (B cells) and thymus (T cells) and acquire certain genetic and immune surface characters which determine their type and function; this is based on *cluster of differentiation* (CD) molecule on their surface. CD surface protein molecules belong to immunoglobulin superfamily of cell adhesion molecules (CAMs).

B CELLS   These cells are involved in humoral immunity by inciting antibody response. B cells in circulation comprise about 10-15% of lymphocytes. Common B cell markers are: CD 19, 20, 21, 23. These cells also possess B cell receptors (BCR) for surface immunoglobulins (IgM and IgG) and Fc receptor for attaching to antibody molecule.

T CELLS   These cells are implicated in inciting cell-mediated immunity and delayed type of hypersensitivity. T cells in circulation comprise 75-80% of lymphocytes. Pan T cell markers are CD3, CD7 and CD2. Besides, T cells also carry receptor (TCR) for recognition of MHC molecules. Depending upon functional activity, T cells have two major subtypes: *T helper(or CD4+) cells* and *T suppressor(or CD8+) cells.*
◈   CD4+ cells are predominantly involved in cell-mediated reactions to viral infections (e.g. in HIV), tissue transplant reactions and tumour lysis.
◈   CD8+ cells are particularly involved in destroying cells infected with viruses, foreign cells and tumour cells.

NATURAL KILLER (NK) CELLS   NK cells comprise about 10-15% of circulating lymphocytes. NK cells are morphologically distinct from B and T cells in being *large granular lymphocytes*. NK cells are part of the natural or innate immunity. These cells recognise antibody-coated target cells and bring about killing of the target directly; this process is termed as *antibody-dependent cell-mediated cytotoxicity (ADCC)*.

MONOCYTES AND MACROPHAGES

Circulating monocytes are immature macrophages and constitute about 5% of peripheral leucocytes.
    Salient features and important immune functions of macrophages are as follows:
1.   Antigen recognition
2.   Phagocytosis
3.   Secretory function e.g. (i) *Cytokines* (IL-1, IL-2, IL-6, IL-8, IL-10, IL-12, tumour necrosis factor-α) and *prostaglandins* (PGE, thromboxane-A, leukotrienes); (ii) *Secretion of proteins involved in wound healing* e.g. collagenase, elastase, fibroblast growth factor, angiogenesis factor; (iii) *Acute phase reactants* e.g. fibronectin, microglobulin, complement components.
4.   Antigen presentation

BASOPHILS AND MAST CELLS

Basophils are a type of circulating granulocytes (0-1%) while mast cells are their counterparts seen in tissues, especially in connective tissue around blood vessels and in submucosal location. Basophils and mast cells have IgE surface receptor. Mast cells and basophils are involved in mediating inflammation in allergic reactions and have a role in wound healing.

CYTOKINES *(p. 48)*

Cytokines are immunomodulating agents composed of soluble proteins, peptides and glycoproteins secreted by haematopoietic and non-haematoopoietic cells in response to various stimuli. Their main role is in molecular interaction between various cells of the immune system and are critical in innate as well as in adaptive immune responses.

CLASSIFICATION   Based on structural similarity, cytokines are grouped in following 3 main categories:
i)   *Haematopoietin family*: G-CSF, GM-CSF, erythropoietin, thrombopoietin. Various interleukins (IL) such as IL-2, IL-3, IL-4, IL-5, IL-6, IL-6, IL-7, IL-9.

ii)   IL-1α and IL-1 β, tumour necrosis factor (TNF, cachectin), platelet-derived growth factor (PDGF), transforming growth factor (TGF)-β family.

iii)   Chemokine family: These regulate movement of cells and act through G-protein-derived receptors e.g. IL-8, monocyte chemokine protein (MCP), eotaxin, platelet factor (PF) 4.

CYTOKINE RECEPTORS   There are 5 members of family of cytokine receptors:

i)   Immunoglogulin (Ig) superfamily is the largest group composed of cell surface receptors and extracellular secreted proteins e.g. IL-1 receptors type 1, type 2 etc.

ii)   Haematopoietic growth factor type 1 receptor family includes receptors or their subunits shared with several interleukins.

iii)   IFN type II receptor family includes receptors for IFN-γ, IFN-β.

iv)   TNF receptor family members are TNF-R1 and TNF-R2, CD40 (B cell marker), CD27 and CD30 (found on activated T and B cells).

v)   Trans-membrane helix receptor family is linked to GTP-binding proteins and includes two important chemokines, chemokine receptor type 4 (CXCR4) and β-chemokine receptor type 5 (CCR5).

MODE OF ACTION OF CYTOKINES   Cytokines may act in one of the following 3 ways:

1)   *Autocrine* when a cytokine acts on the cell which produced it.

2)   *Paracrine* when it acts on another target cell in the vicinity.

3)   *Endocrine* when the cytokine secreted in circulation acts on a distant target.

Cytokines are involved in following actions:

1.   Regulation of growth
2.   Inflammatory mediators
3.   Activation of immune system
4.   Cytokine storm

HLA SYSTEM AND MAJOR HISTOCOMPATIBILITY COMPLEX *(p. 48)*

HLA stands for *Human Leucocyte Antigens* because these are antigens or genetic proteins in the body that determine one's own tissue from non-self (histocompatibility) and were first discovered on the surface of leucocytes. Subsequently, it was found that HLA are actually gene complexes of proteins on the surface of all nucleated cells of the body and platelets. Since these complexes are of immense importance in matching donor and recipient for organ transplant, they are called *major histocompatibility complex (MHC) or HLA complex.*

Out of various genes for histocompatibility, most of the transplantation antigens or MHC are located on short arm (p) of *chromosome 6*; these genes occupy four regions or loci—A, B, C and D, and exhibit marked variation in allelic genes at each locus. Therefore, the product of HLA antigens is highly polymorphic.

Depending upon the characteristics of MHC, they have been divided into 3 classes:

◈   **Class I MHC antigens** have loci as HLA-A, HLA-B and HLA-C. CD8+ (i.e. T suppressor) lymphocytes carry receptors for class I MHC; these cells are used to identify class I antigen on them.

◈   **Class II MHC antigens** have single locus as HLA-D. These antigens have further 3 loci: DR, DQ and DP. Class II MHC is identified by B cells and CD4+ (i.e. T helper) cells.

◈   **Class III MHC antigens** are some components of the complement system (C2 and C4) coded on HLA complex but are not associated with HLA expression and are not used in antigen identification.

ROLE OF HLA COMPLEX

1.   Organ transplantation
2.   Regulation of the immune system
3.   Association of diseases with HLA e.g. autoimmune disorders, spondyloarthropathies, endocrinopathies and neurologic diseases.

According to the genetic relationship between donor and recipient, transplantation of tissues is classified into 4 groups:

1. *Autografts* are grafts in which the donor and recipient is the same individual.

2. *Isografts* are grafts between the donor and recipient of the same genotype.

3. *Allografts* are those in which the donor is of the same species but of a different genotype.

4. *Xenografts* are those in which the donor is of a different species from that of the recipient.

Presently, surgical skills exist for skin grafts and for organ transplants such as kidney, heart, lungs, liver, pancreas, cornea and bone marrow. For any successful tissue transplant without immunological rejection, matched major histocompatibility locus antigens (HLA) between the donor and recipient are of paramount importance as discussed already. The greater the genetic disparity between donor and recipient in HLA system, the stronger and more rapid will be the rejection reaction.

Besides the rejection reaction, a peculiar problem occurring especially in bone marrow transplantation is *graft-versus-host (GVH) reaction*. In humans, GVH reaction results when immunocompetent cells are transplanted to an immunodeficient recipient e.g. treating severe combined immunodeficiency by bone marrow transplantation.

MECHANISMS OF GRAFT REJECTION

Except for autografts and isografts, an immune response against allografts is inevitable. The development of immunosuppressive drugs has made the survival of allografts in recipients possible. Rejection of allografts involves both cell-mediated and humoral immunity.

1. CELL-MEDIATED IMMUNE REACTIONS These are mainly responsible for graft rejection and are mediated by T cells.

2. HUMORAL IMMUNE REACTIONS These include: *preformed circulating antibodies* due to *pre-sensitisation* of the recipient before transplantation e.g. by blood transfusions and previous pregnancies.

TYPES OF REJECTION REACTIONS

Based on the underlying mechanism and time period, rejection reactions are classified into 3 types: hyperacute, acute and chronic.

DISEASES OF IMMUNITY *(p. 50)*

While normal function of immunity is for body defense, its failure or derangement in any way results in diseases of the immune system which are broadly classified into the following 4 groups:

1. Immunodeficiency disorders are characterised by deficient or absent cellular and/or humoral immune functions. This group is comprised by a list of *primary and secondary immunodeficiency diseases* including the dreaded *acquired immunodeficiency syndrome (AIDS)*.

2. Hypersensitivity reactions are characterised by hyperfunction or inappropriate response of the immune system and cover the various mechanisms of *immunologic tissue injury*.

3. Autoimmune diseases occur when the immune system fails to recognise 'self' from 'non-self'. A growing number of *autoimmune and collagen diseases* are included in this group.

4. Possible immune disorders in which the immunologic mechanisms are suspected in their etiopathogenesis. Classical example of this group is *amyloidosis*.

EPIDEMIOLOGY AIDS is pandemic in distribution and is seen in all continents. Regionwise, besides Sub-Saharan Africa, other countries in order of decreasing incidence of AIDS are South and South-East Asia, Latin America, Eastern Europe, Central Asia, North America, while Oceania region has the lowest incidence. The burden of AIDS in India is estimated at 2.4 million cases; epicentre of the epidemic lies in the states of Maharashtra, Tamil Nadu and Andhra Pradesh which together comprise about 50% of all HIV positive cases (mostly contracted heterosexually), while North-East state of Manipur accounts for 8% of all cases (more often among intravenous drug abusers).

ETIOLOGIC AGENT AIDS is caused by an RNA (retrovirus) virus called human immunodeficiency virus (HIV).

HIV-I virion or virus particle is spherical in shape and 100-140 nm in size:

◈ It contains a *core* having *core proteins*, chiefly p24 and p18, two strands of genomic RNA and the enzyme, reverse transcriptase.

◈ The core is covered by a *double layer of lipid membrane* derived from the outer membrane of the infected host cell during budding process of virus. The membrane is studded with *2 envelope glycoproteins, gp120 and gp41.*

ROUTES OF TRANSMISSION Transmission of HIV infection occurs by one of following three routes and it varies in different populations:

1. Sexual transmission Sexual contact in the main mode of spread and constitutes 75% of all cases of HIV transmission. Most cases of AIDS in the industrialised world such as in the US occur in *homosexual* or *bisexual males* while *heterosexual promiscuity* seems to be the dominant mode of HIV infection in Africa and Asia.

2. Transmission via blood and blood products This mode of transmission is the next largest group (25%) and occurs in 3 types of high-risk populations:
i) Intravenous drug abusers
ii) Haemophiliacs
iii) Recipients of HIV-infected blood and blood products.

3. Perinatal transmission HIV infection occurs from infected mother to the newborn during pregnancy *transplacentally.*

It should also be appreciated that HIV contaminated waste products can be *sterilised and disinfected* by most of the chemical germicides used in laboratories at a much lower concentration. These are: sodium hypochlorite (liquid chlorine bleach) (1-10% depending upon amount of contamination with organic material such as blood, mucus), formaldehyde (5%), ethanol (70%), glutaraldehyde (2%), β-propionolactone. HIV is also heat-sensitive and can be inactivated at 56°C for 30 min.

PATHOGENESIS The pathogenesis of HIV infection is largely related to the *depletion of CD4+ T cells (helper T cells) resulting in profound immunosuppression.*

1. Selective tropism for CD4 molecule receptor gp120 envelope glycoprotein of HIV has selective tropism for cells containing CD4 molecule receptor on their surface. These cells most importantly are CD4+ T cells (T helper cells); other such cells include monocyte-macrophages, microglial cells, epithelial cells of the cervix, Langerhans cells of the skin and follicular dendritic cells.

2. Internalisation gp120 of the virion combines with CD4 receptor, but for fusion of virion with the host cell membrane, a chemokine coreceptor (CCR) is necessary.

3. Uncoating and viral DNA formation Once the virion has entered the T cell cytoplasm, reverse transcriptase of the viral RNA forms a single-stranded DNA. Using the single-stranded DNA as a template, DNA polymerase copies it to make it double-stranded DNA, while destroying the original RNA strands.

4. Viral integration The viral DNA so formed may initially remain *unintegrated* in the affected cell but later viral integrase protein inserts the viral DNA into nucleus of the host T cell and *integrates* in the host cell DNA.

5. Viral replication HIV provirus having become part of host cell DNA, host cell DNA transcripts for viral RNA with presence of *tat* gene. Multiplication of viral particles is further facilitated by release of cytokines from T helper cells (CD4+ T cells).

6. Latent period and immune attack In an inactive infected T cell, the infection may remain in latent phase for a long time, accounting for the long incubation period.

7. CD4+ T cell destruction Viral particles replicated in the CD4+ T cells start forming *buds* from the cell wall of the host cell.

8. Viral dissemination Release of viral particles from infected host cell spreads the infection to more CD4+ host cells and produces viraemia.

9. Impact of HIV infection on other immune cells HIV infects other cells of the host immune system and also affects non-infected lymphoid cells.

10. HIV infection of nervous system Out of non-lymphoid organ involvement, HIV infection of nervous system is the most serious and 75-90% of AIDS patients may demonstrate some form of neurological involvement at autopsy. It infects microglial cells, astrocytes and oligodendrocytes.

NATURAL HISTORY HIV infection progresses from an early acute syndrome to a prolonged asymptomatic state to advanced disease. Thus there are different clinical manifestations at different stages. Generally, in an immunocompetent host, the biologic course passes through following 3 phases:

1. Acute HIV syndrome Entry of HIV into the body is heralded by the following sequence of events:
i) High levels of plasma *viraemia*.
ii) Virus-specific immune response by formation of anti-HIV antibodies (*seroconversion*) after 3-6 weeks of initial exposure to HIV.
iii) Initially, sudden marked reduction in *CD4+ T cells* (helper T cells) followed by return to normal levels.
iv) Rise in *CD8+ T cells* (cytotoxic T cells).
v) Appearance of self-limited non-specific *acute viral illness* (flu-like or infectious mononucleosis-like) in 50-70% of adults within 3-6 weeks of initial infection.

2. Middle chronic phase The initial acute seroconversion illness is followed by a phase of competition between HIV and the host immune response.

3. Final crisis phase This phase is characterised by profound immuno-suppression and onset of full-blown AIDS.

REVISED CDC HIV CLASSIFICATION SYSTEM The Centers for Disease Control and Prevention (CDC), US in 1993 revised the classification system for HIV infection in adults and children based on 2 parameters: clinical manifestations and CD4+ T cell counts.

According to this system, irrespective of presence of symptoms, any HIV-infected individual having CD4+ T cell count of <200/µl is labelled as AIDS:

Clinical category A Includes a variety of conditions: asymptomatic case, persistent generalised lymphadenopathy (PGL), and acute HIV syndrome.

Clinical category B Includes symptomatic cases and includes conditions secondary to impaired cell-mediated immunity e.g. bacillary dysentery, mucosal candidiasis, fever, oral hairy leukoplakia, ITP, pelvic inflammatory disease, peripheral neuropathy, cervical dysplasia and carcinoma in situ cervix etc.

Clinical category C This category includes conditions listed for AIDS surveillance case definition. These are mucosal candidiasis, cancer uterine cervix, bacterial infections (e.g. tuberculosis), fungal infections (e.g. histoplasmosis), parasitic infections (e.g. *Pneumocystis* pneumonia), malnutrition and wasting of muscles etc.

PATHOLOGICAL LESIONS AND CLINICAL MANIFESTATIONS OF HIV/ AIDS HIV/AIDS affects all body organs and systems. In general, clinical manifestations and pathological lesions in different organs and systems are owing to progressive deterioration of body's immune system. Disease progression occurs in all untreated patients, even if the disease is apparently latent. Antiretroviral treatment blocks and slows the progression of the disease.

Pathological lesions and clinical manifestations in HIV disease can be explained by 4 mechanisms:

i)   Due to viral infection directly: The major targets are immune system, central nervous system and lymph nodes (persistent generalised lymphadenopathy).

ii)   Due to opportunistic infections: Deteriorating immune system provides the body an opportunity to harbour microorganisms.

iii) Due to secondary tumours: End-stage of HIV/AIDS is characterised by development of certain secondary malignant tumours.

iv)   Due to drug treatment: Drugs used in the treatment produce toxic effects. These include antiretroviral treatment, aggressive treatment of opportunistic infections and tumours.

Multisystem changes are as under:
1.   Wasting syndrome
2.   Persistent generalised lymphadenopathy
3.   GI lesions and manifestations
4.   Pulmonary lesions and manifestations
5.   Mucocutaneous lesions and manifestations
6.   Haematologic lesions and manifestations
7.   CNS lesions and manifestations
8.   Gynaecologic lesions and manifestations
9.   Renal lesions and manifestations
10. Hepatobiliary lesions and manifestations
11. Cardiovascular lesions and manifestations
12. Ophthalmic lesions
13. Musculoskeletal lesions
14. Endocrine lesions

DIAGNOSIS OF HIV/AIDS The investigations of a suspected case of HIV/ AIDS are categorised into 3 groups:

1.   Tests for establishing HIV infection These include antibody tests and direct detection of HIV.

i)   Antibody tests These tests are:
a)   *ELISA*
b)   *Western blot*

ii)   Direct detection of HIV
a) *p24* antigen capture assay.
b) *HIV RNA* assay methods by reverse transcriptase (RT) PCR, branched DNA, nucleic acid sequence-based amplification (NucliSens).
c) *DNA-PCR* by amplification of proviral DNA.
d) *Culture* of HIV from blood monocytes and CD4+ T cells.

2.   Tests for defects in immunity These tests are used for diagnosis as well as for monitoring treatment of cases.
i)   *CD4+ T cell counts.* Progressive fall in number of CD4+ T cells is of paramount importance in diagnosis and staging as CDC categories as described above.
ii)   Rise in CD8+ T cells.
iii) Reversal of CD4+ to CD8+ T cell ratio.
iv)   Lymphopenia.
v)   Polyclonal hypergammaglobulinaemia.
vi)   Increased β-2 microglobulin levels.
vii) Platelet count revealing thrombocytopenia.

3. Tests for detection of opportunistic infections and secondary tumours Diagnosis of organs involved in opportunistic infection and specific tumours secondary to HIV/AIDS is made by aspiration or biopsy methods as for the corresponding primary disease.

HYPERSENSITIVITY REACTIONS (IMMUNOLOGIC TISSUE INJURY) (p. 57)

Hypersensitivity is defined as an exaggerated or inappropriate state of normal immune response with onset of adverse effects on the body. The lesions of hypersensitivity are a form of antigen-antibody reaction. Depending upon the *rapidity, duration and type* of the immune response, these 4 types of hypersensitivity reactions are grouped into either immediate or delayed type:

1. Immediate type in which on administration of antigen, the reaction occurs immediately (within seconds to minutes). Immune response in this type is mediated largely by *humoral antibodies* (B cell mediated). Immediate type of hypersensitivity reactions include *type I, II and III*.

2. Delayed type in which the reaction is slower in onset and develops within 24-48 hours and the effect is prolonged. It is mediated by *cellular response* (T cell mediated) and it includes *Type IV reaction*.

TYPE I: ANAPHYLACTIC (ATOPIC) REACTION

Type I hypersensitivity is defined as a state of rapidly developing or anaphylactic type of immune response to an antigen (i.e. allergen) to which the individual is previously sensitised (anaphylaxis is the opposite of prophylaxis). The reaction appears within 15-30 minutes of exposure to antigen.

ETIOLOGY AND PATHOGENESIS Type I reaction is mediated by *humoral antibodies of IgE type or reagin antibodies* in response to antigen. Type I reaction includes participation by B lymphocytes and plasma cells, mast cells and basophils, neutrophils and eosinophils.

EXAMPLES OF TYPE I REACTION The manifestations of type I reaction may be variable in severity and intensity. It may manifest as a local irritant (skin, nose, throat, lungs etc), or sometimes may be severe and life-threatening anaphylaxis.

Systemic anaphylaxis:
i) Administration of antisera e.g. anti-tetanus serum (ATS).
ii) Administration of drugs e.g. penicillin.
iii) Sting by wasp or bee.

Local anaphylaxis:
i) Hay fever (seasonal allergic rhinitis) due to pollen sensitisation of conjunctiva and nasal passages.
ii) Bronchial asthma due to allergy to inhaled allergens like house dust.
iii) Food allergy to ingested allergens like fish, cow's milk, eggs etc.
iv) Cutaneous anaphylaxis due to contact of antigen with skin characterised by urticaria, wheal and flare.
v) Angioedema, an autosomal dominant inherited disorder characterised by laryngeal oedema, oedema of eyelids, lips, tongue and trunk.

TYPE II: ANTIBODY-MEDIATED (CYTOTOXIC) REACTION

Type II or cytotoxic reaction is defined as reaction by humoral antibodies that attack cell surface antigens on the specific cells and tissues and cause lysis of target cells. Type II reaction too appears generally within 15-30 minutes after exposure to antigen but in myasthenia gravis and thyroiditis it may appear after longer duration.

ETIOLOGY AND PATHOGENESIS In general, type II reactions have participation by complement system, tissue macrophages, platelets, natural killer cells, neutrophils and eosinophils while main antibodies are IgG and IgM class. Type II hypersensitivity is tissue-specific and reaction occurs after antibodies bind to tissue specific antigens, most often on blood cells.

EXAMPLES OF TYPE II REACTION Examples of type II reaction are mainly on blood cells and some other body cells and tissues.

1. Cytotoxic antibodies to blood cells e.g.
i)   Autoimmune haemolytic anaemia
ii) Transfusion reactions
iii) Haemolytic disease of the newborn (erythroblastosis foetalis)
iv) Idiopathic thrombocytopenic purpura (ITP)
v)   Leucopenia with agranulocytosis
vi) Drug-induced cytotoxic antibodies

2. Cytotoxic antibodies to tissue components e.g.
i)   In *Graves' disease* (primary hyperthyroidism),
ii) In *myasthenia gravis*,
iii) In *male sterility*, antisperm antibody is formed
iv) In *type 1 diabetes mellitus*, islet cell autoantibodies are formed
v)   In *hyperacute rejection reaction*, antibodies are formed against donor antigen.

TYPE III: IMMUNE COMPLEX MEDIATED (ARTHUS) REACTION

Type III reactions result from deposition of antigen-antibody complexes on tissues, which is followed by activation of the complement system and inflammatory reaction, resulting in cell injury. The onset of type III reaction takes place about 6 hours after exposure to the antigen.

ETIOLOGY AND PATHOGENESIS Type III reaction is not tissue specific and occurs when antigen-antibody complexes fail to get removed by the body's immune system. There are 3 types of possible etiologic factors precipitating type III reaction:
1. Persistence of low-grade microbial infection
2. Extrinsic environmental antigen
3. Autoimmune process

It may be mentioned here that both type II and type III reactions have antigen-antibody complex formation but the two can be distinguished— antigen in type II is tissue specific while in type III it is not so. Moreover the mechanism of cell injury in type II is direct but in type III it is by deposition of antigen-antibody complex on tissues and subsequent sequence of cell injury takes place. Type III reaction has participation by IgG and IgM antibodies, neutrophils, mast cells and complement.

EXAMPLES OF TYPE III REACTION These are as under:
i)   Immune complex glomerulonephritis in which the antigen may be glomerular basement membrane (GBM) or exogenous agents (e.g. Streptococcal antigen).
ii) Goodpasture syndrome having GBM as antigen.
iii) SLE in which there is nuclear antigen (DNA, RNA) and there is formation of anti-nuclear and anti-DNA autoantibodies.
iv) Rheumatoid arthritis in which there is nuclear antigen.
v)   Farmer's lung in which actinomycetes-contaminated hay acts as antigen.
vi) Polyarteritis nodosa and Wegener's granulomatosis with antineutrophil cytoplasmic antigen.
vii) Henoch-Schönlein purpura in which respiratory viruses act as antigen.
viii) Drug-induced vasculitis in which the drug acts as antigen.

TYPE IV: DELAYED HYPERSENSITIVITY (T CELL-MEDIATED) REACTION

Type IV or delayed hypersensitivity reaction is tissue injury by T cell-mediated immune response without formation of antibodies (contrary to type I, II and III) but is instead a slow and prolonged response. The reaction occurs about 24 hours after exposure to antigen and the effect is prolonged which may last up to 14 days.

ETIOLOGY AND PATHOGENESIS Type IV reaction involves role of mast cells and basophils, macrophages and CD8+ T cells.

EXAMPLES OF TYPE IV REACTION These are as follows:
1.   Reaction against mycobacterial infection e.g. tuberculin reaction, granulomatous reaction in tuberculosis, leprosy.
2.   Reaction against virally infected cells.
3.   Reaction against malignant cells in the body.
4.   Reaction against organ transplantation e.g. transplant rejection, graft versus host reaction.

AUTOIMMUNE DISEASES *(p. 61)*

Autoimmunity is a state in which the body's immune system fails to distinguish between 'self' and 'non-self' and reacts by formation of auto-antibodies against one's own tissue antigens. In other words, there is loss of tolerance to one's own tissues; *autoimmunity is the opposite of immune tolerance.*

PATHOGENESIS (THEORIES) OF AUTOIMMUNITY

Normally, the body's response to self antigens (autoimmunity) is prevented by three major processes:
1.   *Sequestration* of autoantigens
2.   *Generation and maintenance* of tolerance or anergy by T and B lymphocytes in the body.
3.   *Regulatory mechanisms* limiting response by the immune system.
      The mechanisms by which the immune tolerance of the body is broken causes autoimmunity. These are as under:

1.   Immunological factors Failure of immunological mechanisms of tolerance initiates autoimmunity as follows:
i)   Polyclonal activation of B cells
ii)   Generation of self-reacting B cell clones
iii) Decreased T suppressor and increased T helper cell activity.
iv)   Fluctuation of anti-idiotype network control
v)   Sequestered antigen released from tissues.

2.   Genetic factors e.g.
i)   There is increased expression of *Class II HLA antigens* on tissues involved in autoimmunity.
ii)   There is increased *familial incidence* of some forms of the autoimmune disorders.
iii) There is higher incidence of autoimmune diseases in *twins* favouring genetic basis.

3.   Microbial factors Infection with microorganisms, particularly viruses (e.g. EBV infection), and less often bacteria (e.g. streptococci, *Klebsiella*) and mycoplasma, has been implicated.

TYPES AND EXAMPLES OF AUTOIMMUNE DISEASES

Autoimmune diseases are a growing number of such diseases in which autoimmunity is either mediated by formation of immune complexes or they are mediated by T cells.
      Depending upon the type of autoantibody formation, the autoimmune diseases are broadly classified into 2 groups:

1.   Organ specific (Localised) diseases In these, the autoantibodies formed react specifically against an organ or target tissue component and cause its chronic inflammatory destruction. The tissues affected are endocrine glands (e.g. thyroid, pancreatic islets of Langerhans, adrenal cortex), alimentary tract, blood cells and various other tissues and organs.

2.   Organ non-specific (Systemic) diseases These are diseases in which a number of autoantibodies are formed which react with antigens in many tissues and thus cause systemic lesions. The examples of this group are various systemic collagen diseases.
      However, a few autoimmune diseases overlap between these two main categories. Common examples are described here.

SLE is the classical example of systemic autoimmune or collagen diseases. 2 forms of lupus erythematosus are described:

1. Systemic or disseminated form is characterised by acute and chronic inflammatory lesions widely scattered in the body and there is presence of various nuclear and cytoplasmic autoantibodies in the plasma.

2. Discoid form is characterised by chronic and localised skin lesions involving the bridge of nose and adjacent cheeks without any systemic manifestations. Rarely, discoid form may develop into disseminated form.

ETIOLOGY AND PATHOGENESIS The exact etiology of SLE is not known. However, there is role of heredity and certain environmental factors. Interaction between susceptibility genes and environmental factors results in abnormal immune responses by formation of various autoantibodies as under:

i) Antinuclear antibodies (ANA) These are the antibodies against common nuclear antigen that includes DNA as well as RNA. These are demonstrable in about 98% cases and are used as screening test.

ii) Antibodies to double-stranded (anti-dsDNA) This is the most specific for SLE, especially in high titres, and is present in 70% cases.

iii) Anti-Smith antibodies (anti-Sm) These antibodies appear against Smith antigen which is part of ribonucleoproteins. It is also specific for SLE but is seen in about 25% cases.

iv) Other non-specific antibodies Besides above, there are several other antibody tests which lack specificity for SLE e.g.
a) Anti-ribonucleoproteins (anti-RNP)
b) Anti-histone antibody
c) Antiphospholipid antibodies (APLA) or lupus anticoagulant
d) Anti-ribosomal P antibody.

The source of these autoantibodies as well as hypergamma-globulinaemia seen in SLE is the **polyclonal activation of B cells**.

Two types of immunologic tissue injury can occur in SLE:

1. *Type II hypersensitivity* is characterised by formation of autoantibodies against blood cells (red blood cells, platelets, leucocytes) and results in haematologic derangement in SLE.

2. *Type III hypersensitivity* is characterised by antigen-antibody complex (commonly DNA-anti-DNA antibody; sometimes Ig-anti-Ig antibody complex) which is deposited at sites such as renal glomeruli, walls of small blood vessels etc.

LE CELL PHENOMENON This was the first diagnostic laboratory test described for SLE. The test is based on the principle that ANAs cannot penetrate the intact cells and thus cell nuclei should be exposed to bind them with the ANAs.

LE cell is a phagocytic leucocyte, commonly polymorphonuclear neutrophil, and sometimes a monocyte, which engulfs the homogeneous nuclear material of the injured cell. A few other conditions may also show positive LE test e.g. rheumatoid arthritis, lupoid hepatitis, penicillin sensitivity etc.

MORPHOLOGIC FEATURES The manifestations of SLE are widespread in different visceral organs and as erythematous cutaneous eruptions. The principal lesions are renal, vascular, cutaneous and cardiac; other organs and tissues involved are serosal linings (pleuritis, pericarditis), joints (synovitis), spleen (vasculitis), liver (portal triaditis), lungs (interstitial pneumonitis, fibrosing alveolitis), CNS (vasculitis) and in blood (autoimmune haemolytic anaemia, thrombocytopaenia).

M/E The characteristic lesion in SLE is *fibrinoid necrosis* which may be seen in the connective tissue, beneath the endothelium in small blood vessels, under the mesothelial lining of pleura and pericardium, under the endothelium in endocardium, or under the synovial lining cells of joints.

SCLERODERMA (SYSTEMIC SCLEROSIS)

Just like SLE, scleroderma was initially described as a skin disease characterised by progressive fibrosis. But now, 2 main types are recognised:

1. *Diffuse scleroderma* in which the skin shows widespread involvement and may progress to involve visceral structures.

2. *CREST syndrome* characterised by Calcinosis (C), Raynaud's phenomenon (R), Esophageal hypomotility (E), Sclerodactyly (S) and Telangiectasia (T).

ETIOPATHOGENESIS There is role of following 2 factors in its etiology:
1. *Susceptibility genes* as seen in occurrence of disease in families and in twins.
2. *Certain environmental factors* e.g. CMV infection, and role of common shared environmental exposure of certain agents as seen by prevalence of disease in some geographic location.

MORPHOLOGIC FEATURES Disseminated visceral involvement as well as cutaneous lesions are seen in systemic sclerosis.

INFLAMMATORY MYOPATHIES

This group includes three conditions having common clinical feature of progressive skeletal muscle weakness: polymyositis, dermatomyositis and inclusion body myositis. All the three forms of inflammatory myositis appear to have an autoimmune etiology.

SJÖGREN'S SYNDROME

Sjögren's syndrome is characterised by the *triad* of dry eyes *(keratoconjunctivitis sicca)*, dry mouth *(xerostomia)*, and *rheumatoid arthritis*. The combination of the former two symptoms is called *sicca syndrome*. Both humoral and cellular immune mechanisms have been implicated in the etiopathogenesis of lesions in Sjögren's syndrome.

AMYLOIDOSIS (p. 66)

Amyloidosis is the term used for a group of diseases characterised by extracellular deposition of fibrillar insoluble proteinaceous substance called amyloid having common morphological appearance, staining properties and physical structure but with variable protein (or biochemical) composition.

PHYSICAL AND CHEMICAL NATURE OF AMYLOID (p. 67)

Ultrastructural examination and chemical analysis reveal the complex nature of amyloid. *It emerges that on the basis of morphology and physical characteristics, all forms of amyloid are similar in appearance, but they are chemically heterogeneous.* Based on analysis, amyloid is composed of 2 main types of complex proteins:
I. *Fibril proteins* comprise about 95% of amyloid.
II. *Non-fibrillar components* which include *P-component* predominantly; and there are several other different proteins which together constitute the remaining 5% of amyloid.

I. FIBRIL PROTEINS

By electron microscopy, it became apparent that major component of all forms of amyloid (about 95%) consists of meshwork of fibril proteins. These consist of delicate, randomly dispersed, non-branching amyloid fibres having 4-6 fibrils, each measuring 7.5-10 nm in diameter and having indefinite length.

Chemical analysis of fibril proteins of amyloid reveals heterogeneous nature of amyloid. These proteins can be categorised as under:
i) AL (amyloid light chain) protein
ii) AA (amyloid associated) protein
iii) Other proteins

AL PROTEIN AL amyloid fibril protein is derived from immunoglobulin light chain, which may be complete light chain, or may include amino-terminal segment and part of C region of the immunoglobulin light chain. AL fibril protein is more frequently derived from the lambda (λ) light chain (twice more common) than kappa (κ). However, in any given case, there is amino acid sequence homology.

AL type of fibril protein is produced by immunoglobulin-secreting cells and is therefore seen in association with plasma cell dyscrasias and is included in primary systemic amyloidosis.

AA PROTEIN AA fibril protein is composed of protein with molecular weight of 8.5-kD which is derived from larger precursor protein in the serum called SAA (serum amyloid-associated protein) with a molecular weight of 12.5-kD. Unlike AL amyloid, the deposits of AA amyloid do not have sequence homology. In the plasma, SAA circulates in association with HDL3 (high-density lipoprotein). SAA is an acute phase reactant protein synthesised in the liver, in response to chronic inflammatory and traumatic conditions, and thus the level of SAA is high in these conditions.

AA fibril protein is found in secondary amyloidosis which is seen in association with several examples of chronic infectious and autoimmune inflammatory diseases and disseminated malignancies.

OTHER PROTEINS Apart from the two major forms of amyloid fibril proteins, a few other forms of proteins are found in different clinical states:

1. **Transthyretin (TTR)** It is a serum protein synthesised in the liver and normally *transports thy*roxine and *retino*l (trans-thy-retin). ATTR is the most common form of heredofamilial amyloidosis seen in familial amyloid poly-neuropathies.

2. **Aβ2-microglobulin (Aβ2M)** This form of amyloid is seen in cases of long-term haemodialysis (for 10-12 years). As the name suggests, β2M is a small protein which is a normal component of major histocompatibility complex (MHC) class I and has β-pleated sheet structure.

3. **Amyloid β-peptide (Aβ)** Aβ is distinct from Aβ2M and is deposited in cerebral amyloid angiopathy and neurofibrillary tangles in Alzheimer's disease. Aβ is derived from amyloid beta precursor protein (AβPP).

4. **Endocrine amyloid from hormone precursor proteins** e.g. amyloid derived from pro-calcitonin (ACal), islet amyloid polypeptide (AIAPP, amylin), pro-insulin (AIns), prolactin (APro) etc.

5. **Amyloid of prion protein (APrP)** It is derived from precursor prion protein which is a plasma membrane glycoprotein. Prion proteins are proteinaceous infectious particles lacking in RNA or DNA.

II. NON-FIBRILLAR COMPONENTS

Non-fibrillar components comprise about 5% of the amyloid material. These components include the following:

1. **Amyloid P (AP)-component** It is synthesised in the liver and is present in all types of amyloid. It is derived from circulating serum amyloid P-component, a glycoprotein resembling the normal serum α1-glycoprotein and is PAS-positive. It is structurally related to C-reactive protein, an acute phase reactant, but is not similar to it. By electron microscopy, it has a penta-gonal profile (P-component) or doughnut-shape with an external diameter of 9 nm and internal diameter of 4 nm.

2. **Apolipoprotein-E (apoE)** It is a regulator of lipoprotein metabolism and is found in all types of amyloid.

3. **Sulfated glycosaminoglycans (GAGs)** These are constituents of matrix proteins, particularly associated is heparan sulfate in all types of tissue amyloid.

PATHOGENESIS OF AMYLOIDOSIS (p. 69)

Irrespective of the type of amyloid, amyloidogenesis in general *in vivo*, occurs in the following sequence:

1. *Pool of amyloidogenic precursor protein* is present in circulation in different clinical settings and in response to stimuli e.g. increased hepatic synthesis of AA or ATTR, increased synthesis of AL etc.

2. *A nidus for fibrillogenesis,* meaning thereby an alteration in microenvironment, to stimulate deposition of amyloid protein is formed.

3. *Partial degradation or proteolysis* occurs prior to deposition of fibrillar protein which may occur in macrophages or reticuloendothelial cells.

4. The role of *non-fibrillar components* (e.g. AP, apoE and GAGs) in amyloidosis is fibril stabilisation by protein aggregation and protein folding in a way that it is protected from soulbilsation or degradation.

DEPOSITION OF AL AMYLOID

1. The stimulus for production of AL amyloid is some disorder of *immunoglobulin synthesis* e.g. multiple myeloma, B cell lymphoma, other plasma cell dyscrasias.

2. Excessive immunoglobulin production is in the form of *monoclonal gammopathy* i.e. there is production of either intact immunoglobulin, or λ light chain, or κ light chain, or rarely heavy chains. This takes place by monoclonal proliferation of plasma cells, B lymphocytes, or their precursors.

3. *Partial degradation* in the form of limited proteolysis of larger protein molecules occurs in macrophages that are anatomically closely associated with AL amyloid.

4. *Non-fibrillar components* like AP and GAGs play role in folding and aggregation of fibril proteins.

DEPOSITION OF AA AMYLOID

1. AA amyloid is directly related to *SAA levels,* a high-density lipoprotein. SAA is synthesised by the liver in response to *cytokines,* notably interleukin 1 and 6, released from activated macrophages.

2. The levels of SAA are elevated in *long-standing tissue destruction* e.g. in chronic inflammation, cancers. However, SAA levels in isolation do not always lead to AA amyloid.

3. As in AL amyloid, *partial degradation* in the form of limited proteolysis takes place in reticuloendothelial cells.

4. In AA amyloid, a significant role is played by another glycoprotein, *amyloid enhancing factor (AEF)*.

5. As in AL amyloid, there is a role of *AP component* and *glycosamino-glycans* in the fibril protein aggregation and its protection from disaggregation again.

CLASSIFICATION OF AMYLOIDOSIS *(p. 70)*

A *clinicopathologic classification* has been proposed which is widely accepted and is as under:

A. *Systemic (generalised) amyloidosis:*
1. Primary (AL)
2. Secondary/reactive/ inflammatory (AA)
3. Haemodialysis-associated (Aβ2M)
4. Heredofamilial (ATTR, AA, Others)

B. *Localised amyloidosis:*
1. Senile cardiac (ATTR)
2. Senile cerebral (Aβ, APrP)
3. Endocrine (Hormone precursors)
4. Tumour-forming (AL)

A. SYSTEMIC AMYLOIDOSIS

1. PRIMARY SYSTEMIC (AL) AMYLOIDOSIS

Primary amyloidosis consisting of AL fibril proteins is systemic or generalised in distribution. About 30% cases of AL amyloid have some form of plasma cell dyscrasias, most commonly multiple myeloma (in about 15-20% cases), and less often other monoclonal gammopathies such as Waldenström's macroglobulinaemia, heavy chain disease, solitary plasmacytoma and B cell lymphoma. The remaining 70% cases of AL amyloid do not have evident B-cell proliferative disorder or any other associated diseases and thus are cases of true 'primary' (idiopathic) amyloidosis.

AL amyloid is most prevalent type of systemic amyloidosis in North America and Europe and is seen in individuals past the age of 40 years and is rapidly progressive disease if not treated. Primary amyloidosis is often severe in the heart, kidney, bowel, skin, peripheral nerves, respiratory tract, skeletal muscle and tongue (macroglossia).

2. SECONDARY/REACTIVE (AA) SYSTEMIC AMYLOIDOSIS

The second form of systemic or generalised amyloidosis is reactive or inflammatory or secondary in which the fibril proteins contain AA amyloid. Secondary or reactive amyloidosis occurs typically as a complication of chronic infectious (e.g. tuberculosis, bronchiectasis, chronic osteomyelitis, chronic pyelonephritis, leprosy, chronic skin infections), non-infectious chronic inflammatory conditions associated with tissue destruction (e.g. autoimmune disorders such as rheumatoid arthritis, lupus, inflammatory bowel disease), some tumours (e.g. renal cell carcinoma, Hodgkin's disease) and in familial Mediterranean fever, an inherited disorder (discussed below).

Secondary amyloidosis is typically distributed in solid abdominal viscera like the kidney, liver, spleen and adrenals. Secondary reactive amyloidosis is seen less frequently in developed countries due to containment of infections before they become chronic but this is the more common type of amyloidosis in underdeveloped and developing countries of the world.

Secondary systemic amyloidosis can occur at any age and is the only form of amyloid which can even occur in children.

3. HAEMODIALYSIS-ASSOCIATED (Aβ2M) AMYLOIDOSIS

Patients on long-term dialysis for more than 10 years for chronic renal failure may develop systemic amyloidosis derived from β2-microglobulin which is normal component of MHC. The amyloid deposits are preferentially found in the vessel walls at the synovium, joints, tendon sheaths and subchondral bones.

4. HEREDOFAMILIAL AMYLOIDOSIS

A few rare examples of genetically-determined amyloidosis having familial occurrence and seen in certain geographic regions have been described e.g.
i)   Hereditary polyneuropathic (ATTR) amyloidosis
ii)   Amyloid in familial Mediterranean fever (AA)
iii) Rare hereditary forms by mutations of normal proteins.

B. LOCALISED AMYLOIDOSIS

1.   **Senile cardiac amyloidosis (ATTR)** Senile cardiac amyloidosis is seen in 50% of people above the age of 70 years. The deposits are seen in the heart and aorta.

2.   **Senile cerebral amyloidosis (Aβ, APrP)** Senile cerebral amyloidosis is heterogeneous group of amyloid deposition of varying etiologies that includes sporadic, familial, hereditary and infectious. Some of the important diseases associated with cerebral amyloidosis and the corresponding amyloid proteins are: Alzheimer's disease (Aβ), Down's syndrome (Aβ) and transmissible spongiform encephalopathies (APrP).

In Alzheimer's disease, deposit of amyloid is seen as Congophilic angiopathy (amyloid material in the walls of cerebral blood vessels), neurofibrillary tangles and in senile plaques.

3.   **Endocrine amyloidosis (Hormone precursors)** Some endocrine lesions are associated with microscopic deposits of amyloid e.g.
i)   Medullary carcinoma of the thyroid (from procalcitonin i.e. ACal).

ii) Islet cell tumour of the pancreas (from islet amyloid polypeptide i.e. AIAPP or amylin).

iii) Type 2 diabetes mellitus (from pro-insulin, i.e. AIns).

4. Localised tumour forming amyloid (AL) Sometimes, isolated tumour like formation of amyloid deposits are seen e.g. in lungs, larynx, skin, urinary bladder, tongue, eye, isolated atrial amyloid. In most of these cases, the amyloid type is AL.

STAINING CHARACTERISTICS OF AMYLOID (p. 72)

1. STAIN ON GROSS The oldest method since the time of Virchow for demonstrating amyloid on cut surface of a gross specimen, or on the frozen/ paraffin section is iodine stain. Lugol's iodine imparts *mahogany brown* colour to the amyloid-containing area which on addition of dilute sulfuric acid turns blue.

2. H & E Amyloid by light microscopy with haematoxylin and eosin staining appears as extracellular, homogeneous, structureless and eosinophilic hyaline material, especially in relation to blood vessels.

3. METACHROMATIC STAINS (ROSANILINE DYES) Amyloid has the property of metachromasia i.e. the dye reacts with amyloid and undergoes a colour change. Metachromatic stains employed are rosaniline dyes such as methyl violet and crystal violet which impart *rose-pink* colouration to amyloid deposits.

4. CONGO RED AND POLARISED LIGHT All types of amyloid have affinity for Congo red stain; therefore this method is used for confirmation of amyloid of all types. The stain may be used on both gross specimens and microscopic sections; amyloid of all types stains *pink red colour*. If the stained section is viewed in polarised light, the amyloid characteristically shows *apple-green birefringence* due to cross-β-pleated sheet configuration of amyloid fibrils.

5. FLUORESCENT STAINS Fluorescent stain thioflavin-T binds to amyloid and fluoresces *yellow* under ultraviolet light i.e. amyloid emits secondary fluorescence. Thioflavin-S is less specific.

6. IMMUNOHISTOCHEMISTRY Type of amyloid can be classified by immunohistochemical stains in which corresponding antibody stain is used against the specific amyloid protein acting as antigen. However, for mere confirmation of any type of amyloid, most useful stain is *anti-AP stain* since P component is present in all forms of amyloid.

DIAGNOSIS OF AMYLOIDOSIS (p. 73)

Amyloidosis may be detected as an unsuspected morphologic finding in a case, or the changes may be severe so as to produce symptoms and may even cause death. Routine examination of biopsy or fine needle aspiration, followed by Congo red staining and examination under polarizing microscopy, are the two confirmatory methods of tissue diagnosis of amyloidosis.

◈ **Histologic examination** of biopsy material is the commonest and confirmatory method for diagnosis in a suspected case of amyloidosis. Biopsy of an obviously *affected organ* is likely to offer the best results e.g. *kidney biopsy* in a case on dialysis, sural nerve biopsy in familial polyneuropathy. In systemic amyloidosis, renal biopsy provides the best detection rate, but *rectal biopsy* also has a good pick up rate. However, *gingiva* and *skin biopsy* have poor result.

◈ **Fine needle aspiration** of abdominal *subcutaneous fat* followed by Congo red staining and polarising microscopic examination for confirmation has become an acceptable simple and useful technique with excellent result.

MORPHOLOGY OF AMYLOID IN ORGANS (p. 73)

AMYLOIDOSIS OF KIDNEYS

Amyloidosis of the kidneys is most common and most serious because of ill-effects on renal function. The deposits in the kidneys are found in most cases of secondary amyloidosis and in about one-third cases of primary amyloidosis.

G/A The kidneys may be normal-sized, enlarged or terminally contracted due to ischaemic effect of narrowing of vascular lumina. Cut surface is pale, waxy and translucent.

M/E Following features are seen:

❖ *In the glomeruli,* the deposits initially appear on the basement membrane of the glomerular capillaries, but later extend to produce luminal narrowing and distortion of the glomerular capillary tuft.

❖ *In the tubules,* the amyloid deposits likewise begin close to the tubular epithelial basement membrane.

❖ *Vascular involvement* affects chiefly the walls of small arterioles and venules, producing narrowing of their lumina and consequent ischaemic effects.

❖ *Congo red staining* imparts red pink colour and polarising microscopy shows apple-green birefringence which confirms the presence of amyloid.

AMYLOIDOSIS OF SPLEEN

Amyloid deposition in the spleen, for some unknown reasons, may have one of the following two patterns:

1. SAGO SPLEEN ***G/A*** Splenic enlargement is not marked and cut surface shows characteristic translucent pale and waxy nodules resembling sago grains and hence the name.

M/E The amyloid deposits begin in the walls of the arterioles of the white pulp and may subsequently extend out and replace the follicles.

2. LARDACEOUS SPLEEN ***G/A*** There is generally moderate to marked splenomegaly (weight up to 1 kg). Cut surface of the spleen shows map-like areas of amyloid (lardaceous-lard-like; *lard* means fat of pigs).

M/E The deposits involve the red pulp in the walls of splenic sinuses and the small arteries and in the connective tissue.

AMYLOIDOSIS OF LIVER

In about half the cases of systemic amyloidosis, liver is involved by amyloidosis.

G/A The liver is often enlarged, pale, waxy and firm.

M/E The features are as follows:

❖ The amyloid initially appears in the space of Disse (the space between the hepatocytes and sinusoidal endothelial cells).

❖ Later, as the deposits increases, they compress the cords of hepatocytes so that eventually the liver cells are shrunken and atrophic and replaced by amyloid.

AMYLOIDOSIS OF HEART

Heart is involved in systemic amyloidosis quite commonly, more so in the primary than in secondary systemic amyloidosis. It may also be involved in localised form of amyloidosis (senile cardiac).

G/A The heart may be enlarged. The external surface is pale, translucent and waxy. The epicardium, endocardium and valves show tiny nodular deposits or raised plaques of amyloid.

M/E Following features are seen:

❖ Amyloid deposits are seen in and around the coronaries and their small branches.

❖ In cases of primary amyloidosis of the heart, the deposits of AL amyloid are seen around the myocardial fibres in ring-like formations (ring fibres).

❖ In localised form of amyloid of the heart, the deposits are seen in the left atrium and in the interatrial septum.

Involvement of the gastrointestinal tract by amyloidosis may occur at any level from the oral cavity to the anus. Rectal and gingival biopsies are the common sites for diagnosis of systemic amyloidosis. The deposits are initially located around the small blood vessels but later may involve adjacent layers of the bowel wall. Tongue may be the site for tumour-forming amyloid, producing macroglossia.

SELF ASSESSMENT

1. **Transplantation antigens are located on portion of:**
   A. Chromosome 1
   B. Chromosome 6
   C. Chromosome 9
   D. Chromosome 22

2. **Class I HLA antigens are located on:**
   A. All nucleated cells of the body
   B. B and T lymphocytes
   C. Macrophages
   D. Complement system

3. **HIV contaminated waste products can be decontaminated by the following agents except:**
   A. Sodium hypochlorite
   B. Methanol
   C. Formaldehyde
   D. Glutaraldehyde

4. **CD4 bearing subpopulation of macrophages are attacked by HIV and cause the following except:**
   A. Cytopathic effects
   B. Act as reservoir of HIV infection
   C. Act as source of infection in nervous system
   D. Defects in CD4+ T lymphocytes

5. **In autoimmune haemolytic anaemia, the following type of immunologic tissue injury is involved:**
   A. Type I (anaphylactic)
   B. Type II (cytotoxic)
   C. Type III (immune complex)
   D. Type IV (cell mediated)

6. **Out of various antinuclear antibodies, pathognomonic of SLE is:**
   A. Antibody to single-stranded DNA
   B. Antibody to double-stranded DNA
   C. Antibody to histones
   D. Antibody to nucleolar antigen

7. **In cases of renal failure on long-term haemodialysis, there is development of following type of amyloid:**
   A. Amyloid light chain (AL)
   B. Amyloid-associated protein (AA)
   C. Amyloid β_2 microglobulin (Aβ_2m)
   D. β amyloid protein (Aβ)

8. **The most common form of amyloid in developing countries is:**
   A. Primary
   B. Secondary
   C. Hereditary
   D. Localised

9. **Cardiac amyloidosis often produces:**
   A. Dilated cardiomyopathy
   B. Constrictive cardiomyopathy
   C. Restrictive cardiomyopathy
   D. Ischaemic cardiomyopathy

10. **In senile cardiac amyloidosis, the biochemical form of amyloid is:**
    A. AL
    B. AA
    C. ATTR
    D. Aβ_2M

11. **In Alzheimer's disease, cerebral plaques consist of:**
    A. ATTR protein
    B. Aβ_2M protein
    C. Aβ protein
    D. Prion protein

12. **Amyloid enhancing factor (AEF) plays a significant role in:**
    A. Primary amyloid
    B. Secondary amyloid
    C. Senile cerebral amyloid
    D. Haemodialysis-associated amyloid

13. **Grave's disease is a type of:**
    A. Type I reaction
    B. Type II reaction
    C. Type III reaction
    D. Type IV reaction

14. **Non-fibrillar amyloid components include all <u>except</u>:**
    A. Amyloid P component
    B. Apolipoprotein E
    C. Protein X
    D. Cystatin

15. **Which of the following is heredo-familial form of amyloidosis?**
    A. Polyneuropathic amyloidosis
    B. Cardiac amyloidosis
    C. Cerebral amyloidosis
    D. Endocrine amyloidosis

16. **CD4 T cell count in crisis phase of HIV according to revised HIV/AIDS classification is:**
    A. < 100/ microlitre
    B. < 200/ microlitre
    C. < 250/ microlitre
    D. < 500/ microlitre

17. **Test useful for detection of HIV during window period:**
    A. ELISA
    B. Western blot
    C. CD4+ cell count
    D. p24 antigen capture assay

18. **Haematoxylin body represents:**
    A. Nuclear chromatin material
    B. RNA
    C. Cytosolic components
    D. Cell membrane components

19. **For counting of CD4 + T cells in AIDS, the following technique is often employed:**
    A. In situ hybridisation
    B. Polymerase chain reaction
    C. Flow cytometry
    D. Electron microscopy

20. **For karyotyping, the dividing cells are arrested by addition of colchicine in the following mitotic phase:**
    A. Prophase
    B. Metaphase
    C. Anaphase
    D. Telophase

KEY

1 = B	2 = A	3 = B	4 = A	5 = B
6 = B	7 = C	8 = B	9 = C	10 = C
11 = C	12 = B	13 = B	14 = D	15 = A
16 = B	17 = D	18 = A	19 = C	20 = C

4. Derangements of Homeostasis and Haemodynamics

HOMEOSTASIS (p. 78)

Claude Bernarde (1949) first coined the term *internal environment or milieu interieur* for the state in the body in which the interstitial fluid that bathes the cells and the plasma, together maintain the normal morphology and function of the cells and tissues of the body. The mechanism by which the constancy of the internal environment is maintained and ensured is called the *homeostasis*.

The normal composition of internal environment consists of the following components:

1. WATER Water is the principal and essential constituent of the body. The total body water in a normal adult male comprises 50-70% (average 60%) of the body weight and about 10% less in a normal adult female (average 50%).

i) Intracellular fluid compartment This comprises about 33% of the body weight, the bulk of which is contained in the muscles.

ii) Extracellular fluid compartment This constitutes the remaining 27% of body weight. Included in this are the following 4 subdivisions of extracellular fluid (ECF):

a) Interstitial fluid including lymph fluid constitutes the major proportion of ECF (12% of body weight).

b) Intravascular fluid or blood plasma comprises about 5% of the body weight.

c) Mesenchymal tissues such as dense connective tissue, cartilage and bone contain body water that comprises about 9% of the body weight.

d) Transcellular fluid constitutes 1% of body weight. This is the fluid contained in the secretions of secretory cells of the body.

2. ELECTROLYTES The concentration of cations (positively charged) and anions (negatively charged) is different in intracellular and extracellular fluids:

◈ *In the intracellular fluid,* the main cations are potassium and magnesium and the main anions are phosphates and proteins. It has low concentration of sodium and chloride.

◈ *In the extracellular fluid*, the predominant cation is sodium and the principal anions are chloride and bicarbonate. Besides these, a small proportion of non-diffusible proteins and some diffusible nutrients and metabolites such as glucose and urea are present in the ECF.

The essential difference between the two main subdivisions of ECF is the higher protein content in the plasma than in the interstitial fluid which plays an important role in maintaining fluid balance.

NORMAL WATER AND ELECTROLYTE BALANCE (GIBBS-DONNAN EQUILIBRIUM) (p. 79)

Normally, a state of balance exists between the amount of water absorbed into the body and the amount eliminated from the body. The water and electrolytes are distributed nearly constantly in different body fluid compartments:

1. Water is normally *absorbed* into the body from the bowel or is introduced parenterally; average intake being 2800 ml per day.
2. Water is *eliminated* from the body via:

i) kidneys in the urine (average 1500 ml per day);

ii) via the skin as insensible loss in perspiration or as sweat (average 800 ml per day).

iii) via the lungs in exhaled air (average 400 ml per day); and

iv) minor losses via the faeces (average 100 ml per day) and lacrimal, nasal, oral, sexual and mammary (milk) secretions.

The cell wall as well as capillary endothelium are entirely permeable to water but they differ in their permeability to electrolytes. Capillary wall is completely permeable to electrolytes while the cell membrane is somewhat impermeable.

ACID-BASE BALANCE (p. 79)

A number of acids such as carbonic, phosphoric, sulfuric, lactic, hydrochloric and ketoacids are formed during normal metabolic activity. However, carbonic acid is produced in largest amount as it is the end-product of aerobic tissue activity. In spite of these acids, the pH of the blood is kept constant at 7.4 ± 0.05 in health.

PRESSURE GRADIENTS AND FLUID EXCHANGES (p. 79)

Besides water and electrolytes (or crystalloids), both of which are freely interchanged between the interstitial fluid and plasma, the ECF contains colloids (i.e. proteins) which minimally cross the capillary wall. These substances exert pressures responsible for exchange between the interstitial fluid and plasma.

1. OSMOTIC PRESSURE This is the pressure exerted by the chemical constituents of the body fluids. Accordingly, osmotic pressure may be of the following types:

◈ **Crystalloid osmotic pressure** exerted by electrolytes present in the ECF and comprises the major portion of the total osmotic pressure.

◈ **Colloid osmotic pressure (Oncotic pressure)** exerted by proteins present in the ECF and constitutes a small part of the total osmotic pressure but is more significant physiologically. Since the protein content of the plasma is higher than that of interstitial fluid, oncotic pressure of plasma is higher (average 25 mmHg) than that of interstitial fluid (average 8 mmHg).

◈ **Effective oncotic pressure** is the difference between the higher oncotic pressure of plasma and the lower oncotic pressure of interstitial fluid and is *the force that tends to draw fluid into the vessels.*

2. HYDROSTATIC PRESSURE This is the capillary blood pressure. There is considerable *pressure gradient* at the two ends of capillary loop—being higher at the arteriolar end (average 32 mmHg) than at the venular end (average 12 mmHg).

◈ **Tissue tension** is the hydrostatic pressure of interstitial fluid and is lower than the hydrostatic pressure in the capillary at either end (average 4 mmHg).

◈ **Effective hydrostatic pressure** is the difference between the higher hydrostatic pressure in the capillary and the lower tissue tension; it is *the force that drives fluid through the capillary wall into the interstitial space.*

DISTURBANCES OF BODY WATER (p. 80)

OEDEMA (p. 80)

Oedema is defined as abnormal and excessive accumulation of "free fluid" in the interstitial tissue spaces and serous cavities.

◈ *Free fluid in body cavities:* Commonly called as effusion, it is named according to the body cavity in which the fluid accumulates. For example, ascites (if in the peritoneal cavity), hydrothorax or pleural effusion (if in the pleural cavity), and hydropericardium or pericardial effusion (if in the pericardial cavity).

◈ *Free fluid in interstitial space:* Commonly termed as oedema, the fluid lies free in the interstitial space between the cells and can be displaced from one place to another. In the case of oedema in the subcutaneous tissues, momentary pressure of finger produces a depression known as *pitting oedema*. The other variety is *non-pitting* or *solid oedema* in which no pitting is produced on pressure e.g. in myxoedema, elephantiasis.

Oedema may be of 2 main types:

1. *Localised* when limited to an organ or limb e.g. lymphatic oedema, inflammatory oedema, allergic oedema, pulmonary oedema, cerebral oedema etc.

2. *Generalised (anasarca or dropsy)* when it is systemic in distribution, particularly noticeable in the subcutaneous tissues e.g. renal oedema, cardiac oedema, nutritional oedema.

Depending upon fluid composition, oedema fluid may be:

◈ *transudate* which is more often the case, such as in oedema of cardiac and renal disease; or

◈ *exudate* such as in inflammatory oedema.

PATHOGENESIS OF OEDEMA

Oedema is caused by mechanisms that interfere with normal fluid balance of plasma, interstitial fluid and lymph flow. The following mechanisms may be operating singly or in combination to produce oedema:

1. DECREASED PLASMA ONCOTIC PRESSURE A fall in the total plasma protein level (hypoproteinaemia of less than 5 g/dl, mainly hypoalbuminaemia), results in lowering of plasma oncotic pressure in a way that it can no longer counteract the effect of hydrostatic pressure of blood. This results in increased outward movement of fluid from the capillary wall and decreased inward movement of fluid from the interstitial space causing oedema e.g.

i) *Oedema of renal disease* e.g. in nephrotic and nephritic syndrome.

ii) *Ascites* of liver disease e.g. in cirrhosis of the liver.

iii) *Oedema due to other causes* of hypoproteinaemia e.g. in protein-losing enteropathy.

2. INCREASED CAPILLARY HYDROSTATIC PRESSURE A rise in the hydrostatic pressure at the venular end of the capillary which is normally low (average 12 mmHg) to a level more than the plasma oncotic pressure results in minimal or no reabsorption of fluid at the venular end, consequently leading to oedema e.g.

i) *Oedema of cardiac disease* e.g. in congestive cardiac failure, constrictive pericarditis.

ii) *Ascites of liver disease* e.g. in cirrhosis of the liver.

iii) *Passive congestion* e.g. in mechanical obstruction due to thrombosis of veins of the lower legs, varicosities, pressure by pregnant uterus, tumours etc.

iv) *Postural oedema* e.g. transient oedema of feet and ankles due to increased venous pressure seen in individuals whose job involves standing for long hours such as traffic constables and nurses.

3. LYMPHATIC OBSTRUCTION Obstruction to outflow of these channels causes localised oedema, known as lymphoedema e.g.

i) *Removal of axillary lymph nodes* in radical mastectomy for carcinoma of the breast causing lymphoedema of the affected arm.

ii) *Pressure from outside* on the main abdominal or thoracic duct such as due to tumours, effusions in serous cavities etc may produce lymphoedema.

iii) *Inflammation of the lymphatics* as seen in filariasis (infection with *Wuchereria bancrofti*) results in chronic lymphoedema of scrotum and legs known as elephantiasis, a form of non-pitting oedema.

iv) *Occlusion of lymphatic channels* by malignant cells may result in lymphoedema.

v) *Milroy's disease or hereditary lymphoedema* is due to abnormal development of lymphatic channels.

4. TISSUE FACTORS In some situations, the tissue factors in combination with other mechanisms play a role in causation of oedema e.g.

i) *Elevation of oncotic pressure of interstitial fluid* as occurs due to increased vascular permeability and inadequate removal of proteins by lymphatics.

ii) Lowered tissue tension as seen in *loose subcutaneous tissues* of eyelids and external genitalia.

5. INCREASED CAPILLARY PERMEABILITY When the capillary endothelium is injured by various 'capillary poisons' such as toxins and their products (e.g. histamine, anoxia, venoms, certain drugs and chemicals), the capillary permeability to plasma proteins is enhanced due to development of gaps between the endothelial cells, causing leakage of plasma proteins into interstitial fluid e.g.

i) *Generalised oedema* occurring in systemic infections, poisonings, certain drugs and chemicals, anaphylactic reactions and anoxia.

ii) *Localised oedema* A few examples are as under:

◈ *Inflammatory oedema* as seen in infections, allergic reactions, insect-bite, irritant drugs and chemicals. It is generally exudate in nature.

◈ *Angioneurotic oedema* is an acute attack of localised oedema occurring on the skin of face and trunk and may involve lips, larynx, pharynx and lungs. It is possibly neurogenic or allergic in origin.

6. SODIUM AND WATER RETENTION It is best described in relation to normal mechanism of sodium and water balance.

◈ **Intrinsic renal mechanism** is activated in response to sudden reduction in the effective arterial blood volume (hypovolaemia) e.g. in severe haemorrhage. As a result of this, renal ischaemia occurs which causes reduction in the glomerular filtration rate, decreased excretion of sodium in the urine and consequent retention of sodium.

◈ **Extra-renal mechanism** involves the secretion of aldosterone, a sodium-retaining hormone, by the *renin-angiotensin-aldosterone system*. Angiotensin II stimulates the adrenal cortex to secrete aldosterone hormone. Aldosterone increases sodium reabsorption in the renal tubules and sometimes causes a rise in the blood pressure.

◈ **ADH mechanism** Retention of sodium leads to retention of water secondarily under the influence of anti-diuretic hormone (ADH) or vasopressin.

Thus, the possible factors responsible for causating oedema by excessive retention of sodium and water in the extravascular compartment via stimulation of intrinsic renal and extra-renal mechanisms as well as via release of ADH are as under:

i) Reduced glomerular filtration rate in response to hypovolaemia.

ii) Enhanced tubular reabsorption of sodium and consequently its decreased renal excretion.

iii) Increased filtration factor i.e. increased filtration of plasma from the glomerulus.

iv) Decreased capillary hydrostatic pressure associated with increased renal vascular resistance.

The **examples** of oedema by these mechanisms are as under:

i) *Oedema of cardiac disease* e.g. in congestive cardiac failure.

ii) *Ascites* of liver disease e.g. in cirrhosis of liver.

iii) *Oedema of renal disease* e.g. in nephrotic and nephritic syndrome.

IMPORTANT TYPES OF OEDEMA

RENAL OEDEMA

1. Oedema in nephrotic syndrome Since there is persistent and heavy proteinuria (albuminuria) in nephrotic syndrome, there is hypoalbuminaemia causing decreased plasma oncotic pressure resulting in severe generalised oedema *(nephrotic oedema)*. The *nephrotic oedema* is classically more severe, generalised and marked and is present in the subcutaneous tissues as well as in the visceral organs.

2. Oedema in nephritic syndrome Oedema occuring in conditions with diffuse glomerular disease such as in acute diffuse glomerulonephritis and rapidly progressive glomerulonephritis is termed *nephritic oedema*. In contrast to nephrotic oedema, nephritic oedema is primarily not due to hypoproteinaemia because of low albuminuria but is largely due to excessive reabsorption of sodium and water in the renal tubules via renin-angiotensin-aldosterone mechanism.

The *nephritic oedema* is usually mild as compared to nephrotic oedema and begins in the loose tissues such as on the face around eyes, ankles and genitalia.

3. Oedema in acute tubular injury Acute tubular injury following shock or toxic chemicals results in gross oedema of the body. The damaged tubules lose their capacity for selective reabsorption and concentration of the glomerular filtrate, resulting in excessive retention of water and electrolytes, and consequent oliguria.

CARDIAC OEDEMA

Generalised oedema develops in right-sided and congestive cardiac failure. Pathogenesis of cardiac oedema is explained on the basis of the following mechanisms:

1. Reduced cardiac output causes hypovolaemia which stimulates intrinsic-renal and extra-renal hormonal (renin-angiotensin-aldosterone) mechanisms as well as ADH secretion resulting in *sodium and water retention* (as discussed above) and consequent oedema.

2. Due to heart failure, there is elevated central venous pressure which is transmitted backward to the venous end of the capillaries, raising the capillary hydrostatic pressure and consequent transudation.

3. Chronic hypoxia may injure the capillary endothelium causing increased capillary permeability and result in oedema; this is called *forward pressure hypothesis*.

Cardiac oedema is influenced by gravity and is thus characteristically *dependent oedema*.

PULMONARY OEDEMA

Acute pulmonary oedema is the most important form of local oedema as it causes serious functional impairment.

ETIOPATHOGENESIS Pulmonary oedema can result from either the elevation of pulmonary hydrostatic pressure or the increased capillary permeability.

1. Elevation in pulmonary hydrostatic pressure (Haemodynamic oedema) In heart failure, there is increase in the pressure in pulmonary veins which is transmitted to pulmonary capillaries. This results in imbalance between pulmonary hydrostatic pressure and the plasma oncotic pressure so that excessive fluid moves out of pulmonary capillaries into the interstitium of the lungs.

Examples of pulmonary oedema by this mechanism are seen in left heart failure, mitral stenosis, pulmonary vein obstruction, thyrotoxicosis, cardiac surgery, nephrotic syndrome and obstruction to the lymphatic outflow by tumour or inflammation.

2. Increased vascular permeability (Irritant oedema) The vascular endothelium as well as the alveolar epithelial cells (alveolo-capillary membrane) may be damaged causing increased vascular permeability so that excessive fluid and plasma proteins leak out, initially into the interstitium and subsequently into the alveoli.

3. Acute high altitude oedema Individuals climbing to high altitude suddenly without halts and without waiting for acclimatisation to set in, suffer from serious circulatory and respiratory ill-effects.

G/A The lungs in pulmonary oedema are heavy, moist and subcrepitant. Cut surface exudes frothy fluid (mixture of air and fluid).

M/E The alveolar capillaries are congested. Initially, the excess fluid collects in the interstitial lung spaces in the septal walls (interstitial oedema). Later, the fluid fills the alveolar spaces (alveolar oedema).

CEREBRAL OEDEMA

Cerebral oedema or swelling of the brain is the most life-threatening example of oedema. The mechanism of fluid exchange in the brain differs from elsewhere in the body since there are no draining lymphatics in the brain but instead, the function of fluid-electrolyte exchange is performed by the blood-brain barrier located at the endothelial cells of the capillaries.

Cerebral oedema can be of 3 types:

1. VASOGENIC OEDEMA This is the most common type and its mechanism is similar to oedema in other body sites from increased filtration pressure or increased capillary permeability.

2. CYTOTOXIC OEDEMA The underlying mechanism is disturbance in the cellular osmoregulation as occurs in some metabolic derangements, acute hypoxia and with some toxic chemicals.

3. INTERSTITIAL OEDEMA This type of cerebral oedema occurs when the excessive fluid crosses the ependymal lining of the ventricles and accumulates in the periventricular white matter.

HEPATIC OEDEMA

Briefly the mechanisms involved in causation of oedema of the legs and ascites in cirrhosis of the liver is as under:

i) There is *hypoproteinaemia* due to impaired synthesis of proteins by the diseased liver.

ii) Due to portal hypertension, there is increased venous pressure in the abdomen, and hence *raised hydrostatic pressure*.

iii) Failure of inactivation of aldosterone in the diseased liver and hence *hyperaldosteronism*.

iv) Secondary stimulation of renin-angiotensin mechanism promoting *sodium and water retention*.

NUTRITIONAL OEDEMA

Oedema due to nutritional deficiency of proteins (kwashiorkor, prolonged starvation, famine, fasting), vitamins (beri-beri due to vitamin B_1 deficiency) and chronic alcoholism occurs on legs but sometimes may be more generalised. The main contributing factors are hypoproteinaemia and sodium-water retention related to metabolic abnormalities.

MYXOEDEMA

Myxoedema from hypothyroidism is a form of non-pitting oedema occurring on skin of face and other parts of the body as also in the internal organs due to excessive deposition of glycosaminoglycans in the interstitium.

DEHYDRATION *(p. 87)*

Dehydration is a state of pure deprivation of water leading to sodium retention and hence a state of hypernatraemia. In other words, there is only loss of water without loss of sodium.

Pure water deficiency is less common than salt depletion but can occur in the following conditions:

1. GI excretion:
i) Severe vomitings
ii) Diarrhoea
iii) Cholera

2. Renal excretion:
i) Acute renal failure in diuretic phase
ii) Extensive use of diuretics
iii) Endocrine diseases e.g. diabetes insipidus, Addison's disease

3. Loss of blood and plasma:
i) Severe injuries, severe burns
ii) During childbirth

4. Loss through skin:
i) Excessive perspiration
ii) Hyperthermia

5. Accumulation in third space:
i) Sudden development of ascites
ii) Acute intestinal obstruction with accumulation of fluid in the bowel.

OVERHYDRATION *(p. 87)*

Overhydration is increased extracellular fluid volume due to pure water excess or water intoxication.

Overhydration is generally an induced condition and is encountered in the following situations:

1. Excessive unmonitored intravascular infusion:
i) Normal saline (0.9% sodium chloride)
ii) Ringer lactate

2. Renal retention of sodium and water:
i) Congestive heart failure
ii) Acute glomerulonephritis
iii) Cirrhosis
iv) Cushing's syndrome
v) Chronic renal failure

DISTURBANCES OF ELECTROLYTES AND pH OF BLOOD *(p. 88)*

ELECTROLYTE IMBALANCE

Intracellular compartment has higher concentration of potassium, calcium, magnesium and phosphate ions than the blood, while extracellular fluid (including serum) has higher concentration of sodium, chloride, and bicarbonate ions. In health, for *electrolyte homeostasis*, the concentration of electrolytes in both these compartments should be within normal limits. Normal serum levels of electrolytes are maintained in the body by a careful balance of 4 processes: their intake, absorption, distribution and excretion. Disturbance in any of these processes in diverse pathophysiologic states may cause *electrolyte imbalance*.

Among the important components in electrolyte imbalance, abnormalities in serum levels of sodium (hypo- and hypernatraemia), potassium (hypo- and hyperkalaemia), calcium (hypo- and hypercalcaemia) and magnesium (hypo- and hypermagnesaemia) are clinically more important.

pH OF BLOOD

During metabolism of cells, carbon dioxide and metabolic acids are produced. CO_2 combines with water to form carbonic acid.

The disorders of the pH of the blood, termed as acidosis (blood pH below 7.4) and alkalosis (blood pH above 7.4), can be of 2 types:
1. *Alterations in the blood bicarbonate levels:* These are metabolic acidosis and alkalosis.
2. *Alteration in Pco_2* (which depends upon the ventilatory function of the lungs): These are respiratory acidosis and alkalosis.

ACID BASE IMBALANCE *(p. 89)*

Abnormalities in acid-base homeostasis produce following 4 principal metabolic states which have diverse clinical manifestations due to pathophysiologic derangements:

METABOLIC ACIDOSIS

A fall in the blood pH due to metabolic component is brought about by fall of bicarbonate level and excess of H^+ ions in the blood. This occurs in the following situations:

i) Production of large amounts of lactic acid (lactic acidosis) e.g. in vigorous exercise, shock.
ii) Uncontrolled diabetes mellitus (diabetic ketoacidosis).
iii) Starvation.
iv) Chronic renal failure.
v) Therapeutic administration of ammonium chloride or acetazolamide (diamox).

METABOLIC ALKALOSIS

A rise in the blood pH due to rise in the bicarbonate levels of plasma and loss of H^+ ions is called metabolic alkalosis. This is seen in the following conditions:
i) Severe and prolonged vomitings.
ii) Administration of alkaline salts like sodium bicarbonate.
iii) Hypokalaemia such as in Cushing's syndrome, increased secretion of aldosterone.

RESPIRATORY ACIDOSIS

A fall in the blood pH occurring due to raised Pco_2 consequent to hypoventilation of lungs (CO_2 retention) causes respiratory acidosis. This can occur in the following circumstances:
i) Air obstruction as occurs in chronic bronchitis, emphysema, asthma.
ii) Restricted thoracic movement e.g. in pleural effusion, ascites, pregnancy, kyphoscoliosis.
iii) Impaired neuromuscular function e.g. in poliomyelitis, polyneuritis.

RESPIRATORY ALKALOSIS

A rise in the blood pH occurring due to lowered Pco_2 consequent to hyperventilation of the lungs (excess removal of CO_2) is called respiratory alkalosis. This occurs in the following conditions:
i) Hysterical overbreathing.
ii) Working at high temperature.
iii) At high altitude.
iv) Meningitis, encephalitis.
v) Salicylate intoxication.

HAEMODYNAMIC DERANGEMENTS (p. 89)

Derangements of blood flow or haemodynamic disturbances are considered under 2 broad headings:
I. *Disturbances in the volume of the circulating blood* These include: hyperaemia and congestion, haemorrhage and shock.
II. *Circulatory disturbances of obstructive nature* These are: thrombosis, embolism, ischaemia and infarction.

DISTURBANCES IN THE VOLUME OF CIRCULATING BLOOD (p. 90)

HYPERAEMIA AND CONGESTION

Hyperaemia and congestion are the terms used for localised increase in the volume of blood within dilated vessels of an organ or tissue. If the condition develops rapidly it is called *acute*, while more prolonged and gradual response is known as *chronic*.

ACTIVE HYPERAEMIA

The dilatation of arteries, arterioles and capillaries is effected either through sympathetic neurogenic mechanism or via the release of vasoactive substances. The affected tissue or organ is pink or red in appearance (erythema) e.g.
i) Inflammation e.g. congested vessels in the walls of alveoli in pneumonia
ii) Blushing i.e. flushing of the skin of face in response to emotions
iii) Menopausal flush

iv)   Muscular exercise
v)   High grade fever
vi)   Goitre
vii) Arteriovenous malformations

PASSIVE HYPERAEMIA (VENOUS CONGESTION)

The dilatation of veins and capillaries due to impaired venous drainage results in passive hyperaemia or venous congestion, commonly referred to as *passive congestion*. Congestion may be acute or chronic, the latter being more common and is called *chronic venous congestion* (CVC).

◈   *Local venous congestion* results from obstruction to the venous outflow from an organ or part of the body e.g. portal venous obstruction in cirrhosis of the liver, outside pressure on the vessel wall as occurs in tight bandage, plasters, tumours, pregnancy, hernia etc, or intraluminal occlusion by thrombosis.

◈   *Systemic (General) venous congestion* is engorgement of veins e.g. in left-sided and right-sided heart failure and diseases of the lungs which interfere with pulmonary blood flow like pulmonary fibrosis, emphysema etc.

MORPHOLOGY OF CVC OF ORGANS

CVC LUNG

Chronic venous congestion of the lung occurs in left heart failure (e.g. in rheumatic mitral stenosis) resulting in rise in pulmonary venous pressure.

G/A   The lungs are heavy and firm in consistency. The sectioned surface is dark and rusty brown in colour, referred to as *brown induration* of the lungs.

M/E   It shows following features:
i)   The alveolar septa are widened due to presence of interstitial oedema and dilated and congested capillaries in the septal wall.
ii)   Rupture of dilated and congested capillaries may result in minute intra-alveolar haemorrhages. The breakdown of erythrocytes liberates haemosiderin pigment which is taken up by alveolar macrophages, called as *heart failure cells,* seen in the alveolar lumina. The brown induration observed on the cut surface of the lungs is due to the pigmentation and fibrosis.

CVC LIVER

Chronic venous congestion of the liver occurs in right heart failure and sometimes due to occlusion of inferior vena cava and hepatic vein.

G/A   The liver is enlarged and tender and the capsule is tense. Cut surface shows characteristic *nutmeg* appearance due to red and yellow mottled appearance, corresponding to congested centre of lobules and fatty peripheral zone respectively.

M/E   The changes of passive congestion are more marked in the centrilobular zone (zone 3) which is farthest from blood supply (periportal zone, zone 1) and thus bears the brunt of hypoxia the most.
i) The central veins as well as the adjacent sinusoids are distended and filled with blood. The centrilobular hepatocytes undergo degenerative changes, and eventually *centrilobular haemorrhagic necrosis* occurs.
ii) Long-standing cases may show fine centrilobular fibrosis and regeneration of hepatocytes, resulting in cardiac cirrhosis.
iii) The peripheral zone of the lobule is less severely affected by chronic hypoxia and shows some *fatty change* in the hepatocytes.

CVC SPLEEN

Chronic venous congestion of the spleen occurs in right heart failure and in portal hypertension from cirrhosis of liver.

G/A   The spleen in early stage is slightly to moderately enlarged (up to 250 g as compared to normal 150 g), while in long-standing cases there is progressive enlargement and may weigh up to 500 to 1000 g. Sectioned surface is gray tan.

M/E Following features are seen:

i) *Red pulp* is enlarged due to congestion and marked sinusoidal dilatation and there are areas of recent and old haemorrhages.

ii) There is *hyperplasia* of *reticuloendothelial cells* in the red pulp of the spleen (splenic macrophages).

iii) There is *fibrous thickening* of the capsule and of the trabeculae.

iv) Some of haemorrhages overlying fibrous tissue get deposits of haemosiderin pigment and calcium salts; these organised structures are termed as *Gamna-Gandy bodies* or siderofibrotic nodules.

v) Firmness of the spleen in advanced stage is seen more commonly in hepatic cirrhosis (*congestive splenomegaly*) and is the commonest cause of hypersplenism.

HAEMORRHAGE

Haemorrhage is the escape of blood from a blood vessel. The bleeding may occur *externally, or internally* into the serous cavities (e.g. haemothorax, haemoperitoneum, haemopericardium), or into a hollow viscus. Extravasation of blood into the tissues with resultant swelling is known as *haematoma*. Large extravasations of blood into the skin and mucous membranes are called *ecchymoses*. *Purpuras* are small areas of haemorrhages (upto 1 cm) into the skin and mucous membrane, whereas *petechiae* are minute pinhead-sized haemorrhages. Microscopic escape of erythrocytes into loose tissues may occur following marked congestion and is known as *diapedesis*.

The effects of blood loss depend upon 3 main factors:

i)   the amount of blood loss;

ii) the speed of blood loss; and

iii) the site of haemorrhage.

SHOCK

Shock is a life-threatening clinical syndrome of cardiovascular collapse characterised by:

◈   an acute reduction of effective circulating blood volume (hypotension); and

◈   an inadequate perfusion of cells and tissues (hypoperfusion).

Thus, by definition "*true (or secondary) shock*" is a circulatory imbalance between oxygen supply and oxygen requirements at the cellular level, and is also called as circulatory shock and is the type which is commonly referred to as 'shock' if not specified.

CLASSIFICATION AND ETIOLOGY

Although in a given clinical case, two or more factors may be involved in causation of true shock, a simple etiologic classification of shock syndrome divides it into following 3 major types and a few other variants:

1.   **Hypovolaemic shock**   This form of shock results from inadequate circulatory blood volume by various etiologic factors that may be *either* from the loss of red cell mass and plasma due to haemorrhage, *or* from the loss of plasma volume alone.

2.   **Cardiogenic shock**   Acute circulatory failure with sudden fall in cardiac output from acute diseases of the heart without actual reduction of blood volume (normovolaemia) results in cardiogenic shock.

3.   **Septic (Toxaemic) shock**   Severe bacterial infections or septicaemia induce septic shock. It may be the result of Gram-negative septicaemia (endotoxic shock) which is more common, or less often from Gram-positive septicaemia (exotoxic shock).

4. **Other types**   These include: (i) Traumatic shock; (ii) Neurogenic shock; (iii) Hypoadrenal shock.

PATHOGENESIS

In general, all forms of shock involve following 3 derangements:

i)   Reduced effective circulating blood volume.

ii) Reduced supply of oxygen to the cells and tissues with resultant anoxia.
iii) Inflammatory mediators and toxins released from shock-induced cellular injury.

These derangements initially set in compensatory mechanisms (discussed below) but eventually a vicious cycle of cell injury and severe cellular dysfunction lead to breakdown of organ function.

PATHOGENESIS OF HYPOVOLAEMIC SHOCK Hypovolaemic shock occurs from inadequate circulating blood volume due to various causes, most often from loss of red cell mass due to haemorrhage and, therefore, also called as haemorrhagic shock. The major effects in this are due to decreased cardiac output and low intracardiac pressure.

PATHOGENESIS OF CARDIOGENIC SHOCK Cardiogenic shock results from a severe left ventricular dysfunction from various causes such as acute myocardial infarction. The resultant decreased cardiac output has its effects in the form of decreased tissue perfusion and movement of fluid from pulmonary vascular bed into pulmonary interstitial space initially (*interstitial pulmonary oedema*) and later into alveolar spaces (*alveolar pulmonary oedema*).

PATHOGENESIS OF SEPTIC SHOCK Septic shock results most often from Gram-negative bacteria entering the body from genitourinary tract, alimentary tract, respiratory tract or skin, and less often from Gram-positive bacteria. In septic shock, there is immune system activation and severe systemic inflammatory response to infection.

The net result of above mechanisms is vasodilatation and increased vascular permeability in septic shock. Profound peripheral vasodilatation and pooling of blood causes hyperdynamic circulation in septic shock, in contrast to hypovolaemic and cardiogenic shock. Increased vascular permeability causes development of inflammatory oedema. Disseminated intravascular coagulation (DIC) is prone to develop in septic shock due to endothelial cell injury by toxins.

PATHOPHYSIOLOGY (STAGES OF SHOCK)

Although deterioration of the circulation in shock is a progressive and continuous phenomenon and compensatory mechanisms become progressively less effective, historically shock has been divided arbitrarily into 3 stages:

COMPENSATED (NON-PROGRESSIVE, INITIAL, REVERSIBLE) SHOCK In the early stage of shock, an attempt is made to maintain adequate cerebral and coronary blood supply by redistribution of blood so that the vital organs (brain and heart) are adequately perfused and oxygenated. This is achieved by activation of various neurohormonal mechanisms causing *widespread vasoconstriction* and by *fluid conservation by the kidney*.

PROGRESSIVE DECOMPENSATED SHOCK This is a stage when the patient suffers from some other stress or risk factors (e.g. pre-existing cardiovascular and lung disease) besides persistence of the shock condition; this causes progressive deterioration. The effects of resultant tissue hypoperfusion in progressive decompensated shock are:
i) Pulmonary hypoperfusion
ii) Tissue ischaemia

IRREVERSIBLE DECOMPENSATED SHOCK When the shock is so severe that in spite of compensatory mechanisms and despite therapy and control of etiologic agent which caused the shock, no recovery takes place, it is called decompensated or irreversible shock. Its effects due to widespread cell injury are as follows:
i) Progressive vasodilatation
ii) Increased vascular permeability
iii) Release of myocardial depressant factor (MDF)
iv) Worsening pulmonary hypoperfusion
v) Anoxic damage to heart, kidney and brain
vi) Hypercoagulability of blood

Chapter 4

Derangements of Homeostasis and Haemodynamics

MORPHOLOGIC FEATURES

Eventually, shock is characterised by multisystem failure. The morphologic changes in shock are due to hypoxia resulting in degeneration and necrosis in various organs. The major organs affected are the brain, heart, lungs and kidneys. Morphologic changes are also noted in the adrenals, gastrointestinal tract, liver and other organs.

CLINICAL FEATURES AND COMPLICATIONS

The classical features of decompensated shock are characterised by *depression of 4 vital processes:*

i)   Very low blood pressure
ii)   Subnormal temperature
iii)   Feeble and irregular pulse
iv)   Shallow and sighing respiration

In addition, the patients in shock have pale face, sunken eyes, weakness, cold and clammy skin.

Life-threatening complications in shock are due to hypoxic cell injury resulting in immuno-inflammatory responses and activation of various cascades (clotting, complement, kinin). These include the following:

1.   Acute respiratory distress syndrome (ARDS)
2.   Disseminated intravascular coagulation (DIC)
3.   Acute renal failure (ARF)
4.   Multiple organ dysfunction syndrome (MODS)

With progression of the condition, the patient may develop stupor, coma and death.

CIRCULATORY DISTURBANCES OF OBSTRUCTIVE NATURE *(p. 99)*

THROMBOSIS

Thrombosis is the process of formation of solid mass in circulation from the constituents of flowing blood; the mass itself is called a *thrombus*. A term commonly used erroneously synonymous with thrombosis is blood clotting. While *thrombosis* is characterised by events that essentially involve activation of platelets, the process of *clotting* involves only conversion of soluble fibrinogen to insoluble polymerised fibrin. Besides, clotting is also used to denote coagulation of blood *in vitro* e.g. in a test tube. *Haematoma* is the extravascular accumulation of blood e.g. into the tissues. *Haemostatic plugs* are the blood clots formed in healthy individuals at the site of bleeding e.g. in injury to the blood vessel. Thrombi developing in the unruptured cardiovascular system may be life-threatening by causing one of the following harmful effects:

1.   *Ischaemic injury* Thrombi may decrease or stop the blood supply to part of an organ or tissue and cause ischaemia which may subsequently result in infarction.

2.   *Thromboembolism* Thrombus or its part may get dislodged and be carried along in the bloodstream as embolus to lodge in a distant vessel.

PATHOPHYSIOLOGY

Human beings possess inbuilt system by which the blood remains in fluid state normally and guards against the hazards of thrombosis and haemorrhage. However, injury to the blood vessel initiates haemostatic repair mechanism or thrombogenesis.

Virchow described three primary events which predispose to thrombus formation *(Virchow's triad):* endothelial injury, altered blood flow, and hypercoagulability of blood. To this are added the activation processes that follow these primary events: activation of platelets and of clotting system.

1.   ENDOTHELIAL INJURY   The integrity of blood vessel wall is important for maintaining normal blood flow. An intact endothelium has the following functions:

i)   It *protects* the flowing blood from thrombogenic influence of subendothelium.

ii) It elaborates a few *anti-thrombotic* factors (thrombosis inhibitory factors) e.g. Heparin-like substance, thrombomodulin, inhibitors of platelet aggregation, tissue plasminogen activator.

iii) It releases a few *prothrombotic factors* which have procoagulant properties (thrombosis favouring factors) e.g. thromboplastin, von Willebrand factor, platelet activating factor, inhibitor of plasminogen activator.

Vascular injury exposes the subendothelial extracellular matrix or ECM (e.g. collagen, elastin, fibronectin, laminin and glycosaminoglycans) which is thrombogenic and thus plays an important role in initiating haemostasis as well as thrombosis.

2. ROLE OF PLATELETS Following endothelial cell injury, platelets come to play a central role in normal haemostasis as well as in thrombosis. The sequence of events is as under:

i) Platelet adhesion Glycoprotein Ib (GpIb) receptor on the platelets recognises the site of endothelial injury and the circulating platelets adhere to exposed subendothelial ECM *(primary aggregation).*

ii) Platelet release reaction Activated platelets then undergo release reaction by which the platelet granules are released to the exterior. Two main types of platelet granules are released:
a) Dense bodies
b) Alpha granules

iii) Platelet aggregation Following release of ADP, a potent platelet aggregating agent, aggregation of additional platelets takes place *(secondary aggregation).*

3. ROLE OF COAGULATION SYSTEM Coagulation mechanism is the conversion of the plasma fibrinogen into solid mass of fibrin. The coagulation system is involved in both haemostatic process and thrombus formation.

i) In the intrinsic pathway, contact with abnormal surface (e.g. ECM in the subendothelium) leads to activation of factor XII and the sequential interactions of factors XI, IX, VIII and finally factor X, along with calcium ions (factor IV) and platelet factor 3.

ii) In the extrinsic pathway, tissue damage results in release of tissue factor or thromboplastin. Tissue factor on interaction with factor VII activates factor X.

iii) The common pathway begins where both intrinsic and extrinsic pathways converge to activate factor X which forms a complex with factor Va and platelet factor 3, in the presence of calcium ions. This complex activates prothrombin (factor II) to thrombin (factor IIa) which, in turn, converts fibrinogen to fibrin. Initial monomeric fibrin is polymerised to form insoluble fibrin by activation of factor XIII.

Regulation of coagulation system Normally, the blood is kept in fluid state and the coagulation system is kept in check by controlling mechanisms. These are as under:
i) *Protease inhibitors*
ii) *Fibrinolytic system* Two types of plasminogen activators (PA) are identified:
a) Tissue-type PA
b) Urokinase-like PA

4. ALTERATION OF BLOOD FLOW It is described in relation to normal blood flow.
i) *Normally,* there is axial flow of blood.
ii) *Turbulence and stasis* occur in thrombosis in which the normal axial flow of blood is disturbed.

5. HYPERCOAGULABLE STATES (THROMBOPHILIA) Thrombophilia or hypercoagulable states are a group of conditions having increased risk or predisposition to develop venous thrombosis. These conditions may be hereditary (or primary) or acquired (or secondary) causes.

Hereditary (Primary) factors These include deficiency or mutation of some factors e.g.
i) Deficiency of antithrombin III
ii) Deficiency of protein C and S

iii) Mutation in factor V Leiden

iv) Defects in fibrinolysis

v) Increased levels of coagulations factors (II and VIII).

Secondary (acquired) factors Thrombosis is favoured by certain risk factors, some predisposing clinical conditions and antiphospholipid antibody (APLA) syndrome. There are 2 types of APLA: lupus anticoagulant antibody and anti-cardiolipin antibody.

ORIGIN OF THROMBI AT DIFFERENT SITES

Thrombi may arise from the heart, arteries, veins or in microcirculation by different mechanisms.

CARDIAC THROMBI Thrombi may form in any of the chambers of the heart and on the valve cusps. They are more common in the atrial appendages, especially of the right atrium, and on mitral and aortic valves such as vegetations seen in infective endocarditis and non-bacterial thrombotic endocarditis.

ARTERIAL THROMBI e.g.

i) *Aorta:* aneurysms, arteritis.

ii) *Coronary arteries:* atherosclerosis.

iii) *Mesenteric artery:* atherosclerosis, arteritis.

iv) *Arteries of limbs:* atherosclerosis, diabetes mellitus, Buerger's disease, Raynaud's disease.

v) *Renal artery:* atherosclerosis, arteritis.

vi) *Cerebral artery:* atherosclerosis, vasculitis.

VENOUS THROMBI e.g.

i) *Veins of lower limbs:* deep veins of legs, varicose veins.

ii) *Popliteal, femoral and iliac veins:* postoperative stage, postpartum.

iii) *Pulmonary veins:* CHF, pulmonary hypertension.

iv) *Hepatic and portal vein:* portal hypertension.

v) *Superior vena cava:* infections in head and neck.

vi) *Inferior vena cava:* extension of thrombus from hepatic vein.

vii) *Mesenteric veins:* volvulus, intestinal obstruction.

viii) *Renal vein:* renal amyloidosis.

CAPILLARY THROMBI Minute thrombi composed mainly of packed red cells are formed in the capillaries in acute inflammatory lesions, vasculitis and in disseminated intravascular coagulation (DIC).

MORPHOLOGIC FEATURES

G/A Arterial thrombi tend to be white and mural while the venous thrombi are red and occlusive. Mixed or laminated thrombi are also common and consist of alternate white and red layers called lines of Zahn. Red thrombi are soft, red and gelatinous whereas white thrombi are firm and pale.

M/E The composition of thrombus is determined by the rate of flow of blood i.e. whether it is formed in the rapid arterial and cardiac circulation, or in the slow moving flow in veins. The lines of Zahn are formed by alternate layers of light-staining aggregated platelets admixed with fibrin meshwork and dark-staining layer of red cells.

FATE OF THROMBUS

1. RESOLUTION Thrombus activates the fibrinolytic system with consequent release of plasmin which may dissolve the thrombus completely resulting in resolution.

2. ORGANISATION If the thrombus is not removed, it starts getting organised. Phagocytic cells (neutrophils and macrophages) appear and begin to phagocytose fibrin and cell debris.

3. PROPAGATION The thrombus may enlarge in size due to more and more deposition from the constituents of flowing blood.

4. THROMBOEMBOLISM The thrombi in early stage and infected thrombi are quite friable and may get detached from the vessel wall. These are released in part or completely in blood-stream as emboli.

1. CARDIAC THROMBI Large thrombi in the heart may cause sudden death by mechanical obstruction of blood flow or through thromboembolism to vital organs.

2. ARTERIAL THROMBI These cause ischaemic necrosis of the deprived part (infarct) which may lead to gangrene. Sudden death may occur following thrombosis of coronary artery.

3. VENOUS THROMBI (PHLEBOTHROMBOSIS) These may cause following effects:
i) Thromboembolism
ii) Oedema of area drained
iii) Poor wound healing
iv) Skin ulcer
v) Painful thrombosed veins (thrombophlebitis)
vi) Painful white leg (phlegmasia alba dolens) due to ileofemoral venous thrombosis in postpartum cases
vii) Thrombophlebitis migrans in cancer.

4. CAPILLARY THROMBI Microthrombi in microcirculation may give rise to disseminated intravascular coagulation (DIC).

EMBOLISM

Embolism is the process of partial or complete obstruction of some part of the cardiovascular system by any mass carried in the circulation; the transported intravascular mass detached from its site of origin is called an *embolus*. Most usual forms of emboli (90%) are thromboemboli i.e. originating from thrombi or their parts detached from the vessel wall.

Emboli may be of various types:

A. Depending upon the matter in the emboli:
i) Solid
ii) Liquid
iii) Gaseous

B. Depending upon whether infected or not:
i) Bland
ii) Septic

C. Depending upon the source of the emboli:
i) Cardiac emboli
ii) Arterial emboli
iii) Venous emboli
iv) Lymphatic emboli.

D. Depending upon the flow of blood, two special types of emboli are mentioned:
i) *Paradoxical embolus* An embolus which is carried from the venous side of circulation to the arterial side or vice versa, is called paradoxical or crossed embolus.
ii) *Retrograde embolus* An embolus which travels against the flow of blood is called retrograde embolus.

THROMBOEMBOLISM

A detached thrombus or part of thrombus constitutes the most common type of embolism. These may arise in the arterial or venous circulation.

Arterial (systemic) thromboembolism e.g.
A. *Causes within the heart* (80-85%): These are mural thrombi in the left atrium or left ventricle, vegetations on the mitral or aortic valves, prosthetic heart valves and cardiomyopathy.
B. *Causes within the arteries:* These include emboli developing in relation to atherosclerotic plaques, aortic aneurysms, pulmonary veins and paradoxical arterial emboli from the systemic venous circulation.

The *effects* of arterial emboli depend upon their size, site of lodgement, and adequacy of collateral circulation. If the vascular occlusion occurs, the following ill-effects may result:

i)   *Infarction* of the organ or its affected part e.g. ischaemic necrosis in the lower limbs (70-75%), spleen, kidneys, brain, intestine.

ii)   *Gangrene* following infarction in the lower limbs if the collateral circulation is inadequate.

iii) *Arteritis and mycotic aneurysm* formation from bacterial endocarditis.

iv)   *Myocardial infarction* may occur following coronary embolism.

v)   *Sudden death* may result from coronary embolism or embolism in the middle cerebral artery.

Venous thromboembolism e.g.

i)   Deep vein thrombosis (DVT) of the lower legs, the most common cause of venous thrombi.

ii)   Thrombi in the pelvic veins.

iii) Thrombi in the veins of the upper limbs.

iv)   Thrombosis in cavernous sinus of the brain.

v)   Thrombi in the right side of heart.

The most significant *effect* of venous embolism is obstruction of pulmonary arterial circulation leading to pulmonary embolism.

PULMONARY THROMBOEMBOLISM

DEFINITION   Pulmonary embolism is the most common and fatal form of venous thromboembolism in which there is occlusion of pulmonary arterial tree by thromboemboli. In contrast, pulmonary thrombosis is uncommon and may occur in pulmonary atherosclerosis and pulmonary hypertension.

ETIOLOGY   Pulmonary emboli are more common in hospitalised or bed-ridden patients, though they can occur in ambulatory patients as well. The causes are as follows:

i)   Thrombi originating from large veins of lower legs (such as popliteal, femoral and iliac) are the cause in 95% of pulmonary emboli.

ii)   Less common sources include thrombi in varicosities of superficial veins of the legs, and pelvic veins such as peri-prostatic, periovarian, uterine and broad ligament veins.

PATHOGENESIS   The risk factors for pulmonary thromboembolism are stasis of venous blood and hypercoagulable states.

◈   If the thrombus is large, it is impacted at the bifurcation of the main pulmonary artery *(saddle embolus),* or may be found in the right ventricle or its outflow tract.

◈   More commonly, there are *multiple emboli*, or a large embolus may be fragmented into many smaller emboli which are then impacted in a number of vessels.

◈   Rarely, *paradoxical embolism* may occur by passage of an embolus from right heart into the left heart through atrial or ventricular septal defect. In this way, pulmonary emboli may reach systemic circulation.

CONSEQUENCES OF PULMONARY EMBOLISM   Pulmonary embolism occurs more commonly as a complication in patients of acute or chronic debilitating diseases who are immobilised for a long duration. Women in their reproductive period are at higher risk such as in late pregnancy, following delivery and with use of contraceptive pills. Natural history of pulmonary embolism may have following consequences:

i)   Sudden death

ii)   Acute cor pulmonale

iii) Pulmonary infarction

iv)   Pulmonary haemorrhage

v)   Resolution

vi)   Pulmonary hypertension, chronic cor pulmonale and pulmonary arteriosclerosis.

SYSTEMIC EMBOLISM

This is the type of arterial embolism that originates commonly from thrombi in the diseased heart, especially in the left ventricle. These heart diseases include myocardial infarction, cardiomyopathy, RHD, congenital heart disease, infective endocarditis, and prosthetic cardiac valves.

FAT EMBOLISM

Obstruction of arterioles and capillaries by fat globules constitutes fat embolism.

ETIOLOGY It may occur from following causes:

Traumatic causes:
i) Trauma to bones is the most common cause of fat embolism e.g. in fractures of long bones leading to passage of fatty marrow in circulation, concussions of bones, after orthopaedic surgical procedures etc.
ii) Trauma to soft tissue e.g. laceration of adipose tissue and in puerperium due to injury to pelvic fatty tissue.

Non-traumatic causes:
i) Extensive burns
ii) Diabetes mellitus
iii) Fatty liver
iv) Pancreatitis
v) Sickle cell anaemia
vi) Decompression sickness
vii) Inflammation of bones and soft tissues
viii) Extrinsic fat or oils introduced into the body
ix) Hyperlipidaemia
x) Cardiopulmonary bypass surgery

PATHOGENESIS Pathogenesis of fat embolism is explained by following mechanisms:

i) Mechanical theory Mobilisation of fluid fat may occur following trauma to the bone or soft tissues.

ii) Emulsion instability theory This theory explains the pathogenesis of fat embolism in non-traumatic cases. According to this theory, fat emboli are formed by aggregation of plasma lipids (chylomicrons and fatty acids) due to disturbance in natural emulsification of fat.

iii) Intravascular coagulation theory In stress, release of some factor activates disseminated intravascular coagulation (DIC) and aggregation of fat emboli.

iv) Toxic injury theory According to this theory, the small blood vessels of lungs are chemically injured by high plasma levels of free fatty acid.

CONSEQUENCES OF FAT EMBOLISM The effects of fat embolism depend upon the size and quantity of fat globules.

i) Pulmonary fat embolism In patients dying after fractures of bones, presence of numerous fat emboli in the capillaries of the lung is a frequent autopsy finding.

ii) Systemic fat embolism Some of the fat globules may pass through the pulmonary circulation.

AIR EMBOLISM

Air embolism occurs when air is introduced into venous or arterial circulation.

VENOUS AIR EMBOLISM Air may be sucked into systemic veins under the following circumstances:
i)   Operations on the head and neck, and trauma
ii) Obstetrical operations and trauma
iii) Intravenous infusion of blood and fluid
iv) Angiography

  The *effects* of venous air embolism depend upon the following factors:
i)   Amount of air
ii) Rapidity of entry
iii) Position of the patient
iv) General condition of the patient

Derangements of Homeostasis and Haemodynamics

The mechanism of death is by entrapment of air emboli in the pulmonary arterial trunk in the right heart.

ARTERIAL AIR EMBOLISM Entry of air into pulmonary vein or its tributaries may occur in the following conditions:
i)   Cardiothoracic surgery and trauma
ii)   Paradoxical air embolism
iii) Arteriography

The *effects* of arterial air embolism are in the form of certain characteristic features:
i)   Marble skin due to blockage of cutaneous vessels.
ii)   Air bubbles in the retinal vessels seen ophthalmoscopically.
iii) Pallor of the tongue due to occlusion of a branch of lingual artery.
iv)   Coronary or cerebral arterial air embolism may cause sudden death.

DECOMPRESSION SICKNESS

This is a specialised form of gas embolism known by various names such as caisson's disease, divers' palsy or aeroembolism.

PATHOGENESIS Decompression sickness is produced when the individual decompresses suddenly, either from high atmospheric pressure to normal level, or from normal pressure to low atmospheric pressure.
❖   In divers, workers in caissons (diving-bells), offshore drilling and tunnelers, who *descend* to high atmospheric pressure, increased amount of atmospheric gases (mainly nitrogen; others are O_2, CO_2) are dissolved in blood and tissue fluids. When such an individual ascends too rapidly i.e. comes to normal level suddenly from high atmospheric pressure, the gases come out of the solution as minute bubbles.
❖   In aeroembolism, seen in those who *ascend* to high altitudes or air flight in unpressurised cabins, the individuals are exposed to sudden decompression from low atmospheric pressure to normal levels.
Pathologic changes are more pronounced in sudden decompression from high pressure to normal levels than in those who decompress from low pressure to normal levels.

EFFECTS Clinical effects of decompression sickness are of 2 types:
❖   **Acute form** occurs due to acute obstruction of small blood vessels in the vicinity of joints and skeletal muscles. The condition is clinically characterised by: (i) *The bends* (ii) *The chokes* and (iii) *Cerebral effects*.
❖   **Chronic form** is due to foci of ischaemic necrosis throughout body, especially the skeletal system. Ischaemic necrosis may be due to embolism *per se*, but other factors such as platelet activation, intravascular coagulation and hypoxia might contribute. The features of chronic form are as under:
i)   Avascular necrosis of bones
ii)   Neurological symptoms
iii) Lung involvement
iv)   Skin manifestations

AMNIOTIC FLUID EMBOLISM

This is the most serious, unpredictable and unpreventable cause of maternal mortality. During labour and in the immediate postpartum period, the contents of amniotic fluid may enter the uterine veins and reach right side of the heart resulting in fatal complications. The amniotic fluid components which may be found in uterine veins, pulmonary artery and vessels of other organs are: epithelial squames, vernix caseosa, lanugo hair, bile from meconium, and mucus.

The *clinical syndrome* of amniotic fluid embolism is characterised by the following features:
i)   Sudden respiratory distress and dyspnoea
ii)   Deep cyanosis
iii) Cardiovascular shock
iv)   Convulsions
v)   Coma
vi)   Unexpected death

Derangements of Homeostasis and Haemodynamics

ATHEROEMBOLISM

Atheromatous plaques, especially from aorta, may get eroded to form atherosclerotic emboli which are then lodged in medium-sized and small arteries.

TUMOUR EMBOLISM

Malignant tumour cells invade the local blood vessels and may form tumour emboli to be lodged elsewhere, producing metastatic tumour deposits.

ISCHAEMIA

Ischaemia is defined as deficient blood supply to part of a tissue relative to its metabolic needs. The cessation of blood supply may be *complete* (complete ischaemia) or *partial* (partial ischaemia). The adverse effects of ischaemia may result from 3 ways:

1. **Hypoxia** due to deprivation of oxygen to tissues relative to its needs.

2. **Malnourishment of cells** due to inadequate supply of nutrients to the tissue (i.e. glucose, amino acids); this is less important.

3. **Inadequate clearance of metabolites** which results in accumulation of metabolic waste-products in the affected tissue.

ETIOLOGY A number of causes may produce ischaemia. These causes are discussed below with regard to different levels of blood vessels:

1. **Causes in the heart** Inadequate cardiac output resulting from heart block, ventricular arrest and fibrillation from various causes may cause variable degree of hypoxic injury to the brain as under:
   i)   If the arrest continues for 15 seconds, consciousness is lost.
   ii) If the condition lasts for more than 4 minutes, irreversible ischaemic damage to the brain occurs.
   iii) If it is prolonged for more than 8 minutes, death is inevitable.

2. **Causes in the arteries** The commonest and most important causes of ischaemia are due to obstruction in arterial blood supply as under:
   i) *Luminal occlusion of artery (intraluminal):*
      a)   Thrombosis
      b)   Embolism
   ii) *Causes in the arterial walls (intramural):*
      a)   Vasospasm (e.g. in Raynaud's disease)
      b)   Hypothermia, ergotism
      c)   Arteriosclerosis
      d)   Polyarteritis nodosa
      e)   Thromboangiitis obliterans (Buerger's disease)
      f)   Severed vessel wall
   iii) *Outside pressure on an artery (extramural):*
      a)   Ligature
      b)   Tourniquet
      c)   Tight plaster, bandages
      d)   Torsion.

3. **Causes in the veins** Blockage of venous drainage may lead to engorgement and obstruction to arterial blood supply resulting in ischaemia.
   i) *Luminal occlusion of vein (intraluminal):*
      a)   Thrombosis of mesenteric veins
      b)   Cavernous sinus thrombosis
   ii) *Causes in the vessel wall of vein (intramural):*
      a)   Varicose veins of the legs
   iii) *Outside pressure on vein (extramural):*
      a) Strangulated hernia
      b) Intussusception
      c) Volvulus

4. **Causes in the microcirculation** Ischaemia may result from occlusion of arterioles, capillaries and venules.
   i) *Luminal occlusion in microvasculature (intraluminal):*
   a)   By red cells e.g. in sickle cell anaemia, red cells parasitised by malaria, acquired haemolytic anaemia, sludging of the blood.

b) By white cells e.g. in chronic myeloid leukaemia
c) By fibrin e.g. defibrination syndrome
d) By precipitated cryoglobulins
e) By fat embolism
f) In decompression sickness.

ii) *Causes in the microvasculature wall (intramural)*:
a) Vasculitis e.g. in polyarteritis nodosa, Henoch-Schönlein purpura, Arthus reaction, septicaemia.
b) Frost-bite injuring the wall of small blood vessels.

iii) *Outside pressure on microvasculature (extramural)*:
a) Bedsores.

FACTORS DETERMINING SEVERITY OF ISCHAEMIC INJURY The extent of damage produced by ischaemia due to occlusion of arterial or venous blood vessels depends upon a number of factors as under:

1. **Anatomic pattern** The extent of injury by ischaemia depends upon the anatomic pattern of arterial blood supply of the organ or tissue affected.

i) *Single arterial supply without anastomosis* e.g.
a) Central artery of the retina
b) Interlobular arteries of the kidneys.

ii) *Single arterial supply with rich anastomosis* e.g.
a) Superior mesenteric artery supplying blood to the small intestine.
b) Inferior mesenteric artery supplying blood to distal colon.
c) Arterial supply to the stomach by 3 separate vessels derived from coeliac axis.
d) Interarterial anastomoses in the 3 main trunks of the coronary arterial system.

iii) *Parallel arterial supply* e.g.
a) Blood supply to the brain in the region of circle of Willis.
b) Arterial supply to forearm by radial and ulnar arteries.

iv) *Double blood supply* The effect of occlusion of one set of vessels is modified if an organ has dual blood supply e.g.
a) Lungs are perfused by bronchial circulation as well as by pulmonary arterial branches.
b) Liver is supplied by both portal circulation and hepatic arterial flow.

2. **General and cardiovascular status** The general status of an individual as regards cardiovascular function is an important determinant to assess the effect of ischaemia.

3. **Type of tissue affected** Vulnerability of the tissue of the body to the effect of ischaemia is variable. The following tissues are more vulnerable to ischaemia:
i) Brain (cerebral cortical neurons, in particular).
ii) Heart (myocardial cells).
iii) Kidney (especially epithelial cells of proximal convoluted tubules).

4. **Rapidity of development** Sudden vascular obstruction results in more severe effects of ischaemia than if it is gradual.

5. **Degree of vascular occlusion** Complete vascular obstruction results in more severe ischaemic injury than the partial occlusion.

EFFECTS The effects of ischaemia are variable and range from 'no change' to 'sudden death'.

INFARCTION

Infarction is the process of tissue necrosis, usually coagulative type, resulting from ischaemia; the localised area of necrosis so developed is called an *infarct*.

ETIOLOGY All the causes of ischaemia discussed above can cause infarction. However, there are a few other noteworthy features in infarction:
i) Most commonly, infarcts are caused by interruption in arterial blood supply, called *ischaemic necrosis*.

ii) Less commonly, venous obstruction can produce infarcts termed *stagnant hypoxia*.

iii) Generally, *sudden, complete, and continuous occlusion* (e.g. thrombosis or embolism) produces infarcts.

iv) Infarcts may be produced by *nonocclusive circulatory insufficiency* as well e.g. incomplete atherosclerotic narrowing of coronary arteries may produce myocardial infarction due to acute coronary insufficiency.

TYPES OF INFARCTS Infarcts are classified depending upon different features:

1. According to their colour:
i) *Pale or anaemic*
ii) *Red or haemorrhagic.*

2. According to their age:
i) *Recent or fresh*
ii) *Old or healed*

3. According to presence or absence of infection:
i) *Bland*, when free of bacterial contamination
ii) *Septic*, when infected.

PATHOGENESIS The process of infarction takes place as follows:
i) *Localised hyperaemia*
ii) Within a few hours, the affected part becomes swollen due to *oedema and haemorrhage*.
iii) *Cellular changes* such as cloudy swelling and degeneration appear early (reversible cell injury).
iv) There is progressive *proteolysis*.
v) An acute inflammatory reaction and hyperaemia follow.
vi) *Blood pigments*, haematoidin and haemosiderin, liberated by lysis of RBCs are deposited in the infarct.
vii) Following this, there is progressive *ingrowth of granulation tissue* from the margin of the infarct.

INFARCTS OF DIFFERENT ORGANS

INFARCT LUNG Embolism of the pulmonary arteries may produce pulmonary infarction, though not always. This is because lungs receive blood supply from bronchial arteries as well, and thus occlusion of pulmonary artery ordinarily does not produce infarcts.

G/A Pulmonary infarcts are classically wedge-shaped with base on the pleura, haemorrhagic, variable in size, and most often in the lower lobes. Fibrinous pleuritis usually covers the area of infarct. Cut surface is dark purple and may show the blocked vessel near the apex of the infarcted area.

M/E The characteristic histologic feature is coagulative necrosis of the alveolar walls. Initially, there is infiltration by neutrophils and intense alveolar capillary congestion, but later their place is taken by haemosiderin, phagocytes and granulation tissue.

INFARCT KIDNEY Renal infarction is common, found in up to 5% of autopsies. Majority of them are caused by thromboemboli, most commonly originating from the heart such as in mural thrombi in the left atrium, myocardial infarction, vegetative endocarditis and from aortic aneurysm.

G/A Renal infarcts are often multiple and may be bilateral. Characteristically, they are pale or anaemic and wedge-shaped with base resting under the capsule and apex pointing towards the medulla. Generally, a narrow rim of preserved renal tissue under the capsule is spared because it draws its blood supply from the capsular vessels.

M/E The affected area shows characteristic coagulative necrosis of renal parenchyma i.e. there are ghosts of renal tubules and glomeruli without intact nuclei and cytoplasmic content. The margin of the infarct shows inflammatory reaction—initially acute but later macrophages and fibrous tissue predominate.

INFARCT SPLEEN Spleen is one of the common sites for infarction. Splenic infarction results from occlusion of the splenic artery or its branches.

G/A Splenic infarcts are often multiple. They are characteristically pale or anaemic and wedge-shaped with their base at the periphery and apex pointing towards hilum.

M/E The features are similar to those found in anaemic infarcts in kidney. Coagulative necrosis and inflammatory reaction are seen.

INFARCT LIVER Just as in lungs, infarcts in the liver are uncommon due to dual blood supply—from portal vein and from hepatic artery.

G/A Ischaemic infarcts of the liver are usually anaemic but sometimes may be haemorrhagic due to stuffing of the site by blood from the portal vein. Infarcts of Zahn (non-ischaemic infarcts) produce sharply defined red-blue area in liver parenchyma.

M/E Ischaemic infarcts show characteristics of pale or anaemic infarcts as in kidney or spleen. Infarcts of Zahn occurring due to reduced portal blood flow over a long duration result in chronic atrophy of hepatocytes and dilatation of sinusoids.

SELF ASSESSMENT

1. The essential difference between plasma and interstitial fluid compartment is:
   A. Glucose is higher in the former
   B. Urea is higher in the former
   C. Protein content is higher in the former
   D. Potassium is higher in the former

2. Osmotic pressure exerted by the chemical constituents of the body fluids has the following features <u>except</u>:
   A. Crystalloid osmotic pressure comprises minor portion of total osmotic pressure
   B. Oncotic pressure constitutes minor portion of total osmotic pressure
   C. Oncotic pressure of plasma is higher
   D. Oncotic pressure of interstitial fluid is lower

3. For causation of oedema by decreased osmotic pressure, the following factor is most important:
   A. Fall in albumin as well as globulin
   B. Fall in globulin level
   C. Fall in albumin level
   D. Fall in fibrinogen level

4. Transudate differs from exudate in having the following <u>except</u>:
   A. No inflammatory cells   B. Low glucose content
   C. Low protein content   D. Low specific gravity

5. Nephritic oedema differs from nephrotic oedema in having the following <u>except</u>:
   A. Mild oedema
   B. Distributed on face, eyes
   C. Heavy proteinuria
   D. Occurs in acute glomerulonephritis

6. The following type of oedema is characteristically dependent oedema:
   A. Nephrotic oedema   B. Nephritic oedema
   C. Pulmonary oedema   D. Cardiac oedema

7. Pulmonary oedema appears due to elevated pulmonary hydrostatic pressure when the fluid accumulation is:
   A. Two fold   B. Four fold
   C. Eight fold   D. Ten fold

8. **Active hyperaemia is the result of:**
   A. Dilatation of capillaries
   B. Dilatation of arterioles
   C. Venous engorgement
   D. Lymphatic obstruction

9. **Sectioned surface of lung shows brown induration in:**
   A. Pulmonary embolism
   B. Pulmonary haemorrhage
   C. Pulmonary infarction
   D. CVC lung

10. **In septic shock, pathogenesis of endothelial cell injury involves the following mechanisms except:**
    A. Lipopolysaccharide from lysed bacteria injures the endothelium
    B. Interleukin-1 causes endothelial cell injury
    C. TNF-α causes direct cytotoxicity
    D. Adherence of PMNs to endothelium causes endothelial cell injury

11. **An intact endothelium elaborates the following anti-thrombotic factors except:**
    A. Thrombomodulin
    B. ADPase
    C. Tissue plasminogen activator
    D. Thromboplastin

12. **The most common cause of arterial thromboemboli is:**
    A. Cardiac thrombi
    B. Aortic aneurysm
    C. Pulmonary veins
    D. Aortic atherosclerotic plaques

13. **Venous emboli are most often lodged in:**
    A. Intestines
    B. Kidneys
    C. Lungs
    D. Heart

14. **Pathologic changes between sudden decompression from high pressure to normal levels and decompression from low pressure to normal levels are:**
    A. More marked in the former
    B. More marked in the latter
    C. No difference between the two
    D. Acute form is more marked in the latter

15. **The infarct of following organ is invariably haemorrhagic:**
    A. Infarct kidney
    B. Infarct spleen
    C. Infarct lung
    D. Infarct heart

16. **Milroy's disease is:**
    A. Cerebral oedema
    B. Pulmonary oedema
    C. Hereditary lymphoedema
    D. Postural oedema

17. **Pick the correct sequence:**
    A. Renin-Angiotensin II-Angiotensin I-Angiotensinogen-Aldosterone
    B. Angiotensinogen-Renin-Angiotensin II-Angiotensin I-Aldosterone
    C. Renin-Angiotensinogen-Angiotensin I-Angiotensin II-Aldosterone
    D. Aldosterone-Renin-Angiotensinogen-Angiotensin II-Angiotensin I

18. **Which of the following is true?**
    A. Arterial thrombi are white and occlusive
    B. Venous thrombi are white and occlusive
    C. Arterial thrombi are white and mural
    D. Venous thrombi are red and mural.

KEY

1 = C	2 = A	3 = C	4 = B	5 = C
6 = D	7 = D	8 = B	9 = D	10 = A
11 = D	12 = A	13 = C	14 = A	15 = C
16 = C	17 = C	18 = C		

5   Inflammation and Healing

INTRODUCTION

DEFINITION AND CAUSES   Inflammation is defined as the local response of living mammalian tissues to injury from any agent. It is a body defense reaction in order to eliminate or limit the spread of injurious agent, followed by removal of the necrosed cells and tissues.

The injurious agents causing inflammation may be as under:

1. *Infective agents* like bacteria, viruses and their toxins, fungi, parasites.
2. *Immunological agents* like cell-mediated and antigen-antibody reactions.
3. *Physical agents* like heat, cold, radiation, mechanical trauma.
4. *Chemical agents* like organic and inorganic poisons.
5. *Inert materials* such as foreign bodies.

SIGNS OF INFLAMMATION   The Roman writer Celsus in 1st century A.D. named the famous 4 *cardinal signs of inflammation* as:

i)   *rubor* (redness);
ii)   *tumor* (swelling);
iii)   *calor* (heat); and
iv)   *dolor* (pain).

To these, fifth sign *functio laesa* (loss of function) was later added by Virchow.

TYPES OF INFLAMMATION   Depending upon the defense capacity of the host and duration of response, inflammation can be classified as acute and chronic.

A.   *Acute inflammation* is of short duration (lasting less than 2 weeks) and represents the early body reaction, resolves quickly and is usually followed by healing.

The main features of acute inflammation are:

1. accumulation of fluid and plasma at the affected site;
2. intravascular activation of platelets; and
3. polymorphonuclear neutrophils as inflammatory cells.

B.   *Chronic inflammation* is of longer duration and occurs after delay, either after the causative agent of acute inflammation persists for a long time, or the stimulus is such that it induces chronic inflammation from the beginning.

ACUTE INFLAMMATION *(p. 116)*

Acute inflammatory response by the host to any agent is a continuous process but for the purpose of discussion, it can be divided into following two events:

I.   Vascular events
II.   Cellular events

VASCULAR EVENTS

Alteration in the microvasculature (arterioles, capillaries and venules) is the earliest response to tissue injury. These alterations include: haemodynamic changes and changes in vascular permeability.

HAEMODYNAMIC CHANGES

The earliest features of inflammatory response result from changes in the vascular flow and calibre of small blood vessels in the injured tissue. The sequence of these changes is as under:

1. Irrespective of the type of cell injury, immediate vascular response is of **transient vasoconstriction** of arterioles.

2. Next follows **persistent progressive vasodilatation** which involves mainly the arterioles, but to a lesser extent, affects other components of the microcirculation like venules and capillaries.

3. Progressive vasodilatation, in turn, may elevate the **local hydrostatic pressure** resulting in transudation of fluid into the extracellular space.

4. **Slowing or stasis** of microcirculation follows which causes increased concentration of red cells, and thus, raised blood viscosity.

5. Stasis or slowing is followed by **leucocytic margination** or peripheral orientation of leucocytes (mainly neutrophils) along the vascular endothelium.

TRIPLE RESPONSE The features of haemodynamic changes in inflammation are best demonstrated by the **Lewis experiment**. Lewis induced the changes in the skin of inner aspect of forearm by firm stroking with a blunt point. The reaction so elicited is known as *triple response* or *red line response* consisting of the following:

i) *Red line* appears within a few seconds after stroking and is due to local vasodilatation of capillaries and venules.

ii) *Flare* is the bright reddish appearance or flush surrounding the red line and results from vasodilatation of the adjacent arterioles.

iii) *Wheal* is the swelling or oedema of the surrounding skin occurring due to transudation of fluid into the extravascular space.

ALTERED VASCULAR PERMEABILITY

PATHOGENESIS In and around the inflamed tissue, there is accumulation of oedema fluid in the interstitial compartment which comes from blood plasma by its escape through the endothelial wall of peripheral vascular bed. In the initial stage, the escape of fluid is due to vasodilatation and consequent elevation in hydrostatic pressure. This is transudate in nature. But subsequently, the characteristic inflammatory oedema, exudate, appears by increased vascular permeability of microcirculation.

The appearance of inflammatory oedema due to increased vascular permeability of microvascular bed is explained on the basis of **Starling's hypothesis**. According to this, normally the fluid balance is maintained by two opposing sets of forces:

i) Forces that cause **outward movement** of fluid from microcirculation: These are *intravascular hydrostatic pressure* and *colloid osmotic pressure of interstitial fluid*.

ii) Forces that cause **inward movement** of interstitial fluid into circulation: These are *intravascular colloid osmotic pressure* and *hydrostatic pressure of interstitial fluid*.

Whatever little fluid is left in the interstitial compartment is drained away by lymphatics and, thus, no oedema results normally.

However, in inflamed tissues, the endothelial lining of microvasculature becomes more leaky. Consequently, intravascular colloid osmotic pressure decreases and osmotic pressure of the interstitial fluid increases resulting in excessive outward flow of fluid into the interstitial compartment which is exudative inflammatory oedema.

PATTERNS OF INCREASED VASCULAR PERMEABILITY Increased vascular permeability in acute inflammation by which normally non-permeable endothelial layer of microvasculature becomes leaky can have following patterns and mechanisms which may be acting singly or more often in combination:

i) **Contraction of endothelial cells** An example of such *immediate transient response* is mild thermal injury of skin of forearm.

ii) **Contraction or mild endothelial damage** Classic example of *delayed and prolonged leakage* is appearance of sunburns mediated by ultraviolet radiation.

iii) Direct injury to endothelial cells The examples of *immediate sustained leakage* are severe bacterial infections while delayed prolonged leakage may occur following moderate thermal injury and radiation injury.

iv) Leucocyte-mediated endothelial injury The examples are seen in sites where leucocytes adhere to the vascular endothelium e.g. in pulmonary venules and capillaries.

v) Leakiness in neovascularisation In addition, the newly formed capillaries under the influence of vascular endothelial growth factor (VEGF) during the process of repair and in tumours are excessively leaky.

CELLULAR EVENTS

The cellular phase of inflammation consists of 2 processes:
1. exudation of leucocytes; and
2. phagocytosis.

EXUDATION OF LEUCOCYTES

The escape of leucocytes from the lumen of microvasculature to the interstitial tissue is the most important feature of inflammatory response. In acute inflammation, polymorphonuclear neutrophils (PMNs) comprise the first line of body defense, followed later by monocytes and macrophages.

The changes leading to migration of leucocytes are as follows:

1. CHANGES IN THE FORMED ELEMENTS OF BLOOD In the early stage of inflammation, the rate of flow of blood is increased due to vasodilatation. But subsequently, there is slowing or stasis of bloodstream. Due to slowing and stasis, the central stream of cells widens and peripheral plasma zone becomes narrower because of loss of plasma by exudation. This phenomenon is known as *margination*. As a result of this redistribution, neutrophils of the central column come close to the vessel wall; this is known as *pavementing*.

2. ROLLING AND ADHESION Peripherally marginated and pavemented neutrophils slowly roll over the endothelial cells lining the vessel wall *(rolling phase)*. This is followed by transient bond between the leucocytes and endothelial cells becoming firmer *(adhesion phase)*. The following cell adhesion molecules (CAMs) bring about rolling and adhesion phases:

i) **Selectins** These are a group of CAMs expressed on the surface of activated endothelial cells and are structurally composed of lectins or lectin-like protein molecules the most important of which is s-Lewis X molecule. There are 3 types of selectins:
◈ P-selectin
◈ E-selectin
◈ L-selectin

ii) **Integrins** These are a family of endothelial cell surface proteins having alpha (or CD11) and beta (CD18) subunits, which are activated during the process of loose and transient adhesions between endothelial cells and leucocytes.

iii) **Immunoglobulin gene superfamily adhesion molecules.** This group consists of a variety of immunoglobulin molecules present on most cells of the body. These partake in cell-to-cell contact through various other CAMs and cytokines.

3. EMIGRATION After sticking of neutrophils to endothelium, the former move along the endothelial surface till a suitable site between the endothelial cells is found where the neutrophils throw out cytoplasmic pseudopods. Neutrophils are the dominant cells in acute inflammatory exudate in the first 24 hours, and monocyte-macrophages appear in the next 24-48 hours. However, neutrophils are short-lived (24-48 hours) while monocyte-macrophages survive much longer.

4. CHEMOTAXIS The transmigration of leucocytes after crossing several barriers (endothelium, basement membrane, perivascular myofibroblasts and matrix) to reach the interstitial tissues is a chemotactic factor-mediated process called chemotaxis. The concept of chemotaxis is well illustrated by *Boyden's chamber experiment*.

The following agents act as potent chemotactic substances for neutrophils:

i) Leukotriene B4 (LT-B4)
ii) Components of complement system (C5a and C3a in particular)
iii) Cytokines (Interleukins, in particular IL-8)
iv) Soluble bacterial products (such as formylated peptides).

PHAGOCYTOSIS

Phagocytosis is defined as the process of engulfment of solid particulate material by the cells (cell-eating). The cells performing this function are called *phagocytes*.

Neutrophils and macrophages on reaching the tissue spaces produce several proteolytic enzymes—lysozyme, protease, collagenase, elastase, lipase, proteinase, gelatinase, and acid hydrolases. These enzymes degrade collagen and extracellular matrix. Phagocytosis of the microbe by polymorphs and macrophages involves the following 3 steps:

1. RECOGNITION AND ATTACHMENT Phagocytosis is initiated by the expression of cell surface receptors on macrophages which recognise microorganisms: *mannose receptor* and *scavenger receptor*. The process of phagocytosis is further enhanced when the microorganisms are coated with specific proteins, *opsonins*, from the serum and the process is called opsonisation (meaning preparing for eating).

2. ENGULFMENT The opsonised particle or microbe bound to the surface of phagocyte is ready to be engulfed. This is accomplished by formation of cytoplasmic pseudopods around the particle due to activation of actin filaments beneath cell wall, enveloping it in a phagocytic vacuole.

3. KILLING AND DEGRADATION Next comes the stage of killing and degradation of microorganism to dispose it off which is the major function of phagocytes as scavenger cells.

In general, following mechanisms are involved in disposal of microorganisms:

A. INTRACELLULAR MECHANISMS Intracellular metabolic pathways are involved in killing microbes, more commonly by oxidative mechanism and less often by non-oxidative pathways.

i) Oxidative bactericidal mechanism by oxygen free radicals An important mechanism of microbicidal killing is by oxidative damage by the production of reactive oxygen metabolites (O'_2, H_2O_2, OH', $HOCl$, HOI, $HOBr$).

This type of bactericidal activity is carried out either via enzyme myeloperoxidase (MPO) present in the azurophilic granules of neutrophils and monocytes, or independent of enzyme MPO.

ii) Oxidative bactericidal mechanism by lysosomal granules In this mechanism, the preformed granule-stored products of neutrophils and macrophages are discharged or secreted into the phagosome and the extracellular environment.

iii) Non-oxidative bactericidal mechanism Some agents released from the granules of phagocytic cells do not require oxygen for bactericidal activity. These include:

a) Granules
b) Nitric oxide

B. EXTRACELLULAR MECHANISMS These include the following:

i) Granules Degranulation of macrophages and neutrophils explained above continues to exert its effects of proteolysis outside the cells as well.

ii) Immune mechanisms Immune-mediated lysis of microbes takes place outside the cells by mechanisms of cytolysis, antibody-mediated lysis and by cell-mediated cytotoxicity.

These are a large and increasing number of endogenous chemical substances which mediate the process of acute inflammation.

Mediators of inflammation have some common properties as under:

1) These mediators are released either *from the cells or are derived from plasma proteins.*

2) All mediators are *released in response to certain stimuli.* These stimuli may be a variety of injurious agents, dead and damaged tissues, or even one mediator stimulating release of another.

3) Mediators *act on different targets.* They may have similar action on different target cells or differ in their action on different target cells. They may act on cells which formed them or on other body cells.

4) *Range of actions* of different mediators are: increased vascular permeability, vasodilatation, chemotaxis, fever, pain and tissue damage.

5) Mediators have *short lifespan* after their release.

I. *CELL-DERIVED MEDIATORS*

1. VASOACTIVE AMINES Two important pharmacologically active amines that have role in the early inflammatory response (first one hour) are histamine and 5-hydroxytryptamine (5-HT) or serotonin; another addition to this group is neuropeptides.

i) Histamine It is stored in the granules of mast cells, basophils and platelets.

The main *actions* of histamine are: vasodilatation, increased vascular (venular) permeability, itching and pain.

ii) 5-Hydroxytryptamine (5-HT or serotonin) It is present in tissues like chromaffin cells of GIT, spleen, nervous tissue, mast cells and platelets. The actions of 5-HT are similar to histamine but it is a less potent mediator of increased vascular permeability and vasodilatation than histamine.

iii) Neuropeptides Another class of vasoactive amines is tachykinin neuropeptides such as substance P, neurokinin A, vasoactive intestinal polypeptide (VIP) and somatostatin.

2. ARACHIDONIC ACID METABOLITES (EICOSANOIDS) Arachidonic acid is a fatty acid, eicosatetraenoic acid. Arachidonic acid is a constituent of the phospholipid cell membrane, besides its presence in some constituents of diet. Arachidonic acid is released from the cell membrane by phospholipases. It is then activated to form arachidonic acid metabolites or eicosanoids by one of the following 2 pathways.

i) Metabolites via cyclo-oxygenase pathway: Prostaglandins, thromboxane A_2, prostacyclin The name 'prostaglandin' was first given to a substance found in human seminal fluid.

Cyclo-oxygenase (COX), a fatty acid enzyme present as COX-1 and COX-2, acts on activated arachidonic acid to form prostaglandin endoperoxide (PGG_2). PGG_2 is enzymatically transformed into PGH_2 with generation of free radical of oxygen. PGH_2 is further acted upon by enzymes and results in formation of the following 3 metabolites:

a) Prostaglandins (PGD_2, PGE_2 and PGF_2-α)
b) Thromboxane A_2 (TXA_2)
c) Prostacyclin (PGI_2)
d) Resolvins

ii) Metabolites via lipo-oxygenase pathway: 5-HETE, leukotrienes, lipoxins The enzyme, lipo-oxygenase, a predominant enzyme in neutrophils, acts on activated arachidonic acid to form hydroperoxy eicosatetraenoic acid (5-HPETE) which on further peroxidation forms following 3 metabolites:

a) *5-HETE* (hydroxy compound), an intermediate product, is a potent chemotactic agent for neutrophils.

b) *Leukotrienes* (LT) Firstly, unstable leukotriene A_4 (LTA_4) is formed which is acted upon by enzymes to form LTB_4 (chemotactic for phagocytic cells and stimulates phagocytic cell adherence) while LTC_4, LTD_4 and LTE_4 have common actions by causing smooth muscle contraction and thereby induce vasoconstriction, bronchoconstriction and increased vascular permeability.

c) *Lipoxins* (LX) act to regulate and counterbalance actions of leukotrienes.

3. LYSOSOMAL COMPONENTS The inflammatory cells—neutrophils and monocytes, contain lysosomal granules which on release elaborate a variety of mediators of inflammation e.g.

i) Granules of neutrophils Neutrophils have 3 types of granules:
a) Primary or azurophil granules
b) Secondary or specific granules
c) Tertiary granules or C particles

ii) Granules of monocytes and tissue macrophages These cells on degranulation also release mediators of inflammation like acid proteases, collagenase, elastase and plasminogen activator.

4. PLATELET ACTIVATING FACTOR (PAF) It is released from IgE-sensitised basophils or mast cells, other leucocytes, endothelium and platelets. Apart from its action on platelet aggregation and release reaction, the actions of PAF as mediator of inflammation are:
i) increased vascular permeability;
ii) vasodilatation in low concentration and vasoconstriction otherwise;
iii) bronchoconstriction;
iv) adhesion of leucocytes to endothelium; and
v) chemotaxis.

5. CYTOKINES Cytokines are polypeptide substances produced by activated lymphocytes *(lymphokines)* and activated monocytes *(monokines)*.
a) Interleukins (IL-1, IL-6, IL-8, IL-12, IL-17) While IL-1 and IL-6 are active in mediating acute inflammation, IL-12 and IL-17 play a potent role in chronic inflammation. IL-8 is a chemokine for acute inflammatory cells.

b) Tumour necrosis factor (TNF-α and β) TNF-α is a mediator of acute inflammation while TNF-β is involved in cellular cytotoxicity and in development of spleen and lymph nodes.

c) Interferon (IFN)-γ It is produced by T cells and NK cells and may act on all body cells. It acts as mediator of acute inflammation.

d) Other chemokines (IL-8, MCP-1, eotaxin, PF-4) Besides IL-8, a few other chemoattractants for various cells are **MCP-1**, **Eotaxin**, **PF-4**.

6. FREE RADICALS: OXYGEN METABOLITES AND NITRIC OXIDE Free radicals act as potent mediator of inflammation:
i) *Oxygen-derived metabolites* are released from activated neutrophils and macrophages and include superoxide oxygen (O'_2), H_2O_2, OH' and toxic NO products. These oxygen-derived free radicals have the following actions in inflammation:
a) Endothelial cell damage and thereby increased vascular permeability.
b) Activation of protease and inactivation of antiprotease causing tissue matrix damage.
c) Damage to other cells.
ii) *Nitric oxide (NO)* NO plays the following roles in mediating inflammation:
a) Vasodilatation
b) Anti-platelet activating agent
c) Possibly microbicidal action.

II. *PLASMA PROTEIN-DERIVED MEDIATORS (PLASMA PROTEASES)*

These include various products derived from activation and interaction of 4 interlinked systems: kinin, clotting, fibrinolytic and complement.

Hageman factor (factor XII) of clotting system plays a key role in interactions of the four systems.

1. THE KININ SYSTEM This system on activation by factor XIIa generates bradykinin, so named because of the slow contraction of smooth muscle induced by it. Bradykinin acts in the early stage of inflammation and its effects include:
i) smooth muscle contraction;

ii) vasodilatation;

iii) increased vascular permeability; and

iv) pain.

2. THE CLOTTING SYSTEM Factor XIIa initiates the cascade of the clotting system resulting in formation of fibrinogen which is acted upon by thrombin to form fibrin.

The actions of fibrinopeptides in inflammation are:

i) increased vascular permeability;

ii) chemotaxis for leucocyte; and

iii) anticoagulant activity.

3. THE FIBRINOLYTIC SYSTEM This system is activated by plasminogen activator, the sources of which include kallikrein of the kinin system, endothelial cells and leucocytes.

The actions of plasmin in inflammation are as follows:

i) activation of factor XII to form prekallikrein activator that stimulates the kinin system to generate bradykinin;

ii) splits off complement C3 to form C3a which is a permeability factor; and

iii) degrades fibrin to form fibrin split products which increase vascular permeability and are chemotactic to leucocytes.

4. THE COMPLEMENT SYSTEM The activation of complement system can occur either:

i) by *classic pathway* through antigen-antibody complexes; or

ii) by *alternate pathway* via non-immunologic agents such as bacterial toxins, cobra venoms and IgA.

Complement system on activation by either of these two pathways yields activated products which include anaphylatoxins (C3a, C4a and C5a), and membrane attack complex (MAC) i.e. C5b,C6,7,8,9.

The actions of activated complement system in inflammation are as under:

◈ C3a, C5a, C4a (anaphylatoxins) activate mast cells and basophils to release of histamine, cause increased vascular permeability causing oedema in tissues, augments phagocytosis.

◈ C3b is an opsonin.

◈ C5a is chemotactic for leucocytes.

◈ Membrane attack complex (MAC) (C5b-C9) is a lipid dissolving agent and causes holes in the phospholipid membrane of the cell.

REGULATION OF INFLAMMATION (p. 127)

Self-damaging effects are kept in check by the host regulatory mechanisms in order to resolve inflammation. These mechanisms are as follows:

i) Acute phase reactants A variety of acute phase reactant (APR) proteins are released in plasma in response to tissue trauma and infection.

The APR are synthesised mainly in the liver, and to some extent in macrophages. APR along with systemic features of fever and leucocytosis is termed 'acute phase response'. Deficient synthesis of APR leads to severe form of disease in the form of chronic and repeated inflammatory responses.

ii) Glucosteroids The endogenous glucocorticoids act as anti-inflammatory agents. Their levels are raised in infection and trauma by self-regulating mechanism.

iii) Free cytokine receptors The presence of freely circulating soluble receptors for cytokines in the serum correlates directly with disease activity.

iv) Anti-inflammatory chemical mediators As already described, PGE_2 or prostacyclin have both pro-inflammatory as well as anti-inflammatory actions.

THE INFLAMMATORY CELLS (p. 128)

The cells participating in acute and chronic inflammation are circulating leucocytes, plasma cells, tissue macrophages and inflammatory giant cells.

POLYMORPHONUCLEAR NEUTROPHILS (PMNS)

Commonly called as neutrophils or polymorphs, these cells along with basophils and eosinophils are together known as granulocytes due to the presence of granules in their cytoplasm. These cells comprise 40-75% of circulating leucocytes and their number is increased in blood (neutrophilia) and tissues in acute bacterial infections.

The functions of neutrophils in inflammation are as follows:

i)   **Initial phagocytosis** of microorganisms

ii) **Engulfment** of antigen-antibody complexes and non-microbial material.

iii) **Harmful effect** of neutrophils are by causing basement membrane destruction of the glomeruli and small blood vessels in immunologic cell injury.

EOSINOPHILS

These are slightly larger than neutrophils but are fewer in number, comprising 1 to 6% of total blood leucocytes. However, granules of eosinophils are richer in myeloperoxidase than neutrophils and lack lysozyme. High level of steroid hormones leads to fall in number of eosinophils and even disappearance from blood.

The absolute number of eosinophils is increased in the following conditions and, thus, they partake in inflammatory responses associated with these conditions:

i)   allergic conditions;

ii) parasitic infestations;

iii) skin diseases; and

iv) certain malignant lymphomas.

BASOPHILS AND MAST CELLS

The basophils comprise about 1% of circulating leucocytes and are morphologically and functionally similar to their tissue counterparts, mast cells. Basophils and mast cells have receptors for IgE and degranulate when cross-linked with antigen.

The role of these cells in inflammation are:

i)   in immediate and delayed type of hypersensitivity reactions; and

ii) release of histamine by IgE-sensitised basophils.

LYMPHOCYTES

Next to neutrophils, these cells are the most numerous of the circulating leucocytes in adults (20-45%). Apart from blood, lymphocytes are present in large numbers in spleen, thymus, lymph nodes and mucosa-associated lymphoid tissue (MALT).

These cells participate in the following types of inflammatory responses:

i)   *In tissues*, they are dominant cells in chronic inflammation and late stage of acute inflammation.

ii) *In blood*, their number is increased (lymphocytosis) in chronic infections like tuberculosis.

PLASMA CELLS

These cells are larger than lymphocytes with more abundant cytoplasm and an eccentric nucleus which has cart-wheel pattern of chromatin. They develop from B lymphocytes and are rich in RNA and γ-globulin in their cytoplasm. There is an interrelationship between plasmacytosis and hyperglobulinaemia. These cells are most active in antibody synthesis.

Their number is increased in the following conditions:

i)   prolonged infection with immunological responses e.g. in syphilis, rheumatoid arthritis, tuberculosis;

ii) hypersensitivity states; and

iii) multiple myeloma.

MONONUCLEAR-PHAGOCYTE SYSTEM (RETICULOENDOTHELIAL SYSTEM)

This cell system includes cells derived from 2 sources with common morphology, function and origin.

A. Blood monocytes These comprise 4-8% of circulating leucocytes.

B. Tissue macrophages These include the following cells in different tissues:

  i) Macrophages or phagocytes in inflammation.
  ii) Histiocytes which are macrophages present in connective tissues.
  iii) Epithelioid cells are modified macrophages seen in granulomatous inflammation.
  iv) Kupffer cells are macrophages of the liver.
  v) Alveolar macrophages (type II pneumocytes) in the lungs.
  vi) Reticulum cells are macrophages/histiocytes of the bone marrow.
  vii) Tingible body macrophages of germinal centres of the lymph nodes.
  viii) Littoral cells of the splenic sinusoids.
  ix) Osteoclasts in the bones.
  x) Microglial cells of the brain.
  xi) Langerhans' cells/dendritic histiocytes of the skin.
  xii) Hoffbauer cells of the placenta.
  xiii) Mesangial cells of the glomerulus.

The mononuclear phagocytes are the scavenger cells of the body as well as participate in immune system of the body; their functions in inflammation are as under:

i) *Phagocytosis* (cell eating) and *pinocytosis* (cell drinking).

ii) *Macrophages on activation* by lymphokines released by T lymphocytes or by non-immunologic stimuli elaborate a variety of biologically active substances as under:

a) Proteases like collagenase and elastase which degrade collagen and elastic tissue.

b) Plasminogen activator which activates the fibrinolytic system.

c) Products of complement.

d) Some coagulation factors (factor V and thromboplastin) which convert fibrinogen to fibrin.

e) Chemotactic agents for other leucocytes.

f) Metabolites of arachidonic acid.

g) Growth promoting factors for fibroblasts, blood vessels and granulocytes.

h) Cytokines like interleukin-1 and TNF-α.

i) Oxygen-derived free radicals.

GIANT CELLS

A few examples of multinucleate giant cells exist in normal tissues (e.g. osteoclasts in the bones, trophoblasts in placenta, megakaryocytes in the bone marrow). However, in chronic inflammation when the macrophages fail to deal with particles to be removed, they fuse together and form multinucleated giant cells. Some of the common types of giant cells are described below:

A. Giant cells in inflammation:

i) *Foreign body giant cells* These contain numerous nuclei (up to 100) which are uniform in size and shape and resemble the nuclei of macrophages. These nuclei are scattered throughout the cytoplasm. These are seen in chronic infective granulomas, leprosy and tuberculosis.

ii) *Langhans' giant cells* These are seen in tuberculosis and sarcoidosis. Their nuclei are like the nuclei of macrophages and epithelioid cells. These nuclei are arranged either around the periphery in the form of horseshoe or ring, or are clustered at the two poles of the giant cell.

iii) *Touton giant cells* These multinucleated cells have vacuolated cytoplasm due to lipid content e.g. in xanthoma.

iv) *Aschoff giant cells* These multinucleate giant cells are derived from cardiac histiocytes and are seen in rheumatic nodule.

B. Giant cells in tumours:

i) *Anaplastic cancer giant cells* These are larger, have numerous nuclei which are hyperchromatic and vary in size and shape. These are formed from dividing nuclei of the neoplastic cells e.g. carcinoma of the liver, various soft tissue sarcomas etc.

ii) Reed-Sternberg cells These are also malignant tumour giant cells which are generally binucleate and are seen in various histologic types of Hodgkin's lymphomas.

iii) Osteoclastic giant cells of bone tumour Giant cell tumour of the bones or osteoclastoma has uniform distribution of osteoclastic giant cells spread in the stroma.

ACUTE INFLAMMATION—FACTORS, MORPHOLOGY, EFFECTS, FATE *(p. 131)*

FACTORS DETERMINING VARIATION IN INFLAMMATORY RESPONSE

Although acute inflammation is typically characterised by vascular and cellular events with emigration of neutrophilic leucocytes, not all examples of acute inflammation show infiltration by neutrophils. On the other hand, some chronic inflammatory conditions are characterised by neutrophilic infiltration. For example, *typhoid fever* is an example of acute inflammatory process but the cellular response in it is lymphocytic; *osteomyelitis* is an example of chronic inflammation but the cellular response in this condition is mainly neutrophilic.

The variation in inflammatory response depends upon a number of factors and processes.

FACTORS INVOLVING THE ORGANISMS:

i)   Type of injury and infection
ii)   Virulence
iii) Dose
iv)   Portal of entry
v)   Product of organisms

FACTORS INVOLVING THE HOST:

i)   Systemic diseases
ii)   Immune status of host
iii) Congenital neutrophil defects
iv)   Leukopenia
v)   Site or type of tissue involved
vi)   Local host factors

MORPHOLOGY OF ACUTE INFLAMMATION

Inflammation of an organ is usually named by adding the suffix-*itis* to its Latin name e.g. appendicitis, hepatitis, cholecystitis, meningitis etc. A few morphologic varieties of acute inflammation are described below:

1.   TYPES OF EXUDATE The appearance of escaped plasma determines the morphologic type of inflammation as under:

i)   Serous, when the fluid exudate resembles serum or is watery e.g. pleural effusion in tuberculosis, blister formation in burns.

ii)   Fibrinous, when the fibrin content of the fluid exudate is high e.g. in pneumococcal and rheumatic pericarditis.

iii)   Purulent or suppurative exudate is formation of creamy pus as seen in infection with pyogenic bacteria e.g. abscess, acute appendicitis.

iv)   Haemorrhagic, when there is vascular damage e.g. acute haemorrhagic pneumonia in influenza.

v)   Catarrhal, when the surface inflammation of epithelium produces increased secretion of mucus e.g. common cold.

2.   PSEUDOMEMBRANOUS INFLAMMATION It is inflammatory response of mucous surface (oral, respiratory, bowel) to toxins of diphtheria or irritant gases.

3.   ULCER Ulcers are local defects on the surface of an organ produced by inflammation. Some common sites for ulcerations are the stomach, duodenum, intestinal ulcers in typhoid fever, intestinal tuberculosis, bacillary and amoebic dysentery, ulcers of legs due to varicose veins etc. In the acute stage, there is infiltration by polymorphs with vasodilatation.

4. SUPPURATION (ABSCESS FORMATION) When acute bacterial infection is accompanied by intense neutrophilic infiltrate in the inflamed tissue, it results in tissue necrosis. The bacteria which cause suppuration are called pyogenic.

Some of the common examples of abscess formation are as under:
i)   Boil or furuncle
ii) Carbuncle

5. CELLULITIS It is a diffuse inflammation of the soft tissues resulting from spreading effects of substances like hyaluronidase released by some bacteria.

6. BACTERIAL INFECTION OF THE BLOOD This includes the following 3 conditions:

i) Bacteraemia is defined as presence of small number of bacteria in the blood which do not multiply significantly.

ii) Septicaemia means presence of rapidly multiplying, highly pathogenic bacteria in the blood e.g. pyogenic cocci, bacilli of plague etc. Septicaemia is generally accompanied by systemic effects like toxaemia, multiple small haemorrhages, neutrophilic leucocytosis and disseminated intravascular coagulation (DIC).

iii) Pyaemia is the dissemination of small septic thrombi in the blood which cause their effects at the site where they are lodged. This can result in pyaemic abscesses or septic infarcts.

SYSTEMIC EFFECTS OF ACUTE INFLAMMATION

Acute inflammation is associated with systemic effects as well. These include fever, leucocytosis, lymphangitis-lymphadenitis and shock.

FATE OF ACUTE INFLAMMATION

The acute inflammatory process can culminate in one of the following outcomes:
1. Resolution
2. Healing
3. Suppuration
4. Chronic inflammation

CHRONIC INFLAMMATION (p. 134)

DEFINITION AND CAUSES Chronic inflammation is defined as prolonged process in which tissue destruction and inflammation occur at the same time.

Chronic inflammation may occur by one of the following 3 ways:

1. Chronic inflammation following acute inflammation When the tissue destruction is extensive, or the bacteria survive and persist in small numbers at the site of acute inflammation e.g. in osteomyelitis, pneumonia terminating in lung abscess.

2. Recurrent attacks of acute inflammation When repeated bouts of acute inflammation culminate in chronicity of the process e.g. in recurrent urinary tract infection leading to chronic pyelonephritis, repeated acute infection of gallbladder leading to chronic cholecystitis.

3. Chronic inflammation starting *de novo* When the infection with organisms of low pathogenicity is chronic from the beginning e.g. infection with *Mycobacterium tuberculosis*.

GENERAL FEATURES OF CHRONIC INFLAMMATION

Though there may be differences in chronic inflammatory response depending upon the tissue involved and causative organisms, there are some basic similarities amongst various types of chronic inflammation. Following general features characterise any chronic inflammation:

1. MONONUCLEAR CELL INFILTRATION Chronic inflammatory lesions are infiltrated by mononuclear inflammatory cells like phagocytes and lymphoid cells.

The blood monocytes on reaching the extravascular space transform into tissue macrophages. Besides the role of macrophages in phagocytosis, they may get activated in response to stimuli such as cytokines (lymphokines) and bacterial endotoxins.

Other chronic inflammatory cells include lymphocytes, plasma cells, eosinophils and mast cells.

2. TISSUE DESTRUCTION OR NECROSIS Tissue destruction and necrosis are central features of most forms of chronic inflammatory lesions. This is brought about by activated macrophages which release a variety of biologically active substances.

3. PROLIFERATIVE CHANGES As a result of necrosis, proliferation of small blood vessels and fibroblasts is stimulated resulting in formation of inflammatory granulation tissue. Eventually, healing by fibrosis and collagen laying takes place.

SYSTEMIC EFFECTS OF CHRONIC INFLAMMATION

Chronic inflammation is associated with following systemic features:
1. Fever
2. Anaemia
3. Leucocytosis
4. ESR is elevated
5. Amyloidosis

TYPES OF CHRONIC INFLAMMATION

Conventionally, chronic inflammation is subdivided into 2 types:

1. Chronic non-specific inflammation When the irritant substance produces a non-specific chronic inflammatory reaction with formation of granulation tissue and healing by fibrosis, it is called chronic non-specific inflammation e.g. chronic osteomyelitis, chronic ulcer, lung abscess.

2. Chronic granulomatous inflammation In this, the injurious agent causes a characteristic histologic tissue response by formation of granulomas e.g. tuberculosis, leprosy, syphilis, actinomycosis, sarcoidosis etc.

GRANULOMATOUS INFLAMMATION (p. 135)

Granuloma is defined as a circumscribed, tiny lesion, about 1 mm in diameter, composed predominantly of collection of modified macrophages called epithelioid cells, and rimmed at the periphery by lymphoid cells.

PATHOGENESIS OF GRANULOMA Formation of granuloma is a type IV granulomatous hypersensitivity reaction. It is a protective defense reaction by the host but eventually causes tissue destruction because of persistence of the poorly digestible antigen e.g. *Mycobacterium tuberculosis, M. leprae,* suture material, particles of talc etc.

The sequence in evolution of granuloma is briefly outlined below:

1. Engulfment by macrophages Macrophages and monocytes engulf the antigen and try to destroy it.

2. CD4+ T cells Macrophages, being antigen-presenting cells, having failed to deal with the antigen, present it to CD4+ T lymphocytes.

3. Cytokines Various cytokines formed by activated CD4+ T cells and also by activated macrophages perform the following roles:
i) IL-1 and IL-2 stimulate proliferation of more T cells.
ii) Interferon-γ activates macrophages.
iii) TNF-α promotes fibroblast proliferation and activates endothelium to secrete prostaglandins which have a role in vascular response in inflammation.
iv) Growth factors (transforming growth factor-β, platelet-derived growth factor) elaborated by activated macrophages stimulate fibroblast growth.

Thus, a granuloma is formed having macrophages modified as epithelioid cells in the centre, with some interspersed multinucleate giant cells, surrounded peripherally by lymphocytes (mainly T cells), and healing by fibroblasts or collagen depending upon the age of granuloma.

COMPOSITION OF GRANULOMA In general, a granuloma has the following structural composition:

1. Epithelioid cells These are so called because of their epithelial cell-like appearance. They are modified macrophages/histiocytes which are somewhat elongated cells having slipper-shaped nucleus.

2. Multinucleate giant cells Multinucleate giant cells are formed by fusion of adjacent epithelioid cells and may have 20 or more nuclei. These nuclei may be arranged at the periphery like the horseshoe or as a ring, or may be clustered at the two poles (Langhans' giant cells), or they may be present centrally (foreign body giant cells).

3. Lymphoid cells As a cell-mediated immune reaction to antigen, the host response by lymphocytes is integral to composition of a granuloma.

4. Necrosis Necrosis may be a feature of some granulomatous conditions e.g. central caseation necrosis in tuberculosis, so called because of its dry cheese-like appearance.

5. Fibrosis Fibrosis is a feature of healing by proliferating fibroblasts at the periphery of granuloma.

The classical example of granulomatous inflammation is the tissue response to tubercle bacilli which is called *tubercle* seen in tuberculosis. A fully-developed tubercle is about 1 mm in diameter with central area of caseation necrosis, surrounded by epithelioid cells and one to several multinucleated giant cells (commonly Langhans' type), surrounded at the periphery by lymphocytes and bounded by fibroblasts and fibrous tissue.

EXAMPLES OF GRANULOMATOUS INFLAMMATION *(p. 137)*

Granulomatous inflammation is typical of reaction to poorly digestible agents elicited by tuberculosis, leprosy, fungal infections, schistosomiasis, foreign particles etc.

TUBERCULOSIS

INCIDENCE In spite of great advances in chemotherapy and immunology, tuberculosis still continues to be a major public health problem in the entire world, more common in developing countries of Asia, Africa and Latin America.

HIV-ASSOCIATED TUBERCULOSIS HIV-infected individuals have very high incidence of tuberculosis all over the world. Vice-versa, rate of HIV infection in patients of tuberculosis is very high. Infection with *M. avium-intracellulare* (avian or bird strain) is common in patients with HIV/AIDS.

CAUSATIVE ORGANISM Tubercle bacillus or Koch's bacillus (named after discovery of the organism by Robert Koch in 1882) called *Mycobacterium tuberculosis* causes tuberculosis in the lungs and other tissues of the human body. *The organism is a strict aerobe and thrives best in tissues with high oxygen tension such as in the apex of the lung.*

M. tuberculosis hominis is a slender rod-like bacillus, 0.5 μm by 3 μm, is neutral on Gram staining, and can be demonstrated by the following methods:
1. *Acid fast (Ziehl-Neelsen) staining*
2. *Fluorescent methods*
3. *Culture of the organism from sputum or from any other material*
4. *Guinea pig inoculation*
5. *Molecular methods such as nucleic acid amplification (e.g. PCR)*
6. *Immunohistochemical stain with anti-MBP 64 antibody.*

ATYPICAL MYCOBACTERIA (NON-TUBERCULOUS MYCOBACTERIA)
The term atypical mycobacteria or non-tuberculous mycobacteria (NTM) is used for mycobacterial species other than *M. tuberculosis* complex and *M. leprae*. NTM are widely distributed in the environment and are, therefore, also

called as *environmental mycobacteria*. They too are acid fast. Occasionally, human tuberculosis may be caused by NTM which are non-pathogenic to guinea pigs and resistant to usual anti-tubercular drugs.

Conventionally, NTM are classified on the basis of colour of colony produced in culture and the speed of growth in media:

Rapid growers These organisms grow fast on solid media (within 7 days) but are less pathogenic than others. Examples include *M. abscessus, M. fortuitum, M. chelonae*.

Slow growers These species grow mycobacteria on solid media (in 2-3 weeks). Based on the colour of colony formed, they are further divided into following:

Photochromogens: These organisms produce yellow pigment in the culture grown in light.

Scotochromogens: Pigment is produced, whether the growth is in light or in dark.

Non-chromogens: No pigment is produced by the bacilli and the organism is closely related to avium bacillus.

MODE OF TRANSMISSION Human beings acquire infection with tubercle bacilli by one of the following routes:
1. Inhalation
2. Ingestion
3. Inoculation
4. Transplacental route

SPREAD OF TUBERCULOSIS The disease spreads in the body by various routes:

1. Local spread This takes place by macrophages carrying the bacilli into the surrounding tissues.

2. Lymphatic spread Tuberculosis is primarily an infection of lymphoid tissues. The bacilli may pass into lymphoid follicles of pharynx, bronchi, intestines or regional lymph nodes resulting in regional tuberculous lymphadenitis which is typical of childhood infections.

3. Haematogenous spread This occurs either as a result of tuberculous bacillaemia because of the drainage of lymphatics into the venous system or due to caseous material escaping through ulcerated wall of a vein. This produces millet seed-sized lesions in different organs of the body like lungs, liver, kidneys, bones and other tissues and is known as miliary tuberculosis.

4. By the natural passages Infection may spread from:
i) lung lesions into pleura (tuberculous pleurisy);
ii) transbronchial spread into the adjacent lung segments;
iii) tuberculous salpingitis into peritoneal cavity (tuberculous peritonitis);
iv) infected sputum into larynx (tuberculous laryngitis);
v) swallowing of infected sputum (ileocaecal tuberculosis); and
vi) renal lesions into ureter and down to trigone of bladder.

PATHOGENESIS (HYPERSENSITIVITY AND IMMUNITY) Tissue changes seen in tuberculosis are not the result of any exotoxin or endotoxin but are instead the result of host response to the organism which is by way of development of delayed type hypersensitivity (or type IV hypersensitivity) and immunity. Both these host responses develop as a consequence of several lipids present in the microorganism as under:

1. Mycosides such as 'cord factor' which are essential for growth and virulence of the organism in the animals.

2. Glycolipids present in the mycobacterial cell wall like 'Wax-D' which acts as an adjuvant acting along with tuberculoprotein.

In the primary infection, intradermal injection of tubercle bacilli into the skin of a healthy guinea pig evokes no visible reaction for 10-14 days. After this period, a nodule develops at the inoculation site which subsequently ulcerates and heals poorly as the guinea pig, unlike human beings, does not possess any natural resistance. The regional lymph nodes also develop tubercles. This process is a manifestation of delayed type hypersensitivity (type IV reaction) and is comparable to primary tuberculosis in children although healing invariably occurs in children.

In the secondary infection, the sequence of changes is different. When the tubercle bacilli are injected into the skin of the guinea pig who has been previously infected with tuberculosis 4-6 weeks earlier, the sequence and duration of development of lesions is different. In 1-2 days, the site of inoculation is indurated and dark, attaining a diameter of about 1 cm. The skin lesion ulcerates which heals quickly and the regional lymph nodes are not affected. This is called *Koch's phenomenon* and is indicative of hypersensitivity and immunity in the host which is guinea pig in this case.

Immunisation against tuberculosis Protective immunisation against tuberculosis is induced by injection of attenuated strains of bovine type of tubercle bacilli, *Bacille Calmette-Guérin* (BCG).

Tuberculin (Mantoux) skin test (TST) This test is done by intradermal injection of 0.1 ml of tuberculoprotein, purified protein derivative (PPD). Delayed type of hypersensitivity develops in individuals who are having or have been previously infected with tuberculous infection which is identified as an indurated area of more than 15 mm in 72 hours; reaction larger than 15 mm is unlikely to be due to previous BCG vaccination. Patients having disseminated tuberculosis may show negative test due to release of large amount of tuberculoproteins from the endogenous lesions masking the hypersensitivity test.

EVOLUTION OF TUBERCLE The sequence of events which take place when tubercle bacilli are introduced into the tissue culminating in development of a tubercle are as under:

1. When the tubercle bacilli are injected intravenously into the guinea pig, the bacilli are lodged in pulmonary capillaries where an *initial response of neutrophils* is evoked which are rapidly destroyed by the organisms.

2. After about 12 hours, there is *progressive infiltration by macrophages*. This is due to coating of tubercle bacilli with serum complement factors C2a and C3b which act as opsonins and attract the macrophages.

3. The macrophages start *phagocytosing* the tubercle bacilli and either try to kill the bacteria or die away themselves.

4. As a part of body's immune response, T and B cells are activated. Activated CD4+T cells elaborate cytokines, IFN-γ and IL-2. These cytokines and their regulators determine the host's response by infiltrating macrophages-monocytes and develop the cell-mediated *delayed type hypersensitivity reaction*.

5. B cells form antibodies but *humoral immunity* has plays little role in body's defense against tubercle bacilli.

6. In 2-3 days, the macrophages undergo structural changes as a result of immune mechanisms—the cytoplasm becomes pale and eosinophilic and their nuclei become elongated and vesicular. These modified macrophages resemble epithelial cells and are called *epithelioid cells* (i.e. epithelial like).

7. The epithelioid cells in time aggregate into tight clusters or *granulomas*.

8. Some macrophages, unable to destroy tubercle bacilli, fuse together and form *multinucleated giant cells*.

9. Around the mass or cluster of epithelioid cells and a few giant cells, a zone of lymphocytes and plasma cells is formed which is further surrounded by fibroblasts. The lesion at this stage is called *hard tubercle*.

10. Within 10-14 days, the centre of the cellular mass begins to undergo caseation necrosis, characterised by cheesy appearance and high lipid content. This stage is called *soft tubercle* which is the hallmark of tuberculous lesions.

The **fate of a granuloma** is variable:

i)   The caseous material may undergo liquefaction and extend into surrounding soft tissues, discharging the contents on the surface. This is called *cold abscess*.

ii)   In tuberculosis of tissues like bones, joints, lymph nodes and epididymis, sinuses are formed and the *sinus tracts* are lined by tuberculous granulation tissue.

iii) The adjacent granulomas may *coalesce* together enlarging the lesion which is surrounded by progressive fibrosis.

iv) In the granuloma enclosed by fibrous tissue, calcium salts may get deposited in the caseous material *(dystrophic calcification)*.

TYPES OF TUBERCULOSIS

Lung is the main organ affected in tuberculosis while amongst the extra-pulmonary sites, lymph node involvement is most common. Depending upon the type of tissue response and age, the infection with tubercle bacilli is of 2 main types: primary and secondary tuberculosis.

A. PRIMARY TUBERCULOSIS

The infection of an individual who has not been previously infected or immunised is called *primary tuberculosis* or *Ghon's complex* or *childhood tuberculosis*.

Primary complex or Ghon's complex is the lesion produced in the tissue of portal of entry with foci in the draining lymphatic vessels and lymph nodes. The most commonly involved tissues for primary complex are lungs and hilar lymph nodes. *Primary complex or Ghon's complex* in lungs consists of 3 components:

1. Pulmonary component Lesion in the lung is the primary focus or Ghon's focus. It is 1-2 cm solitary area of tuberculous pneumonia located peripherally under a patch of pleurisy, in any part of the lung but more often in subpleural focus in the upper part of lower lobe.

2. Lymphatic vessel component The lymphatics draining the lung lesion contain phagocytes containing bacilli and may develop beaded, miliary tubercles along the path of hilar lymph nodes.

3. Lymph node component This consists of enlarged hilar and tracheo-bronchial lymph nodes in the area drained. The affected lymph nodes are matted and show caseation necrosis.

FATE OF PRIMARY TUBERCULOSIS Primary complex may have one of the following sequelae:

1. The lesions of primary tuberculosis of the lung commonly do not progress but instead heal by *fibrosis*, and in time undergo *calcification* and even *ossification*.

2. In some cases, the primary focus in the lung continues to grow and the caseous material is disseminated through bronchi to the other parts of the same lung or the opposite lung. This is called *progressive primary tuberculosis*.

3. At times, bacilli may enter the circulation through erosion in a blood vessel and spread by haematogenous route to other tissues and organs. This is called *primary miliary tuberculosis* and the lesions may be seen in organs like the liver, spleen, kidney, brain and bone marrow.

4. In certain circumstances like in lowered resistance and increased hypersensitivity of the host, the healed lesions of primary tuberculosis may get reactivated. The bacilli lying dormant in acellular caseous material or healed lesion are activated and cause *progressive secondary tuberculosis*. It affects children more commonly but immunocompromised adults may also develop this kind of progression.

B. SECONDARY TUBERCULOSIS

The infection of an individual who has been previously infected or sensitised is called *secondary*, or *post-primary* or *reinfection*, or *chronic tuberculosis*.

The infection may occur from:

◈ *Endogenous source* such as reactivation of dormant primary complex.

◈ *Exogenous source* such as fresh dose of reinfection by the tubercle bacilli.

The lesions in secondary pulmonary tuberculosis usually begin as 1-2 cm apical area of consolidation of the lung, which, in time, may develop a small area of central caseation necrosis and peripheral fibrosis. It occurs by lymphohaematogenous spread of infection from primary complex to the apex of the affected lung where the oxygen tension is high and favourable for growth of aerobic tubercle bacilli.

Patients with HIV infection previously exposed to tuberculous infection have particularly high incidence of reactivation of primary tuberculosis.

FATE OF SECONDARY PULMONARY TUBERCULOSIS The subapical lesions in lungs can have the following course:

1. The lesions may *heal* with fibrous scarring and calcification.

2. The lesions may *coalesce* together to form larger area of tuberculous pneumonia and produce progressive secondary pulmonary tuberculosis with the following pulmonary and extrapulmonary involvements:

FIBROCASEOUS TUBERCULOSIS The original area of tuberculous pneumonia undergoes peripheral healing and massive central caseation necrosis which may:

❖ either break into a bronchus from a cavity *(cavitary or open fibrocaseous tuberculosis)*; or

❖ remain, as a soft caseous lesion without drainage into a bronchus or bronchiole to produce a non-cavitary lesion *(chronic fibrocaseous tuberculosis)*.

The cavity provides favourable environment for proliferation of tubercle bacilli due to high oxygen tension. The cavity may communicate with bronchial tree and becomes the source of spread of infection *('open tuberculosis')*. Ingestion of sputum containing tubercle bacilli from endogenous pulmonary lesions may produce *laryngeal and intestinal tuberculosis.*

G/A Tuberculous cavity is spherical with thick fibrous wall, lined by yellowish, caseous, necrotic material and the lumen is traversed by thrombosed blood vessels. Around the wall of cavity are seen foci of consolidation. The overlying pleura may also be thickened.

M/E The wall and lumen of cavity shows eosinophilic, granular, caseous material which may show foci of dystrophic calcification. Widespread coalesced tuberculous granulomas composed of epithelioid cells, Langhans' giant cells and peripheral mantle of lymphocytes and having central caseation necrosis are seen. The outer wall of cavity shows fibrosis.

TUBERCULOUS CASEOUS PNEUMONIA The caseous material from a case of secondary tuberculosis in an individual with high degree of hypersensitivity may spread to rest of the lung producing caseous pneumonia.

MILIARY TUBERCULOSIS This is lymphohaematogenous spread of tuberculous infection from primary focus or later stages of tuberculosis. The spread may occur to systemic organs or isolated organ. The spread is either by entry of infection into pulmonary vein producing disseminated or isolated organ lesion in different extra-pulmonary sites (e.g. liver, spleen, kidney, brain, meninges, genitourinary tract and bone marrow), or into pulmonary artery restricting the development of miliary lesions within the lung.

G/A The miliary lesions are millet seed-sized (1 mm diameter), yellowish, firm areas without grossly visible caseation necrosis.

M/E The lesions show the structure of tubercles with minute areas of caseation necrosis.

TUBERCULOUS EMPYEMA The caseating pulmonary lesions of tuberculosis may be associated with pleurisy (pleuritis, pleural effusion) as a reaction and is expressed as a serous or fibrinous exudates. Pleural effusion may heal by fibrosis and obliterate the pleural space (thickened pleura by chronic pleuritis). Occasionally, pleural cavity may contain caseous material and develop into tuberculous empyema.

The clinical manifestations in tuberculosis may be variable depending upon the location, extent and type of lesions. However, in secondary pulmonary tuberculosis which is the common type, the usual clinical features are as under:

1.   Referable to lungs—such as productive cough (may be with haemoptysis), pleural effusion, dyspnoea, orthopnoea etc. Chest X-ray may show typical apical changes like pleural effusion, nodularity, and miliary or diffuse infiltrates in the lung parenchyma.

2.   Systemic features—such as fever, night sweats, fatigue, loss of weight and appetite. Long-standing and untreated cases of tuberculosis may develop systemic secondary amyloidosis.

The *diagnosis* is made by the following tests:

i) *AFB microscopy* of diagnostic specimen such as sputum, aspirated material.

ii) *Mycobacterial culture* (traditional method on LJ medium for 4-8 weeks, newer rapid method by HPLC of mycolic acid with result in 2-3 weeks).

iii) *Molecular methods* such as PCR.

iv) *Complete haemogram* (lymphocytosis and raised ESR).

v) *Radiographic procedures* e.g. chest X-ray showing characteristic hilar nodules and other parenchymal changes).

vi) *Mantoux skin test.*

vii) *Serologic tests* based on detection of antibodies are not useful although these are being advocated in some developing countries.

viii) *Fine needle aspiration cytology* of an enlarged peripheral lymph node is quite useful and easy way for confirmation of diagnosis and has largely replaced the biopsy diagnosis of tuberculosis.

LEPROSY

Leprosy or Hansen's disease (after discovery of the causative organism by Hansen in 1874), was first described in ancient Indian text going back to 6th Century BC, is a chronic non-fatal infectious disease. It affects mainly the cooler parts of the body such as the skin, mouth, respiratory tract, eyes, peripheral nerves, superficial lymph nodes and testis. The earliest and main involvement in leprosy is of the skin and nerves.

CAUSATIVE ORGANISM

The disease is caused by *Mycobacterium leprae* which closely resembles *Mycobacterium tuberculosis* but is less acid-fast. The organisms in tissues appear as compact rounded masses *(globi)* or are arranged in parallel fashion like *cigarettes-in-pack.*

M. leprae can be demonstrated in tissue sections, in split skin smears by splitting the skin, scrapings from cut edges of dermis, and in nasal smears by the following techniques: .

1.   Acid-fast (Ziehl-Neelsen or ZN) staining

2.   Fite-Faraco staining

3.   Gomori methenamine silver (GMS)

4.   Molecular methods e.g. PCR.

5.   IgM antibodies to PGL-1 antigen.

INCIDENCE

The disease is endemic in areas with hot and moist climates and in poor tropical countries. Leprosy is almost exclusively a disease of a few developing countries in Asia, Africa and Latin America. According to the WHO, 8 countries—India, China, Nepal, Brazil, Indonesia, Myanmar (Burma), Madagascar and Nigeria, together constitute about 80% of leprosy cases, of which India accounts for one-third of all registered leprosy cases globally.

Chapter 5

Inflammation and Healing

Leprosy is a slow communicable disease and the incubation period between first exposure and appearance of signs of disease varies from 2 to 20 years (average about 3 years). The infectivity may be from the following sources:
1. *Direct contact* with untreated leprosy patients.
2. *Materno-foetal transmission* across the placenta.
3. Transmission from *milk* of leprosy affected mother to infant.

IMMUNOLOGY OF LEPROSY

Like in tuberculosis, the immune response in leprosy is also T cell-mediated delayed hypersensitivity (type IV reaction) but the two diseases are quite dissimilar as regards immune reactions and lesions.

1. Antigens of leprosy bacilli Lepra bacilli have several antigens. The bacterial cell wall contains large amount of *M. leprae*-specific phenolic glycolipid (PGL-1) and another surface antigen, lipo-arabinomannan (LAM).

2. Genotype of the host Genetic composition of the host as known by MHC class (or HLA type) determines which antigen of leprosy bacilli shall interact with host immune cells.

3. T cell response There is variation in T cell response in two main forms of leprosy:
i) Unlike tubercle bacilli, there is not only *activation* of CD4+ T cells but also of CD8+ T cells.
ii) CD4+ T cells in lepra bacilli infected persons act not only as helper and promoter cells but also assume the role of *cytotoxicity*.
iii) The two subpopulations of CD4+ T cells (or T helper cells)—T_H 1 cells and T_H 2 cells, elaborate different types of *cytokines* in response to stimuli from the lepra bacilli and macrophages.
iv) In tuberculoid leprosy, the response is largely by CD4+ T cells, while in lepromatous leprosy although there is excess of CD8+ T cells (suppressor T) but the macrophages and suppressor T cells fail to destroy the bacilli due to *CD8+ T cell defect*.

4. Humoral response Though the patients of lepromatous leprosy have humoral components such as high levels of immunoglobulins (IgG, IgA, IgM) and antibodies to mycobacterial antigens but these antibodies do not have any protective role against lepra bacilli.

LEPROMIN TEST It is not a diagnostic test but is used for classifying leprosy on the basis of immune response. Intradermal injection of lepromin, an antigenic extract of *M. leprae*, reveals delayed hypersensitivity reaction in patients of tuberculoid leprosy:
1) An early positive reaction appearing as an indurated area in 24-48 hours is called *Fernandez reaction*.
2) A delayed granulomatous lesion appearing after 3-4 weeks is called *Mitsuda reaction*.
    Patients of lepromatous leprosy are negative by the lepromin test.

CLASSIFICATION

RIDLEY AND JOPLING'S CLASSIFICATION Traditionally, two main forms of leprosy are distinguished:
1. Lepromatous type representing *low resistance*; and
2. Tuberculoid type representing *high resistance*.
    Since both these types of leprosy represent two opposite poles of host immune response, these are also called *polar forms* of leprosy.
    Based on clinical, histologic and immunologic features, modified Ridley and Jopling's classification divides leprosy into 5 groups as under:
    TT—Tuberculoid Polar *(High resistance)*
    BT—Borderline Tuberculoid
    BB—Mid Borderline (dimorphic)
    BL—Borderline Lepromatous
    LL—Lepromatous Polar *(Low resistance)*

VARIANTS In addition, not included in Ridley-Jopling's classification are following types:

◈ *Indeterminate leprosy* This is an initial non-specific stage of any type of leprosy.

◈ *Pure neural leprosy* In these cases, skin lesions which are the cardinal feature of leprosy are absent but instead neurologic involvement is the main feature.

◈ *Histoid leprosy* Described by Wade in 1963, this is a variant of LL in which the skin lesions resemble nodules of dermatofibroma and is the lesions are highly positive for lepra bacilli.

REACTIONAL LEPROSY Based on shift in immune status or in patients of leprosy on treatment, two types of reactional leprosy are distinguished:

Type I: Reversal reactions The borderline groups are unstable and may move across the spectrum in either direction with upgrading or downgrading of patient's immune state.

Type II: Erythema nodosum leprosum (ENL) ENL occurs in lepromatous patients after treatment.

HISTOPATHOLOGY OF LEPROSY

M/E In general, for histopathologic evaluation in all suspected cases of leprosy the following general *features* should be looked for:
i) Cell type of granuloma
ii) Nerve involvement
iii) Bacterial load
iv) Presence and absence of lymphocytes
v) Relation of granuloma with epidermis and adenexa.
The salient features in major types of leprosy are as follows.

Lepromatous leprosy The features are as follows:
i) In the dermis, there is proliferation of macrophages with foamy change, particularly around the blood vessels, nerves and dermal appendages. The foamy macrophages are called *'lepra cells' or Virchow cells*.
ii) The lepra cells are heavily laden with acid-fast bacilli demonstrated with AFB staining. The AFB may be seen as compact globular masses *(globi)* or arranged in parallel fashion like *'cigarettes-in-pack'*.
iii) The dermal infiltrate of lepra cells characteristically does not encroach upon the basal layer of epidermis and is separated from epidermis by a subepidermal uninvolved *clear zone*.
iv) The *epidermis* overlying the lesions is thinned out, flat and may even ulcerate.

Tuberculoid leprosy It shows following features:
i) The dermal lesions show granulomas resembling *hard tubercles* composed of epithelioid cells, Langhans' giant cells and peripheral mantle of lymphocytes.
ii) Lesions of tuberculoid leprosy have predilection for *dermal nerves* which may be destroyed and infiltrated by epithelioid cells and lymphocytes.
iii) The granulomatous infiltrate erodes the basal layer of epidermis i.e. there is *no clear zone*.
iv) The *lepra bacilli* are few and seen in destroyed nerves.

Pure neural leprosy Histopathologic features described in skin lesion of various forms of leprosy may be seen in the nerve biopsy specimens. Pure neural leprosy may be AFB positive or AFB negative.

Histoid leprosy It shows following features:
i) Whorls and fascicles of spindle cells in the upper dermis after a clear subepidermal space.
ii) On close scrutiny, these cells have foamy cytoplasm.
iii) The cytoplasm of these cells is laden with lepra bacilli.

Reactional leprosy It has 2 types:
Type I reaction: Reversal reactions. These may be upgrading or downgrading type of reaction:

Upgrading reaction shows an increase of lymphocytes, oedema of the lesions, necrosis in the centre and reduced B.I.

Downgrading reaction shows dispersal and spread of the granulomas and increased presence of lepra bacilli.

Type II: ENL The lesions in ENL show infiltration by neutrophils and eosinophils and prominence of vasculitis. Inflammation often extends deep into the subcutaneous fat causing panniculitis. Bacillary load is increased.

CLINICAL FEATURES

1. **Lepromatous leprosy** The features are:
i)   The skin lesions in LL are generally symmetrical, multiple, slightly hypopigmented and erythematous macules, papules, nodules or diffuse infiltrates. The nodular lesions may coalesce to give *leonine facies* appearance.
ii)   The lesions are hypoaesthetic or anaesthetic but the sensory disturbance is not as distinct as in TT.

2. **Tuberculoid leprosy** It shows following features:
i)   The skin lesions in TT occur as either single or as a few asymmetrical lesions which are hypopigmented and erythematous macules.
ii)   There is a distinct sensory impairment.

SYPHILIS

Syphilis is a venereal (sexually-transmitted) disease caused by spirochaetes, *Treponema pallidum.*

CAUSATIVE ORGANISM

T. pallidum is a coiled spiral filament 10 μm long that moves actively in fresh preparations. The organism cannot be stained by the usual methods and can be demonstrated in the exudates and tissues by:
1.   *dark ground illumination (DGI)* in fresh preparation;
2.   *fluorescent antibody technique;*
3.   *silver impregnation techniques;* and
4.   *nucleic acid amplification* technique by PCR.

INCIDENCE

Most commonly affected regions in the world are in Sub-Saharan Africa, South America, and South East Asia. Male homosexuals are at greater risk.

IMMUNOLOGY

There are two types of serological tests for syphilis: treponemal and non-treponemal.

A.   Treponemal serological tests These tests measure antibody to *T. pallidum* antigen and are more useful and sensitive for the diagnosis of syphilis:
i)   *Fluorescent treponemal antibody-absorbed (FTA-ABS) test.*
ii) *Agglutinin assays* e.g. microhaemagglutination assay for *T. pallidum* (MHA-TP), and Serodia TP-PA.
iii) *T. pallidum passive haemagglutination (TPHA) test.*

B. Non-treponemal serological tests These tests measure non-specific reaginic antibodies IgM and IgG immunoglobulins directed against cardiolipin-lecithin-cholesterol complex and are more commonly used. These tests are as under:
i) *Reiter protein complement fixation (RPCF) test*: test of choice for rapid diagnosis.
ii)   *Venereal Disease Research Laboratory (VDRL)* or *Rapid Plasma Reagin (RPR) test*: This antigen is used in the Standard Test for Syphilis (STS) in Wassermann complement fixing test and VDRL test.

MODE OF TRANSMISSION

1. *Sexual intercourse* is the most common route of infection and results in lesions on glans penis, vulva, vagina and cervix.
2. *Intimate person-to-person contact* with lesions on lips, tongue or fingers.
3. *Transfusion* of infected blood.
4. *Materno-foetal transmission* in congenital syphilis if the mother is infected.

STAGES OF ACQUIRED SYPHILIS

Acquired syphilis is divided into 3 stages depending upon the period after which the lesions appear and the type of lesions.

PRIMARY SYPHILIS Typical lesion of primary syphilis is *chancre* which appears on genitals or at extra-genital sites in 2-4 *weeks* after exposure to infection. Initially, the lesion is a painless papule which ulcerates in the centre.

M/E Its features are:
i) Dense infiltrate of mainly plasma cells, some lymphocytes and a few macrophages.
ii) Perivascular aggregation of mononuclear cells, particularly plasma cells (periarteritis and endarteritis).
iii) Proliferation of vascular endothelium.

SECONDARY SYPHILIS Inadequately treated patients of primary syphilis develop *mucocutaneous lesions* and painless lymphadenopathy in *2-3 months* after the exposure. Mucocutaneous lesions may be in the form of the mucous patches on mouth, pharynx and vagina.

TERTIARY SYPHILIS After a latent period of appearance of secondary lesions and about *2-3 years* following first exposure, tertiary lesions of syphilis appear. Lesions of tertiary syphilis are much less infective than the other two stages and spirochaetes can be demonstrated with great difficulty. These lesions are of 2 main types:
i) **Syphilitic gumma** It is a solitary, localised, rubbery lesion with central necrosis, seen in organs like liver, testis, bone and brain. In the liver, the gumma is associated with scarring of hepatic parenchyma *(hepar lobatum)*.
ii) **Diffuse lesions of tertiary syphilis** The lesions appear following widespread dissemination of spirochaetes in the body. The diffuse lesions are predominantly seen in cardiovascular and nervous systems.

CONGENITAL SYPHILIS Congenital syphilis may develop in a foetus of more than 16 weeks gestation who is exposed to maternal spirochaetaemia. The major morphologic features as under:
i) Saddle-shaped nose deformity due to destruction of bridge of the nose.
ii) The characteristic 'Hutchinson's teeth' which are small, widely spaced, peg-shaped permanent teeth.
iii) Mucocutaneous lesions of acquired secondary syphilis.
iv) Bony lesions like epiphysitis and periostitis.
v) Interstitial keratitis with corneal opacity.
vi) Diffuse fibrosis in the liver.
vii) Interstitial fibrosis of lungs.

ACTINOMYCOSIS

Actinomycosis is a chronic suppurative disease caused by anaerobic bacteria, *Actinomycetes israelii*. The disease is worldwide in distribution. The organisms are commensals in the oral cavity, alimentary tract and vagina. The infection is always endogeneous in origin and not by person-to-person contact. The organisms invade, proliferate and disseminate in favourable conditions like break in mucocutaneous continuity, some underlying disease etc.

MORPHOLOGIC FEATURES Depending upon the anatomic location of lesions, actinomycosis is of 4 types: cervicofacial, thoracic, abdominal, and pelvic.

1. **Cervicofacial actinomycosis** This is the commonest form (60%) and has the best prognosis.

2. **Thoracic actinomycosis** The infection in the lungs is due to aspiration of the organism from oral cavity or extension of infection from abdominal or hepatic lesions.

3. **Abdominal actinomycosis** This type is common in appendix, caecum and liver.

4. **Pelvic actinomycosis** Infection in the pelvis occurs as a complication of intrauterine contraceptive devices (IUCDs).

M/E The main features are as under:

i) The inflammatory reaction is a granuloma with central suppuration. There is formation of abscesses in the centre of lesions and at the periphery chronic inflammatory cells, giant cells and fibroblasts are seen.

ii) The centre of each abscess contains the bacterial colony, 'sulphur granule', characterised by radiating filaments (hence previously known as *ray fungus*) with hyaline, eosinophilic, club-like ends representing secreted immunoglobulins.

iii) Bacterial stains reveal the organisms as gram-positive filaments, nonacid-fast, which stain positively with Gomori's methenamine silver (GMS) staining.

SARCOIDOSIS (BOECK'S SARCOID)

Sarcoidosis is a multisystem disease of unknown etiology. It is worldwide in distribution and affects adults 20-40 years of age. The disease may be asymptomatic or may have organ dysfunction such as respiratory complaints or cutaneous or ocular lesions. The disease is characterised by the presence of non-caseating epithelioid cell granulomas ('sarcoid granuloma') in the affected tissues and organs, notably lymph nodes, lungs and skin. Other sites are the uvea of the eyes, spleen, salivary glands, liver and bones of hands and feet.

ETIOLOGY AND PATHOGENESIS The cause of sarcoidosis remains unknown. However, the disease has immune pathogenesis but the antigenic trigger that stimulates the disease process is still unknown. However, the disease appears to involve 3 interlinked factors:

1. Disturbed immune system
2. Genetic predisposition
3. Exposure to environmental agent

KVEIM'S TEST It is a useful intradermal diagnostic test based on immune pathogenesis of disease. The antigen prepared from involved lymph node or spleen is injected intradermally. In a positive test, nodular lesion appears in 3-6 weeks at the inoculation site which on microscopic examination shows presence of non-caseating granulomas.

M/E The main features are as under:

1. The diagnostic feature in sarcoidosis of any organ or tissue is the *non-caseating sarcoid granuloma*, composed of epithelioid cells, Langhans' and foreign body giant cells and surrounded peripherally by fibroblasts.

2. Typically, granulomas of sarcoidosis are *'naked'* i.e. either devoid of peripheral rim of lymphocytes or there is paucity of lymphocytes.

3. In late stage, the granuloma is either *enclosed by hyalinised fibrous tissue* or is replaced by hyalinised fibrous mass.

4. The giant cells in sarcoid granulomas contain certain *cytoplasmic inclusions* as follows:

i) *Asteroid bodies* which are eosinophilic and stellate-shaped structures.

ii) *Schaumann's bodies or conchoid (conch like) bodies* which are concentric laminations of calcium and of iron salts, complexed with proteins.

iii) *Birefringent cytoplasmic crystals* which are colourless.

Similar types of inclusions are also observed in chronic berylliosis.

HEALING *(p. 155)*

Healing is the body's response to injury in an attempt to restore normal structure and function. It involves 2 processes:

◈ *Regeneration* when healing takes place by proliferation of parenchymal cells and usually results in complete restoration of the original tissues.
◈ *Repair* when healing takes place by proliferation of connective tissue resulting in fibrosis and scarring.
At times, both these processes take place simultaneously.

REGENERATION AND REPAIR (p. 155)

REGENERATION

Some parenchymal cells are short-lived while others have a longer lifespan. In order to maintain proper structure of tissues, these cells are under the constant regulatory control of their cell cycle.

Depending upon their capacity to divide, the cells of the body can be divided into 3 groups.

1. **Labile cells** These cells continue to multiply throughout life under normal physiologic conditions. These include: surface epithelial cells of the epidermis, alimentary tract, respiratory tract, urinary tract, vagina, cervix, uterine endometrium, haematopoietic cells of bone marrow and cells of lymph nodes and spleen.

2. **Stable cells** These cells decrease or lose their ability to proliferate after adolescence but retain the capacity to multiply in response to stimuli throughout adult life. These include: parenchymal cells of organs like liver, pancreas, kidneys, adrenal and thyroid; mesenchymal cells like smooth muscle cells, fibroblasts, vascular endothelium, bone and cartilage cells.

3. **Permanent cells** These cells lose their ability to proliferate around the time of birth. These include: neurons of nervous system, skeletal muscle and cardiac muscle cells.

REPAIR

Repair is the replacement of injured tissue by fibrous tissue. Two processes are involved in repair:
◈ Granulation tissue formation
◈ Contraction of wounds

GRANULATION TISSUE FORMATION

The following 3 phases are observed in the formation of granulation tissue:

1. **PHASE OF INFLAMMATION** Following trauma, blood clots at the site of injury. There is acute inflammatory response with exudation of plasma, neutrophils and some monocytes within 24 hours.

2. **PHASE OF CLEARANCE** Combination of proteolytic enzymes liberated from neutrophils, autolytic enzymes from dead tissues cells, and phagocytic activity of macrophages clear off the necrotic tissue, debris and red blood cells.

3. **PHASE OF INGROWTH OF GRANULATION TISSUE** This phase consists of 2 main processes:

i) **Angiogenesis (neovascularisation)** Formation of new blood vessels at the site of injury takes place by proliferation of endothelial cells from the margins of severed blood vessels. Initially, the proliferated endothelial cells are solid buds but within a few hours develop a lumen and start carrying blood.

The process of angiogenesis is stimulated with proteolytic destruction of basement membrane. Angiogenesis takes place under the influence of following factors:
a) Vascular endothelial growth factor (VEGF)
b) Platelet-derived growth factor (PDGF), transforming growth factor-β (TGF-β), basic fibroblast growth factor (bFGF) and surface integrins.

ii) **Fibrogenesis** The newly formed blood vessels are present in an amorphous ground substance or matrix. The new fibroblasts have features intermediate between those of fibroblasts and smooth muscle cells (*myofibroblasts*). Collagen fibrils begin to appear by about 6th day.

HEALING OF SKIN WOUNDS (p. 158)

Healing of skin wounds provides a classical example of combination of regeneration and repair described above. Wound healing can be accomplished in one of the following two ways.

HEALING BY FIRST INTENTION (PRIMARY UNION)

This is defined as healing of a wound which has the following characteristics:
i)   clean and uninfected;
ii) surgically incised;
iii) without much loss of cells and tissue; and
iv) edges of wound are approximated by surgical sutures.
     The sequence of events in primary union is described below:

1.   Initial haemorrhage   Immediately after injury, the space between the approximated surfaces of incised wound is filled with blood which then clots and seals the wound against dehydration and infection.

2.   Acute inflammatory response   This occurs within 24 hours with appearance of polymorphs from the margins of incision. By 3rd day, polymorphs are replaced by macrophages.

3.   Epithelial changes   The basal cells of epidermis from both the cut margins start proliferating and migrating towards incisional space in the form of epithelial spurs. A well-approximated wound is covered by a layer of epithelium in 48 hours. The migrated epidermal cells separate the underlying viable dermis from the overlying necrotic material and clot.

4.   Organisation   By 3rd day, fibroblasts also invade the wound area. By 5th day, new collagen fibrils start forming which dominate till healing is completed. In 4 weeks, the scar tissue with scanty cellular and vascular elements, a few inflammatory cells and epithelialised surface is formed.

5.   Suture tracks   Each suture track is a separate wound and incites the same phenomena as in healing of the primary wound i.e. filling the space with haemorrhage, some inflammatory cell reaction, epithelial cell proliferation along the suture track from both margins, fibroblastic proliferation and formation of young collagen. When sutures are removed around 7th day, much of epithelialised suture track is avulsed and the remaining epithelial tissue in the track is absorbed.

     Thus, the scar formed in a sutured wound is neat due to close apposition of the margins of wound.

HEALING BY SECOND INTENTION (SECONDARY UNION)

This is defined as healing of a wound having the following characteristics:
i)   open with a large tissue defect, at times infected;
ii) having extensive loss of cells and tissues; and
iii) the wound is not approximated by surgical sutures but is left open.

     The basic events in secondary union are similar to primary union but differ in having a larger tissue defect which has to be bridged. Hence, healing takes place from the base upward and also from the margins inwards. Healing by second intention is slow and results in a large, at times ugly, scar as compared to rapid healing and neat scar of primary union.

     The sequence of events in secondary union is described below:

1.   Initial haemorrhage   As a result of injury, the wound space is filled with blood and fibrin clot which dries.

2.   Inflammatory phase   There is an initial acute inflammatory response followed by appearance of macrophages which clear off the debris as in primary union.

3.   Epithelial changes   As in primary healing, the epidermal cells from both the margins of wound proliferate and migrate into the wound in the form of epithelial spurs till they meet in the middle and re-epithelialise the gap completely. However, the proliferating epithelial cells do not cover the surface fully until granulation tissue from base has started filling the wound space.

4. Granulation tissue Main bulk of secondary healing is by granulations. Granulation tissue is formed by proliferation of fibroblasts and neovascularisation from the adjoining viable elements. The newly-formed granulation tissue is deep red, granular and very fragile. With time, the scar on maturation becomes pale and white due to increase in collagen and decrease in vascularity.

5. Wound contraction Contraction of wound is an important feature of secondary healing, not seen in primary healing.

6. Presence of infection Bacterial contamination of an open wound delays the process of healing due to release of bacterial toxins that provoke necrosis, suppuration and thrombosis.

COMPLICATIONS OF WOUND HEALING

During the course of healing, following complications may occur:
1. Infection
2. Implantation (epidermal) cyst
3. Pigmentation
4. Deficient scar formation
5. Incisional hernia
6. Hypertrophied scars and keloid formation
7. Excessive contraction
8. Neoplasia

EXTRACELLULAR MATRIX— WOUND CONTRACTION AND STRENGTH

The wound starts contracting after 2-3 days and the process is completed by the 14th day. During this period, the wound is reduced by approximately 80% of its original size. The wound is strengthened by proliferation of fibroblasts and myofibroblasts which get structural support from the extracellular matrix (ECM).

ECM has five main components: collagen, adhesive glycoproteins, basement membrane, elastic fibres, and proteoglycans.

1. COLLAGEN The collagens are a family of proteins which provide structural support to the multicellular organism. It is the main component of tissues such as fibrous tissue, bone, cartilage, valves of heart, cornea, basement membrane etc.

Collagen is synthesised and secreted by a complex biochemical mechanism on ribosomes. The collagen synthesis is stimulated by various growth factors and is degraded by collagenase.

Depending upon the biochemical composition, 18 types of collagen have been identified called collagen *type I to XVIII*, many of which are unique for specific tissues. Type I collagen is normally present in the skin, bone and tendons and accounts for 90% of collagen in the body:

Type I, III and V are *true fibrillar collagen* which form the main portion of the connective tissue during healing of wounds in scars.

2. ADHESIVE GLYCOPROTEINS Various adhesive glycoproteins act as glue for the ECM and the cells. These consist of fibronectin, tenascin (cytotactin) and thrombospondin.

3. BASEMENT MEMBRANE Basement membranes are periodic acid-Schiff (PAS)-positive amorphous structures that lie underneath epithelia of different organs and endothelial cells. They consist of collagen type IV and laminin.

4. ELASTIC FIBRES While the tensile strength in tissue comes from collagen, the ability to recoil is provided by elastic fibres. Elastic fibres consist of 2 components—elastin glycoprotein and elastic microfibril.

5. PROTEOGLYCANS These are a group of molecules having 2 components—an essential carbohydrate polymer (called polysaccharide or glycosaminoglycan), and a protein bound to it, and hence the name proteoglycan. Various proteoglycans are distributed in different tissues as under:

i)   *Chondroitin sulphate*—abundant in cartilage, dermis
ii)   *Heparan sulphate*—in basement membranes
iii) *Dermatan sulphate*—in dermis
iv) *Keratan sulphate*—in cartilage
v)   *Hyaluronic acid*—in cartilage, dermis.

FACTORS INFLUENCING HEALING

Two types of factors influence the wound healing: those acting locally, and those acting in general.

A. Local Factors:
1.   *Infection*
2.   *Poor blood supply*
3.   *Foreign bodies*
4.   *Movement*
5.   Exposure to *ionising radiation*
6.   Exposure to *ultraviolet light*
7.   *Type, size and location* of injury.

B. Systemic Factors:
1.   *Age.* Wound healing is rapid in young and somewhat slow in aged and debilitated people.
2.   *Nutrition.* Deficiency of constituents like protein, vitamin C (scurvy), vitamin A and zinc delays the wound healing.
3.   *Systemic infection* delays wound healing.
4.   *Administration of glucocorticoids* has anti-inflammatory effect.
5.   *Uncontrolled diabetics* are more prone to develop infections and hence delay in healing.
6.   *Haematologic abnormalities* like defect of neutrophil functions (chemotaxis and phagocytosis), and neutropenia and bleeding disorders slow the process of wound healing.

HEALING IN SPECIALISED TISSUES *(p. 161)*

FRACTURE HEALING

Healing of fracture by callus formation depends upon some clinical considerations whether the fracture is:
◈   *traumatic* (in previously normal bone), or *pathological* (in previously diseased bone);
◈   *complete or incomplete* like green-stick fracture; and
◈   *simple* (closed), *comminuted* (splintering of bone), or *compound* (communicating to skin surface).

◈   **Primary union of fractures** occurs when the ends of fracture are approximated surgically by application of compression clamps or metal plates. In these cases, bony union takes place with formation of medullary callus without periosteal callus formation. The patient can be made ambulatory early but there is more extensive bone necrosis and slow healing.

◈   **Secondary union** is more common form of fracture healing when the plaster casts are applied for immobilisation of a fracture. Though it is a continuous process, secondary bone union is described under the following 3 headings:

I.   **PROCALLUS FORMATION** Steps involved in the formation of procallus are as follows:
1.   **Haematoma** forms due to bleeding from torn blood vessels, filling the area surrounding the fracture.
2.   **Local inflammatory response** occurs at the site of injury with exudation of fibrin, polymorphs and macrophages.
3.   **Ingrowth of granulation tissue** begins with neovascularisation and proliferation of mesenchymal cells from periosteum and endosteum.
4.   **Callus composed of woven bone and cartilage** starts within the first few days. The cells of inner layer of the periosteum have osteogenic

potential and lay down collagen as well as osteoid matrix in the granulation tissue. The osteoid undergoes calcification and is called *woven bone callus*.

II. OSSEOUS CALLUS FORMATION The procallus acts as scaffolding on which osseous callus composed of lamellar bone is formed. The woven bone is cleared away by incoming osteoclasts and the calcified cartilage disintegrates.

III. REMODELLING During the formation of lamellar bone, osteoblastic laying and osteoclastic removal are taking place remodelling the united bone ends, which after sometime, is indistinguishable from normal bone.

COMPLICATIONS OF FRACTURE HEALING

1. Fibrous union may result instead of osseous union if the immobilisation of fractured bone is not done.

2. Non-union may result if some soft tissue is interposed between the fractured ends.

3. Delayed union may occur from causes of delayed wound healing in general such as infection, inadequate blood supply, poor nutrition, movement and old age.

HEALING OF NERVOUS TISSUE

CENTRAL NERVOUS SYSTEM The nerve cells of the brain, spinal cord and ganglia are permanent cells, and therefore once destroyed are not replaced.

PERIPHERAL NERVOUS SYSTEM In contrast to the cells of CNS, the peripheral nerves show limited regeneration, mainly from proliferation of Schwann cells and fibrils from distal end.

i) Myelin sheath and axon of the intact distal nerve undergo Wallerian degeneration up to the next node of Ranvier towards the proximal end.

ii) Degenerated debris are cleared away by macrophages.

iii) Regeneration in the form of sprouting of fibrils takes place from the viable end of axon. These fibrils grow along the track of degenerated nerve so that in about 6-7 weeks, the peripheral stump consists of tube filled with elongated Schwann cells.

iv) One of the fibrils from the proximal stump enters the old neural tube and develops into new functional axon.

HEALING OF MUSCLE

SKELETAL MUSCLE The regeneration of striated muscle is similar to peripheral nerves. On injury, the cut ends of muscle fibres retract but are held together by stromal connective tissue. The injured site is filled with fibrinous material, polymorphs and macrophages.

◈ If the muscle sheath is intact, sarcolemmal tubes containing histiocytes appear along the endomysial tube which, in about 3 months time, restores properly oriented muscle fibres e.g. in Zenker's degeneration of muscle in typhoid fever.

◈ If the muscle sheath is damaged, it forms a disorganised multinucleate mass and scar composed of fibrovascular tissue e.g. in Volkmann's ischaemic contracture.

SMOOTH MUSCLE Non-striated muscle has limited regenerative capacity e.g. appearance of smooth muscle in the arterioles in granulation tissue. However, in large destructive lesions, the smooth muscle is replaced by permanent scar tissue.

CARDIAC MUSCLE Destruction of heart muscle is replaced by fibrous tissue.

HEALING OF MUCOSAL SURFACES

The cells of mucosal surfaces have very good regeneration and are normally being lost and replaced continuously e.g. mucosa of alimentary tract, respiratory tract, urinary tract, uterine endometrium etc. This occurs by proliferation from margins, migration, multilayering and differentiation of epithelial cells.

HEALING OF SOLID EPITHELIAL ORGANS

Following gross tissue damage to organs like the kidney, liver and thyroid, the replacement is by fibrous scar e.g. in chronic pyelonephritis and cirrhosis of liver. However, in parenchymal cell damage with intact basement membrane or intact supporting stromal tissue, regeneration may occur.

STEM CELL CONCEPT OF HEALING—REGENERATIVE MEDICINE (p. 163)

Currently, the field of stem cell biology has emerged at the forefront of healing of injured tissue, treatment of diseases and holds promise for tissue transplantation in future.

Stem cells are the primitive cells which have 2 main properties:
i)   They have capacity for self renewal.
ii) They can be coaxed into multilineage differentation (i.e. into any of about 220 types of cells e.g. red cells, myocardial fibres, neurons etc).

Stem cells exist in both embryos and in adult tissues:
◈   In embryos, they function to generate new organs and tissues; their presence for organogenesis has been an established fact.
◈   In adults, they normally function to replace cells during the natural course of cell turnover. For example, stem cells in the bone marrow which sponateously differentiate into mature haematopoietic cells has been known for a long time.

Some of the major clinical trials on applications of stem cells underway are in the following directions:

1. **Bone marrow stem cells**   Haematopoieitc stem cells, marrow stromal cells and stem cells sourced from umbilical cord blood have been used for treatment of various forms of blood cancers and other blood disorders for about three decades.

2. **Neuron stem cells**   These cells are capable of generating neurons, astrocytes and oligodendroglial cells. It may be possible to use these cells in neurodegenerative diseases such as Parkinsonism and Alzheimer's disease, and in spinal cord injury.

3. **Islet cell stem cells**   Clinical trials are under way for use of adult mesenchymal stem cells for islet cells in type 1 diabetes.

4. **Cardiac stem cells**   It is now known that the heart has cardiac stem cells which have capacity to repair myocardium after infarction.

5. **Skeletal muscle stem cells**   Although skeletal muscle cells do not divide when injured, stem cells of muscle have capacity to regenerate.

6. **Adult eye stem cells**   The cornea of the eye contains stem cells in the region of limbus. These limbal stem cells have a potential therapeutic use in corneal opacities and damage to the conjunctiva.

7. **Skin stem cells**   In the skin, the stem cells are located in the region of hair follicle and sebaceous glands. These stem cells contribute to repair of damaged epidermis.

SELF ASSESSMENT

1. **Which of the complement components act as chemokines?**
    A. C3b   B. C4b
    C. C5a   D. C4a
2. **All are types of tissue macrophages except:**
    A. Littoral cells   B. Hofbauer cells
    C. Osteoclasts   D. Osteoblasts
3. **Formation of granuloma is:**
    A. Type I hypersensitivity reaction
    B. Type II hypersensitivity reaction

C. Type III hypersensitivity reaction

D. Type IV hypersensitivity reaction

4. **Which of the following is a type of non-tuberculous mycobacteria?**
   A. *Mycobacterium microti*
   B. *Mycobacterium canetti*
   C. *Mycobacterium africanum*
   D. *Mycobacterium ulcerans*

5. **IgM antibody against PGL-1 antigen is used for the diagnosis of:**
   A. Leprosy
   B. Tuberculosis
   C. Syphilis
   D. Brucellosis

6. **Which of the following type of leprosy is not included in Ridley-Jopling classification?**
   A. Mid-borderline leprosy
   B. Borderline tuberculoid leprosy
   C. Indeterminate leprosy
   D. Tuberculoid polar leprosy

7. **Hepar lobatum is seen in:**
   A. Primary syphilis
   B. Secondary syphilis
   C. Tertiary syphilis
   D. Congenital syphilis

8. **Killing of *M. tuberculosis* that grows within the macrophage is brought about by the following mechanisms:**
   A. By reactive oxygen species
   B. By oxygen-independent bactericidal mechanism
   C. By nitric oxide mechanism
   D. By hydrolytic enzymes

9. **Main cytokines acting as mediators of inflammation are as under except:**
   A. Interleukin-1 (IL-1)
   B. Tumour necrosis factor α (TNF-α)
   C. Nitric oxide (NO)
   D. Interferon-γ (IF-γ)

10. **Receptor for IgE is present on:**
    A. Polymorphs
    B. Eosinophil
    C. Basophil
    D. Plasma cell

11. **Typhoid fever is an example of:**
    A. Acute inflammation
    B. Chronic nonspecific inflammation
    C. Chronic granulomatous inflammation
    D. Chronic suppurative inflammation

12. **Tubercle bacilli cause lesions by the following mechanisms:**
    A. Elaboration of endotoxin
    B. Elaboration of exotoxin
    C. Type IV hypersensitivity
    D. Direct cytotoxicity

13. **The following statements are correct for tubercle bacilli except:**
    A. Tubercle bacilli can be cultured
    B. Tubercle bacilli are anaerobe
    C. Tubercle bacilli thrive best in the apex of lung
    D. *M. smegmatis* is not pathogenic to man

14. **Tubercle bacilli in caseous lesions are best demonstrated in:**
    A. Caseous centre
    B. Margin of necrosis with viable tissue
    C. Epithelioid cells
    D. Langhans' giant cells

15. **Leprosy bacilli are:**
    A. Not acid fast
    B. As acid fast as tubercle bacilli
    C. Less acid fast compared to tubercle bacilli
    D. More acid fast compared to tubercle bacilli

16. **Lepromin test is always positive in:**
    A. Lepromatous leprosy
    B. Borderline lepromatous leprosy
    C. Tuberculoid leprosy
    D. Indeterminate leprosy

17. **Spirochaetes are most difficult to demonstrate in:**
    A. Primary syphilis
    B. Secondary syphilis
    C. Tertiary syphilis
    D. Congenital syphilis

18. **Actinomycosis is caused by:**
    A. Fungus
    B. Gram-negative bacteria
    C. Anaerobic bacteria
    D. Acid fast bacteria

19. **Typically, sarcoid granuloma has the following features <u>except</u>:**
    A. Non caseating granuloma
    B. Giant cells have cytoplasmic inclusions
    C. Peripheral mantle of lymphocytes
    D. Fibroblastic proliferation at the periphery of a granuloma

20. **The following holds true for stable cells in cell cycle:**
    A. They remain in cell cycle from one mitosis to the next
    B. They are in resting phase but can be stimulated to enter the cell cycle
    C. They have left the cell cycle
    D. They do not have capacity to multiply in response to stimuli throughout adult life

21. **Connective tissue in scar is formed by the following types of fibrillar collagen:**
    A. Type II, III, IV
    B. Type I, III, V
    C. Type I, II, V
    D. Type III, V, VII

22. **Basement membrane consists of:**
    A. Type I collagen
    B. Type II collagen
    C. Type III collagen
    D. Type IV collagen

23. **The following adhesion molecules play a significant role in rolling of PMNs over endothelial cells <u>except</u>:**
    A. Selectins
    B. Integrins
    C. Opsonins
    D. Immunoglobulin molecules

24. **Which of the following is non-fibrillar collagen?**
    A. Type V
    B. Type I
    C. Type III
    D. Type VI

25. **Which is false about primary union?**
    A. Exuberant granulation tissue to fill the gap
    B. Clear margins
    C. Uninfected
    D. Lead to neat linear scar.

KEY

1 = C	2 = D	3 = D	4 = D	5 = A
6 = C	7 = C	8 = A	9 = C	10 = C
11 = A	12 = C	13 = B	14 = B	15 = C
16 = C	17 = C	18 = C	19 = C	20 = B
21 = B	22 = D	23 = C	24 = D	25 = A

6 Infectious and Parasitic Diseases

INTRODUCTION (p. 165)

In general, tropical and developing countries are particularly affected more by infectious diseases than the developed countries.

❖ There are several examples of certain *infectious diseases* which are not so common in the developed world now but they continue to be major health problems in the developing countries e.g. tuberculosis, leprosy, typhoid fever, cholera, measles, pertussis, malaria, amoebiasis, pneumonia etc.

❖ *Vaccines* have been successful in controlling or eliminating some diseases all over the world e.g. smallpox, poliomyelitis, measles, pertussis etc. Similarly, insecticides have helped in controlling malaria to an extent.

❖ Infections still rank very high *as a cause of death* in the world.

Following is the range of *host-organism inter-relationship,* which may vary quite widely:

1. *Symbiosis* i.e. cooperative association between two dissimilar organisms beneficial to both.

2. *Commensalism* i.e. two dissimilar organisms living together benefitting one without harming the other.

3. *True parasitism* i.e. two dissimilar organisms living together benefitting the parasite but harming the host.

4. *Saprophytism* i.e. organisms thriving on dead tissues.

Besides microorganisms, a modified infectious host protein present in the mammalian CNS has been identified called *prion protein*. Prions are transmissible agents similar to infectious particles but lack nucleic acid.

CHAIN IN TRANSMISSION OF INFECTIOUS DISEASES

Transmission of infections occurs following a chain of events pertaining to various parameters as under:

i) Reservoir of pathogen Infection occurs from the source of reservoir of pathogen. It may be a human being (e.g. in influenza virus), animal (e.g. dog for rabies), insect (e.g. mosquito for malaria), or soil (e.g. enterobiasis).

ii) Route of infection Infection is transmitted from the reservoir to the human being by different routes, usually from breach in the mucosa or the skin, at the portal of exit from the reservoir as well as the portal of entry in the susceptible host.

iii) Mode of transmission The organism may be transmitted directly by physical contact or by faecal contamination (e.g. spread of eggs in hookworm infestation), or indirectly by fomites (e.g. insect bite).

iv) Susceptible host The organism would colonise the host if the host has good immunity but such a host can pass on infection to others. However, if the host is old, debilitated, malnourished, or immunosuppressed due any etiology, he is susceptible to have manifestations of infection.

FACTORS RELATING TO INFECTIOUS AGENTS

1. Mode of entry
2. Spread of infection
3. Virulence of organisms
4. Production of toxins
5. Product of organisms

1. Physical barrier
2. Chemical barrier
3. Effective drainage
4. Immune defense mechanisms

METHODS OF IDENTIFICATION

The organisms causing infections and parasitic diseases may be identified by routine H & E stained sections in many instances. However, confirmation in most cases requires either application of special staining techniques or is confirmed by molecular biologic methods as under:

1. BACTERIA
    i. Gram stain: Most bacteria
    ii. Acid fast stain: Mycobacteria, Nocardia
    iii. Giemsa: Campylobacteria
2. FUNGI
    i. Silver stain: Most fungi
    ii. Periodic acid-Schiff (PAS): Most fungi
    iii. Mucicarmine: Cryptococci
3. PARASITES
    i. Giemsa: Malaria, Leishmania
    ii. Periodic acid-Schiff: Amoebae
    iii. Silver stain: Pneumocystis
4. ALL CLASSES INCLUDING VIRUSES
    i. Culture
    ii. *In situ* hybridisation
    iii. DNA analysis
    iv. Polymerase chain reaction (PCR)

DISEASES CAUSED BY BACTERIA, SPIROCHAETES AND MYCOBACTERIA (p. 167)

PLAGUE (p. 167)

Plague has been a great killer since 14th century (black death) and is known to have wiped out populations of cities. World over, presently about 1000 to 3000 cases are reported annually.

ETIOPATHOGENESIS Plague is caused by *Yersinia (Pasteurella) pestis* which is a small Gram-negative coccobacillus that grows rapidly on most culture media. Direct identification of the organism in tissues is possible by fluorescence antisera methods.

Plague is a zoonotic disease and spreads by rodents, primarily by rats, both wild and domestic; others being squirrels and rabbits. Humans are incidental hosts other than rodents. Infection to humans occurs by rat-flea or by inhalation. Virulence of the organism *Y. pestis* is attributed to the elaboration of plague toxins: pesticin and lipopolysaccharide endotoxin.

M/E Following forms of plague are recognised:

BUBONIC PLAGUE This form is characterised by rapid appearance of tender, fluctuant and enlarged regional lymph nodes, several centimeters in diameter, and may have discharging sinuses on the skin.

SEPTICAEMIC PLAGUE This is a form of progressive, fulminant bacterial infection associated with profound septicaemia in the absence of apparent regional lymphadenitis.

TYPHOIDAL PLAGUE This form of plague is unassociated with regional lymphadenopathy.

PNEUMONIC PLAGUE This is the most dreaded form of plague that occurs by inhalation of bacilli from air-borne particles of carcasses of animals or from affected patient's cough. It is characterised by occurrence of bronchopneumonia.

Anthrax is a bacterial disease of antiquity that spreads from animals to man. The disease is widely prevalent in cattle and sheep but human infection is rare. However, much of knowledge on human anthrax has been gained owing to fear of use of these bacteria for military purpose by rogue countries or for "bio-terrorism" (other microbial diseases in the CDC category A list in this group include: botulism, pneumonic plague, smallpox, tularaemia, and viral haemorrhagic fevers).

ETIOPATHOGENESIS The causative organism, *Bacillus anthracis*, is a gram-positive, aerobic bacillus, 4.5 μm long. It is a spore-forming bacillus and the spores so formed outside the body are quite resistant. The disease occurs as an exogenous infection by contact with soil or animal products contaminated with spores.

Depending upon the portal of entry, three types of human anthrax is known to occur:

i) **Cutaneous form** by direct contact with skin and is most common.

ii) **Pulmonary form** by inhalation, also called as "wool-sorters' disease" and is most fatal.

iii) **Gastrointestinal form** by ingestion and is rare.

LABORATORY DIAGNOSIS Anthrax can be diagnosed by a few simple techniques as under:

i) Smear examination

ii) Culture

WHOOPING COUGH (PERTUSSIS) *(p. 169)*

Whooping cough is a highly communicable acute bacterial disease of childhood caused by *Bordetella pertussis*. The use of DPT vaccine has reduced the prevalence of whooping cough in different populations.

The causative organism, *B. pertussis*, has strong tropism for the brush border of the bronchial epithelium. The organisms proliferate here and stimulate the bronchial epithelium to produce abundant tenacious mucus. Within 7-10 days after exposure, catarrhal stage begins which is the most infectious stage. There is low grade fever, rhinorrhoea, conjunctivitis and excess tear production. Paroxysms of cough occur with characteristic 'whoop'. *B. pertussis* produces a heat-labile toxin, a heat-stable endotoxin, and a lymphocytosis-producing factor called histamine-sensitising factor.

DONOVANOSIS *(p. 170)*

Donovanosis also called granuloma inguinale or granuloma venereum is a sexually-transmitted disease affecting the genitalia, inguinal and perianal regions caused by *Calymmatobacterium donovani*. The infection is transmitted through vaginal or anal intercourse and by autoinoculation.

M/E The ulcer bed shows neutrophilic abscesses. The dermis and subcutaneous tissues are infiltrated by numerous histiocytes containing many bacteria called *Donovan bodies*, and lymphocytes, plasma cells and neutrophils.

LYMPHOGRANULOMA VENEREUM *(p. 170)*

Lymphogranuloma venereum (LGV) is a sexually-transmitted disease caused by *Chlamydia trachomatis* and is characterised by mucocutaneous lesions and regional lymphadenopathy. Chlamydia are no more considered as filterable viruses as was previously thought but are instead intracellular gram-negative bacteria.

M/E The lymph nodes have characteristic stellate-shaped abscesses surrounded by a zone of epithelioid cells (granuloma). Healing stage of the acute lesion takes place by fibrosis and permanent destruction of lymphoid structure.

Another condition related to LGV, cat-scratch disease, is caused by *Bartonella henselae*, an organism linked to rickettsiae but unlike rickettsiae this organism can be grown in culture. The condition occurs more commonly in children (under 18 years of age). There is regional nodal enlargement which appears about 2 weeks after cat-scratch, and sometimes after thorn injury. The lymphadenopathy is self-limited and regresses in 2-4 months.

M/E   Main features are as under:

i)   Initially, there is formation of non-caseating sarcoid-like granulomas.

ii)   Subsequently, there are neutrophilic abscesses surrounded by pallisaded histiocytes and fibroblasts, an appearance simulating LGV discussed above.

STAPHYLOCOCCAL INFECTIONS *(p. 170)*

Staphylococci are gram-positive cocci which are present everywhere—in the skin, umbilicus, nasal vestibule, stool etc. Three species are pathogenic to human beings: *Staph. aureus, Staph. epidermidis* and *Staph. saprophyticus.* Most staphylococcal infections are caused by *Staph. aureus.*

1.   Staphylococcal infections of the skin are quite common e.g. *folliculitis, furuncle, carbuncle* or *cellulitis, styes, impetigo, breast abscess.*
2.   Infections of burns and surgical wounds
3.   Infections of the upper and lower respiratory tract
4.   Bacterial arthritis
5.   Infection of bone (Osteomyelitis)
6.   Bacterial endocarditis
7.   Bacterial meningitis
8.   Septicaemia
9.   Toxic shock syndrome

STREPTOCOCCAL INFECTIONS *(p. 171)*

Streptococci are also gram-positive cocci but unlike staphylococci, they are more known for their non-suppurative autoimmune complications than suppurative inflammatory responses.

The following groups and subtypes of streptococci have been identified and implicated in different streptococcal diseases:

1.   *Group A or Streptococcus pyogenes,* also called β-haemolytic streptococci, are involved in causing upper respiratory tract infection and cutaneous infections (erysipelas). In addition, β-haemolytic streptococci are involved in autoimmune reactions in rheumatic heart disease (RHD).

2.   *Group B or Streptococcus agalactiae* produces infections in the newborn and is involved in non-suppurative post-streptococcal complications such as RHD and acute glomerulonephritis.

3.   *Group C and G streptococci* are responsible for respiratory infections.

4.   *Group D or Streptococcus faecalis,* also called enterococci are important in causation of urinary tract infection, bacterial endocarditis, septicaemia etc.

5.   *Untypable* α-haemolytic streptococci such as *Streptococcus viridans* constitute the normal flora of the mouth and may cause bacterial endocarditis.

6.   *Pneumococcus or Streptococcus pneumoniae* are etiologic agents for bacterial pneumonias, meningitis and septicaemia.

CLOSTRIDIAL DISEASES *(p. 172)*

Clostridia are gram-positive spore-forming anaerobic microorganisms found in the gastrointestinal tract of herbivorous animals and man. On degeneration of these microorganisms, the plasmids are liberated which produce many toxins responsible for the following clostridial diseases depending upon the species:

1.   Gas gangrene by *C. perfringens*
2.   Tetanus by *C. tetani*
3.   Botulism by *C. botulinum*
4.   Clostridial food poisoning by *C. perfringens*
5.   Necrotising enterocolitis by *C. perfringens.*

Of the large number of known fungi, only a few are infective to human beings. Many of the human fungal infections are opportunistic i.e. they occur in conditions with impaired host immune mechanisms.

MYCETOMA (p. 173)

Mycetoma is a chronic suppurative infection involving a limb, shoulder or other tissues and is characterised by draining sinuses. The material discharged from the sinuses is in the form of grains consisting of colonies of fungi or bacteria. Mycetomas are of 2 main types:

◈ *Mycetoma* caused by actinomyces (higher bacteria) also called actinomycetoma comprises about 60% of cases.

◈ *Eumycetoma* caused by true fungi, *Madurella mycetomatis* or *Madurella grisea*, comprises the remaining 40% of the cases.

G/A After several months of infection, the affected site, most commonly foot, is swollen and hence the name 'madura foot'. The lesions extend deeply into the subcutaneous tissues, along the fascia and eventually invade the bones.

M/E They drain through sinus tracts which discharge purulent material and black grains. The surrounding tissue shows granulomatous reaction.

CANDIDIASIS (p. 173)

Candidiasis is an opportunistic fungal infection caused most commonly by *Candida albicans* and occasionally by *Candida tropicalis*. In human beings, Candida species are present as normal flora of the skin and mucocutaneous areas, intestines and vagina. The organism becomes pathogenic when the balance between the host and the organism is disturbed e.g.

1. Oral thrush
2. Candidal vaginitis
3. Cutaneous candidiasis
4. Systemic candidiasis

CUTANEOUS SUPERFICIAL MYCOSIS (p. 174)

Dermatophytes cause superficial mycosis of the skin, the important examples being *Microsporum*, *Trichophyton* and *Epidermophyton*. These superficial fungi are spread by direct contact or by fomites and infect tissues such as the skin, hair and nails e.g.

◈ *Tinea capitis*
◈ *Tinea barbae*
◈ *Tinea corporis*.

DISEASES CAUSED BY VIRUSES (p. 174)

Viral diseases are the most common cause of human illness. Depending upon their nucleic acid genomic composition, they may be single-stranded or double-stranded, RNA or DNA viruses.

VIRAL HAEMORRHAGIC FEVERS (p. 175)

Viral haemorrhagic fevers are a group of acute viral infections which have common features of causing haemorrhages, shock and sometimes death. Viruses causing haemorrhagic fevers were earlier called *arthropod-borne (or arbo)* viruses since their transmission to humans was considered to be from arthropods. However, now it is known that all such viruses are not transmitted by arthropod vectors alone and hence now such haemorrhagic fevers are classified according to the routes of transmission and other epidemiologic features into 4 groups:

1. Mosquito-borne (e.g. yellow fever, dengue fever, Rift Valley fever)
2. Tick-borne (e.g. Crimean haemorrhagic fever, Kyasanur Forest disease)

3. Zoonotic (e.g. Korean haemorrhagic fever, Lassa fever)
4. Marburg virus disease and Ebola virus disease by unknown route.

Of these, mosquito-borne viral haemorrhagic fevers in which *Aedes aegypti* mosquitoes are vectors, are the most common problem the world over, especially in developing countries. Two important examples of Aedes mosquito-borne viral haemorrhagic fevers are yellow fever and dengue fever.

CHIKUNGUNYA VIRUS INFECTION

The word chikungunya means "that which bends up" and is derived from the language in Africa where this viral disease was first found in human beings. Chikungunya virus infection is primarily a disease in nonhuman primates but the infection is transmitted to humans by *A. aegypti* mosquito. The disease is endemic in parts of Africa and Asia and occurs sporadically elsewhere.

INFLUENZA VIRUS INFECTIONS *(p. 176)*

Influenza virus infection is an important and common form of communicable disease, especially prevalent as a seasonal infection in the developed countries. Its general clinical features range from a mild afebrile illness similar to common cold by appearance of sudden fever, headache, myalgia, malaise, chills and respiratory tract manifestations such as cough, soar throat to a more severe form of acute respiratory illness and lymphadenopathy.

ETIOLOGIC AGENT Influenza virus is a single-stranded RNA virus belonging to coronaviruses. Depending upon its antigenic characteristics of the nucleoprotein and matrix, 3 distinct types are known: A, B and C. Out of these, influenza type A is responsible for most serious and severe forms of outbreaks in human beings while types B and C cause a milder form of illness.

Two of the known subtypes of influenza A viruses which have affected the human beings in recent times are as under:

❖ Avian influenza virus A/H5N1 commonly called "bird flu".
❖ Swine influenza virus A/H1N1 commonly called "swine flu".

VARICELLA ZOSTER VIRUS INFECTION *(p. 177)*

Varicella zoster virus is a member of herpes virus family and causes chickenpox (varicella) in non-immune individuals and herpes zoster (shingles) in those who had chickenpox in the past.

HERPES SIMPLEX VIRUS INFECTION *(p. 177)*

Two of the herpes simplex viruses (HSV)—type 1 and 2, cause 'fever blisters' and herpes genitalis respectively.

HSV-1 causes vesicular lesions on the skin, lips and mucous membranes.

HSV-2 causes herpes genitalis characterised by vesicular and necrotising lesions on the cervix, vagina and vulva.

RABIES *(p. 178)*

Rabies is a fatal form of encephalitis in humans caused by rabies virus. The virus is transmitted into the human body by the bite of infected carnivores e.g. dog, wolf, fox and bats. The virus spreads from the contaminated saliva of these animals. The organism enters a peripheral nerve and then travels to the spinal cord and brain.

DISEASES CAUSED BY PARASITES *(p. 178)*

Diseases caused by parasites (protozoa and helminths) are quite common and comprise a very large group of infestations and infections in human beings. Parasites may cause disease due to their presence in the lumen of the intestine, due to infiltration into the blood stream, or due to their presence inside the cells.

AMOEBIASIS *(p. 178)*

Amoebiasis is caused by *Entamoeba histolytica*, named for its lytic action on tissues. It is the most important intestinal infection of man. The condition is particularly more common in tropical and subtropical areas with poor sanitation.

The parasite occurs in 2 forms:

❖ a *trophozoite form* which is active adult form seen in the tissues and diarrhoeal stools; and

❖ a *cystic form* seen in formed stools but not in the tissues.

M/E The lesions of amoebiasis include amoebic colitis, amoeboma, amoebic liver abscess and spread of lesions to other sites.

MALARIA *(p. 179)*

Malaria is a protozoal disease caused by any one or combination of four species of plasmodia: *Plasmodium vivax*, *Plasmodium falciparum*, *Plasmodium ovale* and *Plasmodium malariae*. While *Plasmodium falciparum* causes malignant malaria, the other three species produce benign form of illness. These parasites are transmitted by bite of female *Anopheles* mosquito. The disease is endemic in several parts of the world, especially in tropical Africa, parts of South and Central America, India and South-East Asia.

The main clinical features of malaria are cyclic peaks of high fever accompanied with chills, anaemia and splenomegaly.

Major complications occur in severe falciparum malaria which may have manifestations of cerebral malaria (coma), hypoglycaemia, renal impairment, severe anaemia, haemoglobinuria, jaundice, pulmonary oedema, and acidosis followed by congestive heart failure and hypotensive shock.

FILARIASIS *(p. 180)*

Wuchereria bancrofti and *Brugia malayi* are responsible for causing Bancroftian and Malayan filariasis in different geographic regions. The lymphatic vessels inhabit the adult worm, especially in the lymph nodes, testis and epididymis. Microfilariae seen in the circulation are produced by the female worm. Majority of infected patients remain asymptomatic. Symptomatic cases may have two forms of disease—an acute form and a chronic form.

❖ *Acute form* of filariasis presents with fever, lymphangitis, lymphadenitis, epididymo-orchitis, urticaria, eosinophilia and microfilariaemia.

❖ *Chronic form* of filariasis is characterised by lymphadenopathy, lymphoedema, hydrocele and elephantiasis.

CYSTICERCOSIS *(p. 181)*

Cysticercosis is an infection by the larval stage of *Taenia solium*, the pork tapeworm. The adult tapeworm resides in the human intestines. The eggs are passed in human faeces which are ingested by pigs or they infect vegetables. These eggs then develop into larval stages in the host, spread by blood to any site in the body and form cystic larvae termed *cysticercus cellulosae*.

M/E The cysticercus may be single or there may be multiple cysticerci in the different tissues of the body. The cysts may occur virtually anywhere in body and accordingly produce symptoms; most common sites are the brain, skeletal muscle and skin. Cysticercus consists of a round to oval white cyst, about 1 cm in diameter, contains milky fluid and invaginated scolex with birefringent hooklets.

Acronym 'TORCH' complex refers to development of common complex of symptoms in infants due to infection with different microorganisms that include: *T*oxoplasma, *O*thers, *R*ubella, *C*ytomegalovirus, and *H*erpes simplex virus; category of 'Others' refers to infections such as hepatitis B, coxsackievirus B, mumps and poliovirus. The infection may be acquired by the foetus during intrauterine life, or perinatally and damage the foetus or infant. Since the symptoms produced by TORCH group of organisms are indistinguishable from each other, it is a common practice to test for all the four main TORCH agents in a suspected pregnant mother or infant.

SELF ASSESSMENT

1. **The causative organisms of plague are:**
   - A. Cocci
   - B. Bacilli
   - C. Coccobacilli
   - D. Nocardia
2. **Lymphocytosis in whooping cough occurs due to:**
   - A. Endotoxin by the microorganism
   - B. Exotoxin by the microorganism
   - C. Cytokine
   - D. Histamine-sensitising factor
3. **Granuloma inguinale is characterised by the following <u>except</u>:**
   - A. It is caused by Donovan bacilli
   - B. It is characterised by lymphadenopathy
   - C. It is a sexually transmitted disease
   - D. There are neutrophilic abscesses in the dermis
4. **Prion proteins are implicated in the etiology of:**
   - A. Spongiform encephalopathy
   - B. Viral encephalitis
   - C. Perivenous encephalomyelitis
   - D. Progressive multifocal leucoencephalopathy
5. **Streptococci are commonly implicated in the etiology of the following <u>except</u>:**
   - A. Rheumatic heart disease
   - B. Glomerulonephritis
   - C. Breast abscess
   - D. Subacute bacterial endocarditis
6. **Clostridia are implicated in the following <u>except</u>:**
   - A. Botulism
   - B. Necrotising enterocolitis
   - C. Bacillary dysentery
   - D. Pseudomembranous colitis
7. **Fungi in general can be identified by the following stains <u>except</u>:**
   - A. Silver stain
   - B. Periodic acid Schiff
   - C. Giemsa
   - D. Mucicarmine
8. **Mosquito-borne viral haemorrhagic fever include the following examples <u>except</u>:**
   - A. Dengue fever
   - B. Yellow fever
   - C. Rift Valley fever
   - D. Kyasanur Forest fever
9. **Dengue haemorrhagic fever is characterised by following laboratory findings <u>except</u>:**
   - A. Leucopenia
   - B. Lymphocytosis
   - C. Decreased haematocrit
   - D. Thrombocytopenia
10. **Granuloma inguinale and lymphogranuloma venereum are similar in following aspects, <u>except</u>:**
    - A. Both are sexually transmitted diseases
    - B. Both are caused by bacteria

C. Both are characterised by lymphadenopathy
D. Both begin as lesions on genitals

11. **Necrotic lesions of *Entamoeba histolytica* are due to:**
    A. Cyst stage
    B. Trophozoite stage
    C. Both cyst and trophozoites
    D. Neither cysts nor trophozoites

12. ***P. falciparum* differs from other plasmodia in following aspects <u>except</u>:**
    A. It does not have exoerythrocytic stage
    B. It parasitises only juvenile red cells
    C. It causes malignant malaria
    D. One red cell may contain more than one parasite

13. **In the case of SARS in human beings, the mode of infection is:**
    A. From mosquito   B. Person to person
    C. Poultry birds   D. Domestic dogs

14. **Swine flu influenza virus is:**
    A. H5N1   B. H1N1
    C. H5N2   D. H1N2

15. **Chikungunya is transmitted to humans by:**
    A. Aedes   B. Anopheles
    C. Culex   D. Tick

KEY

1 = C	2 = D	3 = B	4 = A	5 = C
6 = C	7 = C	8 = D	9 = C	10 = C
11 = B	12 = B	13 = C	14 = B	15 = A

7 — Neoplasia

NOMENCLATURE AND CLASSIFICATION *(p. 184)*

INTRODUCTION The term 'neoplasia' means new growth; the new growth produced is called 'neoplasm' or 'tumour'.

Satisfactory definition of a neoplasm or tumour is *'a mass of tissue formed as a result of abnormal, excessive, uncoordinated, autonomous and purposeless proliferation of cells even after cessation of stimulus for growth which caused it'.* Neoplasms may be 'benign' when they are slow-growing and localised without causing much difficulty to the host, or 'malignant' when they proliferate rapidly, spread throughout the body and may eventually cause death of the host. The common term used for all malignant tumours is cancer. Hippocrates (460-370 BC) coined the term *karkinos* for cancer of the breast. The word 'cancer' means crab, thus reflecting the true character of cancer since 'it sticks to the part stubbornly like a crab'.

All tumours, benign as well as malignant, have 2 basic components:

◈ *'Parenchyma'* comprised by proliferating tumour cells; parenchyma determines the nature and evolution of the tumour.

◈ *'Supportive stroma'* composed of fibrous connective tissue and blood vessels; it provides the framework on which the parenchymal tumour cells grow.

The tumours derive their nomenclature on the basis of the parenchymal component comprising them. The suffix *'-oma'* is added to denote benign tumours. Malignant tumours of epithelial origin are called *carcinomas*, while malignant mesenchymal tumours are named *sarcomas* (*sarcos* = fleshy). However, some cancers are composed of highly undifferentiated cells and are referred to as *undifferentiated malignant tumours*.

Although, this broad generalisation regarding nomenclature of tumours usually holds true in majority of instances, some examples contrary to this concept are: *melanoma* for carcinoma of the melanocytes, *hepatoma* for carcinoma of the hepatocytes, *lymphoma* for malignant tumour of the lymphoid tissue, and *seminoma* for malignant tumour of the testis. *Leukaemia* is the term used for cancer of blood forming cells.

SPECIAL CATEGORIES OF TUMOURS

1. Mixed tumours A few examples are as under:

i) *Adenosquamous carcinoma* is the combination of adenocarcinoma and squamous cell carcinoma in the endometrium.

ii) *Adenoacanthoma* is the mixture of adenocarcinoma and benign squamous elements in the endometrium.

iii) *Carcinosarcoma* is the rare combination of malignant tumour of the epithelium (carcinoma) and of mesenchymal tissue (sarcoma) such as in thyroid.

iv) *Collision tumour* is the term used for morphologically two different cancers in the same organ which do not mix with each other.

v) *Mixed tumour of the salivary gland* (or pleomorphic adenoma) is the term used for benign tumour having combination of both epithelial and mesenchymal tissue elements.

2. Teratomas These tumours are made up of a mixture of various tissue types arising from totipotent cells derived from the three germ cell layers—ectoderm, mesoderm and endoderm. Most common sites for teratomas are ovaries and testis (*gonadal teratomas*). But they occur at *extra-gonadal* sites as well, mainly in the midline of the body such as in the head and

Teratomas may be *benign or mature* (most of the ovarian teratomas) or *malignant or immature* (most of the testicular teratomas).

3. Blastomas (Embryomas) Blastomas or embryomas are a group of malignant tumours which arise from embryonal or partially differentiated cells which would normally form blastema of the organs and tissue during embryogenesis. These tumours occur more frequently in infants and children (under 5 years of age). Some examples of such tumours in this age group are: neuroblastoma, nephroblastoma (Wilms' tumour), hepatoblastoma, retinoblastoma, medulloblastoma, pulmonary blastoma.

4. Hamartoma Hamartoma is benign tumour which is made of mature but disorganised cells of tissues indigenous to the particular organ e.g. hamartoma of the lung consists of mature cartilage, mature smooth muscle and epithelium.

5. Choristoma Choristoma is the name given to the ectopic islands of normal tissue. Thus, choristoma is heterotopia but is not a true tumour, though it sounds like one.

CHARACTERISTICS OF TUMOURS *(p. 186)*

The characteristics of tumours are described under the following headings:
I.   Rate of growth
II. Cancer phenotype and stem cells
III. Clinical and gross features
IV. Microscopic features
V.   Spread of tumours
     a. Local invasion or direct spread
     b. Metastasis or distant spread.

I. RATE OF GROWTH *(p. 186)*

The tumour cells generally proliferate more rapidly than the normal cells. In general, benign tumours grow slowly and malignant tumours rapidly. However, there are exceptions to this generalisation. The rate at which the tumour enlarges depends upon 2 main factors:
1. Rate of cell production, growth fraction and rate of cell loss
2. Degree of differentiation of the tumour.

The regulation of tumour growth is under the control of growth factors secreted by the tumour cells. Out of various growth factors, important ones modulating tumour biology are listed below and discussed later:
i)   Epidermal growth factor (EGF)
ii)   Fibroblast growth factor (FGF)
iii) Platelet-derived growth factor (PDGF)
iv)   Colony stimulating factor (CSF)
v)   Transforming growth factors-β (TGF-β)
vi)   Interleukins 1 and 6 (IL-1, IL-6)
vii) Vascular endothelial growth factor (VEGF)
viii) Hepatocyte growth factor (HGF)

II. CANCER PHENOTYPE AND STEM CELLS *(p. 188)*

Normally growing cells in an organ are related to the neighbouring cells— they grow under normal growth controls, perform their assigned function and there is a balance between the rate of cell proliferation and the rate of cell death including cell suicide (i.e. apoptosis).
i)   Cancer cells disobey the growth controlling signals in the body and thus *proliferate rapidly*.
ii) Cancer cells escape death signals and achieve *immortality*.
iii) Imbalance between cell proliferation and cell death in cancer causes *excessive growth*.
iv) Cancer cells lose properties of differentiation and thus perform *little or no function*.

v) Due to loss of growth controls, cancer cells are genetically unstable and develop *newer mutations*.

vi) Cancer cells overrun their neighbouring tissue and *invade locally*.

vii) Cancer cells have the ability to travel from the site of origin to other sites in the body where they colonise and establish *distant metastasis*.

Cancer cells originate by clonal proliferation of a single progeny of a cell (monoclonality). Cancer cells arise from stem cells normally present in the tissues in small number and are not readily identifiable.

III. CLINICAL AND GROSS FEATURES (p. 188)

Clinically, benign tumours are generally slow growing, and depending upon the location, may remain asymptomatic (e.g. subcutaneous lipoma), or may produce serious symptoms (e.g. meningioma in the nervous system). On the other hand, malignant tumours grow rapidly, may ulcerate on the surface, invade locally into deeper tissues, may spread to distant sites (metastasis), and also produce systemic features such as weight loss, anorexia and anaemia. In fact, three cardinal clinical features of malignant tumours are: *anaplasia, invasiveness and metastasis* (discussed later).

Gross appearance of benign and malignant tumours may be quite variable and the features may not be diagnostic on the basis of gross appearance alone. However, certain distinctive features characterise almost all tumours compared to neighbouring normal tissue of origin—they have a different colour, texture and consistency.

◈ *Benign tumours* are generally spherical or ovoid in shape. They are encapsulated or well-circumscribed, freely movable, more often firm and uniform, unless secondary changes like haemorrhage or infarction supervene.

◈ *Malignant tumours,* on the other hand, are usually irregular in shape, poorly-circumscribed and extend into the adjacent tissues. Secondary changes like haemorrhage, infarction and ulceration are seen more often. Sarcomas typically have fish-flesh like consistency while carcinomas are generally firm.

IV. MICROSCOPIC FEATURES (p. 188)

1. MICROSCOPIC PATTERN

Some of the common patterns in tumours are as under:

i) The *epithelial tumours* generally consist of acini, sheets, columns or cords of epithelial tumour cells that may be arranged in solid or papillary pattern.

ii) The *mesenchymal tumours* have mesenchymal tumour cells arranged as interlacing bundles, fascicles or whorls, lying separated from each other usually by the intercellular matrix substance such as hyaline material in leiomyoma, cartilaginous matrix in chondroma, osteoid in osteosarcoma, reticulin network in soft tissue sarcomas etc.

2. CYTOMORPHOLOGY OF NEOPLASTIC CELLS (DIFFERENTIATION AND ANAPLASIA)

The neoplastic cell is characterised by morphologic and functional alterations, the most significant of which are '*differentiation*' and '*anaplasia*'.

◈ **Differentiation** is defined as the extent of morphological and functional resemblance of parenchymal tumour cells to corresponding normal cells. If the deviation of neoplastic cell in structure and function is minimal as compared to normal cell, the tumour is described as '*well-differentiated*' such as most benign and low-grade malignant tumours. '*Poorly differentiated*', '*undifferentiated*' or '*dedifferentiated*' are synonymous terms for poor structural and functional resemblance to corresponding normal cell.

◈ **Anaplasia** is lack of differentiation and is a characteristic feature of most malignant tumours. Depending upon the degree of differentiation, the extent of anaplasia is also variable i.e. poorly differentiated malignant tumours have high degree of anaplasia.

As a result of anaplasia, noticeable morphological and functional alterations in the neoplastic cells are observed which are best appreciated under *higher magnification* of the microscope.

i)   Loss of polarity
ii)   Pleomorphism
iii)   Increased N:C ratio
iv)   Anisonucleosis
v)   Hyperchromatism
vi)   Prominent nucleolus or nucleoli
◈   Abnormal or atypical mitotic figures
viii) Tumour giant cells
ix)   Functional (Cytoplasmic) changes
◈   There may be both qualitative and quantitative abnormality of the cellular function in some anaplastic tumours
◈   Ectopic hormone production
x)   Chromosomal abnormalities

3. TUMOUR ANGIOGENESIS AND STROMA

The connective tissue alongwith its vascular network forms the supportive framework on which the parenchymal tumour cells grow and receive nourishment.

TUMOUR ANGIOGENESIS   In order to provide nourishment to growing tumour, new blood vessels are formed from pre-existing ones (angiogenesis).

TUMOUR STROMA   The collagenous tissue in the stroma may be scanty or excessive.
◈   If the epithelial tumour is almost entirely composed of parenchymal cells, it is called *medullary* e.g. medullary carcinoma of the breast, medullary carcinoma of the thyroid.
◈   If there is excessive connective tissue stroma in the epithelial tumour, it is referred to as *desmoplasia* and the tumour is hard or *scirrhous* e.g. infiltrating duct carcinoma breast, linitis plastica of the stomach.

4. INFLAMMATORY REACTION

Some tumours show chronic inflammatory reaction, chiefly of lymphocytes, plasma cells and macrophages, and in some instances granulomatous reaction, as a part of the morphologic features of the tumour, in the absence of ulceration. This is due to cell-mediated immunologic response by the host in an attempt to destroy the tumour. In some cases, such an immune response improves the prognosis.

The *examples* of such reaction are: seminoma testis, malignant melanoma of the skin, lymphoepithelioma of the throat, medullary carcinoma of the breast, choriocarcinoma, Warthin's tumour of salivary glands etc.

V. SPREAD OF TUMOURS *(p. 192)*

One of the cardinal features of malignant tumours is its ability to invade and destroy adjoining tissues (local invasion or direct spread) and disseminate to distant sites (metastasis or distant spread).

LOCAL INVASION (DIRECT SPREAD)

BENIGN TUMOURS   Most benign tumours form encapsulated or circum-scribed masses that *expand and push aside* the surrounding normal tissues without actually invading, infiltrating or metastasising.

MALIGNANT TUMOURS   Malignant tumours also enlarge by expansion and some well-differentiated tumours may be partially encapsulated as well e.g. follicular carcinoma thyroid. But characteristically, they are distinguished from benign tumours by *invasion, infiltration and destruction* of the surrounding tissue, besides spread to distant sites or metastasis.

Metastasis (*meta* = transformation, *stasis* = residence) is defined as spread of tumour by invasion in such a way that discontinuous secondary tumour mass/masses are formed at the site of lodgement. *Besides anaplasia, invasiveness and metastasis are the two other most important features to distinguish malignant from benign tumours.*

ROUTES OF METASTASIS

Cancers may spread to distant sites by following pathways:

1. LYMPHATIC SPREAD *In general, carcinomas metastasise by lymphatic route while sarcomas favour haematogenous route.* However, some sarcomas may also spread by lymphatic pathway. The involvement of lymph nodes by malignant cells may be of two forms:

i) Lymphatic permeation

ii) Lymphatic emboli

◈ Generally, regional lymph nodes draining the tumour are invariably involved producing *regional nodal metastasis*

◈ However, all regional nodal enlargements are not due to nodal metastasis because necrotic products of tumour and antigens may also incite regional lymphadenitis of *sinus histiocytosis.*

◈ Sometimes lymphatic metastases do not develop first in the lymph node nearest to the tumour because of venous-lymphatic anastomoses or due to obliteration of lymphatics by inflammation or radiation, so called *skip metastasis.*

◈ Other times, due to obstruction of the lymphatics by tumour cells, the lymph flow is disturbed and tumour cells spread against the flow of lymph causing *retrograde metastases* at unusual sites e.g. metastasis of carcinoma prostate to the supraclavicular lymph nodes.

◈ *Virchow's lymph node* is nodal metastasis preferentially to supraclavicular lymph node from cancers of abdominal organs e.g. cancer stomach, colon, and gallbladder.

2. HAEMATOGENOUS SPREAD *Blood-borne metastasis is the common route for sarcomas but certain carcinomas also frequently metastasise by this mode,* especially those of the lung, breast, thyroid, kidney, liver, prostate and ovary. The sites where blood-borne metastasis commonly occurs are: the liver, lungs, brain, bones, kidney and adrenals. However, a few organs such as the spleen, heart, and skeletal muscle generally do not allow tumour metastasis to grow.

i) *Systemic veins* drain blood into vena cavae from limbs, head and neck and pelvis. Therefore, cancers of these sites more often metastasise to the lungs.

ii) *Portal veins* drain blood from the bowel, spleen and pancreas into the liver. Thus, tumours of these organs frequently have secondaries in the liver.

iii) *Pulmonary veins* provide another route of spread of not only primary lung cancer but also metastatic growths in the lungs. Blood in the pulmonary veins carrying cancer cells from the lungs reaches left side of the heart and then into systemic circulation and thus may form secondary masses elsewhere in the body.

iv) *Arterial spread* of tumours is less likely because they are thick-walled and contain elastic tissue which is resistant to invasion.

v) *Retrograde spread* by blood route may occur at unusual sites due to retrograde spread after venous obstruction, just as with lymphatic metastases. Important examples are vertebral metastases in cancers of the thyroid and prostate.

3. SPREAD ALONG BODY CAVITIES AND NATURAL PASSAGES Uncommon routes of spread of some cancers are by *seeding* across body cavities and *natural passages* as under:

i) Transcoelomic spread Certain cancers invade through the serosal wall of the coelomic cavity so that tumour fragments or clusters of tumour cells break off to be carried in the coelomic fluid and are implanted elsewhere in the body cavity. Peritoneal cavity is involved most often, but occasionally pleural and pericardial cavities are also affected e.g.

a) *Carcinoma of the stomach* seeding to both ovaries (Krukenberg tumour).

b) *Carcinoma of the ovary* spreading to the entire peritoneal cavity without infiltrating the underlying organs.

c) *Pseudomyxoma peritonei* is the gelatinous coating of the peritoneum from mucin-secreting carcinoma of the ovary or apppendix.

d) *Carcinoma of the bronchus and breast* seeding to the pleura and pericardium.

ii)   Spread along epithelium-lined surfaces   e.g.

a) the fallopian tube from the endometrium to the ovaries or *vice-versa;*

b) through the bronchus into alveoli; and

c) through the ureters from the kidneys into lower urinary tract.

iii)   Spread via cerebrospinal fluid   Malignant tumour of the ependyma and leptomeninges may spread by release of tumour fragments and tumour cells into the CSF and produce metastases at other sites in the central nervous system.

MECHANISM AND BIOLOGY OF INVASION AND METASTASIS

The process of local invasion and distant spread by lymphatic and haematogenous routes (together called lymphovascular spread) discussed above involves passage through barriers before gaining access to the vascular lumen.

1.   Aggressive clonal proliferation and angiogenesis   The first step in the spread of cancer cells is the development of rapidly proliferating clone of cancer cells. This is explained on the basis of *tumour heterogeneity.*

2.   Tumour cell loosening   In epithelial cancers, there is either loss or inactivation of E-cadherin and also other CAMs of immunoglobulin superfamily, all of which results in loosening of cancer cells.

3.   Tumour cell-ECM interaction   Loosened cancer cells are now attached to ECM proteins, mainly *laminin* and *fibronectin.*

4.   Degradation of ECM   Tumour cells overexpress *proteases* and matrix-degrading enzymes, *metalloproteinases* (e.g. collagenases and gelatinase), while the inhibitors of metalloproteinases are decreased.

5.   Entry of tumour cells into capillary lumen   The tumour cells after degrading the basement membrane are ready to migrate into lumen of capillaries or venules.

6.   Thrombus formation   The tumour cells protruding in the lumen of the capillary are now covered with constituents of the circulating blood and form the thrombus.

7.   Extravasation of tumour cells   Tumour cells in the circulation (capillaries, venules, lymphatics) may mechanically block these vascular channels and attach to vascular endothelium and then extravasate to the extravascular space.

8.   Survival and growth of metastatic deposit   The extravasated malignant cells on lodgement in the right environment grow further under the influence of growth factors produced by host tissues, tumour cells and by cleavage products of matrix components.

GRADING AND STAGING OF CANCER *(p. 197)*

'Grading' and 'staging' are the two systems to predict tumour behaviour and guide therapy after a malignant tumour is detected. *Grading is defined as the gross appearance and microscopic degree of differentiation of the tumour, while staging means extent of spread of the tumour within the patient.* Thus, grading is done on patholologic basis while staging is on clinical grounds.

GRADING

Cancers may be graded grossly and microscopically. Gross features like exophytic or fungating appearance are indicative of less malignant growth than diffusely infiltrating tumours. However, grading is largely based on 2 important histologic features: *the degree of anaplasia, and the rate of growth.* Based on these features, cancers are categorised from grade I as the most differentiated, to grade III or IV as the most undifferentiated or anaplastic.

STAGING

The extent of spread of cancers can be assessed by 3 ways—by clinical examination, by investigations, and by pathologic examination of the tissue removed. Two important staging systems currently followed are: TNM staging and AJC staging.

Currently, clinical staging of tumours does not rest on routine radiography (X-ray, ultrasound) and exploratory surgery but more modern techniques are available by which it is possible to 'stage' a malignant tumour by non-invasive techniques.

EPIDEMIOLOGY AND MOLECULAR PATHOGENESIS OF CANCER *(p. 197)*

CANCER INCIDENCE

Worldwide incidence (in descending order) of 5 most common cancers in men, women, and children are as under:

	MEN	WOMEN	CHILDREN (UNDER 20)
1.	Prostate (oral cavity in India)	Breast (cervix in India)	Acute leukaemia
2.	Lung	Lung	Gliomas
3.	Colorectal	Colorectal	Bone sarcoma
4.	Urinary bladder	Endometrial	Endocrine
5.	Lymphoma	Lymphoma	Soft tissue sarcoma

Due to varying etiologic factors, cancers of the cervix and oral cavity are more common in India while cancers of the breast and lung are commoner in the Western populations.

In general, most common cancers in the developed and developing countries are as under:

◈ *Developed countries:* lung, breast, prostate and colorectal.
◈ *Developing countries:* liver, cervix, oral cavity and oesophagus.

About one-third of all cancers worldwide are attributed to 9 *modifiable life-style factors*: tobacco use, alcohol consumption, obesity, physical inactivity, low fiber diet, unprotected sex, polluted air, indoor household smoke, and contaminated injections.

EPIDEMIOLOGIC FACTORS *(p. 198)*

A. PREDISPOSING FACTORS

1. FAMILIAL AND GENETIC FACTORS It has long been suspected that familial predisposition and heredity play a role in the development of cancers. In general, the risk of developing cancer in relatives of a known cancer patient is almost three times higher as compared to control subjects. Some of the cancers with familial occurrence are colon, breast, ovary, brain and melanoma. Familial cancers occur at a relatively early age, appear at multiple sites and occur in 2 or more first-degree blood relatives. The overall estimates suggest that genetic cancers comprise about 5% of all cancers. Some of the common examples are as under:

i)   Retinoblastoma
ii)   Familial polyposis coli develop cancer of the colon
iii) Multiple endocrine neoplasia (MEN)
iv)   Neurofibromatosis or von Recklinghausen's disease

v) *Cancer of the breast* Female relatives of breast cancer patients have 2 to 6 times higher risk of developing breast cancer. Inherited breast cancer comprises about 5-10% of all breast cancers. As discussed later, there are two breast cancer susceptibility genes, *BRCA-1* and *BRCA-2*. Mutations in these genes appear in about 3% cases and these patients have about 85% risk of development of breast cancer.

vi) Congenital chromosomal syndromes

a) Down's syndrome or mongolism

b) Klinefelter syndrome

vii) DNA-chromosomal instability syndromes.

2. RACIAL AND GEOGRAPHIC FACTORS Differences in racial incidence of some cancers may be partly attributed to the role of genetic composition but are largely due to influence of the environment and geographic differences affecting the whole population such as climate, soil, water, diet, habits, customs etc:

i) White Europeans and Americans develop most commonly malignancies of the prostate, lung, breast and colorectal region. Liver cancer is uncommon in these races.

ii) Black Africans, on the other hand, have more commonly cancers of the skin, penis, cervix and liver.

iii) Japanese have five times higher incidence of carcinoma of the stomach than the Americans. Breast cancer is uncommon in Japanese women than American women.

iv) South-East Asians, especially of Chinese origin, develop nasopharyngeal cancer more commonly.

v) Indians of both sexes have higher incidence of carcinoma of the oral cavity and upper aerodigestive tract, while in females carcinoma of uterine cervix and of the breast run parallel in incidence.

3. ENVIRONMENTAL AND CULTURAL FACTORS It may seem rather surprising that through out our life we are surrounded by an environment of carcinogens which we eat, drink, inhale and touch. A few examples are:

i) Cigarette smoking

ii) Alcohol abuse

iii) Synergistic interaction of alcohol and tobacco

iv) Cancer of the cervix

v) Penile cancer

vi) Betel nut cancer

vii) Industrial and environmental substances

viii) Overweight individuals, deficiency of vitamin A and people consuming diet rich in animal fats.

4. AGE The most significant risk factor for cancer is age. Generally, cancers occur in older individuals past 5th decade of life (two-third of all cancers occur above 65 years of age), though there are variations in age incidence in different forms of cancers. Besides acute leukaemias, *other tumours in infancy and childhood* are: neuroblastoma, nephroblastoma (Wilms' tumour), retinoblastoma, hepatoblastoma, rhabdomyosarcoma, Ewing's sarcoma, teratoma and CNS tumours.

5. SEX Apart from the malignant tumours of organs peculiar to each sex, most tumours are generally more common in men than in women except cancer of the breast, gallbladder, thyroid and hypopharynx. Although there are geographic and racial variations, *cancer of the breast* is the commonest cancer in *women* throughout the world while *lung cancer* is the commonest cancer in *men*.

B. CHRONIC PRE-MALIGNANT AND NON-NEOPLASTIC CONDITIONS

Premalignant lesions are a group of conditions which predispose to the subsequent development of cancer. For example:

1. Dysplasia and carcinoma *in situ* (intraepithelial neoplasia)

i) Uterine cervix at the junction of ecto- and endocervix

ii) Bronchus
iii) Bowen's disease of the skin
iv) Actinic or solar keratosis
v) Oral leukoplakia
vi) Barrett's oesophagus developing metaplasia and dysplasia
vii) Intralobular and intraductal carcinoma of the breast.

2. Some benign tumours e.g.
i) Multiple adenomas of the large intestine have high incidence of developing adenocarcinoma.
ii) Neurofibromatosis (von Recklinghausen's disease) may develop into sarcoma.
iii) Pleomorphic adenoma (mixed salivary tumour) may sometimes develop carcinoma (carcinoma ex pleomophic adenoma).

3. Miscellaneous conditions Certain inflammatory (both infectious and non-infectious) and hyperplastic conditions are prone to development of cancer, e.g.
i) HPV-induced chronic cervicitis has high risk of developing cervical cancer.
ii) Patients of long-standing ulcerative colitis are predisposed to develop colorectal cancer.
iii) Cirrhosis of the liver has predisposition to develop hepatocellular carcinoma.
iv) *H. pylori* gastriits developing gastric cancer and lymphoma.
v) Chronic bronchitis in heavy cigarette smokers may develop cancer of the bronchus.
vi) Chronic irritation from jagged tooth or ill-fitting denture may lead to cancer of the oral cavity.
vii) Squamous cell carcinoma developing in an old burn scar (Marjolin's ulcer).

C. HORMONES AND CANCER

Cancer is more likely to develop in organs and tissues which undergo proliferation under the influence of excessive hormonal stimulation. Hormone-sensitive tissues developing tumours are the breast, endometrium, myometrium, vagina, thyroid, liver, prostate and testis.

1. OESTROGEN Women receiving oestrogen therapy and women with oestrogen-secreting granulosa cell tumour of the ovary have increased risk of developing endometrial carcinoma. Adenocarcinoma of the vagina is seen with increased frequency in adolescent daughters of mothers who had received oestrogen therapy during pregnancy.

2. CONTRACEPTIVE HORMONES The sequential types of oral contraceptives increase the risk of developing breast cancer. Other tumours showing a slightly increased frequency in women receiving contraceptive pills for long durations are benign tumours of the liver.

3. ANABOLIC STEROIDS Consumption of anabolic steroids by athletes increases the risk of developing benign and malignant tumours of the liver.

4. HORMONE-DEPENDENT TUMOURS For example:
i) *Prostatic cancer* usually responds to the administration of oestrogens.
ii) *Breast cancer* may regress with oophorectomy, hypophysectomy or on administration of male hormones.
iii) *Thyroid cancer* may slow down in growth with administration of thyroxine that suppresses the secretion of TSH by the pituitary.

MOLECULAR BASIS OF CANCER (p. 201)

1. Monoclonality of tumours There is strong evidence to support that most human cancers arise from a single clone of cells by genetic transformation or mutation. For example:
i) In a case of multiple myeloma (a malignant disorder of plasma cells), there is production of a single type of immunoglobulin.

ii) All the tumour cells in benign uterine tumours (leiomyoma) contain either A or B genotype of G6PD (i.e. the tumour cells are derived from a single progenitor clone of cell), while the normal myometrial cells are mosaic of both types of cells derived from A as well as B isoenzyme.

2. Field theory of cancer In an organ developing cancer, in the backdrop of normal cells, limited number of cells only grow in to cancer after undergoing sequence of changes under the influence of etiologic agents. This is termed as 'field effect'.

3. Multi-step process of cancer growth and progression Carcinogenesis is a gradual multi-step process involving many generations of cells. The various causes may act on the cell one after another (*multi-hit process*). The same process is also involved in further progression of the tumour.

4. Genetic theory of cancer Cell growth of normal as well as abnormal types is under genetic control. In cancer, there are either genetic abnormalities in the cell, or there are normal genes with abnormal expression. Thus the abnormalities in genetic composition may be from inherited or induced mutations (induced by etiologic carcinogenic agents namely: chemicals, viruses, radiation). Eventually, the mutated cells transmit their characters to the next progeny of cells and result in cancer.

5. Genetic regulators of normal and abnormal mitosis In normal cell growth, regulatory genes control mitosis as well as cell ageing, terminating in cell death by apoptosis.

◈ **In normal cell growth,** there are 4 regulatory genes:

i) *Proto-oncogenes* are growth-promoting genes i.e. they encode for cell proliferation pathway.

ii) *Anti-oncogenes* are growth-inhibiting or growth suppressor genes.

iii) *Apoptosis regulatory genes* control the programmed cell death.

iv) *DNA repair genes* are those normal genes which regulate the repair of DNA damage that has occurred during mitosis and also control the damage to proto-oncogenes and anti-oncogenes.

◈ **In cancer,** the transformed cells are produced by abnormal cell growth due to genetic damage to these normal controlling genes. Thus, corresponding abnormalities in these 4 cell regulatory genes are as under:

i) Activation of growth-promoting oncogenes causing transformation of cell (mutant form of normal proto-oncogene in cancer is termed *oncogene*).

ii) Inactivation of cancer-suppressor genes (i.e. inactivation of anti-oncogenes) permitting the cellular proliferation of transformed cells.

iii) Abnormal apoptosis regulatory genes which may act as oncogenes or anti-oncogenes.

iv) Failure of DNA repair genes and thus inability to repair the DNA damage resulting in mutations.

CANCER-RELATED GENES AND CELL GROWTH (HALLMARKS OF CANCER)

Genetic basis of cancer includes following *major genetic properties*, also termed as *molecular hallmarks of cancer*.

1. EXCESSIVE AND AUTONOMOUS GROWTH: GROWTH PROMOTING ONCOGENES

Mutated form of normal protooncogenes in cancer is called oncogenes. In general, overactivity of oncogenes enhances cell proliferation and promotes development of human cancer. Transformation of proto-oncogene (i.e. normal cell proliferation gene) to oncogenes (i.e. cancer cell proliferation gene) may occur by three mechanisms:

i) *Point mutations* i.e. an alteration of a single base in the DNA chain. The most important example is *RAS* oncogene.

ii) *Chromosomal translocations* i.e. transfer of a portion of one chromosome carrying protooncogene to another chromosome and making it independent of growth controls e.g.

◈ Philadelphia chromosome

◈ Burkitt's lymphoma

iii) *Gene amplification* i.e. increasing the number of copies of DNA sequence in protooncogene e.g.

◈ Neuroblastoma having *n-MYC HSR* region.

◈ *ERB-B1* in breast and ovarian cancer.

Most of the oncogenes encode for components of cell signaling system for promoting cell proliferation. Accordingly, these are given below under following 5 groups pertaining to different components of cell proliferation signaling systems:

	TYPE	ASSOCIATED HUMAN TUMOURS
1.	**GROWTH FACTORS**	
	i) *PDGF-β*	Gliomas, sarcoma
	ii) *TGF-α*	Carcinomas, astrocytoma
	iii) *FGF*	Bowel cancers
		Breast cancer
	iv) *c-MET*	Follicular carcinoma thyroid
2.	**RECEPTORS FOR GROWTH FACTORS**	
	i) *EGF* receptors	Squamous cell carcinoma lung, glioblastoma
		Ca breast, ovary, stomach, lungs
	ii) *c-KIT* receptor (Steel factor)	GIST
	iii) RET receptor	MEN type 2A and type 2B, medullary ca thyroid
	iv) FMS-like tyrosine kinase receptor	Acute myeloid leukaemia
3.	**CYTOPLASMIC SIGNAL TRANSDUCTION PROTEINS**	
	GTP-bound	Common in 1/3rd human tumours, Ca lung, colon, pancreas
	Non-GF receptor tyrosine kinase	CML, acute leukaemias
4.	**NUCLEAR TRANSCRIPTION FACTORS**	
	C-MYC	Burkitt's lymphoma
	N-MYC	Neuroblastoma, small cell Ca lung
	L-MYC	Small cell Ca lung
5.	**CELL CYCLE REGULATORY PROTEINS**	
	Cyclins	Ca breast, liver, mantle cell lymphoma
		Ca breast
	CDKs	Glioblastoma, melanoma, sarcomas

2. REFRACTORINESS TO GROWTH INHIBITION: GROWTH SUPPRESSING ANTI-ONCOGENES

The mutation of normal growth suppressor anti-oncogenes results in removal of the brakes for growth; thus the inhibitory effect to cell growth is removed and the abnormal growth continues unchecked. In other words, mutated anti-oncogenes behave like growth-promoting oncogenes.

Major anti-oncogenes implicated in human cancers are as under:

	GENE	ASSOCIATED HUMAN TUMOURS
1.	*RB*	Retinoblastoma, osteosarcoma
2.	*p53 (TP53)*	Most human cancers, common in Ca lung, head and neck, colon, breast
3.	*TGF–β and its receptor*	Ca pancreas, colon, stomach
4.	*APC and β-catenin proteins*	Ca colon

5. *Others*

i) BRCA 1 and 2	Ca breast, ovary
ii) VHL	Renal cell carcinoma
iii) WT 1 and 2	Wilms' tumour
iv) NF 1 and 2	Neurofibromatosis type 1 and 2

3. *ESCAPING CELL DEATH BY APOPTOSIS: GENES REGULATING APOPTOSIS AND CANCER*

Another mechanism of tumour growth is by escaping cell death by apoptosis. Apoptosis in normal cell is guided by cell death receptor, *CD95*, resulting in DNA damage. Besides, there is role of some other pro-apoptotic factors (*BAD, BAX, BID* and *p53*) and apoptosis-inhibitors (*BCL2, BCL-X*).

In cancer cells, the function of apoptosis is interfered due to mutations in the above genes which regulate apoptosis in the normal cell. For example:

a) **BCL2 gene** seen in normal lymphocytes, but its mutant form with characteristic translocation (t14;18) (q32;q21) was first described in B-cell lymphoma. It is also seen in many other human cancers such as that of breast, thyroid and prostate.

b) **CD95** receptors are depleted in hepatocellular carcinoma and hence the tumour cells escape apoptosis.

4. *AVOIDING CELLULAR AGEING: TELOMERES AND TELOMERASE IN CANCER*

After each mitosis (cell doubling) there is progressive shortening of telomeres which are the terminal tips of chromosomes. Telomerase is the RNA enzyme that helps in repair of such damage to DNA and maintains normal telomere length in successive cell divisions.

Cancer cells in most malignancies have markedly upregulated telomerase enzyme, and hence telomere length is maintained. Thus, cancer cells avoid ageing, mitosis does not slow down or cease, thereby immortalising the cancer cells.

5. *CONTINUED PERFUSION OF CANCER: TUMOUR ANGIOGENESIS*

Cancers can only survive and thrive if the cancer cells are adequately nourished and perfused, as otherwise they cannot grow further.

i) **Promoters of tumour angiogenesis** include the most important *vascular endothelial growth factor (VEGF)* (released from genes in the parenchymal tumour cells) and *basic fibroblast growth factor (bFGF)*.

ii) **Anti-angiogenesis factors** inhibiting angiogenesis include *thrombospondin-1* (also produced by tumour cells themselves), *angiostatin, endostatin and vasculostatin*.

6. *INVASION AND DISTANT METASTASIS: CANCER DISSEMINATION*

One of the most important characteristic of cancers is invasiveness and metastasis.

7. *DNA DAMAGE AND REPAIR SYSTEM: MUTATOR GENES AND CANCER*

p53 gene is held responsible for detection and repair of DNA damage. However, if this system of DNA repair is defective as happens in some inherited mutations (mutator genes), the defect in unrepaired DNA is passed to the next progeny of cells and cancer results. For example:

i) Hereditary non-polyposis colon cancer (HNPCC or Lynch syndrome)
ii) Ataxia telangiectasia (AT)
iii) Xeroderma pigmentosum
iv) Bloom syndrome
v) Hereditary breast cancer patients having mutated BRCA1 and BRCA2 genes.

8. CANCER PROGRESSION AND HETEROGENEITY: CLONAL AGGRESSIVENESS

Another feature of note in biology of cancers is that with passage of time cancers become more aggressive; this property is termed *tumour progression*. In terms of molecular biology, this attribute of cancer is due to the fact that with passage of time cancer cells acquire more and more *heterogeneity*.

9. CANCER—A SEQUENTIAL MULTISTEP MOLECULAR PHENOMENON: MULTISTEP THEORY

It needs to be appreciated that cancer occurs following several sequential steps of abnormalities in the target cell e.g. initiation, promotion and progression in proper sequence. Similarly, multiple steps are involved at genetic level by which cell proliferation of cancer cells is activated: by activation of growth promoters, loss of growth suppressors, inactivation of intrinsic apoptotic mechanisms and escaping cellular ageing. A classic example of this sequential genetic abnormalities in cancer is seen in adenoma-carcinoma sequence in development of colorectal carcinoma.

10. MICRO-RNAs IN CANCER: ONCOMIRS

◈   Normally, microRNAs function as the post-translational gene regulators of cell proliferation, differentiation and survival.

◈   In cancer, microRNAs have an oncogenic role in initiation and progression and are termed as oncogenic microRNAs, abbreviated as *oncomiRs*. These oncogenic microRNAs influence various cellular processes in cancer such as control of proliferation, cell cycle regulation, apoptosis, differentiation, metastasis and metabolism.

CARCINOGENS AND CARCINOGENESIS *(p. 209)*

Based on implicated causative agents, etiology and pathogenesis of cancer can be discussed under following 3 headings:
A.   Chemical carcinogens and chemical carcinogenesis
B.   Physical carcinogens and radiation carcinogenesis
C.   Biologic carcinogens and viral oncogenesis.

A. CHEMICAL CARCINOGENESIS *(p. 210)*

The first ever evidence of any cause for neoplasia came from the observation of Sir Percival Pott in 1775 that there was higher incidence of cancer of the scrotal skin in boys enganged in sweeping industrial chimneys in London. Similar other observations in occupational wokers who have skin soaked in industrial oils and reporting higher incidence of cancer of the skin invoked wide interest in soot and coal tar and its constituents as possible carcinogenic agents. Since then the list of chemical carcinogens which can experimentally induce cancer in animals and have epidemiological evidence in causing human neoplasia, is ever increasing.

STAGES IN CHEMICAL CARCINOGENESIS

Chemical carcinogenesis occurs by induction of mutation in the proto-oncogenes and anti-oncogenes. The phenomena of cellular transformation by chemical carcinogens (as also other carcinogens) is a progressive process involving 3 sequential stages:

INITIATION OF CARCINOGENESIS

Initiation is the first stage in carcinogenesis induced by initiator chemical carcinogens. The change can be produced by a single dose of the initiating agent for a short time, though larger dose for longer duration is more effective. The change so induced is sudden, irreversible and permanent.

1.   **Metabolic activation** Vast majority of chemical carcinogens are indirect-acting or procarcinogens requiring metabolic activation, while

direct-acting carcinogens do not require this activation. The indirect-acting carcinogens are activated in the liver by the mono-oxygenases of the cytochrome P-450 system in the endoplasmic reticulum.

2. Reactive electrophiles While direct-acting carcinogens are intrinsically electrophilic, indirect-acting substances become electron-deficient after metabolic activation i.e. they become reactive electrophiles.

3. Target molecules The primary target of electrophiles is DNA, producing mutagenesis. The change in DNA may lead to 'the initiated cell' or some form of cellular enzymes may be able to repair the damage in DNA.

It has been observed that most frequently affected growth promoter oncogene is *RAS* gene mutation and anti-oncogene (tumour suppressor) is *p53* gene mutation.

4. The initiated cell The unrepaired damage produced in the DNA of the cell becomes permanent and fixed only if the altered cell undergoes at least one cycle of proliferation. This results in transferring the change to the next progeny of cells so that the DNA damage becomes *permanent* and *irreversible*.

PROMOTION OF CARCINOGENESIS

Promotion is the next sequential stage in the chemical carcinogenesis. Promoters of carcinogenesis are substances such as phorbol esters, phenols, hormones, artificial sweeteners and drugs like phenobarbital. They differ from initiators in the following respects:

i) They do not produce sudden change.

ii) They require application or administration, as the case may be, *following* initiator exposure, for sufficient time and in sufficient dose.

iii) The change induced may be reversible.

iv) They do not damage the DNA *per se* and are thus not mutagenic but instead enhance the effect of direct-acting carcinogens or procarcinogens.

v) Tumour promoters act by further clonal proliferation and expansion of initiated (mutated) cells, and have reduced requirement of growth factor, especially after *RAS* gene mutation.

PROGRESSION OF CARCINOGENESIS

Progression of cancer is the stage when mutated proliferated cell shows phenotypic features of malignancy. These features pertain to morphology, biochemical composition and molecular features of malignancy. Such phenotypic features appear only when the initiated cell starts to proliferate rapidly and in the process acquires more and more mutations.

CARCINOGENIC CHEMICALS IN HUMANS

The list of diverse chemical compounds which can produce cancer in experimental animals is a long one but only some of them have sufficient epidemiological evidence in human neoplasia. Depending upon the mode of action of carcinogenic chemicals, they are divided into 2 broad groups: initiators and promoters.

INITIATOR CARCINOGENS

Chemical carcinogens which can initiate the process of neoplastic transformation are further categorised into 2 subgroups—

1. DIRECT-ACTING CARCINOGENS These chemical carcinogens do not require metabolic activation and fall into 2 classes:

i) **Alkylating agents** This group includes mainly various anti-cancer drugs (e.g. cyclophosphamide, chlorambucil, busulfan, melphalan, nitrosourea etc), β-propiolactone and epoxides. They are weakly carcinogenic and are implicated in the etiology of the lymphomas and leukaemias in human beings.

ii) **Acylating agents** The examples are acetyl imidazole and dimethyl carbamyl chloride.

2. INDIRECT-ACTING CARCINOGENS (PROCARCINOGENS) These are chemical substances which require prior metabolic activation before becoming potent 'ultimate' carcinogens. This group includes vast majority of carcinogenic chemicals. It includes the following 4 categories:

i) Polycyclic aromatic hydrocarbons They comprise the largest group of common procarcinogens which, after metabolic activation, can induce neoplasia.

Main sources of polycyclic aromatic hydrocarbons are: combustion and chewing of tobacco, smoke, fossil fuel (e.g. coal), soot, tar, mineral oil, smoked animal foods, industrial and atmospheric pollutants. Important chemical compounds included in this group are: anthracenes (benza-, dibenza-, dimethyl benza-), benzapyrene and methylcholanthrene. The following examples have evidence to support the etiologic role of these substances:

a) *Smoking and lung cancer:* There is 20 times higher incidence of lung cancer in smokers of 2 packs (40 cigarettes) per day for 20 years.

b) *Skin cancer:* Direct contact of polycyclic aromatic hydrocarbon compounds with skin is associated with higher incidence of skin cancer.

c) *Tobacco and betel nut chewing and cancer oral cavity:* Cancer of the oral cavity is more common in people chewing tobacco and betel nuts.

ii) Aromatic amines and azo-dyes For example:

a) β-*naphthylamine* in the causation of bladder cancer, especially in aniline dye and rubber industry workers.

b) *Benzidine* in the induction of bladder cancer.

c) *Azo-dyes* used for colouring foods (e.g. butter and margarine to give them yellow colour, scarlet red for colouring cherries etc) in the causation of hepatocellular carcinoma.

iii) Naturally-occurring products Some of the important chemical carcinogens derived from plant and microbial sources are aflatoxin B1, actinomycin D, mitomycin C, safrole and betel nuts. Out of these, aflatoxin B1 implicated in causing human hepatocellular carcinoma is the most important, especially when concomitant viral hepatitis B is present. It is derived from the fungus, *Aspergillus flavus*, that grows in stored grains and plants.

iv) Miscellaneous A variety of other chemical carcinogens having a role in the etiology of human cancer are as under:

a) *Nitrosamines and nitrosamides* are involved in gastric carcinoma.

b) *Vinyl chloride monomer* derived from polyvinyl chloride (PVC) polymer in the causation of haemangiosarcoma of the liver.

c) *Asbestos* in bronchogenic carcinoma and mesothelioma, especially in smokers.

d) *Arsenical compounds* in causing epidermal hyperplasia and basal cell carcinoma.

e) *Metals* like nickel, lead, cobalt, chromium etc in industrial workers causing lung cancer.

f) *Insecticides and fungicides* (e.g. aldrin, dieldrin, chlordane) in carcinogenesis in experimental animals.

g) *Saccharin and cyclomates* in cancer in experimental animals.

PROMOTER CARCINOGENS

Promoters are chemical substances which lack the intrinsic carcinogenic potential but their application subsequent to initiator exposure helps the initiated cell to proliferate further. These substances include phorbol esters, phenols, certain hormones and drugs.

TESTS FOR CHEMICAL CARCINOGENICITY

There are 2 main methods of testing chemical compound for its carcinogenicity:

1. EXPERIMENTAL INDUCTION The chemical is administered repeatedly, the dose varied, and promoting agents are administered subsequently. After many months, the animal is autopsied and results obtained.

2. **TESTS FOR MUTAGENICITY (AMES' TEST)** Ames' test evaluates the ability of a chemical to induce mutation in the mutant strain of *Salmonella typhimurium* that cannot synthesise histidine. Such strains are incubated with the potential carcinogen to which liver homogenate is added to supply enzymes required to convert procarcinogen to ultimate carcinogen. If the chemical under test is mutagenic, it will induce mutation in the mutant strains of *S. typhimurium* in the form of functional histidine gene, which will be reflected by the number of bacterial colonies growing on histidine-free culture medium.

B. PHYSICAL CARCINOGENESIS (p. 214)

Physical agents in carcinogenesis are divided into 2 groups:

RADIATION CARCINOGENESIS

Ultraviolet (UV) light and ionising radiation are the two main forms of radiation carcinogens which can induce cancer in experimental animals and are implicated in causation of some forms of human cancers. A property common between the two forms of radiation carcinogens is the appearance of mutations followed by a long period of latency after initial exposure, often 10-20 years or even later. Also, radiation carcinogens may act to enhance the effect of another carcinogen (co-carcinogens). Ultraviolet light and ionising radiation differ in their mode of action as below:

1. ULTRAVIOLET LIGHT The main source of UV radiation is the sunlight; others are UV lamps and welder's arcs. UV light penetrates the skin for a few millimetres only so that its effect is limited to epidermis. In humans, excessive exposure to UV rays can cause various forms of skin cancers—squamous cell carcinoma, basal cell carcinoma and malignant melanoma. In support of this is the epidemiological evidence of high incidence of these skin cancers in fair-skinned Europeans, albinos who do not tan readily, inhabitants of Australia and New Zealand living close to the equator who receive more sunlight.

2. IONISING RADIATION Ionising radiation of all kinds like X-rays, α-, β- and γ-rays, radioactive isotopes, protons and neutrons can cause cancer in animals and in man. Most frequently, radiation-induced cancers are all forms of leukaemias (except chronic lymphocytic leukaemia); others are cancers of the thyroid (most commonly papillary carcinoma), skin, breast, ovary, uterus, lung, myeloma, and salivary glands.

Damage to the DNA resulting in mutagenesis is the most important action of ionising radiation. It may cause chromosomal breakage, translocation, or point mutation. The effect depends upon a number of factors such as type of radiation, dose, dose-rate, frequency and various host factors such as age, individual susceptibility, immune competence, hormonal influences and type of cells irradiated.

NON-RADIATION PHYSICAL CARCINOGENESIS

A few rare examples of these uncommon associations are as under:

i) Stones in the gallbladder and in the urinary tract having higher incidence of cancers of these organs.

ii) Healed scars following burns or trauma for increased risk of carcinoma of affected skin.

iii) Occupational exposure to asbestos (asbestosis) associated with asbestos-associated tumours of the lung and malignant mesothelioma of the pleura.

iv) Workers engaged in hardwood cutting or engraving having high incidence of adenocarcioma of paranasal sinuses.

C. BIOLOGIC CARCINOGENESIS (p. 216)

The epidemiological studies on different types of cancers indicate the involvement of transmissible biologic agents in their development, chiefly *viruses*. Other microbial agents implicated in carcinogenesis are as follows:

❖ **Parasites** *Schistosoma haematobium* infection of the urinary bladder is associated with high incidence of squamous cell carcinoma of the urinary bladder in some parts of the world such as in Egypt. *Clonorchis sinensis*, the liver fluke, lives in the hepatic duct and is implicated in causation of cholangiocarcinoma.

❖ **Fungus** *Aspergillus flavus* grows in stored grains and liberates aflatoxin; its human consumption, especially by those with HBV infection, is associated with development of hepatocellular carcinoma.

❖ **Bacteria** *Helicobacter pylori*, a gram-positive spiral-shaped micro-organism, colonises the gastric mucosa and has been found in cases of chronic gastritis and peptic ulcer; its prolonged infection may lead to gastric lymphoma and gastric carcinoma.

VIRAL CARCINOGENESIS

It has been estimated that about 20% of all cancers worldwide are due to persistent virus infection. Most of the common viral infections (including oncogenic viruses) can be transmitted by one of the 3 routes:

i) *Horizontal transmission* Commonly, viral infection passes from one to another by direct contact, by ingestion of contaminated water or food, or by inhalation as occurs in most contagious diseases.

ii) *By parenteral route* such as by inoculation as happens in some viruses by inter-human spread and from animals and insects to humans.

iii) *Vertical transmission*, when the infection is genetically transmitted from infected parents to offsprings.

Based on their nucleic acid content, oncogenic viruses fall into 2 broad groups:

1. Those containing deoxyribonucleic acid are called *DNA oncogenic viruses.*

2. Those containing ribonucleic acid are termed *RNA oncogenic viruses or retroviruses.*

VIRAL ONCOGENESIS: GENERAL ASPECTS

Support to the etiologic role of oncogenic viruses in causation of human cancers is based on the following:

1. Epidemiologic data.
2. Presence of viral DNA in the genome of host target cell.
3. Demonstration of virally induced transformation of human target cells in culture.
4. *In vivo* demonstration of expressed specific transforming viral genes in premalignant and malignant cells.
5. *In vitro* assay of specific viral gene products which produce effects on cell proliferation and survival.

1. Mode of DNA viral oncogenesis Host cells infected by DNA oncogenic viruses may have one of the following 2 results:

i) *Replication* The virus may replicate in the host cell with consequent lysis of the infected cell and release of virions.

ii) *Integration* The viral DNA may integrate into the host cell DNA.

The latter event (integration) results in inducing mutation and thus neoplastic transformation of the host cell, while the former (replication) brings about cell death but no neoplastic transformation. A feature essential for host cell transformation is the expression of virus-specific T-(transforming protein) antigens immediately after infection of the host cell by DNA oncogenic virus (discussed later).

2. Mode of RNA viral oncogenesis RNA viruses or retroviruses contain two identical strands of RNA and the enzyme, reverse transcriptase:

i) Reverse transcriptase is RNA-dependent DNA synthetase that acts as a template to synthesise *a single strand of matching viral* DNA i.e. reverse of the normal in which DNA is transcribed into messenger RNA.

ii) The single strand of viral DNA is then copied by DNA-dependent DNA synthetase to form another strand of complementary DNA resulting in *double-stranded viral* DNA or provirus.

iii) The provirus is then integrated into the DNA of the host cell genome and may induce mutation and thus transform the cell into *neoplastic cell.*

iv) Retroviruses are *replication-competent.* The host cells which allow replication of integrated retrovirus are called permissive cells. Non-permissible cells do not permit replication of the integrated retrovirus.

v) Viral replication begins after integration of the provirus into host cell genome. Integration results in transcription of proviral genes or progenes into messenger RNA which then forms *components of the virus particle—* virion core protein from *gag* gene, reverse transcriptase from *pol* gene, and envelope glycoprotein from *env* gene.

DNA ONCOGENIC VIRUSES

DNA oncogenic viruses have direct access to the host cell nucleus and are incorporated into the genome of the host cell. DNA viruses are classified into 5 subgroups, each of which is capable of producing neoplasms in different hosts. These are as under:

	VIRUS & HOST	ASSOCIATED TUMOUR
1.	PAPOVAVIRUSES	
	Human papilloma virus **Humans**	Cervical cancer and its precursor lesions, squamous cell carcinoma at other sites Skin cancer in epidermodysplasia verruciformis Papillomas (warts) on skin, larynx, genitals (genital warts)
	Papilloma viruses Cotton-tail rabbits Bovine	Papillomas (warts) Alimentary tract cancer
	Polyoma virus Mice	Various carcinomas, sarcomas
	SV-40 virus Monkeys Hamsters **Humans**	Harmless Sarcoma ? Mesothelioma
2.	HERPESVIRUSES	
	Epstein-Barr virus **Humans**	Burkitt's lymphoma Nasopharyngeal carcinoma
	Human herpesvirus 8 (Kaposi's sarcoma herpesvirus) **Humans**	Kaposi's sarcoma Pleural effusion lymphoma
	Lucke' frog virus Frog	Renal cell carcinoma
	Marek's disease virus Chickens	T-cell leukaemia-lymphoma
3.	ADENOVIRUSES Hamsters	Sarcomas
4.	POXVIRUSES Rabbits **Humans**	Myxomatosis Molluscum contagiosum, papilloma
5.	HEPADNAVIRUSES	
	Hepatitis B virus **Humans**	Hepatocellular carcinoma

RNA oncogenic viruses are retroviruses i.e. they contain the enzyme reverse transcriptase (RT), though all retroviruses are not oncogenic. The enzyme, reverse transcriptase, is required for reverse transcription of viral RNA to synthesise viral DNA strands i.e. reverse of normal—rather than DNA encoding for RNA synthesis, viral RNA transcripts for the DNA by the enzyme RT present in the RNA viruses. RT is a DNA polymerase and helps to form complementary DNA (cDNA) that moves into host cell nucleus and gets incorporated into it.

Based on their activity to transform target cells into neoplastic cells, RNA viruses are divided into 3 subgroups as under:

VIRUS & HOST	ASSOCIATED TUMOUR
1. ACUTE TRANSFORMING VIRUSES	
Rous sarcoma virus Chickens	Sarcoma
Leukaemia-sarcoma virus Avian, feline, bovine, primate	Leukaemias, sarcomas
2. SLOW TRANSFORMING VIRUSES	
Mice, cats, bovine	Leukaemias, lymphomas
Mouse mammary tumour virus (Bittner milk factor) Daughter mice	Breast cancer
3. HUMAN T-CELL LYMPHOTROPIC VIRUS (HTLV)	
HTLV-I **Human**	Adult T-cell leukaemia lymphoma (ATLL)
HTLV-II **Human**	T-cell variant of hairy cell leukaemia
4. HEPATITIS C VIRUS (HCV)	
Human	Hepatocellular carcinoma

VIRUSES AND HUMAN CANCER: A SUMMARY

In humans, epidemiological as well as circumstantial evidence has been accumulating since the discovery of contagious nature of common human wart (papilloma) in 1907 that cancer may have viral etiology. Presently, about 20% of all human cancers worldwide are virally induced. Different viruses implicated in human tumours are as under:

Benign tumours:
i) Human wart (papilloma) caused by human papilloma virus
ii) Molluscum contagiosum caused by poxvirus

Malignant tumours:
i) *Burkitt's lymphoma* by Epstein-Barr virus.
ii) *Nasopharyngeal carcinoma* by Epstein-Barr virus.
iii) *Primary hepatocellular carcinoma* by hepatitis B virus and hepatitis C virus.
iv) *Cervical cancer* by high risk human papilloma virus types (HPV 16 and 18).
v) *Kaposi's sarcoma* by human herpes virus type 8 (HHV-8).
vi) *Pleural effusion B cell lymphoma* by HHV8.
vii) *Adult T-cell leukaemia and lymphoma* by HTLV-1.
viii) *T-cell variant of hairy cell leukaemia* by HTLV-2.

Current knowledge and understanding of viral carcinogenesis has provided an opportunity to invent specific vaccines and suggest appropriate specific therapy. For example, hepatitis B vaccines is being widely used to control hepatitis B and is expected to lower incidence of HBV-related hepatocellular **129** carcinoma in high risk populltations. HPV vaccine is being used in some countries in young women and is expeted to protect them against HPV-associated precancerous lesions of the cervix.

Chapter 7

Neoplasia

CLINICAL ASPECTS OF NEOPLASIA (p. 222)

HOST RESPONSE AGAINST TUMOUR (TUMOUR IMMUNOLOGY) (p. 222)

It has long been known that body's immune system can recognise tumour cells as 'non-self' and they attempt to destroy them and limit the spread of cancer. The following observations provide basis for this concept:

1. Certain cancers evoke significant *lymphocytic infiltrate* composed of immunocompetent cells and such tumours have somewhat better prognosis e.g. medullary carcinoma breast (as compared with infiltrating ductal carcinoma), seminoma testis (as compared with other germ cell tumours of testis).

2. Rarely, a cancer may *spontaneously regress* partially or completely, probably under the influence of host defense mechanism. For example, rare spontaneous disappearance of malignant melanoma temporarily from the primary site which may then reappear as metastasis.

3. It is highly unusual to have primary and *secondary tumours in the spleen* due to its ability to destroy the growth and proliferation of tumour cells.

4. Existence of immune surveillance is substantiated by increased frequency of *cancers in immunodeficient host* e.g. in AIDS patients, or development of post-transplant lymphoproliferative disease.

1. TUMOUR ANTIGENS

Tumour cells express surface antigens which have been seen in animals and in some human tumours. Presently distinction of tumour antigens is based on their recognition by the host immune cells, i.e. CD8+ T cells (CTL), and by the molecular structure of the tumour antigens. Currently, various groups of tumour antigens are as follows:

i) Oncoproteins from mutated oncogenes e.g. products of *RAS*, *BCL/ RABL* and CDK4.

ii) Protein products of tumour suppressor genes e.g. mutated proteins *p53* and β-catenin.

iii) Overexpressed cellular proteins e.g. in melanoma the tumour antigen is structurally normal melanocyte specific protein, tyrosinase, which is overexpressed. Similarly, *HER2/neu* protein is overexpressed in many cases of breast cancer.

iv) Abnormally expressed cellular proteins e.g. *MAGE* gene silent in normal adult tissues except in male germ line but *MAGE* genes are expressed on surface of many tumours such as melanoma (abbreviation *MAGE* from 'melanoma antigen' in which it was first found), cancers of liver, lung, stomach and oesophagus.

v) Tumour antigens from viral oncoproteins e.g. viral oncoproteins of HPV (E6, E7) in cervical cancer and EBNA proteins of EBV in Burkitt's lymphoma.

vi) Tumour antigens from randomly mutated genes Mutated cells elaborate protein products targeted by CTL.

vii) Cell specific differentiation antigens e.g. various CD markers for various subtypes of lymphomas, prostate specific antigen (PSA) in carcinoma of prostate.

viii) Oncofoetal antigens e.g. AFP in liver cancer and CEA in colon cancer.

ix) Abnormal cell surface molecules e.g. there may be changed blood group antigen, or abnormal expression of mucin in ovarian cancer (CA-125) and in breast cancer (MUC-1).

Although both cell-mediated and humoral immunity is mounted by the host against the tumour, siginificant anti-tumour effector mechanism is mainly cell-mediated.

i)   Cell-mediated   mechanism This   is   the   main   mechanism   of destruction of tumour cells by the host. The following cellular responses can destroy the tumour cells and induce tumour immunity in humans:

a)   *Specifically sensitised cytotoxic T lymphocytes (CTL)* i.e. CD8+ T cells are directly cytotoxic to the target cell and require contact between them and tumour cells.

b)   *Natural killer (NK) cells* are lymphocytes which after activation by IL-2, destroy tumour cells without sensitisation, either directly or by antibody-dependent cellular cytotoxicity (ADCC).

c) *Macrophages* are activated by interferon-γ secreted by T-cells and NK-cells, and therefore there is close collaboration of these two subpopulations of lymphocytes and macrophages.

ii)   Humoral   mechanism As   such   there   are   no   anti-tumour humoral antibodies which are effective against cancer cells *in vivo*. However, *in vitro* humoral antibodies may kill tumour cells by complement activation or by antibody-dependent cytotoxicity.

3. CANCER IMMUNOTHERAPY

It is a generally-accepted hypothesis that the best defense against human diseases is our own immune system. As outlined above, in cancer the immune system starts failing and requires to be boosted to become more effective in fighting against cancer. Immunotherapy has been used as treatment against cancer in combination with other therapies (surgery, radiation, chemotherapy) as under:

i)   Non-specific stimulation of the host immune response.

ii)   Specific stimulation of the immune system.

iii)   Current status of immunotherapy is focussed on following three main approaches:

a)   Cellular immunotherapy

b)   Cytokine therapy

c)   Monoclonal antibody therapy.

EFFECT OF TUMOUR ON HOST *(p. 224)*

Malignant tumours produce more ill-effects than the benign tumours. The effects may be local, or generalised and more widespread.

A. LOCAL EFFECTS

Both benign and malignant tumours cause local effects on the host due to their size or location. Malignant tumours due to rapid and invasive growth potential have more serious effects. Some of the local effects of tumours are as under:

i)   Compression

ii)   Mechanical obstruction

iii)   Tissue destruction

iv)   Infarction, ulceration, haemorrhage

B. SYSTEMIC MANIFESTATIONS

Generalised effects of cancer include cancer cachexia, fever, tumour lysis syndrome and paraneoplastic syndromes.

1.   CANCER CACHEXIA Patients with advanced and disseminated cancers terminally have asthenia (emaciation), and anorexia, together referred to as cancer cachexia (meaning wasting).

2.   FEVER Fever of unexplained origin may be presenting feature in some malignancies such as in Hodgkin's disease, adenocarcinoma kidney, osteogenic sarcoma and many other tumours.

3. TUMOUR LYSIS SYNDROME This is a condition caused by extensive destruction of a large number of rapidly proliferating tumour cells. The condition is seen more often in cases of lymphomas and leukaemias than solid tumours and may be due to large tumour burden (e.g. in Burkitt's lymphoma), chemotherapy, administration of glucocorticoids or certain hormonal agents (e.g. tamoxifen).

4. PARANEOPLASTIC SYNDROMES Paraneoplastic syndromes (PNS) are a group of conditions developing in patients with advanced cancer which are neither explained by direct and distant spread of the tumour, nor by the usual hormone elaboration by the tissue of origin of the tumour.

The various clinical syndromes included in the PNS are as under:

i) **Endocrine syndrome** e.g.
a) Hypercalcaemia
b) Cushing's syndrome
c) Polycythaemia
d) Hypoglycaemia

ii) **Neuromyopathic syndromes** e.g. peripheral neuropathy, cortical cerebellar degeneration, myasthenia gravis syndrome, polymyositis.

iii) **Effects on osseous, joints and soft tissue** e.g. hypertrophic pulmonary osteoarthropathy and clubbing of fingers.

iv) **Haematologic and vascular syndrome** e.g. venous thrombosis (Trousseau's phenomenon), non-bacterial thrombotic endocarditis, disseminated intravascular coagulation (DIC), leukemoid reaction and normocytic normochromic anaemia occurring in advanced cancers.

v) **Gastrointestinal syndromes** e.g. Malabsorption, hypoalbuminaemia .

vi) **Renal syndromes** e.g. Renal vein thrombosis, systemic amyloidosis

vii) **Cutaneous syndromes** e.g. Acanthosis nigricans, seborrheic dermatitis, exfoliative dermatitis.

viii) **Amyloidosis** Primary amyloid deposits may occur in multiple myeloma whereas renal cell carcinoma and other solid tumours may be associated with secondary systemic amyloidosis.

PATHOLOGIC DIAGNOSIS OF CANCER *(p. 226)*

1. HISTOLOGICAL METHODS

These methods are most valuable in arriving at the accurate diagnosis and are based on microscopic examination of excised tumour mass or open/needle biopsy from the mass supported with complete clinical and investigative data. The tissue must be fixed in 10% formalin for light microscopic examination and in glutaraldehyde for electron microscopic studies, while quick-frozen section and hormonal analysis are carried out on fresh unfixed tissues. These methods are as under:

i) Paraffin-embedding technique The represesentative tissue piece from larger tumour mass or biopsy is processed through a tissue processor having an overnight cycle, embedded in molten paraffin wax for making tissue blocks. These blocks are trimmed followed by fine-sectioning into 3-4 μm sections using rotary microtome for which either fixed knife or disposable blades are used for cutting. These sections are then stained with haematoxylin and eosin (H & E) and examined microscopically.

ii) Frozen section In this technique, unfixed tissue is used and the procedure is generally carried out when the patient is undergoing surgery and is still under anaesthesia. Here, instead of tissue processor and paraffin-embedding, cryostat machine is used and fresh unfixed tissue is used. The tissue biopsy is quickly frozen to ice at about −25°C that acts as embedding medium and then sectioned. Sections are then ready for rapid H & E or toluidine blue staining.

2. CYTOLOGICAL METHODS

Cytological methods for diagnosis consist of 2 types of methods: study of cells shed off into body cavities (exfoliative cytology) and study of cells by

3. HISTOCHEMISTRY AND CYTOCHEMISTRY

Histochemistry and cytochemistry are additional diagnostic tools which help the pathologist in identifying the chemical composition of cells, their constituents and their products by special staining methods. Though immunohistochemical techniques are more useful for tumour diagnosis, histochemical and cytochemical stains (also called as special stains) are still employed for this purpose. Some of the common examples are as under:

	SUBSTANCE	STAIN
1.	Basement membrane/ collagen	Periodic acid-Schiff (PAS) Reticulin Van Gieson Masson's trichrome
2.	Glycogen	PAS with diastase loss
3.	Acid mucin (mesenchymal origin)	Alcian blue
4.	Mucin (in general)	Combined Alcian blue-PAS
5.	Argyrophilic/ argentaffin granules	Silver stains
6.	Cross striations	PTAH stain
7.	Enzymes	Myeloperoxidase Acid phosphatase Alkaline phosphatase
8.	Nucleolar organiser regions (NORs)	Colloidal silver stain

4. IMMUNOHISTOCHEMISTRY

With current technology, it is possible to use routinely processed paraffin-embedded tissue blocks for immunohistochemistry (IHC), thus making profound impact on diagnostic surgical pathology. Earlier, diagnostic surgical pathology used to be considered a subjective science with inter-observer variation, particularly in borderline lesions and lesions of undetermined origin, but use of IHC has added *objectivity, specificity* and *reproducibility* to the surgical pathologist's diagnosis.

IHC is an immunological method of recognising a cell by one or more of its specific components in the cell membrane, cytoplasm or nucleus and are accordingly interpreted.

Various applications of IHC in tumour diagnosis are as under:

i)   Tumours of uncertain histogenesis Towards this, IHC stains for *intermediate filaments* (keratin, vimentin, desmin, neurofilaments, and glial fibrillary acidic proteins) expressed by the tumour cells are of immense value besides other common IHC stains.

ii)   Prognostic markers in cancer e.g. proto-oncogenes (e.g. HER-2/ neu overexpression in carcinoma breast), tumour suppressor genes or antioncogenes (e.g. *Rb* gene, *p53*), growth factor receptors (e.g. epidermal growth factor receptor or *EGFR*), and tumour cell proliferation markers (e.g. *Ki67*, proliferation cell nuclear antigen *PCNA*).

iii)   Prediction of response to therapy IHC is widely used to predict therapeutic response in two important tumours—ER and PR in carcinoma of the breast and androgen receptors in carcinoma prostate.

iv)   Infections e.g. detection of viruses (HBV, CMV, HPV, herpesviruses), bacteria (e.g. *Helicobacter pylori*), and parasites (*Pneumocystis carinii*) etc.

5. ELECTRON MICROSCOPY

Ultrastructural examination of tumour cells offers selective role in diagnostic pathology. A few general features of malignant tumour cells by EM examination can be appreciated:

i) Cell junctions, their presence and type.
ii) Cell surface, e.g. presence of microvilli.
iii) Cell shape and cytoplasmic extensions.
iv) Shape of the nucleus and features of nuclear membrane.
v) Nucleoli, their size and density.
vi) Cytoplasmic organelles—their number is generally reduced.
vii) Dense bodies in the cytoplasm.
viii) Any other secretory product in the cytoplasm e.g. melanosomes in melanoma and membrane-bound granules in endocrine tumours.

6. TUMOUR MARKERS (BIOCHEMICAL ASSAYS)

In order to distinguish from the preceding techniques of tumour diagnosis in which 'stains' are imparted on the tumour cells in section or smear, tumour markers are biochemical assays of products elaborated by the tumour cells in blood or other body fluids.

Tumour markers include: cell surface antigens (or oncofoetal antigens), cytoplasmic proteins, enzymes, hormones and cancer antigens. Two of the best known examples of oncofoetal antigens secreted by foetal tissues as well as by tumours are as under:

i) **Alpha-foetoprotein (AFP)** This is a glycoprotein synthesised normally by foetal liver cells. Their serum levels are elevated in hepatocellular carcinoma and non-seminomatous germ cell tumours of the testis. Certain non-neoplastic conditions also have increased serum levels of AFP e.g. in hepatitis, cirrhosis, toxic liver injury and pregnancy.

ii) **Carcino-embryonic antigen (CEA)** CEA is also a glycoprotein normally synthesised in embryonic tissue of the gut, pancreas and liver. Their serum levels are high in cancers of the gastrointestinal tract, pancreas and breast. As in AFP, CEA levels are also elevated in certain non-neoplastic conditions e.g. in ulcerative colitis, Crohn's disease, hepatitis and chronic bronchitis.

7. OTHER MODERN AIDS IN PATHOLOGIC DIAGNOSIS OF TUMOURS

In addition to the methods described above, some other modern diagnostic techniques have emerged for tumour diagnostic pathology but their availability as well as applicability are limited.

i) **Flow cytometry** This is a computerised technique by which the detailed characteristics of individual tumour cells are recognised and quantified and the data can be stored for subsequent comparison too.

ii) **In situ hybridisation** This is a molecular technique by which nucleic acid sequences (cellular/viral DNA and RNA) can be localised by specifically-labelled nucleic acid probe directly in the intact cell (in situ) rather than by DNA extraction.

iii) **Cell proliferation analysis** Besides flow cytometry, the degree of proliferation of cells in tumours can be determined by various other methods e.g.
a) Mitotic count
b) Radioautography
c) Microspectrophotometric analysis
d) IHC proliferation markers
e) Nucleolar organiser region (NOR)

iv) **Image analyzer and morphometry** The system is used to perform measurement of architectural, cellular and nuclear features of tumour cells.

v) **Molecular diagnostic techniques** The group of molecular biologic methods in the tumour diagnostic laboratory are a variety of DNA/RNA-based molecular techniques in which the DNA/RNA are extracted (compared from in situ above) from the cell and then analysed. Molecular diagnostic techniques include: DNA analysis by Southern blot, RNA analysis by northern blot, and polymerase chain reaction (PCR).

vi) DNA microarray analysis of tumours Currently, it is possible to perform molecular profiling of a tumour by use of gene chip technology which allows measurement of levels of expression of several thousand genes (up-regulation or down-regulation) simultaneously.

SELF ASSESSMENT

1. **Hamartoma refers to:**
   A. Tumour differentiating towards more than one cell line
   B. Tumour arising from totipotent cells
   C. Mass of disorganised but mature cells indigenous to the part
   D. Mass of ectopic rests of normal tissue

2. **Increased number of normal mitoses may be present in the following tissues <u>except</u>:**
   A. Bone marrow cells   B. Nails
   C. Hepatocytes   D. Intestinal epithelium

3. **A tumour is termed medullary when it is almost entirely composed of:**
   A. Amyloid stroma   B. Large areas of necrosis
   C. Abundant lymphoid tissue   D. Parenchymal cells

4. **All the following malignant tumours metastasise <u>except</u>:**
   A. Synovial sarcoma   B. Malignant mesothelioma
   C. Glioma   D. Neuroblastoma

5. **The following malignant tumours frequently spread through haematogenous route <u>except</u>:**
   A. Bronchogenic carcinoma   B. Renal cell carcinoma
   C. Follicular carcinoma thyroid   D. Seminoma testis

6. **Degradation of ECM is brought about by the following <u>except</u>:**
   A. Proteases   B. Metalloproteinases
   C. Free radicals   D. Cathepsin D

7. **Grading of tumours depends upon the following <u>except</u>:**
   A. Degree of anaplasia   B. Metastatic spread
   C. Rate of growth of cells   D. Degree of differentiation

8. **Patients of xeroderma pigmentosum are prone to develop the following cancers <u>except</u>:**
   A. Basal cell carcinoma   B. Sweat gland carcinoma
   C. Malignant melanoma   D. Squamous cell carcinoma

9. **The primary target of reactive electrophiles is as under:**
   A. Cytochrome P-450   B. RNA
   C. DNA   D. Mitochondria

10. **Carcinogenic influence of radiation appears after:**
    A. < 2 years   B. 2-5 years
    C. 5-10 years   D. > 10 years

11. **The following hereditary diseases have higher incidence of cancers due to inherited defect in DNA repair mechanism <u>except</u>:**
    A. Ataxia telangiectasia   B. Xeroderma pigmentosum
    C. Familial polyposis coli   D. Bloom's syndrome

12. **The following form of ionising radiation exposure is associated with highest risk of cancer:**
    A. α-rays   B. β-rays
    C. γ-rays   D. X-rays

13. **Women receiving oestrogen therapy have an increased risk of developing the following cancers <u>except</u>:**
    A. Breast cancer   B. Endometrial carcinoma
    C. Gallbladder cancer   D. Hepatocellular carcinoma

14. **Important cyclins in cell cycle include the following <u>except</u>:**
    A. Cyclin A
    B. Cyclin B
    C. Cyclin C
    D. Cyclin D
15. **Bittner milk factor is a transmissible agent belonging to the following category:**
    A. Acute transforming virus
    B. Slow transforming virus
    C. HTLV-I
    D. HTLV-II
16. **Important examples of tumour suppressor genes implicated in human cancers include the following <u>except</u>:**
    A. *RB gene*
    B. *TP53*
    C. *APC*
    D. *ERB-B*
17. **An example of tumour-associated antigen (TAA) is:**
    A. Testis specific antigen (MAGE)
    B. Alpha-fetoprotein (AFP)
    C. Carcinoembryonic antigen (CEA)
    D. Prostate specific antigen (PSA)
18. **Hypercalcaemia as a paraneoplastic syndrome is observed in the following tumours <u>except</u>:**
    A. Squamous cell carcinoma lung
    B. Small cell carcinoma lung
    C. Renal cell carcinoma
    D. Breast cancer
19. **Lymphocytic infiltrate is frequently present in the following tumours indicative of host immune response <u>except</u>:**
    A. Seminoma testis
    B. Medullary carcinoma breast
    C. Papillary carcinoma thyroid
    D. Malignant melanoma
20. **The following antibody-stain is used in immunohistochemistry to identify epithelial cells:**
    A. Desmin
    B. Vimentin
    C. Cytokeratin
    D. Neurofilaments
21. **Which of the following viral infection is not known to produce any human tumour?**
    A. Polyoma virus
    B. EBV
    C. HSV
    D. HTLV
22. **All are autosomal dominant inherited cancer syndromes <u>except</u>:**
    A. Retinoblastoma
    B. Xeroderma pigmentosum
    C. HNPCC
    D. Neurofibromatosis
23. **Phosphorylation of retinoblastoma gene:**
    A. Inhibits cell replication
    B. Promotes cellular quiescence
    C. Stops cell cycle progression
    D. Promotes cell division
24. **p53:**
    A. Activates cyclins
    B. Activates BAX
    C. Activates CDKs
    D. Activates bcl2
25. **All are matrix metalloproteinases <u>except</u>:**
    A. Collagenase
    B. Gelatinase
    C. Stromelysin
    D. Elastase
26. **All are anti-angiogenesis factors <u>except</u>:**
    A. Thrombospondin-1
    B. Basic fibroblast growth factor (bFGF)
    C. Endostatin
    D. Angiostatin
27. **Which of the following is a test for mutagenicity?**
    A. Kveim's test
    B. Ame's test
    C. Schilling's test
    D. Mantoux test

28. **All are autosomal dominant inherited cancer syndromes except:**
    A. Retinoblastoma
    B. Xeroderma pigmentosum
    C. HNPCC
    D. Neurofibromatosis

29. **DNA extraction is a pre-requisite for the following molecular techniques except:**
    A. PCR technique
    B. In situ hybridisation
    C. Western blot technique
    D. Southern blot technique

30. **All are methods of cell proliferation analysis except:**
    A. Microspectrophotometry
    B. Flow cytometry
    C. PCR
    D. Immunohistochemistry

KEY

1 = C	2 = B	3 = D	4 = C	5 = D
6 = C	7 = B	8 = B	9 = C	10 = D
11 = C	12 = A	13 = C	14 = C	15 = B
16 = D	17 = D	18 = B	19 = C	20 = C
21 = A	22 = B	23 = D	24 = B	25 = D
26 = B	27 = B	28 = B	29 = B	30 = C

8 Environmental and Nutritional Diseases

ENVIRONMENTAL DISEASES (p. 231)

The subject of environmental hazards to health has assumed great significance in the modern world. Currently, the field of 'environmental pathology' encompasses all such diseases caused by progressive deterioration in the environment, most of which is man-made. Some of the important factors which have led to the alarming environmental degradation are as under:

1. Population explosion
2. Urbanisation of rural and forest land to accommodate the increasing numbers
3. Accumulation of wastes
4. Unsatisfactory disposal of radioactive and electronic waste
5. Industrial effluents and automobile exhausts.

But the above atmospheric pollutants appear relatively minor compared with *voluntary intake of three pollutants*—use of tobacco, consumption of alcohol and intoxicant drugs. The WHO estimates that 80% cases of cardiovascular disease and type 2 diabetes mellitus, and 40% of all cancers are preventable through 'three pillars of prevention': avoidance of tobacco, healthy diet and physical activity. The WHO has further determined that about a quarter of global burden of diseases and 23% of all deaths are related to modifiable environmental factors. Infant mortality related to environmental factors in developing countries is 12 times higher than in the developed countries.

ENVIRONMENTAL POLLUTION (p. 231)

Environment is air we collectively breathe and share with others at all places—outside, inside homes and at work place. *Pollution* is the contamination of the natural environment which determines adverse effects on health.

AIR POLLUTION

For survival of mankind, it is important to prevent depletion of ozone layer (O_3) in the outer space from pollutants such as chlorofluorocarbons and nitrogen dioxide produced in abundance by day-to-day activities on our planet earth due to industrial effluent and automobile exhausts.

A vast variety of pollutants are inhaled daily, some of which may cause trivial irritation to the upper respiratory pathways, while others may lead to acute or chronic injury to the lungs, and some are implicated in causation of lung cancer. Whereas some pollutants are prevalent in certain industries (such as coal dust, silica, asbestos), others are general pollutants present widespread in the ambient atmosphere (e.g. sulphur dioxide, nitrogen dioxide, carbon monoxide).

The adverse effects of air pollutants on lung depend upon a few variables that include:

i) longer duration of exposure;
ii) total dose of exposure;
iii) impaired ability of the host to clear inhaled particles; and
iv) particle size of 1-5 μm capable of getting impacted in the distal airways to produce tissue injury.

Our environment gets affected by long-term or accidental exposure to certain man-made or naturally-occurring chemicals. A large number of chemicals are found as contaminants in the ecosystem, food and water supply and find their way into the food chain of man. These substances exert their toxic effects depending upon their mode of absorption, distribution, metabolism and excretion. Some of the substances are directly toxic while others cause ill-effects via their metabolites.

A few common examples of environmental chemicals are as follows:

1. Agriculture chemicals Modern agriculture thrives on pesticides, fungicides, herbicides and organic fertilisers which may pose a potential acute poisoning as well as long-term hazard. The problem is particularly alarming in developing countries like India, China and Mexico where farmers and their families are unknowingly exposed to these hazardous chemicals during aerial spraying of crops.

◈ Acute poisoning by organophosphate insecticides

◈ Chronic human exposure to low level agricultural chemicals.

2. Volatile organic solvents e.g. methanol, chloroform, petrol, kerosene, benzene, ethylene glycol, toluene etc.

3. Metals e.g. mercury, arsenic, cadmium, iron, nickel and aluminium.

4. Aromatic hydrocarbons containing polychlorinated biphenyl which are contaminant in several preservatives, herbicides and antibacterial agents.

5. Cyanide Cyanide in the environment is released by combustion of plastic, silk and is also present in cassava and the seeds of apricots and wild cherries. Cyanide is a very toxic chemical and kills by blocking cellular respiration by binding to mitochondrial cytochrome oxidase.

6. Environmental dusts These substances cause pneumoconioses while others are implicated in cancer.

TOBACCO SMOKING

HABITS

Tobacco smoking is the most prevalent and preventable cause of disease and death. Cigarette smoking is a major health problem all over the world. In India, a country of 1.25 billion people, a quarter (300 million) are tobacco users in one form or the other. Smoking *bidis* and chewing *pan masala*, *zarda* and *gutka* are more widely practiced than cigarettes. Another habit prevalent in Indian states of Uttar Pradesh and Bihar is chewing of tobacco alone or mixed with slaked lime as a bolus of *paan* kept in mouth for long hours which is the major cause of cancer of upper aerodigestive tract and oral cavity.

Besides the harmful effects of smoking on active smokers themselves, involuntary exposure of smoke to bystanders (passive smoking) is also injurious to health, particularly to infants and children.

DOSE AND DURATION

Tobacco contains several harmful constituents which include nicotine, many carcinogens, carbon monoxide and other toxins. The harmful effects of smoking are related to a variety of factors, the most important of which is dose of exposure expressed in terms of pack years. For example, one pack of cigarettes daily for 5 years means 5 pack years. It is estimated that a person who smokes 2 packs of cigarettes daily at the age of 30 years reduces his life by 8 years than a non-smoker.

TOBACCO-RELATED DISEASES

Tobacco contains numerous toxic chemicals having adverse effects varying from minor throat irritation to carcinogenesis. The relative risk of major diseases in tobacco smokers compared from non-smokers and accounting for higher mortality include the following (in descending order of frequency):

i) Cancer of the lung: 12 to 23 times
ii) Chronic obstructive pulmonary disease (COPD): 10-13 times
iii) Cancers of upper aerodigestive tract (larynx, pharynx, lip, oral cavity, oesophagus): 6 to 14 times
iv) Aortic aneurysm: 6-7 times
v) Other cancers by systemic effects (kidneys, pancreas, urinary bladder, stomach, cervix): 2-3 times
vi) Cerebrovascular accidents (CVA): 2-4 times
vii) Coronary heart disease: 2 to 3 times relative risk
viii) Sudden infant death syndrome: 2 times
ix) Buerger's disease (thromboangiitis obliterans)
x) Peptic ulcer disease with 70% higher risk in smokers.
xi) Early menopause in smoker women.
xii) In smoking pregnant women, higher risk of lower birth weight of foetus, higher perinatal mortality and intellectual deterioration of newborn.

CHEMICAL AND DRUG INJURY *(p. 233)*

During life, each one of us is exposed to a variety of chemicals and drugs. These are broadly divided into the following two categories:

THERAPEUTIC (IATROGENIC) DRUG INJURY

Though the basis of patient management is rational drug therapy, nevertheless adverse drug reactions do occur in 2-5% of patients. In general, the risk of adverse drug reaction increases with increasing number of drugs administered.

NON-THERAPEUTIC TOXIC AGENTS

1. ALCOHOLISM

Chronic alcoholism is defined as the regular imbibing of an amount of ethyl alcohol (ethanol) that is sufficient to harm an individual socially, psychologically or physically. Generally, 10 gm of ethanol is present in:

❖ one can of beer (or half a bottle of beer);
❖ 120 ml of neat wine; or
❖ 30 ml of 43% liquor (small peg).

A daily consumption of 40 gm of ethanol (4 small pegs or 2 large pegs) is likely to be harmful; intake of 100 gm or more daily is certainly dangerous. Daily and heavy consumption of alcohol is more harmful than moderate social drinking having gap periods, since the liver where ethanol is metabolised, gets time to heal.

METABOLISM

Absorption of alcohol begins in the stomach and small intestine and appears in blood shortly after ingestion. In brief alcohol is metabolised in the liver by the following 3 pathways:

1. By the major rate-limiting pathway of alcohol dehydrogenase (ADH) in the cytosol, which is then quickly destroyed by aldehyde dehydrogenase (ALDH), especially with low blood alcohol levels.
2. Via microsomal P-450 system (microsomal ethanol oxidising system, MEOS) when the blood alcohol level is high.
3. Minor pathway via catalase from peroxisomes.

ILL-EFFECTS OF ALCOHOLISM

A. ACUTE ALCOHOLISM The acute effects of inebriation are most prominent on the central nervous system but it also injures the stomach and liver.

B. CHRONIC ALCOHOLISM Chronic alcoholism produces widespread injury to organs and systems.

Some of the more important organ effects in chronic alcoholism are as under:

1. **Liver** Alcoholic liver disease and cirrhosis are the most common and important effects of chronic alcoholism.

2. **Pancreas** Chronic calcifying pancreatitis and acute pancreatitis are serious complications of chronic alcoholism.

3. **Gastrointestinal tract** Gastritis, peptic ulcer and oesophageal varices associated with fatal massive bleeding may occur.

4. **Central nervous system** Peripheral neuropathies and Wernicke-Korsakoff syndrome, cerebral atrophy, cerebellar degeneration and amblyopia (impaired vision) are seen in chronic alcoholics.

5. **Cardiovascular system** Alcoholic cardiomyopathy and beer-drinkers' myocardiosis with consequent dilated cardiomyopathy may occur. Level of HDL (atherosclerosis-protective lipoprotein), however, has been shown to increase with moderate consumption of alcohol.

6. **Endocrine system** In men, testicular atrophy, feminisation, loss of libido and potency, and gynaecomastia may develop. These effects appear to be due to lowering of testosterone levels.

7. **Blood** Haematopoietic dysfunction with secondary megaloblastic anaemia and increased red blood cell volume may occur.

8. **Immune system** Alcoholics are more susceptible to various infections.

9. **Cancer** There is higher incidence of cancers of upper aerodigestive tract in chronic alcoholics but the mechanism is not clear.

2. LEAD POISONING

Lead poisoning may occur in children or adults due to accidental or occupational ingestion.

In children, following are the main sources of lead poisoning:
i)   Chewing of lead-containing furniture items, toys or pencils.
ii) Eating of lead paint flakes from walls.

In adults, the sources are as follows:
1.   Occupational exposure to lead during spray painting, recycling of automobile batteries (lead oxide fumes), mining, and extraction of lead.
2.   Accidental exposure by contaminated water supply, house freshly coated with lead paint, and sniffing of lead-containing petrol (hence unleaded petrol introduced as fuel).

Lead is absorbed through the gastrointestinal tract or lungs. The absorbed lead is distributed in two types of tissues:

a)   *Bones, teeth, nails and hair* representing relatively harmless pool of lead. About 90% of absorbed lead accumulates in the developing metaphysis of bones in children and appears as areas of increased bone densities ('lead lines') on X-ray. Lead lines are also seen in the gingiva.

b)   *Brain, liver, kidneys and bone marrow* accumulate the remaining 10% lead which is directly toxic to these organs. It is excreted via kidneys.

Lead toxicity occurs in the following organs predominantly:

Nervous system The changes are as under:
i)   *In children*, lead encephalopathy; oedema of brain, flattening of gyri and compression of ventricles.
ii) *In adults*, demyelinating peripheral motor neuropathy which typically affects radial and peroneal nerves resulting in wristdrop and footdrop respectively.

Haematopoietic system These changes are:
i) *Microcytic hypochromic anaemia*
ii) Prominent basophilic stippling of erythrocytes.

Kidneys Lead is toxic to proximal tubular cells of the kidney and produces *lead nephropathy* characterised by accumulation of intranuclear inclusion bodies consisting of lead-protein complex in the proximal tubular cells.

3. CARBON MONOXIDE POISONING

Carbon monoxide (CO) is a colourless and odourless gas produced by
incomplete combustion of carbon. Sources of CO gas are:
i)   automobile exhaust;
ii)   burning of fossil fuel in industries or at home; and
iii) tobacco smoke.

CO is an important cause of accidental death due to systemic oxygen
deprivation of tissues. This is because haemoglobin has about 200-times
higher affinity for CO than for O_2 and thus varying amount of carboxyhaemo-
globin is formed depending upon the extent of CO poisoning.

CO poisoning may present in 2 ways:

◈   **Acute CO poisoning** in which there is sudden development of brain
hypoxia characterised by oedema and petechial haemorrhages.

◈   **Chronic CO poisoning** presents with nonspecific changes of slowly
developing hypoxia of the brain.

4. DRUG ABUSE

Drug abuse is defined as the use of certain drugs for the purpose of 'mood
alteration' or 'euphoria' or 'kick' but subsequently leading to habit-forming,
dependence and eventually addiction. Some of the commonly abused drugs
and substances are as under:
1.   Marijuana or 'pot'
2.   Derivatives of opium
3.   CNS depressants
4.   CNS stimulants
5.   Psychedelic drugs
6.   Inhalants

Following are a few common drug abuse-related infectious
complications:
1.   At the site of injection—cellulitis, abscesses, ulcers, thrombosed veins
2.   Thrombophlebitis
3.   Bacterial endocarditis
4.   High risk for AIDS
5.   Viral hepatitis and its complications
6.   Focal glomerulonephritis
7.   Talc (foreign body) granuloma formation in the lungs.

INJURY BY PHYSICAL AGENTS (p. 237)

THERMAL AND ELECTRICAL INJURY

Thermal and electrical burns, fall in body temperature below 35°C
(hypothermia) and elevation of body temperature above 41°C (hyperthermia),
are all associated with tissue injury.

1.   **Hypothermia** may cause focal injury as in frostbite, or systemic injury
and death as occurs on immersion in cold water for varying time.

2.   **Hyperthermia** likewise, may be localised as in cutaneous burns, and
systemic as occurs in fevers.

3.   **Thermal burns** depending upon severity are categorised into full
thickness (third degree) and partial thickness (first and second degree). The
most serious complications of burns are haemoconcentration, infections and
contractures on healing.

4.   **Electrical burns** may cause damage *firstly,* by electrical dysfunction of
the conduction system of the heart and death by ventricular fibrillation, and
secondly by heat produced by electrical energy.

INJURY BY RADIATION

The most important form of radiation injury is ionising radiation which has
three types of effects on cells:

i) Somatic effects which cause acute cell killing.
ii) Genetic damage by mutations and therefore, passes genetic defects in the next progeny of cells.
iii) Malignant transformation of cells.

Ionising radiation causes damage to the following major organs:
1. *Skin:* radiation dermatitis, cancer.
2. *Lungs:* interstitial pulmonary fibrosis.
3. *Heart:* myocardial fibrosis, constrictive pericarditis.
4. *Kidney:* radiation nephritis.
5. *Gastrointestinal tract:* strictures of small bowel and oesophagus.
6 *Gonads:* testicular atrophy in males and destruction of ovaries.
7. *Haematopoietic tissue:* pancytopenia due to bone marrow depression.
8. *Eyes:* cataract.

Besides ionising radiation, other form of harmful radiation is *solar (u.v.) radiation* which may cause acute skin injury as sunburns, chronic conditions such as solar keratosis and early onset of cataracts in the eyes.

NUTRITIONAL DISEASES *(p. 238)*

NUTRITIONAL REQUIREMENT

Nutritional status of a society varies according to the socioeconomic conditions. In the Western world, nutritional imbalance is more often a problem accounting for increased frequency of obesity, while in developing countries of Africa, Asia and South America, chronic malnutrition is a serious health problem, particularly in children.

For good health, humans require energy-providing nutrients (proteins, fats and carbohydrates), vitamins, minerals, water and some non-essential nutrients.

PATHOGENESIS OF DEFICIENCY DISEASES

The nutritional deficiency disease develops when the essential nutrients are not provided to the cells adequately. The nutritional deficiency may be of 2 types:

1. Primary deficiency This is due to either the lack or decreased amount of essential nutrients in diet.

2. Secondary or conditioned deficiency Secondary or conditioned deficiency is malnutrition occurring as a result of the various factors e.g.
i) Interference with ingestion
ii) Interference with absorption
iii) Interference with utilisation
iv) Increased excretion
v) Increased nutritional demand

Irrespective of the type of nutritional deficiency (primary or secondary), nutrient reserves in the tissues begin to get depleted, which initially result in biochemical alterations and eventually lead to functional and morphological changes in tissues and organs.

OBESITY *(p. 238)*

Dietary imbalance and overnutrition may lead to obesity. *Obesity is defined as an excess of adipose tissue that imparts health risk; a body weight of 20% excess over ideal weight for age, sex and height is considered a health risk.* The most widely used method to gauge obesity is body mass index (BMI) which is equal to weight in kg/height in m^2. A cut-off BMI value of 30 is used for obesity in both men and women.

ETIOLOGY *Obesity results when caloric intake exceeds utilisation.* The imbalance of these two components can occur in the following situations:
1. *Inadequate pushing of oneself away from the dining table* causing overeating.
2. *Insufficient pushing of oneself out of the chair* leading to inactivity and sedentary life style.

3. *Genetic predisposition* to develop obesity.
4. *Diets largely derived from carbohydrates* and fats than protein-rich diet.
5. *Secondary obesity* may result following a number of underlying diseases such as hypothyroidism, Cushing's disease, insulinoma and hypothalamic disorders.

PATHOGENESIS Besides the generally accepted role of adipocytes for fat storage, these cells also release endocrine-regulating molecules. These molecules include: energy regulatory hormone (leptin), cytokines (TNF-α and interleukin-6), insulin sensitivity regulating agents (adiponectin, resistin and RBP4), prothrombotic factors (plasminogen activator inhibitor), and blood pressure regulating agent (angiotensinogen).

Recently, two obesity genes have been found: *ob* gene and its protein product leptin, and *db* gene and its protein product leptin receptor.

EFFECTS OF OBESITY These are as under:
1. Hyperinsulinaemia
2. Type 2 diabetes mellitus
3. Hypertension
4. Hyperlipoproteinaemia
5. Atherosclerosis
6. Nonalcoholic fatty liver disease (NAFLD)
7. Cholelithiasis
8. Hypoventilation syndrome (Pickwickian syndrome)
9. Osteoarthritis
10. Cancer

STARVATION *(p. 240)*

Starvation is a state of overall deprivation of nutrients. Its causes may be the following:
i) deliberate fasting—religious or political;
ii) famine conditions in a country or community; or
iii) secondary undernutrition such as due to chronic wasting diseases (infections, inflammatory conditions, liver disease), cancer etc.

METABOLIC CHANGES The following metabolic changes take place in starvation:

1. Glucose *Glucose stores* of the body are sufficient for one day's metabolic needs only. Hepatic gluconeogenesis from other sources such as breakdown of proteins takes place.

2. Proteins Protein stores and the triglycerides of adipose tissue have enough energy for about 3 months in an individual. *Proteins* breakdown to release amino acids which are used as fuel for hepatic gluconeogenesis.

3. Fats After about one week of starvation, protein breakdown is decreased and *triglycerides* of adipose tissue breakdown to form glycerol and fatty acids.

PROTEIN-ENERGY MALNUTRITION *(p. 240)*

The inadequate consumption of protein and energy as a result of primary dietary deficiency or conditioned deficiency may cause loss of body mass and adipose tissue, resulting in protein energy or protein calorie malnutrition (PEM or PCM).

The spectrum of *clinical syndromes* produced as a result of PEM includes the following:
1. *Kwashiorkor* which is related to protein deficiency though calorie intake may be sufficient.
2. *Marasmus* is starvation in infants occurring due to overall lack of calories.

METALS AND TRACE ELEMENTS *(p. 240)*

Several minerals in trace amounts are essential for health since they form components of enzymes and cofactors for metabolic functions. Besides *calcium* and *phosphorus* required for vitamin D manufacture, others include: *iron, copper, iodine, zinc, selenium, manganese, nickel, chromium, molybdenum, fluorine.* However, out of these, the dietary deficiency of first five trace elements is associated with deficiency states as under:

i)   *Iron:* Microcytic hypochromic anaemia.

ii) *Calcium:* Reduced bone mass, osteoporosis.

iii) *Phosphorus*: Rickets, osteomalacia.

iv) *Copper:* Muscle weakness, neurologic defect, anaemia, growth retardation.

v)   *Iodine:* Goitre and hyperthyroidism, cretinism.

DISORDERS OF VITAMINS *(p. 241)*

Vitamins are organic substances which cannot be synthesised within the body and are essential for maintenance of normal structure and function of cells. Thus, these substances must be provided in the human diet. Most of the vitamins are of plant or animal origin so that they normally enter the body as constituents of ingested plant food or animal food. They are required in minute amounts in contrast to the relatively large amounts of essential amino acids and fatty acids. Vitamins do not play any part in production of energy.

ETIOLOGY OF VITAMIN DEFICIENCIES In the developing countries, *multiple deficiencies* of vitamins and other nutrients are common due to generalised malnutrition of dietary origin. In the developed countries, *individual vitamin deficiencies* are noted more often, particularly in children, adolescent, pregnant and lactating women, and in some due to poverty. A few other noteworthy features about vitamins are as under:

1.   While vitamin deficiency as well as its excess may occur from another disease, the states of excess and deficiency themselves also cause disease.

2.   Vitamins in high dose can be used as drugs.

CLASSIFICATION OF VITAMINS Vitamins are conventionally divided into 2 groups: fat-soluble and water-soluble.

1.   Fat-soluble vitamins There are 4 fat-soluble vitamins: A, D, E and K. They are absorbed from intestine in the presence of bile salts and intact pancreatic function. Beside the deficiency syndromes of these vitamins, a state of *hypervitaminosis* due to excess of vitamin A and D also occurs.

2.   Water-soluble vitamins This group conventionally consists of vitamin C and members of B complex group. Besides, choline, biotin and flavonoids are new additions to this group. Water-soluble vitamins are more readily absorbed from small intestine. Being water soluble, these vitamins are more easily lost due to cooking or processing of food.

Various clinical disorders produced by vitamin deficiencies are as under.

VITAMINS	DEFICIENCY DISORDERS
I. FAT-SOLUBLE VITAMINS	
Vitamin A (Retinol)	Ocular lesions (night blindness, xerophthalmia, keratomalacia, Bitot's spots, blindness) Cutaneous lesions (xeroderma) Other lesions (squamous metaplasia of respiratory epithelium, urothelium and pancreatic ductal epithelium, subsequent anaplasia; retarded bone growth)
Vitamin D (Calcitriol)	Rickets in growing children Osteomalacia in adults Hypocalcaemic tetany
Vitamin E (α-Tocopherol)	Degeneration of neurons, retinal pigments, axons of peripheral nerves; denervation of muscles Reduced red cell lifespan Sterility in male and female animals

| Vitamin K | Hypoprothrombinaemia (in haemorrhagic disease of newborn, biliary obstruction, malabsorption, anticoagulant therapy, antibiotic therapy, diffuse liver disease) |

II. WATER-SOLUBLE VITAMINS

| Vitamin C (Ascorbic acid) | Scurvy (haemorrhagic diathesis, skeletal lesions, delayed wound healing, anaemia, lesions in teeth and gums) |

Vitamin B Complex

(i) Thiamine (Vitamin B_1)	Beriberi ('dry' or peripheral neuritis, 'wet' or cardiac manifestations, 'cerebral' or Wernicke-Korsakoff's syndrome)
(ii) Riboflavin (Vitamin B_2)	Ariboflavinosis (ocular lesions, cheilosis, glossitis, dermatitis)
(iii) Niacin/ Nicotinic acid (Vitamin B_3)	Pellagra (dermatitis, diarrhoea, dementia)
(iv) Pyridoxine (Vitamin B_6)	Vague lesions (convulsions in infants, dermatitis, cheilosis, glossitis, sideroblastic anaemia)
(v) Folate/Folic acid	Megaloblastic anaemia
(vi) Cyanoco-balamin (Vitamin B_{12})	Megaloblastic anaemia Pernicious anaemia
(vii) Biotin	Mental and neurological symptoms
Choline	Fatty liver, muscle damage
Flavonoids	Preventive of neurodegenerative disease, osteoporosis, diabetes

DIET AND CANCER (p. 249)

There are three possible mechanisms on which the story of this relationship of diet on cancer can be built up:

1. DIETARY CONTENT OF EXOGENOUS CARCINOGENS

i) The most important example in this mechanism comes from naturally-occurring carcinogen *aflatoxin* which is strongly associated with high incidence of hepatocellular carcinoma in those consuming grain contaminated with mould, *Aspergillus flavus*.

ii) *Artificial sweeteners* (e.g. saccharine cyclomates), food additives and pesticide contamination of food are implicated as carcinogens derived from diet.

2. ENDOGENOUS SYNTHESIS OF CARCINOGENS OR PROMOTERS

i) In the context of etiology of *gastric carcinoma,* nitrites, nitrates and amines from the digested food are transformed in the body to carcinogens—nitrosamines and nitrosamides.

ii) In the etiology of *colon cancer,* low fibre intake and high animal-derived fats are implicated. High fat diet results in rise in the level of bile acids and their intermediate metabolites produced by intestinal bacteria which act as carcinogens. The low fibre diet, on the other hand, does not provide adequate protection to the mucosa and reduces the stool bulk and thus increases the time the stools remain in the colon.

iii) In the etiology of *breast cancer,* epidemiologic studies have implicated the role of animal proteins, fats and obesity but the evidence is yet unsubstantiated.

3. INADEQUATE PROTECTIVE FACTORS

Some components of diet such as *vitamin C, A, E, selenium,* and β-*carotenes* have protective role against cancer. These substances in normal amounts in the body act as antioxidants and protect the cells against free radical injury.

SELF ASSESSMENT

1. **The harmful effects of smoking of following tobacco products are most severe:**
   A. Cigarettes
   B. *Bidis*
   C. Cigar
   D. Pipe

2. **The major pathway of ethanol metabolism in the liver is via:**
   A. Alcohol dehydrogenase in the SER
   B. Microsomal P-450
   C. Catalase in the peroxisomes
   D. None of the above

3. **Lead poisoning produces the following change in red cells:**
   A. Pappenheimer bodies
   B. Howell-Jolly bodies
   C. Basophilic stippling
   D. Heinz bodies

4. **Between CO and O_2, haemoglobin has:**
   A. Greater affinity for former
   B. Greater affinity for latter
   C. Equal affinity for both
   D. No affinity for the former

5. **1 g of carbohydrate provides:**
   A. 2 Kcal
   B. 4 Kcal
   C. 7 Kcal
   D. 9 Kcal

6. **Health risk in obesity is due to weight in excess of the following for age and sex:**
   A. 10%
   B. 20%
   C. 30%
   D. 40%

7. **Obesity is due to:**
   A. Hyperplasia of adipocytes only
   B. Hypertrophy of adipocytes only
   C. Hyperplasia as well as hypertrophy of adipocytes
   D. Fatty change in liver only

8. **In starvation, first nutrient to be depleted in the body is:**
   A. Fat
   B. Carbohydrate
   C. Protein
   D. Vitamins

9. **State of hypervitaminosis occurs in:**
   A. Vitamin A and B
   B. Vitamin B and C
   C. Vitamin C and D
   D. Vitamin A and D

10. **The main function of vitamin E is:**
    A. Immune regulation
    B. Hepatic microsomal carboxylation
    C. Antioxidant activity
    D. Maintenance of structure and function of epithelia

11. **Most active form of vitamin D is:**
    A. 7-dehydrocholesterol
    B. Ergosterol

C. 25-hydroxy vitamin D
D. 1, 25-dihydroxy vitamin D

12. **Which of the following is the gene for obesity?**
    A. *Rb* gene   B. *db* gene
    C. *p53* gene   D. *p63* gene

KEY

1 = B	2 = A	3 = C	4 = A	5 = C
6 = B	7 = C	8 = B	9 = D	10 = C
11 = D	12 = B			

Genetic and Paediatric Diseases

DEVELOPMENTAL DEFECTS *(p. 251)*

Developmental defects are a group of abnormalities during foetal life due to errors in morphogenesis. The branch of science dealing with the study of developmental anomalies is called *teratology*. Certain chemicals, drugs, physical and biologic agents are known to induce such birth defects and are called *teratogens*. The morphologic abnormality or defect in an organ or anatomic region of the body so produced is called *malformation*.

PATHOGENESIS

The teratogens may result in one of the following outcomes:
i) Intrauterine death
ii) Intrauterine growth retardation (IUGR)
iii) Functional defects
iv) Malformation

The effects of teratogens in inducing developmental defects are related to the following factors:
i) Variable individual susceptibility to teratogen.
ii) Intrauterine stage at which patient is exposed to teratogen.
iii) Dose of teratogen.
iv) Specificity of developmental defect for specific teratogen.

CLASSIFICATION

Various developmental anomalies resulting from teratogenic effects are categorised as under:

Agenesis means the complete absence of an organ e.g. unilateral or bilateral agenesis of kidney.

Aplasia is the absence of development of an organ with presence of rudiment or anlage e.g. aplasia of lung with rudimentary bronchus.

Hypoplasia is incomplete development of an organ not reaching the normal adult size e.g. microglossia.

Atresia refers to incomplete formation of lumen in hollow viscus e.g. oesophageal atresia.

Developmental dysplasia is defective development of cells and tissues resulting in abnormal or primitive histogenetic structures e.g. renal dysplasia.

Dystraphic anomalies are the defects resulting from failure of fusion e.g. spina bifida.

Ectopia or heterotopia refers to abnormal location of tissue at ectopic site e.g. pancreatic heterotopia in the wall of stomach.

EXAMPLES OF DEVELOPMENTAL DEFECTS

A few common clinically important examples are given below:

1. **Anencephaly-spina bifida complex** This is the group of anomalies resulting from failure to fuse (dystraphy).

2. **Thalidomide malformations** Thalidomide is the best known example of teratogenic drug which was used as a sedative by pregnant women and

3. Foetal hydantoin syndrome Babies born to mothers on anti-epileptic treatment with hydantoin have characteristic facial features and congenital heart defects.

4. Foetal alcohol syndrome Ethanol is another potent teratogen. Consumption of alcohol by pregnant mother in first trimester increases the risk of miscarriages, stillbirths, growth retardation and mental retardation in the newborn.

5. TORCH complex Infection with TORCH group of organisms (*T*oxoplasma, *O*thers, *R*ubella, *C*ytomegalovirus, and *H*erpes simplex) during pregnancy is associated with multisystem anomalies and TORCH syndrome in the newborn.

6. Congenital syphilis Vertical transmission of syphilis from mother to foetus is characterised by Hutchinson's triad: interstitial keratitis, sensorineural deafness and deformed Hutchinson's teeth, along with saddle-nose deformity.

CYTOGENETIC (KARYOTYPIC) ABNORMALITIES *(p. 252)*

Human germ cells (ova and sperms) contain 23 chromosomes (haploid or 1N) while all the nucleated somatic cells of the human body contain 23 pairs of chromosomes (diploid or 2N)—44 autosomes and 2 sex chromosomes, being XX in females (46, XX) and XY in males (46, XY). An inactive X chromosome in the somatic cells in females lies condensed in the nucleus and is called as *sex chromatin* seen specifically in the somatic cells in females. *Nuclear sexing* can be done for genetic female testing by preparing and staining the smears of squamous cells scraped from oral cavity, or by identifying the *Barr body* in the circulating neutrophils as drumstick appendage attached to one of the nuclear lobes. A minimum of 30% cells positive for sex chromatin is indicative of genetically female composition.

Based on length of chromosomes, they are divided into 7 groups—A to G, called *Denver classification* adopted at a meeting in Denver, Colorado in US.

Chromosomal banding techniques are employed for study of classes of chromosomes. Chromosomal bands are unique alternate dark and light staining patterns. Banding techniques include:
i) G-banding (Giemsa stain);
ii) Q-banding (quinacrine fluorescence stain);
iii) R-banding (reverse Giemsa staining); and
iv) C-banding (constitutive heterochromatin demonstration).

NUMERICAL ABNORMALITIES

1. Polyploidy is the term used for the number of chromosomes which is a multiple of haploid number e.g. triploid or 3N (69 chromosomes), tetraploid or 4N (92 chromosomes). Polyploidy occurs normally in megakaryocytes and dividing liver cells. Polyploidy in somatic cells of conceptus results in spontaneous abortions.

2. Aneuploidy is the number of chromosomes which is not an exact multiple of haploid number e.g. hypodiploid or 2N-1 (45 chromosomes) monosomy, hyperdiploid or 2 N+1 (47 chromosomes) trisomy.

The most common mechanism of aneuploidy is **nondisjunction.** Nondisjunction is the failure of chromosomes to separate normally during cell division during first or second stage of meiosis, or in mitosis.

Three clinically important syndromes resulting from numerical aberrations of chromosomes due to nondisjunction are as under:

◈ **Down's syndrome** There is trisomy 21 in about 95% cases of Down's syndrome due to nondisjunction during meiosis in one of the parents. Down's syndrome is the most common chromosomal disorder and is the commonest cause of mental retardation. The incidence of producing offspring with Down's syndrome rises in mothers over 35 years of age.

◈ **Klinefelter's syndrome** Klinefelter's syndrome is the most important example of sex chromosome trisomy. About 80% cases have 47, XXY karyotype while others are mosaics. Typically, these patients have testicular dysgenesis. In general, sex chromosome trisomies are more common than trisomies of autosomes.

◈ **Turner's syndrome** Turner's syndrome is an example of monosomy (45, X0) most often due to loss of X chromosome in paternal meiosis.

STRUCTURAL ABNORMALITIES

During cell division (meiosis as well as mitosis), certain structural abnormalities of chromosomes may appear. Structural abnormalities may be balanced or unbalanced.

i) *Balanced structural alteration* means no change in total number of genes or genetic material.

ii) *Unbalanced structural alteration* refers to gene rearrangement resulting in loss or gain of genetic material.

A few examples are as follows:

1. TRANSLOCATIONS Translocation means crossing over or exchange of fragment of chromosome which may occur between non-homologous or homologous chromosomes. There are two main types of translocations: reciprocal in about two-third and Robertsonian in one-third cases:

◈ **Reciprocal translocation** Reciprocal translocation may be balanced (without any loss of genetic material during the exchange) or unbalanced (with some loss of genetic material).

i) *Balanced reciprocal translocation* is more common and the individual is phenotypically normal e.g. translocation between long arm (q) of chromosomes 22 and long arm (q) of chromosome 9 written as t (9;22). This translocation is termed Philadelphia chromosome seen in most cases of chronic myeloid leukaemia.

ii) *Unbalanced reciprocal translocations* are less common and account for repeated abortions and malformed children.

◈ **Robertsonian translocation** In this, there is fusion of two acrocentric chromosomes (having very short arms) at the centromere (centric fusion) with loss of short arms.

2. DELETIONS Loss of genetic material from the chromosome is called deletion. Deletion may be from the terminal or middle portion of the chromosome.

3. INVERSION Inversion is a form of rearrangement involving breaks of a single chromosome at two points.

4. RING CHROMOSOME A ring of chromosome is formed by a break at both the telomeric (terminal) ends of a chromosome followed by deletion of the broken fragment and then end-to-end fusion.

5. ISOCHROMOSOME When centromere, rather than dividing parallel to the long axis, instead divides transverse to the long axis of chromosome, it results in either two short arms only or two long arms only called isochromosomes.

SINGLE-GENE DEFECTS (MENDELIAN DISORDERS) *(p. 254)*

In order to unravel causes of disease at genetic level, spectacular advances have been made in human genetics. With mapping of human genome consisting of about 30,000 genes, it is possible to perform molecular profiling of diseases at genetic level.

MUTATIONS The term mutation is applied to permanent change in the DNA of the cell. Mutations affecting germ cells are transmitted to the next progeny producing *inherited diseases,* while the mutations affecting somatic cells give rise to *various cancers* and *congenital malformations.* Presently, following types of mutations have been described:

i) **Point mutation** is the result of substitution of a single nucleotide base by a different base.

ii) **Stop codon or nonsense mutation** refers to a type of mutation in which the protein chain is prematurely terminated or truncated.

iii) **Frameshift mutation** occurs when there is insertion or deletion of one or two base pairs in the DNA sequence.

iv) **Trinucleotide repeat mutation** is characterised by amplification of a sequence of three nucleotides.

INHERITANCE PATTERN The inheritance pattern of genetic abnormalities may be *dominant or recessive, autosomal or sex-linked:*

A *dominant gene* produces its effects, whether combined with similar dominant or recessive gene. *Recessive genes* are effective only if both genes are similar. However, when both alleles of a gene pair are expressed in heterozygous state, it is called *codominant inheritance*. A single gene may express in multiple allelic forms known as *polymorphism*. *Autosomal diseases* are due to defect in any of 1 to 22 autosomes while *sex-linked disorders* are mostly X-linked.

◈ **Autosomal dominant inheritance** pattern is characterised by one faulty copy of gene (i.e. mutant allele) in any autosome and one copy of normal allele; disease phenotype is seen in all such individuals. Patients having autosomal dominant inheritance disease have 50% chance of passing on the disease to the next generation.

◈ In **autosomal recessive inheritance**, both copies of genes are mutated. Usually, it occurs when both parents are carriers of the defective gene, i.e. having one normal allele and one defective allele in each parent, and each parent passes on their defective gene to the next progeny causing disease. There is 25% chance of transmission of autosomal recessive disease when both parents are carriers.

◈ **X-linked disorders** are caused by mutations in genes on X-chromosome, derived from either one of the two X-chromosomes in females, or from the single X-chromosome of the male.

◈ There are much fewer genes on Y-chromosome and are determinant for testis. **Y-linked diseases** are rare and include male infertility, excessive hair on pinna, retinitis pigmentosa, colour blindness and XYY syndrome.

MULTIFACTORIAL INHERITANCE *(p. 256)*

Multifactorial disorders are those disorders which result from the combined effect of genetic composition and environmental influences e.g.
1. Cleft lip and cleft palate
2. Pyloric stenosis
3. Diabetes mellitus
4. Hypertension
5. Congenital heart disease
6. Coronary heart disease.

STORAGE DISEASES (INBORN ERRORS OF METABOLISM) *(p. 256)*

Storage diseases or inborn errors of metabolism are biochemically distinct groups of disorders occurring due to genetic defect in the metabolism of carbohydrates, lipids, and proteins resulting in intracellular accumulation of metabolites. These substances may collect within the cells throughout the body but most commonly affected organ or site is the one where the stored material is normally found and degraded. Since lysosomes comprise the chief site of intracellular digestion (autophagy as well as heterophagy), the material is naturally stored in the lysosomes, and hence the generic name 'lysosomal storage diseases'. Cells of mononuclear-phagocyte system are particularly rich in lysosomes; therefore, reticuloendothelial organs containing numerous phagocytic cells like the liver and spleen are most commonly involved in storage disease.

Based on the biochemical composition of the accumulated material within the cells, storage diseases are classified into distinct groups, each group containing a number of diseases depending upon the specific enzyme deficiency. A few general comments can be made about all storage diseases:

◈   All the storage diseases occur either as a result of autosomal recessive, or sex-(X-) linked recessive genetic transmission.

◈   Most, but not all, of the storage diseases are lysosomal storage diseases. However, out of the glycogen storage diseases, type II (Pompe's disease) is the only example of lysosomal storage disease.

GLYCOGEN STORAGE DISEASES (GLYCOGENOSES)

These are a group of inherited disorders in which there is defective glucose metabolism resulting in excessive intracellular accumulation of glycogen in various tissues. Based on specific enzyme deficiencies, glycogen storage diseases are divided into 8 main types designated by Roman numerals I to VIII. However, based on pathophysiology, glycogen storage diseases can be divided into 3 main subgroups:
1.   Hepatic forms
2.   Myopathic forms
3.   Other forms.
     A few common examples are given below.

VON GIERKE'S DISEASE (TYPE I GLYCOGENOSIS)   This condition is inherited as an autosomal recessive disorder due to deficiency of enzyme, glucose-6-phosphatase. In the absence of glucose-6-phosphatase, excess of normal type of glycogen accumulates in the liver and also results in hypoglycaemia due to reduced formation of free glucose from glycogen.

     Most prominent feature is enormous hepatomegaly with intracyto-plasmic and intranuclear glycogen. The kidneys are also enlarged and show intracytoplasmic glycogen in tubular epithelial cells. Other features include gout, skin xanthomas and bleeding tendencies due to platelet dysfunction.

POMPE'S DISEASE (TYPE II GLYCOGENOSIS)   This is also an autosomal recessive disorder due to deficiency of a lysosomal enzyme, acid maltase, and is the only example of *lysosomal* storage disease amongst the various types of glycogenoses. Its deficiency, therefore, results in accumulation of glycogen in many tissues, most often in the heart and skeletal muscle, leading to cardiomegaly and hypotonia.

MUCOPOLYSACCHARIDOSES (MPS)

Mucopolysaccharidoses are a group of six inherited syndromes numbered from MPS I to MPS VI. Each of these result from deficiency of specific lysosomal enzyme involved in the degradation of mucopolysaccharides or glycosaminoglycans, and are, therefore, a form of lysosomal storage diseases. Mucopolysaccharides which accumulate in the MPS are: chondroitin sulphate, dermatan sulphate, heparan sulphate and keratan sulphate. All these syndromes are autosomal recessive disorders except MPS II (Hunter's syndrome) which has X-linked recessive transmission.

GAUCHER'S DISEASE

This is an autosomal recessive disorder in which there is mutation in lysosomal enzyme, acid β-glucosidase (earlier called glucocerebrosidase), which normally cleaves glucose from ceramide. This results in lysosomal accumulation of glucocerebroside (ceramide-glucose) in phagocytic cells of the body and sometimes in the neurons.

     Clinically, 3 subtypes of Gaucher's disease are identified based on neuronopathic involvement:

◈   **Type I or classic form** is the adult form of disease in which there is storage of glucocerebrosides in the phagocytic cells of the body, principally involving the spleen, liver, bone marrow, and lymph nodes. This is the most common type comprising 80% of all cases of Gaucher's disease.

◈   **Type II** is the infantile form in which there is progressive involvement of the central nervous system.

◈   **Type III** is the juvenile form of the disease having features in between type I and type II i.e. they have systemic involvement like in type I and progressive involvement of the CNS as in type II.

M/E Shows large number of characteristically distended and enlarged macrophages called *Gaucher cells* which are found in the spleen, liver, bone marrow and lymph nodes, and in the case of neuronal involvement, in the Virchow-Robin space. The cytoplasm of these cells is abundant, granular and fibrillar resembling crumpled tissue paper. They have mostly a single nucleus but occasionally may have two or three nuclei.

NIEMANN-PICK DISEASE

This is also an autosomal recessive disorder characterised by accumulation of sphingomyelin and cholesterol due to defect in acid sphingomyelinase.

Two types have been described:
◆ **Type A** is more common and typically presents in infancy and is characterised by hepatosplenomegaly, lymphadenopathy, rapidly progressive deterioration of CNS and physical underdevelopment.
◆ **Type B** develops later and has a progressive hepatosplenomegaly with development of cirrhosis due to replacement of the liver by foam cells, and impaired lung function due to infiltration in lung alveoli.

M/E Shows storage of sphingomyelin and cholesterol within the lysosomes, particularly in the cells of mononuclear phagocyte system. The cells of Niemann-Pick disease are somewhat smaller than Gaucher cells and their cytoplasm is not wrinkled but is instead foamy and vacuolated which stains positively with fat stains. These cells are widely distributed in the spleen, liver, lymph nodes, bone marrow, lungs, bowel and brain.

OTHER PAEDIATRIC DISEASES *(p. 258)*

1. **Neonatal period** is the period of continuation of dependent intrauterine foetal life to independent postnatal period. Therefore, this is the period of maximum risk to life due to perinatal causes (e.g. prematurity, low birth weight, perinatal infections, respiratory distress syndrome, birth asphyxia, birth trauma etc) and congenital anomalies. If adequate postnatal medical care is not provided, neonatal mortality is high.

2. **In infancy,** the major health problems are related to congenital anomalies, infections of lungs and bowel, and sudden infant death syndrome (often during sleep).

3. **Young children from 1-4 years** are exposed to higher risk of sustaining injuries, and manifest certain congenital anomalies. Some malignant tumours are peculiar to this age group.

4. **Older children from 5-14 years** too have higher risk of injuries from accidents and have other problems related to congenital anomalies and certain malignant tumours at this age.

TUMOURS OF INFANCY AND CHILDHOOD *(p. 259)*

Tumours of infancy and childhood comprise 2% of all malignant tumours but they are the leading cause of death in this age group exceeded only by accidents. Benign tumours are more common than malignant neoplasms but they are generally of little immediate consequence.

HISTOGENESIS Histogenetic evolution of tumours at different age groups takes place as under:
1. Some tumours are *developmental tumours.*
2. Many other tumours originate in abnormally developed organs and organ rests; (*embryonic tumours*).
3. In embryonic tumours, proliferation of embryonic cells occurs which *have not reached the differentiation stage* essential for specialised functions i.e. the cells proliferate as *undifferentiated or as partially differentiated* stem cells and an embryonal tumour (embryoma or blastoma) is formed.
4. Tumours of infancy and childhood have *some features of normal embryonic or foetal cells* in them which proliferate under growth promoting influence of oncogenes.

5. Under appropriate conditions, these malignant embryonal cells may *cease to proliferate* and transform into non-proliferating mature differentiated cells.

BENIGN TUMOURS AND TUMOUR-LIKE CONDITIONS

Many of the benign tumours seen in infancy and childhood are actually growth of displaced cells and masses of tissues and their proliferation takes place along with the growth of the child. Some of these tumours undergo a phase of spontaneous regression subsequently. While some consider such lesions as mere *'tumour-like lesions or malformations'*, others call them benign tumours. A few such examples are as under:

1. **Hamartomas** Hamartomas are focal accumulations of cells normally present in that tissue but are arranged in an abnormal manner.

2. **Choristoma (heterotopia)** Choristoma or heterotopia is collection of normal cells and tissues at aberrant locations.

MALIGNANT TUMOURS

◈ In infants and children under 4 years of age: the most common malignant tumours are various types of *blastomas*.

◈ Children between 5 to 9 years of age: *haematopoietic malignancies* are more common.

◈ In the age range of 10-14 years (prepubertal age): *soft tissue and bony sarcomas* are the prominent tumours.

SELF ASSESSMENT

1. **Teratogens are defined as agents which induce:**
   A. Mitosis
   B. Carcinogenesis
   C. Birth defects
   D. Fallot's tetralogy

2. **For chromosomal study, it is best to use the following nucleated cells:**
   A. Polymorphs
   B. Lymphocytes
   C. Epithelial cells
   D. Fibroblasts

3. **For chromosomal study, the dividing cells are arrested by colchicine in the following phase of cell cycle:**
   A. Prophase
   B. Metaphase
   C. Anaphase
   D. Telophase

4. **Denver classification divides chromosomes based on their length into the following groups:**
   A. A to C (3 groups)
   B. A to E (5 groups)
   C. A to G (7 groups)
   D. A to I (9 groups)

5. **Polyploidy is generally not a feature of dividing cells of the following type:**
   A. Megakaryocytes
   B. Hepatocytes
   C. Tubular cells
   D. Conceptus of abortions

6. **Numeric abnormality in chromosome occurs in the following conditions <u>except</u>:**
   A. Ph chromosome in CML
   B. Turner's syndrome
   C. Klinefelter's syndrome
   D. Down's syndrome

7. **Mutations affecting germ cells produce:**
   A. Cancers
   B. Inherited diseases
   C. Congenital malformations
   D. Aneuploidy

8. **In lysosomal storage diseases, the following cells are particularly involved:**
   A. Hepatocytes
   B. Skeletal muscle
   C. Macrophages
   D. White pulp of spleen

9. **Out of the following glycogenosis, the following is example of lysosomal storage disease:**
   A. von Gierke's disease
   B. Pompe's disease
   C. Forbe's disease
   D. Anderson's disease
10. **Blastomas are childhood tumours seen more often in the age range of:**
    A. <4 years
    B. 5-9 years
    C. 10-14 years
    D. 14-16 years
11. **All of the following are X-linked recessive disorders <u>except</u>:**
    A. Haemophilia A and B
    B. Chronic granulomatous disease
    C. G-6 PD deficiency
    D. Sickle cell anaemia
12. **Gaucher cells are positive for all <u>except</u>:**
    A. PAS
    B. Mucicarmine
    C. Oil red O
    D. Prussian blue

KEY

1 = C	2 = B	3 = B	4 = C	5 = C
6 = A	7 = B	8 = C	9 = B	10 = A
11 = D	12 = B			

10 Introduction to Haematopoietic System and Disorders of Erythroid Series

Haematology and Lymphoreticular Tissues

The section on disorders of the haematopoietic system is concerned with diseases of the blood and the bone marrow. Conventionally, it includes study of constituents of circulating blood and blood-forming organs.

However, currently the WHO classification of malignancies of haematopoietic system and lymphoreticular tissues has been widely accepted and has superseded previous FAB (French-American-British) Cooperative Group classifications. While the criteria for the FAB group classification system was the location of leucocytes (in blood and in tissues), the WHO classification takes into consideration both 'circulating' leucocytes and 'fixed' leucocytes present anywhere in the tissues together since these diseases may disseminate from one pool to the other.

Based on these modifications in classification systems, the section on diseases of blood, bone marrow and lymphoreticular tissues has been structured into three chapters: introduction to haematopoietic system and disorders of erythroid series (Chapter 10), disorders of platelets, bleeding disorders and basic transfusion medicine (Chapter 11) and disorders of leucocytes (myeloid and lymphoid series) and diseases of lymphoreticular tissues (Chapter 12).

BONE MARROW AND HAEMATOPOIESIS (p. 261)

Haematopoiesis is production of formed elements of the blood. Normally, it takes place in the bone marrow. Circulating blood normally contains 3 main types of mature blood cells—the red cells (erythrocytes), the white cells (leucocytes) and the platelets (thrombocytes). These blood cells perform their respective major physiologic functions: *erythrocytes* largely concerned with oxygen transport, *leucocytes* play various roles in body defense against infection and tissue injury, while *thrombocytes* are primarily involved in maintaining integrity of blood vessels and in preventing blood loss. The lifespan of these cells in circulating blood is variable—neutrophils have a short lifespan of 8-12 hours, followed by platelets with a lifespan of 8-10 days, while the RBCs have the longest lifespan of 90-120 days. Their concentration is normally maintained within well-defined limits.

HAEMATOPOIETIC ORGANS (p. 261)

In the human embryo, the *yolk sac* is the main site of haematopoiesis in the first few weeks of gestation. By about 3rd month, however, the *liver and spleen* are the main sites of blood cell formation and continue to do so until about 2 weeks after birth. Haematopoiesis commences in the *bone marrow* by 4th and 5th month and becomes fully active by 7th and 8th month so that at birth practically all the bones contain active marrow. During normal childhood and adult life, therefore, the marrow is the only source of new blood cells. However, during childhood, there is progressive fatty replacement throughout the long bones so that by adult life the haemato-poietic marrow is confined to the central skeleton (vertebrae, sternum, ribs, skull, sacrum and pelvis) and proximal ends of femur, tibia and humerus. Even in these haematopoietic areas, about 50% of the marrow consists of fat.

Haematopoiesis involves two stages: mitotic division or proliferation, and differentiation or maturation.

It is known for a few decades that blood cells develop from a small population of common multipotent haematopoietic stem cells (HSC). HSC express a variety of cell surface proteins such as CD34 and adhesion proteins which help these cells to "home" to the bone marrow when infused.

After a series of divisions, HSC differentiate into two types of progenitors—*lymphoid* (immune system) stem cells, and *non-lymphoid or myeloid* (trilineage) stem cells. The former develop into T, B and NK cells while the latter differentiate into 3 types of cell lines—granulocyte-monocyte progenitors (producing neutrophils, eosinophils, basophils and monocytes), erythroid progenitors (producing red cells), and megakaryocytes (as the source of platelets). Monocytes on entering the tissues form a variety of phagocytic macrophages, both of which together constitute mononuclear-phagocyte system.

Two cardinal functions of HSC are self-renewal and differentiation of their progenitor cells to produce leucocytes, erythroid cells and platelets. Haematopoiesis or myelopoiesis is regulated by certain endogenous glycoproteins called haematopoietic growth factors, cytokines and hormones. For example:
i) Erythropoietin: for red cell formation
ii) Granulocyte colony-stimulating factor (G-CSF): for production of granulocytes
iii) Granulocyte-macrophage colony-stimulating factor (GM-CSF): for production of granulocytes and monocyte-macrophages
iv) Thrombopoietin; for production of platelets.

BONE MARROW EXAMINATION *(p. 262)*

Bone marrow examination may be performed by two methods—*aspiration* and *trephine biopsy*.

BONE MARROW ASPIRATION The method involves suction of marrow via a strong, wide bore, short-bevelled needle fitted with a stylet and an adjustable guard in order to prevent excessive penetration; for instance Salah bone marrow aspiration needle. Smears are prepared immediately from the bone marrow aspirate and are fixed in 95% methanol after air-drying. The usual Romanowsky technique is employed for staining and a stain for iron is performed routinely so as to assess the reticuloendothelial stores of iron.

The marrow film provides assessment of cellularity, details of developing blood cells (i.e. normoblastic or megaloblastic, myeloid, lymphoid, macrophages and megakaryocytic), ratio between erythroid and myeloid cells, storage diseases, and for the presence of cells foreign to the marrow such as secondary carcinoma, granulomatous conditions, fungi (e.g. histoplasmosis) and parasites (e.g. malaria, leishmaniasis, trypanosomiasis).

TREPHINE BIOPSY Trephine biopsy is performed by a simple *Jamshidi trephine needle* by which a core of tissue from periosteum to bone marrow cavity is obtained. The tissue is then fixed, soft decalcified and processed for histological sections and stained with haematoxylin and eosin and for reticulin. Trephine biopsy is useful over aspiration since it provides an excellent view of the overall marrow architecture, cellularity, and presence or absence of infiltrates and in cases with 'dry tap'.

ERYTHROPOIESIS *(p. 264)*

Erythropoiesis is production of mature erythrocytes of the peripheral blood which takes place in the bone marrow from morphologically unrecognisable HSC. Red cell production is influenced by growth factors and hormones, notably erythropoietin.

Erythropoietic activity in the body is regulated by erythropoietin, which is produced in response to anoxia. The principal site of erythropoietin production is the kidney though there is evidence of its extra-renal production in certain unusual circumstances. Its levels are, therefore, lowered in chronic renal diseases, while a case of renal cell carcinoma may be associated with its increased production and erythrocytosis.

SIGNIFICANCE

1. There is an increased production of erythropoietin in most types of anaemias. However, in anaemia of chronic diseases (e.g. in infections and neoplastic conditions) there is no such enhancement of erythropoietin.
2. In polycythaemia rubra vera, there is erythrocytosis but depressed production of erythropoietin. This is because of an abnormality of HSC class which is not under erythropoietin control.

ERYTHROID SERIES *(p. 265)*

1. **PROERYTHROBLAST** The earliest recognisable cell in the marrow is a proerythroblast or pronormoblast. It is a large cell, 15-20 µm in diameter having deeply basophilic cytoplasm and a large central nucleus containing nucleoli. The deep blue colour of the cytoplasm is due to high content of RNA which is associated with active protein synthesis.

2. **BASOPHILIC (EARLY) ERYTHROBLAST** It is a round cell having a diameter of 12-16 µm with a large nucleus which is slightly more condensed than the proerythroblast and contains basophilic cytoplasm.

3. **POLYCHROMATIC (INTERMEDIATE) ERYTHROBLAST** Next maturation stage has a diameter of 12-14 µm. The nucleus at this stage is coarse and deeply basophilic. The cytoplasm is characteristically polychromatic i.e. contains admixture of basophilic RNA and acidophilic haemoglobin. The cell at this stage ceases to undergo proliferative activity.

4. **ORTHOCHROMATIC (LATE) ERYTHROBLAST** The final stage in the maturation of nucleated red cells is the orthochromatic or late erythroblast. The cell at this stage is smaller, 8-12 µm in diameter, containing a small and pyknotic nucleus with dark nuclear chromatin. The cytoplasm is characteristically acidophilic with diffuse basophilic hue due to the presence of large amounts of haemoglobin.

5. **RETICULOCYTE** The reticulocytes are juvenile red cells devoid of nuclei but contain ribosomal RNA so that they are still able to synthesise haemoglobin. The reticulocytes in the peripheral blood are distinguished from mature red cells by slightly basophilic hue in the cytoplasm similar to that of an orthochromatic erythroblast. Reticulocytes can be counted in the laboratory by *vital staining* with dyes such as new methylene blue or brilliant cresyl blue. Reticulocytes are found normally in the peripheral blood. Normal range of reticulocyte count in health is 0.5-2.5% in adults and 2-6% in infants. Their percentage in the peripheral blood is a fairly accurate reflection of erythropoietic activity.

THE RED CELL *(p. 265)*

The normal human erythrocyte is a biconcave disc, 7.2 µm in diameter, and has a thickness of 2.4 µm at the periphery and 1 µm in the centre. The biconcave shape renders the red cells quite flexible so that they can pass through capillaries whose minimum diameter is 3.5 µm. More than 90% of the weight of erythrocyte consists of haemoglobin. The lifespan of red cells is 120 ± 30 days.

RED CELL MEMBRANE The red cell membrane is a trilaminar structure having a bimolecular lipid layer interposed between two layers of proteins.

◈ Important *proteins* in red cell membrane are band 3 protein (named on the basis of the order in which it migrates during electrophoresis), glycophorin and spectrin.

❖ Important *lipids* are glycolipids, phospholipids and cholesterol.
❖ *Carbohydrates* form skeleton of erythrocytes having a lattice-like network which is attached to the internal surface of the membrane and is responsible for biconcave form of the erythrocytes.

NUTRITIONAL REQUIREMENTS FOR ERYTHROPOIESIS (p. 266)

New red cells are being produced each day for which the marrow requires certain essential substances.

1. Metals Iron is essential for red cell production because it forms part of the haem molecule in haemoglobin. Cobalt and manganese are certain other metals required for red cell production.

2. Vitamins Vitamin B_{12} and folate are essential for biosynthesis of nucleic acids. Vitamin C (ascorbic acid) plays an indirect role by facilitating the iron turnover in the body. Vitamin B_6 (pyridoxine), vitamin E (tocopherol) and riboflavin are the other essential vitamins required in the synthesis of red cells.

3. Amino acids Amino acids comprise the globin component of haemoglobin.

HAEMOGLOBIN Haemoglobin consists of a basic protein, *globin*, and the iron-porphyrin complex, *haem*. Normal adult haemoglobin (*HbA*) constitutes 96-98% of the total haemoglobin content and consists of four polypeptide chains, $\alpha_2\beta_2$. Small quantities of 2 other haemoglobins present in adults are: *HbF* containing $\alpha_2\gamma_2$ globin chains comprising 0.5-0.8% of total haemoglobin, and *HbA$_2$* having $\alpha_2\delta_2$ chains and constituting 1.5-3.5% of total haemoglobin.

Synthesis of haem occurs largely in the mitochondria by a series of biochemical reactions. The reaction is stimulated by erythropoietin and inhibited by haem. Each molecule of haem combines with a globin chain synthesised by polyribosomes. A tetramer of 4 globin chains, each having its own haem group, constitutes the haemoglobin molecule.

RED CELL FUNCTIONS The essential function of the red cells is to carry oxygen from the lungs to the tissue and to transport carbon dioxide to the lungs. In order to perform these functions, the red cells have the ability to generate energy as ATP by anaerobic glycolytic pathway (Embden-Meyerhof pathway).

1. Oxygen carrying The normal adult haemoglobin, HbA, is an extremely efficient oxygen-carrier. The four units of tetramer of haemoglobin molecule take up oxygen in succession, which, in turn, results in stepwise rise in affinity of haemoglobin for oxygen. This is responsible for the *sigmoid shape* of the oxygen dissociation curve.

i) Normal adult haemoglobin (HbA) has *lower affinity for oxygen* than foetal haemoglobin and, therefore, releases greater amount of bound oxygen at pO_2 in tissue capillaries.

ii) A *fall in the pH* (acidic pH) lowers affinity of oxyhaemoglobin for oxygen, so called the Bohr effect, thereby causing enhanced release of oxygen from erythrocytes at the lower pH in tissue capillaries.

iii) A *rise in red cell concentration of 2,3-BPG*, an intermediate product of Embden-Meyerhof pathway, as occurs in anaemia and hypoxia, causes decreased affinity of HbA for oxygen. This, in turn, results in enhanced supply of oxygen to the tissue.

2. CO_2 transport Another important function of the red cells is the CO_2 transport. In the tissue capillaries, the pCO_2 is high so that CO_2 enters the erythrocytes where much of it is converted into bicarbonate ions which diffuse back into the plasma. In the pulmonary capillaries, the process is reversed and bicarbonate ions are converted back into CO_2.

RED CELL DESTRUCTION Red cells have a mean lifespan of 120 days, after which red cell metabolism gradually deteriorates as the enzymes are not replaced. The destroyed red cells are removed mainly by the macrophages of the reticuloendothelial (RE) system of the marrow, and to some extent by the macrophages in the liver and spleen. The breakdown of red cells liberates iron for recirculation via plasma transferrin to marrow erythroblasts, and protoporphyrin which is broken down to bilirubin.

1. Mean corpuscular volume (MCV)

$$\frac{\text{PCV in L/L}}{\text{RBC count/L}}$$

The normal value is 85 ± 8 fl (77-93 fl).

2. Mean corpuscular haemoglobin (MCH)

$$\frac{\text{Hb/L}}{\text{RBC count/L}}$$

The normal range is 29.5 ± 2.5 pg (27-32 pg).

3. Mean corpuscular haemoglobin concentration (MCHC)

$$\frac{\text{Hb/dl}}{\text{PCV in L/L}}$$

The normal value is 32.5 ± 2.5 g/dl (30-35 g/dl).

ANAEMIA—GENERAL CONSIDERATIONS (p. 268)

Anaemia is defined as reduced haemoglobin concentration in blood below the lower limit of the normal range for the age and sex of the individual. In adults, the lower extreme of the normal haemoglobin is taken as 13.0 g/dl for males and 11.5 g/dl for females. Although haemoglobin value is employed as the major parameter for determining whether or not anaemia is present, the red cell counts, haematocrit (PCV) and absolute values (MCV, MCH and MCHC) provide alternate means of assessing anaemia.

PATHOPHYSIOLOGY

Subnormal level of haemoglobin causes lowered oxygen-carrying capacity of the blood. This, in turn, initiates compensatory physiologic adaptations such as follows:
i)   Increased release of oxygen from haemoglobin
ii)   Increased blood flow to the tissues
iii) Maintenance of the blood volume
iv)   Redistribution of blood flow to maintain the cerebral blood supply.
      Eventually, however, tissue hypoxia develops causing impaired functions of the affected tissues.

GENERAL CLINICAL FEATURES (p. 268)

The haemoglobin level at which symptoms and signs of anaemia develop depends upon 4 main factors:
1.   The speed of onset of anaemia
2.   The severity of anaemia
3.   The age of the patient
4.   The haemoglobin dissociation curve

SYMPTOMS In symptomatic cases of anaemia, the presenting features are: tiredness, easy fatiguability, generalised muscular weakness, lethargy and headache. In older patients, there may be symptoms of cardiac failure, angina pectoris, intermittent claudication, confusion and visual disturbances.

SIGNS A few general signs common to all types of anaemias are as under:
1.   Pallor
2.   Hyperdynamic circulation
3.   Symptoms referable to the CNS
4.   Retinal haemorrhages
5.   Menstrual disturbances
6.   Mild proteinuria
7.   Anorexia, flatulence, nausea, constipation and weight loss.

GENERAL SCHEME OF INVESTIGATIONS OF ANAEMIA (p. 269)

In order to confirm or deny the presence of anaemia, its type and its cause, the following plan of investigations is generally followed, of which complete blood counts (CBC) with reticulocyte count is the basic test.

A. HAEMOGLOBIN ESTIMATION The first and foremost investigation in any suspected case of anaemia is to carry out a haemoglobin estimation. Several methods are available but most reliable and accurate is the cyanmethaemoglobin (HiCN) method employing Drabkin's solution and a spectrophotometer. If the haemoglobin value is below the lower limit of the normal range for particular age and sex, the patient is said to be anaemic. In pregnancy, there is haemodilution and, therefore, the lower limit in normal pregnant women is less (10.5 g/dl) than in the non-pregnant state.

B. PERIPHERAL BLOOD FILM EXAMINATION The haemoglobin estimation is invariably followed by examination of a peripheral blood film for morphologic features after staining it with the Romanowsky dyes (e.g. Leishman's stain, May-Grünwald-Giemsa's stain, Jenner-Giemsa's stain, Wright's stain etc). The blood smear is evaluated in an area where there is neither Rouleaux formation nor so thin as to cause red cell distortion. Such an area can usually be found at junction of the body with the tail of the film, but not actually at the tail. The following abnormalities in erythroid series of cells are particularly looked for in a blood smear e.g.

1. Variation in size (Anisocytosis) Normally, there is slight variation in diameter of the red cells from 6.7-7.7 μm (mean value 7.2 μm). Increased variation in size of the red cell is termed anisocytosis. Anisocytosis may be due to the presence of *macrocytosis, microcytosis,* or may be *dimorphic.*

2. Variation in shape (Poikilocytosis) Increased variation in shape of the red cells is termed poikilocytosis. The nature of the abnormal shape determines the cause of anaemia. Poikilocytes are produced in various types of abnormal erythropoiesis e.g. in megaloblastic anaemia, iron deficiency anaemia, thalassaemia, myelosclerosis and microangiopathic haemolytic anaemia.

3. Inadequate haemoglobin formation (Hypochromasia) e.g. hypochromasia and hyperchromasia.

4. Compensatory erythropoiesis e.g. polychromasia, erythroblastaemia, punctate basophilia or basophilic stippling and Howell-Jolly bodies.

5. Miscellaneous changes Several morphologic abnormalities of red cells may be found in different haematological disorders e.g. spherocytosis, schistocytosis, irregularly contracted red cells, leptocytosis or target cell, sickle cells or drepanocytes, crenated red cells, acanthocytosis, burr cells, stomatocytosis and ovalocytosis or elliptocytosis.

C. RED CELL INDICES These are as under:
1. In iron deficiency and thalassaemia, MCV, MCH and MCHC are reduced.
2. In anaemia due to acute blood loss and haemolytic anaemias, MCV, MCH and MCHC are all within normal limits.
3. In megaloblastic anaemias, MCV is raised above the normal range.

D. LEUCOCYTE AND PLATELET COUNT Measurement of leucocyte and platelet count helps to distinguish pure anaemia from pancytopenia in which red cells, granulocytes and platelets are all reduced.

E. RETICULOCYTE COUNT Reticulocyte count (normal 0.5-2.5%) is done in each case of anaemia to assess the marrow erythropoietic activity.

F. ERYTHROCYTE SEDIMENTATION RATE It usually gives a clue to the underlying organic disease but anaemia itself may also cause rise in the ESR.

G. BONE MARROW EXAMINATION Bone marrow aspiration is done in cases where the cause for anaemia is not obvious.

CLASSIFICATION OF ANAEMIAS (p. 271)

PATHOPHYSIOLOGIC CLASSIFICATION

I. Anaemia due to blood loss
A. Acute post-haemorrhagic anaemia
B. Anaemia of chronic blood loss

II. **Anaemia due to impaired red cell formation**

A. *Cytoplasmic maturation defects*
   1. Deficient haem synthesis: iron deficiency anaemia
   2. Deficient globin synthesis: thalassaemic syndromes

B. *Nuclear maturation defects*
   Vitamin B_{12} and/or folic acid deficiency: megaloblastic anaemia

C. *Haematopoietic stem cell proliferation and differentiation abnormality*
   1. Aplastic anaemia
   2. Pure red cell aplasia

D. *Bone marrow failure due to systemic diseases* (anaemia of chronic disorders) e.g.
   1. Anaemia of inflammation/infections, disseminated malignancy
   2. Anaemia in renal disease
   3. Anaemia due to endocrine and nutritional deficiencies (hypometabolic states)
   4. Anaemia in liver disease

E. *Bone marrow infiltration* e.g.
   1. Leukaemias
   2. Lymphomas
   3. Myelosclerosis
   4. Multiple myeloma

F. *Congenital anaemia* e.g.
   1. Sideroblastic anaemia
   2. Congenital dyserythropoietic anaemia.

III. **Anaemia due to increased red cell destruction (haemolytic anaemias)**

A. Intracorpuscular defect (hereditary and acquired).
B. Extracorpuscular defect (acquired haemolytic anaemias).

MORPHOLOGIC CLASSIFICATION Based on the red cell size, haemoglobin content and red cell indices, anaemias are classified into 3 types:

1. Microcytic, hypochromic MCV, MCH, MCHC are all reduced e.g. in iron deficiency anaemia and in certain non-iron deficient anaemias (sideroblastic anaemia, thalassaemia, anaemia of chronic disorders).

2. Normocytic, normochromic MCV, MCH, MCHC are all normal e.g. after acute blood loss, haemolytic anaemias, bone marrow failure, anaemia of chronic disorders.

3. Macrocytic MCV is raised e.g. in megaloblastic anaemia due to deficiency of vitamin B_{12} or folic acid.

HYPOCHROMIC ANAEMIAS (p. 272)

Hypochromic anaemias are classified into 2 groups:
I. Hypochromic anaemia due to iron deficiency.
II. Hypochromic anaemias other than iron deficiency.
   The latter category includes 3 groups of disorders—sideroblastic anaemia, thalassaemia and anaemia of chronic disorders.

IRON DEFICIENCY ANAEMIA (p. 272)

The commonest nutritional deficiency disorder present throughout the world is iron deficiency but its prevalence is higher in the developing countries.

IRON METABOLISM

The iron required for haemoglobin synthesis is derived from 2 primary sources—ingestion of foods containing iron (e.g. leafy vegetables, beans, meats, liver etc) and recycling of iron from senescent red cells.

ABSORPTION The average Western diet contains 10-15 mg of iron, out of which only 5-10% is normally absorbed. In pregnancy and in iron deficiency, the proportion of absorption is raised to 20-30%. Iron is absorbed mainly in the duodenum and proximal jejunum. The absorption is regulated by *mucosal block mechanism:*

◈ Absorption of **non-haem iron** is enhanced by factors such as ascorbic acid (vitamin C), citric acid, amino acids, sugars, gastric secretions and hydrochloric acid of the stomach. Iron absorption is impaired by factors like medicinal antacids, milk, pancreatic secretions, phytates, phosphates, ethylene diamine tetra-acetic acid (EDTA) and tannates contained in tea. Non-haem iron is released as ferrous or ferric form but is absorbed almost exclusively as ferrous form.

◈ The mechanism of dietary **haem iron** absorption is not clearly understood yet but it is through a different transport than DMT 1.

TRANSPORT Iron is transported in plasma bound to a β-globulin, *transferrin*, synthesised in the liver. Transferrin-bound iron is made available to the marrow where the developing erythroid cells having *transferrin receptors* utilise iron for haemoglobin synthesis.

EXCRETION The body is unable to regulate its iron content by excretion alone. The amount of iron lost per day is 0.5-1 mg which is independent of iron intake. This loss is nearly twice more (i.e. 1-2 mg/day) in menstruating women.

DISTRIBUTION In an adult, iron is distributed in the body as under:

1. **Haemoglobin**—present in the red cells, contains most of the body iron (65%).

2. **Myoglobin**—comprises a small amount of iron in the muscles (3.5%).

3. **Haem and non-haem enzymes**—e.g. cytochrome, catalase, peroxidases.

4. **Transferrin-bound iron**—circulates in the plasma.

5. **Ferritin and haemosiderin**—are the *storage forms* of excess iron (30%). They are stored in the mononuclear-phagocyte cells of the spleen, liver and bone marrow and in the parenchymal cells of the liver.

PATHOGENESIS

The development of iron deficiency depends upon one or more of the following factors:
1. Increased blood loss
2. Increased requirements
3. Inadequate dietary intake
4. Decreased intestinal absorption.

In general, in developed countries the mechanism of iron deficiency is usually due to chronic occult blood loss, while in the developing countries poor intake of iron or defective absorption are responsible for iron deficiency anaemia.

ETIOLOGY

Based on the above-mentioned pathogenetic mechanisms, following etiologic factors are involved in development of iron deficiency anaemia at different age and sex:

1. **FEMALES IN REPRODUCTIVE PERIOD OF LIFE** The highest incidence of iron deficiency anaemia is in women during their reproductive years of life. It may be from one or more of the following causes:
i) *Blood loss* This is the most important cause of anaemia in women during child-bearing age group.
ii) *Inadequate intake* Inadequate intake of iron is prevalent in women of lower economic status.
iii) *Increased requirements* During pregnancy and adolescence, the demand of body for iron is increased.

2. **POST-MENOPAUSAL FEMALES** e.g.
i) *Post-menopausal uterine bleeding* due to carcinoma of the uterus.
ii) *Bleeding from the alimentary tract* such as due to carcinoma of stomach and large bowel and hiatus hernia.

3. **ADULT MALES** Iron deficiency in males is infrequent. However, it may occur from the following causes:

i) *Gastrointestinal tract* is the usual source of bleeding which may be due to peptic ulcer, haemorrhoids, hookworm infestation, carcinoma of stomach and large bowel, oesophageal varices, hiatus hernia, chronic aspirin ingestion and ulcerative colitis.

ii) *Urinary tract* e.g. due to haematuria and haemoglobinuria.

iii) *Nose* e.g. in repeated epistaxis.

iv) *Lungs* e.g. in haemoptysis from various causes.

4. **INFANTS AND CHILDREN** Iron deficiency anaemia is fairly common during infancy and childhood with a peak incidence at 1-2 years of age.

CLINICAL FEATURES

As already mentioned, iron deficiency anaemia is much more common in women between the age of 20 and 45 years than in men; at periods of active growth in infancy, childhood and adolescence; and is also more frequent in premature infants.

1. ANAEMIA The onset of iron deficiency anaemia is generally slow. The usual symptoms are weakness, fatigue, dyspnoea on exertion, palpitations and pallor of the skin, mucous membranes and sclerae.

2. EPITHELIAL TISSUE CHANGES Long-standing chronic iron deficiency anaemia causes epithelial tissue changes in some patients. The changes occur in the nails (koilonychia or spoon-shaped nails), tongue (atrophic glossitis), mouth (angular stomatitis), and oesophagus.

LABORATORY FINDINGS

The development of anaemia progresses in 3 stages:

◈ Firstly, *storage iron depletion* occurs during which iron reserves are lost.

◈ The next stage is *iron deficient erythropoiesis* during which the erythroid iron supply is reduced.

◈ The final stage is the development of *frank iron deficiency anaemia* when the red cells become microcytic and hypochromic.

1. BLOOD PICTURE AND RED CELL INDICES These are as under:

i) **Haemoglobin** The essential feature is a fall in haemoglobin concentration up to a variable degree.

ii) **Red cells** The red cells in the blood film are hypochromic and microcytic, and there is anisocytosis and poikilocytosis.

iii) **Reticulocyte count** The reticulocyte count is normal or reduced.

iv) **Absolute values** The red cell indices reveal a diminished MCV (below 50 fl), diminished MCH (below 15 pg), and diminished MCHC (below 20 g/dl).

v) **Leucocytes** The total and differential white cell counts are usually normal.

vi) **Platelets** Platelet count is usually normal.

2. BONE MARROW FINDINGS Bone marrow examination is not essential in such cases routinely but is done in complicated cases so as to distinguish from other hypochromic anaemias.

i) **Marrow cellularity** The marrow cellularity is increased due to erythroid hyperplasia (myeloid-erythroid ratio decreased).

ii) **Erythropoiesis** There is normoblastic erythropoiesis with predominance of small polychromatic normoblasts (micronormoblasts). The *cytoplasmic maturation lags behind* so that the late normoblasts have pyknotic nucleus but persisting polychromatic cytoplasm.

iii) **Other cells** Myeloid, lymphoid and megakaryocytic cells are normal in number and morphology.

iv) **Marrow iron** Iron staining (Prussian blue reaction) on bone marrow aspirate smear shows deficient reticuloendothelial iron stores.

3. BIOCHEMICAL FINDINGS These are as under:

i) The *serum iron* level is low (normal 40-140 µg/dl); it is often under 50 µg/dl.

ii) *Total iron binding capacity (TIBC)* is high (normal 250-450 µg/dl) and rises to give less than 10% saturation (normal 33%).

iii) *Serum ferritin* is very low (normal 30-250 ng/ml) indicating poor tissue iron stores.

PRINCIPLES OF TREATMENT

The management of iron deficiency anaemia consists of 2 essential principles: correction of disorder causing the anaemia, and correction of iron deficiency.

SIDEROBLASTIC ANAEMIA *(p. 277)*

The sideroblastic anaemias comprise a group of disorders of diverse etiology in which the nucleated erythroid precursors in the bone marrow, show characteristic 'ringed sideroblasts.'

SIDEROCYTES These are red cells containing granules of non-haem iron. These granules stain positively with Prussian blue reaction as well as stain with Romanowsky dyes when they are referred to as *Pappenheimer bodies.* Siderocytes are normally not present in the human peripheral blood.

SIDEROBLASTS These are nucleated red cells (normo-blasts) containing siderotic granules which stain positively with Prussian blue reaction.

Normal sideroblasts contain a few fine, scattered cytoplasmic granules representing iron which has not been utilised for haemoglobin synthesis.

Abnormal sideroblasts are further of 2 types:

❖ *One type* is a sideroblast containing numerous, diffusely scattered, coarse cytoplasmic granules and are seen in conditions such as dyserythropoiesis and haemolysis.

❖ The other type is *ringed sideroblast* in which haem synthesis is disturbed as occurs in sideroblastic anaemias. Ringed sideroblasts contain numerous large granules, often forming a complete or partial ring around the nucleus.

TYPES OF SIDEROBLASTIC ANAEMIAS

I. HEREDITARY SIDEROBLASTIC ANAEMIA This is a rare X-linked disorder associated with defective enzyme activity of *aminolevulinic acid (ALA) synthetase* required for haem synthesis.

II. ACQUIRED SIDEROBLASTIC ANAEMIA The acquired sideroblastic anaemias are classified into primary and secondary types.

A. Primary acquired sideroblastic anaemia Primary, idiopathic, or refractory acquired sideroblastic anaemia occurs spontaneously in middle-aged and older individuals of both sexes. The disorder has its pathogenesis in disturbed growth and maturation of erythroid precursors at the level of haematopoietic stem cell, possibly due to reduced activity of the enzyme, ALA synthetase.

B. Secondary acquired sideroblastic anaemia Acquired sideroblastic anaemia may develop secondary to a variety of causes:

1. *Drugs, chemicals and toxins:* Isoniazid, an anti-tuberculous drug and a pyridoxine antagonist, is most commonly associated with development of sideroblastic anaemia by producing abnormalities in pyridoxine metabolism.

2. *Haematological disorders:* These include myelofibrosis, polycythaemia vera, acute leukaemia, myeloma, lymphoma and haemolytic anaemia.

3. *Miscellaneous:* Occasionally, secondary sideroblastic anaemia may occur in association with a variety of inflammatory, neoplastic and autoimmune diseases such as carcinoma, myxoedema, rheumatoid arthritis and SLE.

LABORATORY FINDINGS

1. There is generally moderate to severe degree of *anaemia*.

2.   The *blood picture* shows hypochromic anaemia which may be microcytic, or there may be some normocytic red cells as well (dimorphic).

3.   *Absolute values* (MCV, MCH and MCHC) are reduced in hereditary type but MCV is often raised in acquired type.

4.   *Bone marrow examination* shows erythroid hyperplasia with usually macronormoblastic erythropoiesis. Marrow iron stores are raised and pathognomonic ring sideroblasts are present.

5.   *Serum ferritin* levels are raised.

6.   *Serum iron* is usually raised with almost complete saturation of TIBC.

7.   There is increased *iron deposition* in the tissue.

PRINCIPLES OF TREATMENT

The treatment of secondary sideroblastic anaemia is primarily focussed on removal of the offending agent.

ANAEMIA OF CHRONIC DISORDERS *(p. 278)*

One of the commonly encountered anaemia is in patients of a variety of chronic systemic diseases in which anaemia develops secondary to a disease process but there is no actual invasion of the bone marrow.

PATHOGENESIS

In general, 2 factors appear to play significant role in the pathogenesis of anaemia in chronic disorders. These are: *defective red cell production and reduced red cell lifespan.*

ETIOLOGY

1.   Anaemia in chronic infections/inflammation
     a.   *Infections e.g.* tuberculosis, lung abscess, pneumonia, osteomyelitis, subacute bacterial endocarditis, pyelonephritis.
     b.   *Non-infectious inflammations* e.g. rheumatoid arthritis, SLE, vasculitis, dermatomyositis, scleroderma, sarcoidosis, Crohn's disease.
     c.   *Disseminated malignancies* e.g. Hodgkin's disease, disseminated carcinomas and sarcomas.

2.   Anaemia of renal disease e.g.
     uraemia, renal failure

3.   Anaemia of hypometabolic state e.g.
     endocrinopathies (myxoedema, Addison's disease, hyperthyroidism, hypopituitarism, Addison's disease), protein malnutrition, scurvy and pregnancy, liver disease.

LABORATORY FINDINGS

i)   **Haemoglobin**   Anaemia is generally mild to moderate.

ii)   **Blood picture**   The type of anaemia in these cases is generally normocytic normochromic.

iii)   **Absolute values**   MCHC is slightly low.

iv)   **Reticulocyte count**   The reticulocyte count is generally low.

v)   **Red cell survival**   Mild to moderate shortening of their lifespan.

vi)   **Bone marrow**   Examination of the marrow generally reveals normal erythroid maturation. However, the red cell precursors have reduced stainable iron than normal, while macrophages in the marrow usually contain increased amount of iron.

vii)   **Serum iron and TIBC**   Serum iron is characteristically reduced in this group of anaemias while TIBC is low-to-normal.

viii)   **Serum ferritin**   Serum ferritin levels are increased in these patients and is the most distinguishing feature from true iron-deficiency anaemia.

ix)   **Other plasma proteins**   In addition, certain other plasma proteins called '*phase reactants*' are raised in patients with chronic inflammation, probably under the stimulus of interleukin-1 released by activated macrophages.

MEGALOBLASTIC ANAEMIA *(p. 280)*

The megaloblastic anaemias are disorders caused by impaired DNA synthesis. The underlying defect for the asynchronous maturation of the nucleus is defective DNA synthesis due to deficiency of vitamin B_{12} (cobalamin) and/or folic acid (folate).

VITAMIN B_{12} METABOLISM

SOURCES The only dietary sources of vitamin B_{12} are foods of animal protein origin such as kidney, liver, heart, muscle meats, fish, eggs, cheese and milk. Cooking has little effect on its activity. Vitamin B_{12} is synthesised in the human large bowel by microorganisms but is not absorbed from this site and, thus, the humans are entirely dependent upon dietary sources.

ABSORPTION After ingestion, vitamin B_{12} in food is released and forms a stable complex with gastric R-binder. On entering the duodenum, the vitamin B_{12}-R-binder complex is digested releasing vitamin B_{12} which then binds to intrinsic factor (IF). The vitamin B_{12}-IF complex, on reaching the distal ileum, binds to the specific receptors on the mucosal brush border, thereby enabling the vitamin to be absorbed.

TISSUE STORES Normally, the liver is the principal storage site of vitamin B_{12} and stores about 2 mg of the vitamin, while other tissues like the kidney, heart and brain together store about 2 mg.

FUNCTIONS Vitamin B_{12} plays an important role in general cell metabolism, particularly essential for normal haematopoiesis and for maintenance of integrity of the nervous system. Vitamin B_{12} acts as a co-enzyme for 2 main biochemical reactions in the body:

◈ *Firstly, as methyl cobalamin (methyl B_{12})* in the methylation of homocysteine to methionine by methyl tetrahydrofolate (THF).

◈ *Secondly, as adenosyl cobalamin (adenosyl B_{12})* in propionate metabolism for the conversion of methyl malonyl co-enzyme A to succinyl co-enzyme A:

FOLATE METABOLISM

SOURCES Folate exists in different plants, bacteria and animal tissues. Its main dietary sources are fresh green leafy vegetables, fruits, liver, kidney, and to a lesser extent, muscle meats, cereals and milk. Folate is labile and is largely destroyed by cooking and canning. Some amount of folate synthesised by bacteria in the human large bowel is not available to the body.

ABSORPTION AND TRANSPORT Folate is normally absorbed from the duodenum and upper jejunum and to a lesser extent, from the lower jejunum and ileum. Polyglutamate form in the foodstuffs is first cleaved by the enzyme, folate conjugase, in the mucosal cells to mono- and diglutamates which are readily assimilated.

TISSUE STORES The liver and red cells are the main storage sites of folate, largely as methyl THF polyglutamate form. The total body stores of folate are about 10-12 mg enough for about 4 months.

FUNCTIONS It acts as a co-enzyme for 2 important biochemical reactions involving transfer of 1-carbon units (viz. methyl and formyl groups):

◈ *Thymidylate synthetase reaction* Formation of dTMP.

◈ *Methylation of homocysteine to methionine* This reaction is linked to vitamin B_{12} metabolism.

BIOCHEMICAL BASIS OF MEGALOBLASTIC ANAEMIA

The basic biochemical abnormality common to both vitamin B_{12} and folate deficiency is a block in the pathway of DNA synthesis and that there is an inter-relationship between vitamin B_{12} and folate metabolism in the methylation reaction of homocysteine to methionine.

Two of the important folate-dependent (1-carbon transfer) reactions for formation of building blocks in DNA synthesis are as under:

1. Thymidylate synthetase reaction This reaction involves synthesis of deoxy thymidylate monophosphate (dTMP) from deoxy uridylate monophosphate (dUMP).

2. Homocysteine-methionine reaction Homocysteine is converted into methionine by transfer of a methyl group from methylene-THF. After transfer of 1-carbon from methylene-THF, THF is produced. This reaction requires the presence of vitamin B_{12} (methyl-B_{12}).

Deficiency of folate from any cause results in reduced supply of the coenzyme, methylene-THF, and thus interferes with the synthesis of DNA. Deficiency of vitamin B_{12} traps folate as its transport form, methyl-THF, thereby resulting in reduced formation of the active form, methylene-THF, needed for DNA synthesis. This is referred to as *methyl-folate trap hypothesis*.

ETIOLOGY AND CLASSIFICATION OF MEGALOBLASTIC ANAEMIA

1. VITAMIN B_{12} DEFICIENCY In Western countries, deficiency of vitamin B_{12} is more commonly due to pernicious (Addisonian) anaemia. True vegetarians like traditional Indian Hindus and breast-fed infants have dietary lack of vitamin B_{12}.

2. FOLATE DEFICIENCY Folate deficiency is more often due to poor dietary intake. Other causes include malabsorption, excess folate utilisation such as in pregnancy and in various disease states, chronic alcoholism, and excess urinary folate loss.

Patients with tropical sprue are often deficient in both vitamin B_{12} and folate. Combined deficiency of vitamin B_{12} and folate may occur from severe deficiency of vitamin B_{12} because of the biochemical interrelationship with folate metabolism.

3. OTHER CAUSES These include many drugs which interfere with DNA synthesis, acquired defects of haematopoietic stem cells, and rarely, congenital enzyme deficiencies.

CLINICAL FEATURES

1. Anaemia
2. Glossitis
3. Neurologic manifestations
4. Others e.g. mild jaundice, angular stomatitis, purpura, melanin pigmentation, symptoms of malabsorption, weight loss and anorexia.

LABORATORY FINDINGS

A. *GENERAL LABORATORY FINDINGS*

1. BLOOD PICTURE AND RED CELL INDICES These are as under:

i) Haemoglobin Haemoglobin estimation reveals values below the normal range.

ii) Red cells Red blood cell morphology in a blood film shows the characteristic macrocytosis. However, *macrocytosis* can also be seen in several other disorders such as: haemolysis, liver disease, chronic alcoholism, hypothyroidism, aplastic anaemia, myeloproliferative disorders and reticulocytosis.

iii) Reticulocyte count The reticulocyte count is generally low to normal in untreated cases.

iv) Absolute values The red cell indices reveal an elevated MCV (above 120 fl) proportionate to the severity of macrocytosis, elevated MCH (above 50 pg) and normal or reduced MCHC.

v) Leucocytes The total white blood cell count may be reduced. Presence of characteristic hypersegmented neutrophils (having more than 5 nuclear lobes) in the blood film should raise the suspicion of megaloblastic anaemia.

vi) Platelets Platelet count may be moderately reduced in severely anaemic patients. Bizarre forms of platelets may be seen.

2. BONE MARROW FINDINGS These are as under:

i) Marrow cellularity The marrow is hypercellular with a decreased myeloid-erythroid ratio.

ii) Erythropoiesis There is erythroid hyperplasia due to characteristic megaloblastic erythropoiesis. *Megaloblasts* are abnormal, large, nucleated erythroid precursors, having nuclear-cytoplasmic asynchrony i.e. the nuclei are less mature than the development of cytoplasm. The nuclei are large, having fine, sieve-like and open chromatin that stains lightly, while the haemoglobinisation of the cytoplasm proceeds normally or at a faster rate i.e. *nuclear maturation lags behind that of cytoplasm.*

iii) Other cells Granulocyte precursors are also affected to some extent. Giant forms of metamyelocytes and band cells may be present in the marrow.

iv) Marrow iron Prussian blue staining for iron in the marrow shows an increase in the number and size of iron granules in the erythroid precursors.

3. BIOCHEMICAL FINDINGS These are as under:

i) There is rise in *serum unconjugated bilirubin and* LDH as a result of ineffective erythropoiesis causing marrow cell breakdown.

ii) The *serum iron and ferritin* may be normal or elevated.

B. *SPECIAL TESTS FOR CAUSE OF SPECIFIC DEFICIENCY*

TESTS FOR VITAMIN B$_{12}$ DEFICIENCY These are as under:

i) Microbiological assay In this test, the serum sample to be assayed is added to a medium containing all other essential growth factors required for a vitamin B$_{12}$-dependent microorganism. The medium along with microorganism is incubated and the amount of vitamin B$_{12}$ is determined turbimetrically. *E. gracilis is* considered more sensitive and accurate microorganism for this assay.

ii) Radioassay Assays of serum B$_{12}$ by radioisotope dilution (RID) and radioimmunoassay (RIA) have been developed.

iii) Schilling test (24-hour urinary excretion test) Schilling test is done to detect vitamin B$_{12}$ deficiency as well as to distinguish and detect lack of IF and malabsorption syndrome. The results of test also depend upon good renal function and proper urinary collection. Radioisotope used for labeling B$_{12}$ is either ^{58}Co or ^{57}Co. The test is performed in 3 stages:
◈ Stage I: Without IF
◈ Stage II: With IF
◈ Stage III: Test for malabsorption of vitamin B$_{12}$

iv) Serum enzyme levels Serum determination of methylmalonic acid and homocysteine by sophisticated enzymatic assays can be done. Both are elevated in cobalamine deficiency, while in folate deficiency there is only elevation of homocysteine.

TESTS FOR FOLATE DEFICIENCY Measurement of *formiminoglutamic acid (FIGLU) urinary excretion* after histidine load was used formerly for assessing folate status but it is less specific and less sensitive than the serum assays. Currently, there are 3 tests used to detect folate deficiency—urinary excretion of FIGLU, serum and red cell folate assay.

PRINCIPLES OF TREATMENT

Most cases of megaloblastic anaemia need therapy with appropriate vitamin. Severely-anaemic patients in whom a definite deficiency of either vitamin cannot be established with certainty are treated with both vitamins concurrently.

The marrow begins to revert back to normal morphology within a few hours of initiating treatment and becomes normoblastic within 48 hours of start of treatment. Reticulocytosis appears within 4-5 days after therapy is started and peaks at day 7. Haemoglobin should rise by 2-3 g/dl each fortnight.

Pernicious anaemia (PA) was first described by Addison in 1855 as a chronic disorder of middle-aged and elderly individual of either sex in which intrinsic factor (IF) secretion ceases owing to atrophy of the gastric mucosa.

PATHOGENESIS

There is evidence to suggest that the atrophy of gastric mucosa in PA resulting in absence or low level of IF is caused by an autoimmune reaction against gastric parietal cells as under:

1. The incidence of PA is high in patients with *other autoimmune diseases*.
2. Patients with PA have abnormal *circulating autoantibodies* such as anti-parietal cell antibody (90% cases) and anti-intrinsic factor antibody (50% cases).
3. *Relatives* of patients with PA have an increased incidence of the disease.
4. *Corticosteroids* have been reported to be beneficial in curing the disease both pathologically and clinically.
5. PA is more common in patients with *agammaglobulinaemia*.
6. Certain *HLA types* have been reported to be associated with PA.

M/E The findings are as under:

The most characteristic pathologic finding in PA is gastric atrophy affecting the acid- and pepsin-secreting portion of the stomach. Gastric epithelium may show cellular atypia.

CLINICAL FEATURES

The clinical manifestations are mainly due to vitamin B_{12} deficiency and include: anaemia, glossitis, neurological abnormalities, gastrointestinal manifestations hepatosplenomegaly, congestive heart failure and haemor-rhagic manifestations.

PRINCIPLES OF TREATMENT

1. Parenteral vitamin B_{12} replacement therapy.
2. Symptomatic and supportive therapy such as physiotherapy for neurologic deficits and occasionally blood transfusion.
3. Follow-up for early detection of cancer of the stomach.

HAEMOLYTIC ANAEMIAS AND ANAEMIA DUE TO BLOOD LOSS (P. 286)

DEFINITION AND CLASSIFICATION

Haemolytic anaemias are defined as anaemias resulting from an increase in the rate of red cell destruction. The red cell lifespan is shortened in haemolytic anaemia i.e. there is accelerated haemolysis.

The premature destruction of red cells in haemolytic anaemia may occur at either of the following 2 sites:

◈ **Firstly,** the red cells undergo lysis in the circulation and release their contents into plasma *(intravascular haemolysis)*. In these cases the plasma haemoglobin rises substantially and part of it may be excreted in the urine *(haemoglobinuria)*.

◈ **Secondly,** the red cells are taken up by cells of the RE system where they are destroyed and digested *(extravascular haemolysis)*. In extravascular haemolysis, plasma haemoglobin level is, therefore, barely raised.

Extravascular haemolysis is more common than the former.

Clinically, haemolytic anaemias may be acute or chronic, mild to severe, hereditary or acquired. Haemolytic anaemias are broadly classified into 2 main categories:

I. *Acquired haemolytic anaemias* caused by a variety of extrinsic environmental factors *(i.e. extracorpuscular)*.

II. *Hereditary haemolytic anaemias* are usually the result of intrinsic red cell defects *(i.e. intracorpuscular)*.

A simplified classification is given below:

I. ACQUIRED
  A. *Antibody:* Immunohaemolytic anaemias
    1. Autoimmune haemolytic anaemia (AIHA)
       i) Warm antibody AIHA
       ii) Cold antibody AIHA
    2. Drug-induced immunohaemolytic anaemia
    3. Isoimmune haemolytic anaemia
  B. *Mechanical trauma:* Microangiopathic haemolytic anaemia
  C. *Direct toxic effects:* Malaria, bacterial, infection and other agents
  D. *Acquired red cell membrane abnormalities:* Paroxysmal nocturnal haemoglobinuria (PNH)
  E. *Splenomegaly*
II. HEREDITARY
  A. *Abnormalities of red cell membrane*
    1. Hereditary spherocytosis
    2. Hereditary elliptocytosis (hereditary ovalocytosis)
    3. Hereditary stomatocytosis
  B. *Disorders of red cell interior*
    1. *Red cell enzyme defects (Enzymopathies)*
       i) Defects in the hexose monophosphate shunt: G6PD deficiency
       ii) Defects in the Embden-Meyerhof (or glycolytic) pathway: pyruvate kinase deficiency
    2. *Disorders of haemoglobin (Haemoglobinopathies)*
       i) Structurally abnormal haemoglobins: sickle syndromes, other haemoglobinopathies
       ii) Reduced globin chain synthesis: thalassaemias

GENERAL ASPECTS *(p. 287)*

GENERAL CLINICAL FEATURES

1. Presence of pallor of mucous membranes.
2. Positive family history with life-long anaemia in patients with congenital haemolytic anaemia.
3. Mild fluctuating jaundice due to unconjugated hyperbilirubinaemia.
4. Urine turns dark on standing due to excess of urobilinogen in urine.
5. Splenomegaly is found in most chronic haemolytic anaemias, both congenital and acquired.
6. Pigment gallstones are found in some cases.

LABORATORY EVALUATION OF HAEMOLYSIS

I. *TESTS OF INCREASED RED CELL BREAKDOWN*

1. *Serum bilirubin*—unconjugated (indirect) bilirubin is raised.
2. *Urine urobilinogen* is raised but there is no bilirubinuria.
3. *Faecal stercobilinogen* is raised.
4. *Serum haptoglobin* (α-globulin binding protein) is reduced or absent.
5. *Plasma lactic dehydrogenase* is raised.
6. *Evidences of intravascular haemolysis* in the form of haemoglobinaemia, haemoglobinuria, methaemoglobinaemia and haemosiderinuria.

II. *TESTS OF INCREASED RED CELL PRODUCTION*

1. *Reticulocyte count* reveals reticulocytosis.
2. *Routine blood film* shows macrocytosis, polychromasia and presence of normoblasts.
3. *Bone marrow* shows erythroid hyperplasia with usually raised iron stores.
4. *X-ray of bones* shows evidence of expansion of marrow space.

III. *TESTS OF DAMAGE TO RED CELLS*

1. *Routine blood film* shows a variety of abnormal morphological appearances of red cells.

2. *Osmotic fragility* is increased or decreased.
3. *Autohaemolysis test* with or without addition of glucose.
4. *Coombs' antiglobulin test.*
5. *Electrophoresis* for abnormal haemoglobins.
6. *Estimation of HbA₂.*
7. *Estimation of HbF.*
8. *Tests for sickling.*
9. *Screening test for G6PD deficiency* and other enzymes (e.g. Heinz bodies test).

IV. TESTS FOR SHORTENED RED CELL LIFESPAN

A shortened red cell survival is best tested by ^{51}Cr labelling method. Normal RBC lifespan of 120 days is shortened to 20-40 days in moderate haemolysis and to 5-20 days in severe haemolysis.

I. ACQUIRED HAEMOLYTIC ANAEMIAS (p. 288)

A. IMMUNOHAEMOLYTIC ANAEMIAS

Immunohaemolytic anaemias are a group of anaemias occurring due to antibody production by the body against its own red cells.

AUTOIMMUNE HAEMOLYTIC ANAEMIA (AIHA)

'WARM' ANTIBODY AIHA

PATHOGENESIS Warm antibodies reactive at body temperature and coating the red cells are generally IgG class antibodies and occasionally they are IgA. The spleen is particularly efficient in trapping red cells coated with IgG antibodies. It is, thus, the major site of red cell destruction in warm antibody AIHA.

CLINICAL FEATURES Warm antibody AIHA may occur at any age and in either sex. The disease may occur without any apparent cause (idiopathic) but about a quarter of patients develop this disorder as a complication of an underlying disease affecting the immune system.

The usual clinical features are as follows:
1. Chronic anaemia of varying severity with remissions and relapses.
2. Splenomegaly.
3. Occasionally hyperbilirubinaemia.

LABORATORY FINDINGS These are as under:
1. Mild to moderate chronic anaemia.
2. Reticulocytosis.
3. Prominent spherocytosis in the peripheral blood film.
4. Positive direct Coombs' (antiglobulin) test for presence of warm antibodies on the red cell, best detected at 37°C.
5. A positive indirect Coombs' (antiglobulin) test at 37°C
6. Unconjugated (indirect) hyperbilirubinaemia.
7. Co-existent immune thrombocytopenia along with occasional venous thrombosis may be present.
8. In more severe cases, haemoglobinaemia and haemoglobinuria may be present.

'COLD' ANTIBODY AIHA

PATHOGENESIS Antibodies which are reactive in the cold (4°C) may induce haemolysis under 2 conditions:

1. Cold agglutinin disease The antibodies are IgM type which bind to the red cells best at 4°C. These cold antibodies are usually directed against the *I* antigen on the red cell surface.

The etiology of cold antibody remains unknown. It is seen in the course of certain infections (e.g. *Mycoplasma* pneumonia, infectious mononucleosis) and in lymphomas.

2. Paroxysmal cold haemoglobinuria (PCH) In PCH, cold antibody is an IgG antibody (Donath-Landsteiner antibody) which is directed against *P*

blood group antigen and brings about complement-mediated haemolysis.
Attacks of PCH are precipitated by exposure to cold.

PCH is uncommon and may be seen in association with tertiary syphilis or as a complication of certain infections such as *Mycoplasma,* pneumonia, flu, measles and mumps.

CLINICAL FEATURES These are as under:
1. Chronic anaemia which is worsened by exposure to cold.
2. Raynaud's phenomenon.
3. Cyanosis affecting the cold exposed regions such as tips of nose, ears, fingers and toes.
4. Haemoglobinaemia and haemoglobinuria occur on exposure to cold.

LABORATORY FINDINGS These are as follows:
1. Chronic anaemia.
2. Low reticulocyte count since *young red cells are affected more.*
3. Spherocytosis is less marked.
4. Positive direct Coombs' test.
5. The cold antibody titre is very high at 4°C and very low at 37°C (Donath-Landsteiner test).

DRUG-INDUCED IMMUNOHAEMOLYTIC ANAEMIA

Drugs may cause immunohaemolytic anaemia by 3 different mechanisms:
1. α-methyl dopa type antibodies
2. Penicillin-induced immunohaemolysis
3. Innocent bystander immunohaemolysis

In each type of drug-induced immunohaemolytic anaemia, discontinuation of the drug results in gradual disappearance of haemolysis.

ISOIMMUNE HAEMOLYTIC ANAEMIA

Isoimmune haemolytic anaemias are caused by acquiring isoantibodies or alloantibodies by blood transfusions, pregnancies and in haemolytic disease of the newborn. These antibodies produced by one individual are directed against red blood cells of the other.

B. MICROANGIOPATHIC HAEMOLYTIC ANAEMIA

Microangiopathic haemolytic anaemia is caused by abnormalities in the microvasculature. It is generally due to mechanical trauma to the red cells in circulation and is characterised by red cell fragmentation (schistocytosis). There are 3 different ways by which microangiopathic haemolytic anaemia results:

1. EXTERNAL IMPACT e.g. in prolonged marchers, joggers, karate players etc. These patients develop haemoglobinaemia, haemoglobinuria (march haemoglobinuria), and sometimes myoglobinuria as a result of damage to muscles.

2. CARDIAC HAEMOLYSIS A small proportion of patients who receive prosthetic cardiac valves or artificial grafts develop haemolysis.

3. FIBRIN DEPOSIT IN MICROVASCULATURE e.g.
i) Abnormalities of the vessel wall
ii) Thrombotic thrombocytopenic purpura.
iii) Haemolytic-uraemic syndrome.
iv) Disseminated intravascular coagulation (DIC).
v) Vasculitis in collagen diseases.

C. HAEMOLYTIC ANAEMIA FROM DIRECT TOXIC EFFECTS

Haemolysis may result from direct toxic effects of certain agents e.g.
1. Malaria
2. Bartonellosis
3. Septicaemia with *Clostridium welchii*
4. Other microorganisms
5. Copper

6. Lead poisoning
7. Snake and spider bites
8. Extensive burns.

D. PAROXYSMAL NOCTURNAL HAEMOGLOBINURIA (PNH)

PNH is a rare acquired disorder of red cell membrane in which there is chronic intravascular haemolysis due to undue sensitivity of red blood cells to complement due to defective synthesis of a red cell membrane protein.

PATHOGENESIS PNH is considered as an acquired clonal disease of the cell membrane while normal clone also continues to proliferate. The defect is a mutation in the stem cells affecting myeloid progenitor cells that is normally required for the biosynthesis of glycosyl phosphatidyl inositol (GPI) essential for anchoring of the cell.

CLINICAL AND LABORATORY FINDINGS These are as under:
i) Haemolytic anaemia.
ii) Pancytopenia (mild granulocytopenia and thrombocytopenia frequent).
iii) Intermittent clinical haemoglobinuria; acute haemolytic episodes occur at night identified by passage of brown urine in the morning.
iv) Haemosiderinuria very common.
v) Venous thrombosis as a common complication.

The presence of inordinate sensitivity of red blood cells, leucocytes and platelets to complement in PNH can be demonstrated *in vitro* by Ham's test using red cell lysis at acidic pH or by sucrose haemolysis test.

E. HAEMOLYTIC ANAEMIA IN SPLENOMEGALY

Splenomegaly exaggerates the damaging effect to which the red cells are exposed. Besides haemolytic anaemia, splenomegaly is usually associated with pancytopenia. Splenectomy or reduction in size of spleen by appropriate therapy relieves the anaemia as well as improves the leucocyte and platelet counts.

II. HEREDITARY HAEMOLYTIC ANAEMIAS *(p. 291)*

A. HEREDITARY ABNORMALITIES OF RED CELL MEMBRANE

There are 3 important types of inherited red cell membrane defects: hereditary spherocytosis, hereditary elliptocytosis (hereditary ovalocytosis) and hereditary stomatocytosis.

HEREDITARY SPHEROCYTOSIS

Hereditary spherocytosis is a common type of hereditary haemolytic anaemia of autosomal dominant inheritance in which the red cell membrane is abnormal.

PATHOGENESIS The molecular abnormality in hereditary spherocytosis is a defect in proteins which anchor the lipid bilayer to the underlying cytoskeleton. These are:
1. Spectrin deficiency
2. Ankyrin abnormality

Inherited mutation in spectrin or ankyrin causes defect in anchoring of lipid bilayer cell membrane. This results in formation of spheroidal contour and smaller size of red blood cells, termed *microspherocytes*.

CLINICAL FEATURES The family history may be present.
1. *Anaemia* is usually mild to moderate.
2. *Splenomegaly* is a constant feature.
3. *Jaundice* occurs due to increased concentration of unconjugated (indirect) bilirubin.
4. *Pigment gallstones* are frequent.

LABORATORY FINDINGS These are as under:
1. *Anaemia* of mild to moderate degree.
2. *Reticulocytosis*, usually 5-20%.

3. Blood film shows the characteristic abnormality of erythrocytes in the form of microspherocytes.

4. MCV is usually normal or slightly decreased but *MCHC is increased.*

5. *Osmotic fragility is increased.*

6. *Autohaemolysis test* shows increased spontaneous autohaemolysis.

7. *Direct Coombs' (antiglobulin) test* is negative.

HEREDITARY ELLIPTOCYTOSIS (HEREDITARY OVALOCYTOSIS)

Hereditary elliptocytosis or hereditary ovalocytosis is another autosomal dominant disorder involving red cell membrane protein *spectrin*. Acquired causes of elliptocytosis include iron deficiency and myeloproliferative disorders.

HEREDITARY STOMATOCYTOSIS

Stomatocytes are cup-shaped RBCs having one surface concave and the other side as convex. The underlying defect is in membrane protein, *stomatin*, having autosomal dominant pattern of inheritance.

B. HEREDITARY DISORDERS OF RED CELL INTERIOR

RED CELL ENZYME DEFECTS (ENZYMOPATHIES)

G6PD DEFICIENCY

Among the defects in hexose monophosphate shunt, the most common is G6PD deficiency. G6PD gene is located on the X chromosome and its deficiency is, therefore, a sex (X)-linked trait affecting males, while the females are carriers and are asymptomatic. Several variants of G6PD have been described. The most common and significant clinical variant is A– (negative) type found in black males.

PATHOGENESIS Individuals with inherited deficiency of G6PD, an enzyme required for hexose monophosphate shunt for glucose metabolism, fail to develop adequate levels of reduced glutathione in their red cells. This results in oxidation and precipitation of haemoglobin within the red cells forming Heinz bodies.

CLINICAL FEATURES These are as under:

1. **Acute haemolytic anaemia** This develops in males, being X-linked disorder, within hours of exposure to oxidant stress such as drugs like primaquin, infection, favism and metabloc acidosis. It *affects the older red cells only.*

2. **Chronic haemolytic anaemia** Cases having severe enzyme deficiency have chronic persistent haemolysis throughout life.

3. **Neonatal jaundice** Infants born with G6PD deficiency may continue to have unconjugated hyperbilirubinaemia and may even develop kernicterus.

LABORATORY FINDINGS These are as under:

1. **During the period of acute haemolysis,** there is rapid fall in haematocrit by 25-30%, features of intravascular haemolysis such as rise in plasma haemoglobin, haemoglobinuria, rise in unconjugated bilirubin and fall in plasma haptoglobin. Formation of Heinz bodies is visualised by means of supravital stains such as crystal violet, also called *Heinz body haemolytic anaemia.*

2. **Between the crises,** the affected patient generally has no anaemia. The red cell survival is, however, shortened.

The diagnosis of G6PD enzyme deficiency is made by one of the screening tests (e.g. methaemoglobin reduction test or MRT, fluorescent screening test, ascorbate cyanide screening test), or by direct enzyme assay on red cells.

PK DEFICIENCY

Pyruvate kinase (PK) deficiency is the only significant enzymopathy of the Embden-Meyerhof glycolytic pathway. The disorder is inherited as an autosomal recessive pattern.

Haemoglobin in RBCs may be abnormally synthesised due to inherited defects. These disorders may be of two types:

◆ *Qualitative disorders* in which there is structural abnormality in synthesis of haemoglobin e.g. sickle cell syndrome, other haemoglobinopathies.

◆ *Quantitative disorders* in which there quantitatively decreased globin chain synthesis of haemoglobin e.g. thalassaemias.

STRUCTURALLY ABNORMAL HAEMOGLOBINS

SICKLE SYNDROMES

The most important and widely prevalent type of haemoglobinopathy is due to the presence of sickle haemoglobin (HbS) in the red blood cells. The red cells with HbS develop 'sickling' when they are exposed to low oxygen tension. Sickle syndromes have the highest frequency in black race and in Central Africa where *falciparum* malaria is endemic. Patients with HbS are relatively protected against falciparum malaria. Sickle syndromes occur in 3 different forms:

HETEROZYGOUS STATE: SICKLE CELL TRAIT

Sickle cell trait (AS) is a benign heterozygous state of HbS in which only one abnormal gene is inherited. Patients with AS develop no significant clinical problems except when they become severely hypoxic and may develop sickle cell crises.

LABORATORY FINDINGS These patients have no anaemia. The diagnosis is made by:

1. *Demonstration of sickling* done under condition of reduced oxygen tension by an oxygen consuming reagent, sodium metabisulfite.

2. *Haemoglobin electrophoresis* reveals 35-40% of the total haemoglobin as HbS.

HOMOZYGOUS STATE: SICKLE CELL ANAEMIA

Sickle cell anaemia (SS) is a homozygous state of HbS in the red cells in which an abnormal gene is inherited from each parent. SS is a severe disorder associated with protean clinical manifestations and decreased life expectancy.

PATHOGENESIS It can be explained as under:

1. Basic molecular lesion In HbS, basic genetic defect is the *single point mutation* in one amino acid out of 146 in haemoglobin molecule—there is *substitution of valine for glutamic acid* at 6-residue position of the β-globin, producing Hb $\alpha_2\beta_2{}^s$.

2. Mechanism of sickling During deoxygenation, the red cells containing HbS change from biconcave disc shape to an elongated crescent-shaped or sickle-shaped cell.

3. Reversible-irreversible sickling The oxygen-dependent sickling process is usually reversible.

4. Factors determining rate of sickling
i)   Presence of non-HbS haemoglobins
ii) Intracellular concentration of HbS
iii) Total haemoglobin concentration
iv) Extent of deoxygenation
v)   Acidosis and dehydration
vi) Increased concentration of 2, 3-BPG in the red cells.

CLINICAL FEATURES The clinical manifestations of homozygous sickle cell disease are widespread. The symptoms begin to appear after 6th month of life when most of the HbF is replaced by HbS.

1.   **Anaemia** There is usually severe chronic haemolytic anaemia.

2.   **Vaso-occlusive phenomena** Patients of SS develop recurrent vaso-occlusive episodes throughout their lives due to obstruction to capillary blood

flow by sickled red cells upon deoxygenation or dehydration which may be of 2 types:

i) *Microinfarcts* affecting particularly the abdomen, chest, back and joints.

ii) *Macroinfarcts* involving most commonly the spleen (splenic sequestration, autosplenectomy), bone marrow (pains), bones (aseptic necrosis, osteomyelitis), lungs (pulmonary infections), kidneys (renal cortical necrosis), CNS (stroke), retina (damage) and skin (ulcers).

3. Constitutional symptoms Patients with SS have impaired growth and development and increased susceptibility to infection due to markedly impaired splenic function.

LABORATORY FINDINGS These are as under:

1. Moderate to severe anaemia (haemoglobin concentration 6-9 g/dl).

2. The blood film shows sickle cells and target cells.

3. A positive sickling test with a reducing substance such as sodium metabisulfite.

4. Haemoglobin electrophoresis shows no normal HbA but shows predominance of HbS and 2-20% HbF.

DOUBLE HETEROZYGOUS STATES

Double heterozygous conditions involving combination of HbS with other haemoglobinopathies may occur. Most common among these are sickle-β-thalassaemia ($\beta^S\beta^{thal}$), sickle C disease (SC), and sickle D disease (SD).

OTHER STRUCTURAL HAEMOGLOBINOPATHIES

Besides sickle haemoglobin, about 400 structurally different abnormal human haemoglobins have been discovered in different parts of the world. A few important and common variants are:

❖ HbC Haemoglobinopathy
❖ HbD Haemoglobinopathy
❖ HbE Haemoglobinopathy
❖ Haemoglobin O-Arab Disease
❖ Unstable-Hb Haemoglobinopathy

REDUCED GLOBIN CHAIN SYNTHESIS: THALASSAEMIAS

DEFINITION

The thalassaemias are a diverse group of hereditary disorders in which there is reduced synthesis of one or more of the globin polypeptide chains. Thus, thalassaemias, unlike haemoglobinopathies which are qualitative disorders of haemoglobin, are *quantitative abnormalities of polypeptide globin chain synthesis*. In India, thalassaemia is seen through country and an estimated 35 million have β-thalassaemia major. Its incidence is particularly high in some races such as Punjabis who migrated from Pakistan after partition, Bengalis, Gujratis and Parsis.

GENETICS AND CLASSIFICATION

Depending upon whether the genetic defect or deletion lies in transmission of α- or β-globin chain genes, thalassaemias are classified into α- and β-thalas-saemias. Thus, patients with α-thalassaemia have structurally normal α-globin chains but their production is impaired. Similarly, in β-thalassaemia, β-globin chains are structurally normal but their production is decreased. Each of the two main types of thalassaemias may occur as heterozygous (called α- *and β-thalassaemia minor* or *trait*), or as homozygous state (termed α- and *β-thalassaemia major*).

A classification of various types of thalassaemias along with the clinical syndromes produced and salient laboratory findings are given below.

TYPE	HB	CLINICAL SYNDROME
α-THALASSAEMIAS		
1. *Hydrops foetalis*	3-10 gm/dl	Fatal *in utero* or in early infancy
2. *Hb-H disease*	2-12 gm/dl	Haemolytic anaemia

3.	α-*Thalassaemia trait*	10-14 gm/dl	Microcytic hypochromic blood picture but no anaemia

β-THALASSAEMIAS

1.	β-*Thalassaemia major*	< 5 gm/dl	Severe congenital haemolytic anaemia, requires blood transfusions
2.	β-*Thalassaemia intermedia*	5-10 gm/dl	Severe anaemia, but regular blood transfusions not required
3.	β-*Thalassaemia minor*	10-12 gm/dl	Usually asymptomatic

PATHOPHYSIOLOGY OF ANAEMIA IN THALASSAEMIA

A constant feature of all forms of thalassaemia is the presence of anaemia which occurs from following mechanisms:

α-**Thalassaemia** In α-thalassaemia major, the obvious cause of anaemia is the inability to synthesise adult haemoglobin, while in α-thalassaemia trait there is reduced production of normal adult haemoglobin.

β-**Thalassaemia** In β-thalassaemia major, the most important cause of anaemia is premature red cell destruction brought about by erythrocyte membrane damage caused by the precipitated α-globin chains. During their passage through the splenic sinusoids, these red cells are further damaged and develop pitting due to removal of the precipitated aggregates. Thus, such red cells are irreparably damaged and are phagocytosed by the RE cells of the spleen and the liver causing anaemia, hepatosplenomegaly, and excess of tissue iron stores. Patients with β-thalassaemia minor, on the other hand, have very mild ineffective erythropoiesis, haemolysis and shortening of red cell lifespan.

α-THALASSAEMIA

MOLECULAR PATHOGENESIS The α-thalassaemias are most commonly due to deletion of one or more of the α-chain genes located on short arm of chromosome 16. Since there is a pair of α-chain genes, the clinical manifestations of α-thalassaemia depend upon the number of genes deleted:

1. Four α-gene deletion: Hb Bart's hydrops foetalis.
2. Three α-gene deletion: HbH disease.
3. Two α-gene deletion: α-thalassaemia trait.
4. One α-gene deletion: α-thalassaemia trait (carrier).

β-THALASSAEMIAS

MOLECULAR PATHOGENESIS In contrast to α-thalassaemia, gene deletion rarely ever causes β-thalassaemia and is only seen in an entity called *hereditary persistence of foetal haemoglobin (HPFH)*. Instead, most of β-thalassaemias arise from different types of mutations of β-globin gene resulting from single base changes. The symbol β° is used to indicate the complete absence of β-globin chain synthesis while β+ denotes partial synthesis of the β-globin chains. Some of the important ones having effects on β-globin chain synthesis are as under:

i) Transcription defect
ii) Translation defect
iii) mRNA splicing defect

Depending upon the extent of reduction in β-chain synthesis, there are 3 types of β-thalassaemia:

1. Homozygous form: β-Thalassaemia major It is the most severe form of congenital haemolytic anaemia. It is further of 2 types:

i) β° *thalassaemia major* characterised by complete absence of β-chain synthesis.

ii) β+ *thalassaemia major* having incomplete suppression of β-chain synthesis.

2. β-Thalassaemia intermedia It is β-thalassaemia of intermediate degree of severity that does not require regular blood transfusions.

3. Heterozygous form: β-thalassaemia minor (trait) It is a mild asymptomatic condition in which there is moderate suppression of β-chain synthesis.

Besides β-thalassaemia minor, a few uncommon globin chain combinations resulting in β-thalassaemia trait:
i)   δβ-thalassaemia minor
ii) Hb Lepore syndrome

β-THALASSAEMIA MAJOR

β-thalassaemia major, also termed Mediterranean or Cooley's anaemia is the most common form of congenital haemolytic anaemia. β-thalassaemia major is a homozygous state with either complete absence of β-chain synthesis (β° *thalassaemia major*) or only small amounts of β-chains are formed (β+ thalassaemia major). These result in excessive formation of alternate haemoglobins, HbF ($\alpha_2\gamma_2$) and HbA$_2$ ($\alpha_2\delta_2$).

CLINICAL FEATURES   These are as follows:
1.   Anaemia starts appearing within the first 4-6 months of life.
2.   Marked hepatosplenomegaly.
3.   Expansion of bones occurs due to marked erythroid hyperplasia leading to thalassaemic facies and malocclusion of the jaw.
4.   Iron overload due to repeated blood transfusions causes damage to the endocrine organs resulting in slow rate of growth and development, delayed puberty, diabetes mellitus and damage to the liver and heart.

LABORATORY FINDINGS   The haematological investigations reveal the following findings:
1. *Anaemia*, usually severe.
2. *Blood film* shows severe microcytic hypochromic red cell morphology, marked anisopoikilocytosis, basophilic stippling, presence of many target cells, tear drop cells and normoblasts.
3. *Serum bilirubin* (unconjugated) is generally raised.
4. *Reticulocytosis* is generally present.
5. *MCV, MCH and MCHC* are significantly reduced.
6. *WBC count is* often raised with some shift to left.
7. *Platelet count* is usually normal but may be reduced in patients with massive splenomegaly.
8. *Osmotic fragility* reveals *decreased osmotic fragility*.
9. *Haemoglobin electrophoresis* shows presence of increased amounts of HbF, increased amount of HbA$_2$, and almost complete absence or presence of variable amounts of HbA.
10. *Bone marrow aspirate examination* shows normoblastic erythroid hyperplasia with predominance of intermediate and late normoblasts.

PRINCIPLES OF TREATMENT   It is largely supportive.
1.   Anaemia is generally severe and patients require regular blood transfusions (4-6 weekly) to maintain haemoglobin above 8 g/dl.
2.   In order to maintain increased demand of hyperplastic marrow, folic acid supplement is given.
3.   Splenectomy is beneficial in children over 6 years of age.
4.   Prevention and treatment of iron overload is done by chelation therapy (desferrioxamine).
5.   Bone marrow transplantation from HLA-matched donor that provides stem cells which can form normal haemoglobin.

Since these patients require multiple blood transfusions, they are at increased risk of developing AIDS. In general, patients with β-thalassaemia major have short life expectancy. The biggest problem is iron overload and consequent myocardial siderosis leading to cardiac arrhythmias, congestive heart failure, and ultimately death.

The β-thalassaemia minor or β-thalassaemia trait, a heterozygous state, is a common entity characterised by moderate reduction in β-chain synthesis.

CLINICAL FEATURES Clinically, the condition is usually asymptomatic and the diagnosis is generally made when the patient is being investigated for mild chronic anaemia. The spleen may be palpable.

LABORATORY FINDINGS These are as under:
1. *Mild anaemia*; mean haemoglobin level is about 15% lower than in normal person for the age and sex.
2. *Blood film* shows mild anisopoikilocytosis, microcytosis and hypochromia, occasional target cells and basophilic stippling.
3. *Serum bilirubin* may be normal or slightly raised.
4. *Mild reticulocytosis* is often present.
5. *MCV, MCH and MCHC* may be slightly reduced.
6. *Decreased osmotic fragility.*
7. *Haemoglobin electrophoresis* is confirmatory for the diagnosis and shows about two-fold increase in HbA_2 and a slight elevation in HbF (2-3%).

PREVENTION OF THALASSAEMIA
Finally, since thalassaemia is an inheritable disease, its prevention is possible by making an antenatal diagnosis. This is done by chorionic villous biopsy or cells obtained by amniocentesis and foetal DNA studied by PCR amplification technique for presence of genetic mutations of thalassaemias.

ANAEMIA OF BLOOD LOSS (p. 301)

ACUTE BLOOD LOSS The effects are as under:
i) Immediate threat to life due to hypovolaemia which may result in shock and death.
ii) If the patient survives, shifting of interstitial fluid to intravascular compartment with consequent haemodilution with low haematocrit.

LABORATORY FINDINGS These are as under:
i) Normocytic and normochromic anaemia
ii) Low haematocrit
iii) Increased reticulocyte count in peripheral blood (10-15% after one week) reflecting accelerated marrow erythropoiesis.

CHRONIC BLOOD LOSS When the loss of blood is slow and insidious, the effects of anaemia will become apparent only when the rate of loss is more than rate of production and the iron stores are depleted.

APLASTIC ANAEMIA AND OTHER PRIMARY BONE MARROW DISORDERS (p. 301)

'*Bone marrow failure*' is the term used for primary disorders of the bone marrow which result in impaired formation of the erythropoietic precursors and consequent anaemia. It includes the following disorders:
1. *Aplastic anaemia*, most importantly.
2. *Other primary bone marrow disorders* e.g. myelophthisic anaemia, pure red cell aplasia, and myelodysplastic syndromes.

APLASTIC ANAEMIA (p. 301)

Aplastic anaemia is defined as pancytopenia (i.e. simultaneous presence of anaemia, leucopenia and thrombocytopenia) resulting from aplasia of the bone marrow.

ETIOLOGY AND CLASSIFICATION

A. PRIMARY APLASTIC ANAEMIA Primary aplastic anaemia includes 2 entities:
1. Fanconi's anaemia This has an autosomal recessive inheritance and is often associated with other congenital anomalies such as skeletal and renal abnormalities, and sometimes mental retardation.

2. Immune causes In many cases, suppression of haematopoietic stem cells by immunologic mechanisms may cause aplastic anaemia.

B. SECONDARY APLASTIC ANAEMIA Secondary causes are more common.

1. Drugs A number of drugs are cytotoxic to the marrow and cause aplastic anaemia. The association of a drug with aplastic anaemia may be either predictably dose-related or an idiosyncratic reaction.

2. Toxic chemicals These include examples of industrial, domestic and accidental use of substances such as benzene derivatives, insecticides, arsenicals etc.

3. Infections Aplastic anaemia may occur following viral hepatitis, Epstein-Barr virus infection, AIDS and other viral illnesses.

4. Miscellaneous Lastly, aplastic anaemia has been reported in association with certain other illnesses such as SLE, and with therapeutic X-rays.

CLINICAL FEATURES

1. Anaemia and its symptoms like mild progressive weakness and fatigue.
2. Haemorrhage from various sites due to thrombocytopenia such as from the skin, nose, gums, vagina, bowel, and occasionally in the CNS and retina.
3. Infections of the mouth and throat are commonly present.
4. The lymph nodes, liver and spleen are generally not enlarged.

LABORATORY FINDINGS

1. Anaemia Haemoglobin levels are moderately reduced.

2. Leucopenia The absolute granulocyte count is particularly low (below 1500/μl) with relative lymphocytosis.

3. Thrombocytopenia Platelet count is always reduced.

4. Bone marrow examination A bone marrow aspirate may yield a 'dry tap'. A trephine biopsy is generally essential for making the diagnosis which reveals patchy cellular areas in a hypocellular or aplastic marrow due to replacement by fat.

PRINCIPLES OF TREATMENT

In general, younger patients show better response to proper treatment.

A. General management It consists of the following:
1. Identification and elimination of the possible cause.
2. Supportive care consisting of blood transfusions, platelet concentrates, and treatment and prevention of infections.

B. Specific treatment
1. Marrow stimulating agents
2. Immunosuppressive therapy
3. Bone marrow transplantation

MYELOPHTHISIC ANAEMIA *(p. 303)*

Development of severe anaemia may result from infiltration of the marrow termed as myelophthisic anaemia. The causes for marrow infiltrations include the following:
1. Haematologic malignancies (e.g. leukaemia, lymphoma, myeloma).
2. Metastatic deposits from non-haematologic malignancies (e.g. cancer breast, stomach, prostate, lung, thyroid).
3. Advanced tuberculosis.
4. Primary lipid storage diseases (Gaucher's and Niemann-Pick's disease).
5. Osteopetrosis and myelofibrosis may rarely cause myelophthisis.

LABORATORY FINDINGS

The type of anaemia in myelophthisis is generally normocytic normochromic with some fragmented red cells, basophilic stippling and normoblasts in the peripheral blood. Thrombocytopenia is usually present but the leucocyte count is increased with slight shift-to-left of myeloid cells i.e. a picture of *leucoerythroblastic reaction*.

PURE RED CELL APLASIA (p. 303)

Pure red cell aplasia (PRCA) is a rare syndrome involving a selective failure in the production of erythroid elements in the bone marrow but with normal granulopoiesis and megakaryocytopoiesis. Patients have normocytic normochromic anaemia with normal granulocyte and platelet count. Reticulocytes are markedly decreased or are absent.

PRCA exists in the following forms:

1. **Transient self-limited PRCA** It is due to temporary marrow failure in aplastic crisis in haemolytic anaemias and in acute B19 parvovirus infection.

2. **Acquired PRCA** It is seen in middle-aged adults in association with some other diseases, most commonly thymoma; others are connective tissue diseases.

3. **Chronic B19 parvovirus infections** PRCA may occur from chronic B19 parvovirus infection in children and is common and treatable.

4. **Congenital PRCA (Blackfan-Diamond syndrome)** It is a rare chronic disorder detected at birth or in early childhood.

SELF ASSESSMENT

1. **During foetal life, haematopoiesis commences in the bone marrow by:**
   A. 2nd to 3rd month
   B. 4th to 5th month
   C. 6th to 7th month
   D. 7th to 8th month

2. **Bone marrow trephine biopsy has advantage over aspiration since:**
   A. The former method is less time-consuming
   B. Romanowsky stains can be done in the former
   C. Architectural pattern of marrow is better in the former
   D. Cell morphology is better appreciated in the former

3. **Erythroid cells continue to proliferate up to the stage of:**
   A. Reticulocytes
   B. Late normoblasts
   C. Intermediate normoblasts
   D. Early normoblasts

4. **Weight of haemoglobin in RBC is:**
   A. 50%
   B. 70%
   C. 90%
   D. 99%

5. **Red cell membrane defects include the following <u>except</u>:**
   A. Spherocytosis
   B. Ovalocytosis
   C. Leptocytosis
   D. Echinocytosis

6. **The following factors determine the release of oxygen from haemoglobin in tissue capillaries <u>except</u>:**
   A. Nature of globin chains in Hb
   B. Bicarbonate ions in blood
   C. pH of blood
   D. Concentration of 2,3-BPG

7. **Absorption of iron is enhanced by the following <u>except</u>:**
   A. Ascorbic acid
   B. Citric acid
   C. Tannates
   D. Sugars

8. **In iron deficiency anaemia, TIBC is:**
   A. Low
   B. Normal
   C. High
   D. Borderline

9. **Pappenheimer bodies are found in:**
   A. Sideroblasts
   B. Siderocytes
   C. Late normoblasts
   D. Intermediate normoblasts

10. **In anaemia of chronic disorders, serum ferritin is:**
    A. Normal
    B. Low
    C. Increased
    D. Absent

11. **Folate circulates in plasma as:**
    A. Methyl tetrahydrofolate
    B. Polyglutamate
    C. Monoglutamate
    D. Diglutamate

12. **Measurement of formiminoglutamic acid (FIGLU) for folate deficiency is done in:**
    A. Whole blood
    B. Serum
    C. Plasma
    D. Urine

13. **Pernicious anaemia causes pathologic changes in the anatomic region of stomach as under <u>except</u>:**
    A. Antrum
    B. Body
    C. Body-fundic area
    D. Fundus

14. **In warm antibody autoimmune haemolytic anaemias, the antibody is commonly:**
    A. IgA
    B. IgG
    C. IgM
    D. IgD

15. **Cold agglutinin antibody in autoimmune haemolytic anaemia affects:**
    A. Mature erythrocytes
    B. Reticulocytes
    C. Siderocytes
    D. Late erythroblasts

16. **In paroxysmal nocturnal haemoglobinuria (PNH), the undue sensitivity of red cells to complement can be detected by:**
    A. Ham's test
    B. Heinz body test
    C. Direct Coombs' test
    D. Indirect Coombs' test

17. **In hereditary spherocytosis, the following membrane structure is deficient:**
    A. Band 3 protein
    B. Glycophorin
    C. Spectrin
    D. Glycolipid

18. **G6PD deficiency has the following genetic basis of inheritance:**
    A. Autosomal dominant
    B. Autosomal recessive
    C. Sex-linked trait
    D. Sex-linked homozygous

19. **The rate of sickling in sickle cell anaemia is directly correlated with the following factors <u>except</u>:**
    A. Higher concentration of HbS
    B. Lower concentration of HbA
    C. Higher concentration of HbF
    D. Higher deoxygenation

20. **Molecular pathogenesis of α-thalassaemia involves:**
    A. Mutation in transcription promoter sequence
    B. Gene deletion
    C. Codon termination mutation
    D. mRNA splicing defect

21. **The pathognomonic abnormality in β-thalassaemia minor is:**
    A. Marked rise in HbA2
    B. Marked rise in HbF
    C. Marked unconjugated hyperbilirubinaemia
    D. Marked anaemia

22. **In aplastic anaemia, there is generally:**
    A. Relative neutrophilia
    B. Relative lymphocytosis
    C. Microcytosis
    D. Reticulocyte count normal

23. **Erythropoietin is produced by:**
    A. Liver
    B. Lungs
    C. Bone marrow
    D. Kidney

24. **Pappenheimer bodies represent:**
    A. DNA
    B. RNA
    C. Non-haem iron
    D. Mitochondria

25. **In Schilling's test 'hot' B_{12} is given:**
    A. Intramuscular
    B. Subcutaneous
    C. Intravenous
    D. Oral

26. **Antibody in paroxysmal cold haemoglobinuria is against:**
    A. P blood group antigen
    B. I blood group antigen
    C. A blood group antigen
    D. Rh blood group antigen

27. **Which of the following G6PD variant provides protection against malaria?**
    A. Type B
    B. Type A+
    C. Type A –
    D. G6PD Mediterranean

28. **Which of the following is <u>not</u> microangiopathic haemolytic anaemia?**
    A. March haemoglobinuria
    B. TTP
    C. HUS
    D. Lead poisoning

29. **Precipitated gamma chains are known as:**
    A. Heinz bodies
    B. Pappenheimer bodies
    C. Hb Barts
    D. Russel bodies

30. **Which of the following autoantibodies is most likely to be present in a patient with pernicious anemia?**
    A. Antigliadin antibodies
    B. Anti-intrinsic factor antibodies
    C. Antimitochondrial antibodies
    D. Antismooth muscle antibodies

KEY

1 = B	2 = C	3 = C	4 = C	5 = C
6 = B	7 = C	8 = C	9 = B	10 = C
11 = A	12 = D	13 = A	14 = B	15 = B
16 = A	17 = C	18 = C	19 = C	20 = B
21 = A	22 = B	23 = D	24 = C	25 = D
26 = A	27 = C	28 = D	29 = A	30 = B

Disorders of Platelets, Bleeding Disorders and Basic Transfusion Medicine

DISORDERS OF PLATELETS (p. 305)

THROMBOPOIESIS

Platelets are formed in the bone marrow by a process of fragmentation of the cytoplasm of megakaryocytes. Platelet production is under the control of thrombopoietin, the nature and origin of which are not yet established. The stages in platelet production are as under:

MEGAKARYOBLAST The earliest precursor of platelets in the bone marrow is megakaryoblast. It arises from haematopoietic stem cell by a process of differentiation.

PROMEGAKARYOCYTE A megakaryoblast undergoes endo-reduplication of nuclear chromatin i.e. nuclear chromatin replicates repeatedly in multiples of two without division of the cell.

MEGAKARYOCYTE A mature megakaryocyte is a large cell, 30-90 μm in diameter, and contains 4-16 nuclear lobes having coarsely clumped chromatin. The cytoplasm is abundant, light blue in colour and contains red-purple granules. Platelets are formed from pseudopods of megakaryocyte cytoplasm which get detached into the blood stream. Each megakaryocyte may form up to 4000 platelets.

PLATELETS Platelets are small (1-4 μm in diameter), discoid, non-nucleate structures containing red-purple granules. The normal platelet count ranges from 150,000-400,000/μl and the lifespan of platelets is 7-10 days.

The main *functions* of platelets is in haemostasis which includes two closely linked processes:

1. Primary haemostasis This term is used for platelet plug formation at the site of injury. Primary haemostasis involves three steps:

i) *Platelet adhesion:* Platelets adhere to collagen in the subendothelium due to presence of receptor on platelet surface, glycoprotein (Gp) Ia-IIa which is an integrin. The adhesion to the vessel wall is further stabilised by von Willebrand factor, an adhesion glycoprotein.

ii) *Platelet release:* After adhesion, platelets become activated and release three types of granules from their cytoplasm: dense granules, α-granules and lysosomal vesicles.

iii) *Platelet aggregation:* This process is mediated by fibrinogen which forms bridge between adjacent platelets via glycoprotein receptors on platelets, GpIIb-IIIa.

2. Secondary haemostasis This involves plasma coagulation system resulting in fibrin plug formation and takes several minutes for completion.

INVESTIGATIONS OF HAEMOSTATIC FUNCTION (p. 306)

Formation of haemostatic plug is a complex mechanism and involves maintenance of a delicate balance among at least 5 components. Accordingly, there are specific tests for assessing each of these components:

A. *Blood vessel wall:* Tests for disordered vascular haemostasis
B. *Platelets:* Tests for platelets and their functions

C. *Plasma coagulation factors:* Tests for blood coagulation
D. *Fibrinolytic system:* Tests or fibrolysis
E. *Inhibitors:* Tests for coagulation inhibitors

A. INVESTIGATION OF DISORDERED VASCULAR HAEMOSTASIS

Disorders of vascular haemostasis may be due to increased vascular permeability, reduced capillary strength and failure to contract after injury. Tests of defective vascular function are as under:

1. BLEEDING TIME This simple test is based on the principle of formation of haemostatic plug following a standard incision on the volar surface of the forearm and the time the incision takes to stop bleeding is measured. Normal range is 3-8 minutes. A prolonged bleeding time may be due to following causes:
i)   Thrombocytopenia.
ii) Disorders of platelet function.
iii) von Willebrand's disease.

2. HESS CAPILLARY RESISTANCE TEST (TOURNIQUET TEST) This test is done by tying sphygmomanometer cuff to the upper arm and raising the pressure in it between diastolic and systolic for 5 minutes. The test is positive in increased capillary fragility as well as in thrombocytopenia.

B. INVESTIGATION OF PLATELETS AND PLATELET FUNCTION

Haemostatic disorders are commonly due to abnormalities in platelet number, morphology or function.

1. SCREENING TESTS
i)   Peripheral blood platelet count.
ii) Skin bleeding time.
iii) Examination of fresh blood film.

2. SPECIAL TESTS
i)   *Platelet adhesion tests* such as retention in a glass bead column.
ii) *Aggregation tests* which are turbidometric techniques.
iii) *Granular content* of the platelets and their release.
iv) *Platelet coagulant activity* is measured indirectly by prothrombin consumption index.

C. INVESTIGATION OF BLOOD COAGULATION

The normal blood coagulation system consists of cascade of activation of 13 coagulation factors. These form intrinsic, extrinsic and common pathways which culminate in formation of thrombin that acts on fibrinogen to produce fibrin. Coagulation tests include screening and confirmatory special tests as under:

SCREENING TESTS

1. Whole blood coagulation time Normal range is 4-9 minutes at 37°C.

2. Activated partial thromboplastin time (APTT) or partial thromboplastin time with kaolin (PTTK) This test is used to measure the intrinsic system factors (VIII, IX, XI and XII) as well as factors common to both intrinsic and extrinsic systems (factors X, V, prothrombin and fibrinogen). The normal range is 30-40 seconds. The common causes of a prolonged PTTK (or APTT) are as follows:
i)   Parenteral administration of heparin.
ii) Disseminated intravascular coagulation.
iii) Liver disease.
iv) Circulating anticoagulants.

3. One-stage prothrombin time (PT) PT measures the extrinsic system factor VII as well as factors in the common pathway. The normal PT in this test is 10-14 seconds. The common causes of prolonged one-stage PT are as under:
i)   Administration of oral anticoagulant drugs.

ii) Liver disease, especially obstructive liver disease.
iii) Vitamin K deficiency.
iv) Disseminated intravascular coagulation.

4. Measurement of fibrinogen The *screening tests* for fibrinogen deficiency are semiquantitative fibrinogen titre and thrombin time (TT). The normal value of thrombin time is under 20 seconds.

SPECIAL TESTS
1. Coagulation factor assays
2. Quantitative assays

D. INVESTIGATION OF FIBRINOLYTIC SYSTEM
1. Estimation of fibrinogen.
2. Fibrin degradation products (FDP) in the serum.
3. Ethanol gelation test.
4. Euglobin or whole blood lysis time.

E. INVESTIGATION OF COAGULATION INHIBITORS

There is an inbuilt system in the body by which coagulation remains confined as per need and does not become generalised. Important inhibitors are as under:
1. Antithrombin III
2. Protein C and S

BLEEDING DISORDERS (HAEMORRHAGIC DIATHESIS) (p. 309)

The tendency to bleeding may be *spontaneous* in the form of small haemorrhages into the skin and mucous membranes (e.g. petechiae, purpura, ecchymoses), or there may be excessive external or internal bleeding *following trivial trauma* and surgical procedure (e.g. haematoma, haemarthrosis etc).

The causes of haemorrhagic diatheses may or may not be related to platelet abnormalities. These causes are broadly divided into the following groups:
I. Haemorrhagic diathesis due to vascular abnormalities
II. Haemorrhagic diathesis related to platelet abnormalities
III. Disorders of coagulation factors
IV. Haemorrhagic diathesis due to fibrinolytic defects
V. Combination of all these as occurs in disseminated intravascular coagulation (DIC).

HAEMORRHAGIC DIATHESES DUE TO VASCULAR DISORDERS (p. 309)

Vascular bleeding disorders, also called non-thrombocytopenic purpuras or vascular purpuras, are normally mild and characterised by petechiae, purpuras or ecchymoses confined to the skin and mucous membranes.
Vascular bleeding disorders may be *inherited* or *acquired*.

A. INHERITED VASCULAR BLEEDING DISORDERS
1. Hereditary haemorrhagic telangiectasia (Osler-Weber-Rendu disease)
2. Inherited disorders of connective tissue matrix

B. ACQUIRED VASCULAR BLEEDING DISORDERS
1. Henoch-Schönlein purpura
2. Haemolytic-uraemic syndrome
3. Simple easy bruising (Devil's pinches)
4. Infection
5. Drug reactions
6. Steroid purpura
7. Senile purpura
8. Scurvy

A. THROMBOCYTOPENIAS

Thrombocytopenia is defined as a reduction in the peripheral blood platelet count below the lower limit of normal i.e. below 150,000/μl. Thrombocytopenia is associated with abnormal bleeding that includes spontaneous skin purpura and mucosal haemorrhages as well as prolonged bleeding after trauma. However, spontaneous haemorrhagic tendency becomes clinically evident only after severe depletion of the platelet count to level below 20,000/μl.

Thrombocytopenia may result from 4 main groups of causes as under:

I. IMPAIRED PLATELET PRODUCTION

1. *Generalised bone marrow failure e.g.*
   Aplastic anaemia, leukaemia, myelofibrosis, megaloblastic anaemia, marrow infiltrations (carcinomas, lymphomas, multiple myeloma, storage diseases).
2. *Selective suppression of platelet production e.g.*
   Drugs (quinine, quinidine, sulfonamides, PAS, rifampicin, anticancer drugs, thiazide diuretics), (heparin, diclofenac, acyclovir), alcohol intake.

II. ACCELERATED PLATELET DESTRUCTION

1. *Immunologic thrombocytopenias e.g.*
   ITP (acute and chronic), neonatal and post-transfusion (isoimmune), drug-induced, secondary immune thrombocytopenia (post-infection, SLE, AIDS, CLL, lymphoma).
2. *Increased consumption e.g.*
   DIC, TTP, giant haemangiomas, microangiopathic haemolytic anaemia.

III. SPLENIC SEQUESTRATION
Splenomegaly

IV. DILUTIONAL LOSS
Massive transfusion of old stored blood to bleeding patients

A few common types are described below:

DRUG-INDUCED THROMBOCYTOPENIA

Many commonly used drugs cause thrombocytopenia by depressing megakaryocyte production. In most cases, an immune mechanism by formation of drug-antibody complexes is implicated in which the platelet is damaged as an 'innocent bystander'.

HEPARIN-INDUCED THROMBOCYTOPENIA

Thrombocytopenia due to administration of heparin is distinct from that caused by other drugs in following ways:
i) Thrombocytopenia is generally not so severe to fall to level below 20,000/μl.
ii) Unlike drug-induced thrombocytopenia, heparin-induced thrombo-cytopenia is not associated with bleeding but instead these patients are more prone to develop thrombosis.

Diagnosis is made by a combination of laboratory and clinical features with 4 *Ts*: thrombocytopenia, thrombosis, time of fall of platelet count, absence of other causes of thrombocytopenia.

IMMUNE THROMBOCYTOPENIC PURPURA (ITP)

Idiopathic (or immune) thrombocytopenic purpura (ITP), is charac-terised by immunologic destruction of platelets and normal or increased megakaryocytes in the bone marrow.

PATHOGENESIS On the basis of duration of illness, ITP is classified into acute and chronic forms.

Acute ITP This is a self-limited disorder, seen most frequently in children following recovery from a viral illness (e.g. hepatitis C, infectious mononucleosis, CMV infection, HIV infection) or an upper respiratory illness. The onset of acute ITP is sudden and severe thrombocytopenia but recovery occurs within a few weeks to 6 months.

Chronic ITP Chronic ITP occurs more commonly in adults, particularly in women of child-bearing age (20-40 years). The disorder develops insidiously and persists for several years. Though chronic ITP is idiopathic, similar immunologic thrombocytopenia may be seen in association with SLE, AIDS and autoimmune thyroiditis. The pathogenesis of chronic ITP is explained by formation of *anti-platelet autoantibodies,* usually by platelet-associated IgG humoral antibodies synthesised mainly in the spleen.

CLINICAL FEATURES The clinical manifestation of ITP may develop abruptly in cases of acute ITP, or the onset may be insidious as occurs in majority of cases of chronic ITP. The usual manifestations are petechial haemorrhages, easy bruising, and mucosal bleeding such as menorrhagia in women, nasal bleeding, bleeding from gums, melaena and haematuria. Intracranial haemorrhage is, however, rare. Splenomegaly and hepatomegaly may occur in cases with chronic ITP but lymphadenopathy is quite uncommon in either type of ITP.

LABORATORY FINDINGS These are as follows:
1. *Platelet count* is markedly reduced, usually in the range of 10,000-50,000/µl.
2. *Blood film* shows only occasional platelets which are often large in size.
3. *Bone marrow* shows increased number of megakaryocytes which have large non-lobulated single nuclei and may have reduced cytoplasmic granularity and presence of vacuoles.
4. With sensitive techniques, *anti-platelet IgG antibody* can be demonstrated on platelet surface or in the serum of patients.

PRINCIPLES OF TREATMENT Spontaneous recovery occurs in 90% cases of acute ITP, while only less than 10% cases of chronic ITP recover spontaneously. Treatment is directed at reducing the level and source of autoantibodies and reducing the rate of destruction of sensitised platelets.

THROMBOTIC THROMBOCYTOPENIC PURPURA (TTP) AND HAEMOLYTIC-URAEMIC SYNDROME (HUS)

Thrombotic thrombocytopenic purpura (TTP) and haemolytic-uraemic syndrome (HUS) are a group of thrombotic microangiopathies which are essentially characterised by triad of *thrombocytopenia, microangiopathic haemolytic anaemia and formation of hyaline fibrin microthrombi* within the microvasculature throughout the body.

PATHOGENESIS TTP is initiated by endothelial injury followed by release of von Willebrand factor and other procoagulant material from endothelial cells, leading to the formation of microthrombi. Trigger for the endothelial injury comes from immunologic damage by diverse conditions.

CLINICAL FEATURES The clinical manifestations of TTP are due to microthrombi in the arterioles, capillaries and venules throughout the body. Besides features of thrombocytopenia and microangiopathic haemolytic anaemia, characteristic findings include fever, transient neurologic deficits and renal failure. The spleen may be palpable.

LABORATORY FINDINGS These are:
1. Thrombocytopenia.
2. Microangiopathic haemolytic anaemia with negative Coombs' test.
3. Leucocytosis, sometimes with leukaemoid reaction.
4. Bone marrow examination reveals normal or slightly increased megakaryocytes.

B. THROMBOCYTOSIS

Thrombocytosis is defined as platelet count in excess of 4,00,000/μl. While essential or primary thrombocytosis or thrombocythaemia is discussed under myeloproliferative disorders secondary or reactive thrombocytosis can occur following massive haemorrhage, iron deficiency, severe sepsis, marked inflammation, disseminated cancers, haemolysis, or following splenectomy.

C. DISORDERS OF PLATELET FUNCTIONS

HEREDITARY DISORDERS

1. DEFECTIVE PLATELET ADHESION e.g. Bernard-Soulier syndrome, In von Willebrand's disease.

2. DEFECTIVE PLATELET AGGREGATION e.g. thrombasthenia (Glanzmann's disease).

3. DISORDERS OF PLATELET RELEASE REACTION These are due to complex instrinsic deficiencies.

ACQUIRED DISORDERS

1. ASPIRIN THERAPY Prolonged use of aspirin leads to easy bruising and abnormal bleeding time. This is because aspirin inhibits the enzyme cyclooxygenase, and thereby suppresses the synthesis of prostaglandins which are involved in platelet aggregation as well as release reaction.

2. OTHERS These include: uraemia, liver disease, multiple myeloma, Waldenström's macroglobulinaemia and various myeloproliferative disorders.

COAGULATION DISORDERS (p. 313)

The type of bleeding in coagulation disorders is different from that seen in vascular and platelet abnormalities. Instead of spontaneous appearance of petechiae and purpuras, the plasma coagulation defects manifest more often in the form of large ecchymoses, haematomas and bleeding into muscles, joints, body cavities, GIT and urinary tract.

Disorders of plasma coagulation factors may have hereditary or acquired origin.

1. CLASSIC HAEMOPHILIA (HAEMOPHILIA A)

Classic haemophilia or haemophilia A is the most common hereditary coagulation disorder occurring due to deficiency or reduced activity of factor VIII (anti-haemophilic factor). The disorder is inherited as a sex-(X-) linked recessive trait and, therefore, manifests clinically in males, while females are usually the carriers.

Currently, *haemophilia A (classic haemophilia)* is inherited deficiency of factor VIII due to mutation in F8 gene, and *haemophilia B (Christmas disease)* is inherited deficiency of factor IX due to mutation in F9 gene.

PATHOGENESIS Haemophilia A is caused by quantitative reduction of factor VIII in 90% of cases, while 10% cases have normal or increased level of factor VIII with reduced activity. Normal haemostasis requires 25% factor VIII activity. Though occasional patients with 25% factor VIII level may develop bleeding, most symptomatic haemophilic patients have factor VIII levels below 5%.

CLINICAL FEATURES Patients of haemophilia suffer from bleeding for hours or days after the injury. Haemophilic bleeding can involve any organ but occurs most commonly as recurrent painful haemarthroses and muscle haematomas, and sometimes as haematuria.

LABORATORY FINDINGS These are as follows:
i) Whole blood coagulation time is prolonged in severe cases only.
ii) Prothrombin time is usually normal.
iii) Activated partial thromboplastin time (APTT or PTTK) is typically prolonged.

PRINCIPLES OF TREATMENT Symptomatic patients with bleeding episodes are treated with factor VIII replacement therapy, consisting of factor VIII concentrates or plasma cryoprecipitates.

2. CHRISTMAS DISEASE (HAEMOPHILIA B)

Inherited deficiency of factor IX (Christmas factor or plasma thromboplastin component) produces Christmas disease or haemophilia B.

PRINCIPLES OF TREATMENT Therapy in symptomatic haemophilia B consists of infusion of either fresh frozen plasma or a plasma enriched with factor IX.

3. VON WILLEBRAND'S DISEASE

DEFINITION AND PATHOGENESIS von Willebrand's disease (vWD) is the most common hereditary coagulation disorder occurring due to qualitative or quantitative defect in von Willebrand's factor (vWF).
i) vWD is inherited as an autosomal dominant trait which may occur in either sex.
ii) The vWF is *synthesised* in the endothelial cells, megakaryocytes and platelets but not in the liver cells.
iii) The main *function* of vWF is to facilitate the adhesion of platelets to subendothelial collagen.

CLINICAL FEATURES Clinically, the patients of vWD are characterised by spontaneous bleeding from mucous membranes and excessive bleeding from wounds.

Bleeding episodes in vWD are treated with cryoprecipitates or factor VIII concentrates.

LABORATORY FINDINGS These are:
i) Prolonged bleeding time.
ii) Normal platelet count.
iii) Reduced plasma vWF concentration.
iv) Defective platelet aggregation with ristocetin, an antibiotic.
v) Reduced factor VIII activity.

4. VITAMIN K DEFICIENCY

Vitamin K is a fat-soluble vitamin which plays important role in haemostasis since it serves as a cofactor in the formation of 6 prothrombin complex proteins *(vitamin K-dependent coagulation factors)* synthesised in the liver: factor II, VII, IX, X, protein C and protein S.

Vitamin K deficiency may present in the newborn or in subsequent childhood or adult life.

5. COAGULATION DISORDERS IN LIVER DISEASE

Since liver is the major site for synthesis and metabolism of coagulation factors, liver disease often leads to multiple haemostatic abnormalities. The liver also produces inhibitors of coagulation such as antithrombin III and protein C and S and plays a role in the clearance of activated factors and fibrinolytic enzymes. Thus, patients with liver disease may develop hyper-coagulability and are predisposed to develop DIC and systemic fibrinolysis.

Many a times, the haemostatic abnormality in liver disease is complex but most patients have prolonged PT and PTTK, mild thrombocytopenia, normal fibrinogen level and decreased hepatic stores of vitamin K.

OTHER BLEEDING AND COAGULATION DISORDERS (p. 315)

HAEMORRHAGIC DIATHESES DUE TO FIBRINOLYTIC DEFECTS

Unchecked and excessive fibrinolysis may sometimes be the cause of bleeding. The causes of *primary pathologic fibrinolysis* leading to haemorrhagic defects are:

1. Deficiency of α_2-plasmin inhibitor following trauma or surgery.
2. Impaired clearance of tissue plasminogen activator such as in cirrhosis of liver.

HYPERCOAGULABLE STATE

Hypercoagulability or thrombophilia is a state of increased risk of thrombosis due to abnormality in haemostatic equilibrium i.e. reverse of abnormal bleeding. It may occur due to inherited or acquired disorders as under:

I. Inherited factors:

1. Antithrombin III deficiency
2. Protein C deficiency
3. Protein S deficiency
4. Activated protein C resistance (Factor V Leiden)
5. Inherited disorders of fibrinolytic pathways e.g. dysfibrinogenaemia, dysplasminogenaemia
6. Increased prothrombin production

II. Acquired factors:

1. Antiphospholipid antibodies (APLA) e.g. lupus anticoagulant, anticardiolipin antibodies
2. Impaired venous return due to stasis
3. Oral contraceptives
4. Disseminated malignancy
5. Nephrotic syndrome
6. Postoperative cases

DISSEMINATED INTRAVASCULAR COAGULATION (DIC)

Disseminated intravascular coagulation (DIC), also termed defibrination syndrome or consumption coagulopathy, is a complex thrombo-haemorrhagic disorder (intravascular coagulation and haemorrhage) occurring as a secondary complication in some systemic diseases.

ETIOLOGY

Although there are numerous conditions associated with DIC, most frequent causes are listed below:
1. Massive tissue injury
2. Infections
3. Widespread endothelial damage
4. Miscellaneous e.g. snake bite, shock, acute intravascular haemolysis, heat stroke.

PATHOGENESIS

1. Activation of coagulation The etiologic factors listed above initiate widespread activation of coagulation pathway by release of tissue factor.

2. Thrombotic phase Endothelial damage from the various thrombogenic stimuli causes generalised platelet aggregation and adhesion with resultant deposition of small thrombi and emboli throughout the microvasculature.

3. Consumption phase The early thrombotic phase is followed by a phase of consumption of coagulation factors and platelets.

4. Secondary fibrinolysis As a protective mechanism, fibrinolytic system is secondarily activated at the site of intravascular coagulation. Secondary fibrinolysis causes breakdown of fibrin resulting in formation of FDPs in the circulation.

CLINICAL FEATURES

There are 2 main features of DIC—*bleeding* as the most common manifestation, and *organ damage* due to ischaemia caused by the effect of widespread intravascular thrombosis such as in the kidney and brain.

1. The platelet count is low.
2. Blood film shows the features of microangiopathic haemolytic anaemia.
3. Prothrombin time, thrombin time and activated partial thromboplastin time, are all prolonged.
4. Plasma fibrinogen levels are reduced due to consumption in microvascular coagulation.
5. Fibrin degradation products (FDPs) are raised due to secondary fibrinolysis.

BLOOD GROUPS AND BLOOD TRANSFUSION (p. 317)

BLOOD GROUP ANTIGENS AND ANTIBODIES

Karl Landsteiner described the existence of major human blood groups in 1900 and was awarded Nobel Prize in 1930. The term *blood group* is applied to any well-defined system of red blood cell antigens which are inherited characteristics. The ABO and Rhesus (Rh) blood group systems are of major clinical significance. Other minor and clinically less important blood group systems are: Lewis system, P system, I system, MNS system, Kell and Duffy system, and Luthern system.

Individuals who lack the corresponding antigen and have not been previously transfused have *naturally-occurring antibodies* in their serum. The most important are anti-A and anti-B antibodies, usually of IgM class. *Immune antibodies,* on the other hand, are acquired in response to transfusion and by transplacental passage during pregnancy.

ABO SYSTEM This system consists of 3 major allelic genes: A, B and O, located on the long arm of chromosome 9. These genes control the synthesis of blood group antigens A and B. The serum of an individual contains naturally-occurring antibodies to A and/or B antigen, whichever antigen is lacking in the person's red cells. In routine practice, the ABO type is determined by testing the red blood cells with anti-A and anti-B and by testing the serum against A, B and O red blood cells.

Red blood cells of type O and A_2 have large amounts of another antigen called *H substance* which is genetically different from ABO but is a precursor of A and B antigens. An O group individual who inherits A or B genes but fails to inherit H gene from either parent is called O_h *phenotype or Bombay blood group.*

RHESUS SYSTEM The Rh allelic genes are *C or c, D or d* and *E or e,* located on chromosome 1. One set of 3 genes is inherited from each parent giving rise to various complex combinations. The corresponding antigens are similarly named *Cc, Ee* and only *D* since no *d* antigen exists.

However, out of all these, *D* antigen is most strongly immunogenic and, therefore, clinically most important. In practice, Rh grouping is performed with anti-D antiserum. Individuals who are D-positive are referred to as *Rh-positive* and those who lack D antigen are termed *Rh-negative.*

BLOOD TRANSFUSION (p. 318)

Blood transfusion goes through following sequential steps:
1. *Healthy blood donor selection* with haemoglobin more than 12.5 g/dl and free of infectious diseases.
2. *Blood collection by phlebotomy* in a sterile plastic blood bag containing anticoagulant, commonly acid citrate, mixing blood and coagulant gently while blood is flowing in to the bag.
3. *Storage of blood bag* in refrigerator at 2° to 6° C.
4. *Donor testing* for ABO-Rh grouping, and for infectious organism (HBV, HBsAg, HCV, syphilis and malaria).
5. *Blood grouping* (ABO-Rh) of the recipient.
6. *Pre-transfusion compatibility testing* of donor and recipient as under:
i) *Antibody screening* of the patient's serum to detect the presence of clinically significant antibodies.

ii) Cross-matching the patient's serum against donor red cells to confirm donor-recipient compatibility.

7. Supervised blood transfusion to observe reactions if any.

The indications for blood transfusion are acute blood loss and various haematologic disorders.

COMPLICATIONS OF BLOOD TRANSFUSION

A carefully prepared and supervised blood transfusion is quite safe. However, in 5-6% of transfusions, untoward complications occur, some of which are minor while others are more serious and at times fatal.

Transfusion reactions are generally classified into 2 types: immune and non-immune.

A. *IMMUNOLOGIC TRANSFUSION REACTIONS*

1. Haemolytic transfusion reactions Haemolytic transfusion reaction may be *immediate* or *delayed, intravascular* or *extravascular.*

2. Transfusion-related acute lung injury (TRALI) This is an uncommon reaction resulting from transfusion of donor plasma containing high levels of anti-HLA antibodies which bind to leucocytes of recipient. These leucocytes then aggregate in pulmonary micromutation and release mediators of increased vascular permeability resulting in acute pulmonary oedema and signs and symptoms of respiratory failure.

3. Other allergic reactions These are:
i) Febrile reaction
ii) Anaphylactic shock
iii) Allergic reactions
iv) Graft-versus-host disease.

B. *NONIMMUNE TRANSFUSION REACTIONS* These include:

1. Circulatory overload
2. Massive transfusion
3. Transmission of infection
4. Air embolism
5. Thrombophlebitis
6. Transfusion haemosiderosis

BLOOD COMPONENTS

Blood from donors is collected as whole blood in a suitable anticoagulant. Nowadays it is a common practice to divide whole blood into components which include: packed RBCs, platelets, fresh-frozen plasma (FFP) and cryoprecipitate.

The procedure consists of initial centrifugation at low speed to separate whole blood into two parts: *packed RBCs* and *platelet-rich plasma (PRP).* Subsequently, PRP is centrifuged at high speed to yield two parts: *random donor platelets* and *FFP. Cryoprecipitates* are obtained by thawing of FFP followed by centrifugation. *Apheresis* is the technique of direct collection of large excess of platelets from a single donor.

HAEMOLYTIC DISEASE OF NEWBORN (p. 319)

Haemolytic disease of the newborn (HDN) results from the passage of IgG antibodies from the maternal circulation across the placenta into the circulation of the foetal red cells. Besides pregnancy, sensitisation of the mother may result from previous abortions and previous blood transfusion.

HDN can occur from incompatibility of ABO or Rh blood group system. ABO incompatibility is much more common but the HDN in such cases is usually mild, while Rh-D incompatibility results in more severe form of the HDN.

PATHOGENESIS

HDN due to Rh-D incompatibility   Rh incompatibility occurs when a Rh-negative mother is sensitised to Rh-positive blood. This results most often from a Rh-positive foetus by passage of Rh-positive red cells across the placenta into the circulation of Rh-negative mother.

It must be emphasised here that the risk of sensitisation of a Rh-negative woman married to Rh-positive man is small in first pregnancy but increases during successive pregnancies if prophylactic anti-D immuno-globulin is not given within 72 hours after the first delivery.

HDN due to ABO incompatibility   About 20% pregnancies with ABO incompatibility between the mother and the foetus develop the HDN. Naturally-occurring anti-A and anti-B antibodies which are usually of IgM class do not cross the placenta, while immune anti-A and anti-B antibodies which are usually of IgG class may cross the placenta into foetal circulation and damage the foetal red cells.

CLINICAL FEATURES

The HDN due to Rh-D incompatibility in its *severest form* may result in intra-uterine death from *hydrops foetalis. Moderate disease* produces a baby born with severe anaemia and jaundice due to unconjugated hyperbilirubinaemia. When the level of unconjugated bilirubin exceeds 20 mg/dl, it may result in deposition of bile pigment in the basal ganglia of the CNS called *kernicterus* and result in permanent brain damage.

LABORATORY FINDINGS

1. *Cord blood* shows variable degree of anaemia, reticulocytosis, elevated serum bilirubin and a positive direct Coombs' test if the cord blood is Rh-D positive.
2. *Mother's blood* is Rh-D negative with high plasma titre of anti-D.

COURSE AND PROGNOSIS

The course in HDN may range from death, to minimal haemolysis, to mental retardation.

SELF ASSESSMENT

1. **If a patient is on parenteral heparin therapy, the following test is used to monitor the administration:**
   A. Whole blood coagulation time
   B. Prothrombin time
   C. Thrombin time
   D. Activated partial thromboplastin time

2. **Chronic ITP is characterised by the following features <u>except</u>:**
   A. Splenomegaly
   B. Reduced platelet lifespan
   C. Reduced number of megakaryocytes in the bone marrow
   D. Demonstration of anti-platelet IgG antibody

3. **For manifest bleeding haemophilia, the activity of factor VIII is generally:**
   A. More than 75%   B. 50-75%
   C. 25-50%   D. Below 25%

4. **Disseminated intravascular coagulation (DIC) is characterised by the following <u>except</u>:**
   A. Thrombocytopenia
   B. Microangiopathic haemolytic anaemia
   C. Presence of FDPs in the blood
   D. Normal prothrombin time

5. **Naturally-occurring antibodies in the serum of a non-transfused person are:**
   - A. IgA
   - B. IgD
   - C. IgG
   - D. IgM

6. **Tests for platelet function include all <u>except</u>:**
   - A. Platelet adhesion tests
   - B. Ethanol gelation test
   - C. Aggregation test
   - D. Granular content of platelets

7. **Heparin induced thrombocytopenia causes:**
   - A. Bleeding
   - B. Thrombosis
   - C. Both bleeding are thrombosis
   - D. No symptoms

8. **Antibodies in chronic ITP are:**
   - A. IgA
   - B. IgM
   - C. IgE
   - D. IgG

9. **Which of the following is not included in TTP triad?**
   - A. Anti-platelet antibodies
   - B. Thrombocytopenia
   - C. Microangiopathic haemolytic anaemia
   - D. Fibrin microthrombi

10. **Bernard-Soulier Syndrome is a defect in:**
    - A. Platelet aggregation
    - B. Platelet adhesion
    - C. Platelet release reaction
    - D. Platelet morphology

11. **Most common hereditary coagulation disorder is:**
    - A. Haemophilia A
    - B. Haemophilia B
    - C. von Willebrand's disease
    - D. Protein C deficiency

12. **Most common manifestation of DIC is:**
    - A. Bleeding
    - B. Thrombosis
    - C. Microangiopathic haemolytic anaemia
    - D. Organ damage

13. **Bombay blood group is characterised by:**
    - A. Absence of A gene
    - B. Absence of B gene
    - C. Absence of both A & B genes
    - D. Absence of H gene

14. **Hemolytic disease of newborn occurs when:**
    - A. Mother Rh+ve, foetus Rh –ve
    - B. Mother Rh-ve, foetus Rh +ve
    - C. Both mother and foetus Rh –ve
    - D. Both mother and foetus Rh +ve

KEY

1 = D	2 = C	3 = D	4 = D	5 = D
6 = B	7 = B	8 = D	9 = A	10 = B
11 = C	12 = A	13 = D	14 = B	

12 Disorders of Leucocytes and Lymphoreticular Tissues

Haematopoietic stem cells in the bone marrow differentiate into two types of progenitors—*lymphoid* (immune system) stem cells, and *non-lymphoid or myeloid* (trilineage) stem cells. The former develop into T, B and NK cells while the latter differentiate into 3 types of cell lines.

Leucocyte pool in the body lies at two distinct locations: in circulating blood and in the tissues. This concept holds more true for lymphoid cells in particular, which are present in circulation as well as are distributed in the lymphoid tissues of the body (lymph nodes, spleen, mucosa-associated lymphoid tissue—MALT, pharyngeal lymphoid tissue). Current WHO classification of lymphoma-leukaemia does not consider diseases of lymphocytes in the blood and in the lymphoid tissues as separate disorders; instead these diseases are seen to represent different stages of the same biologic process. Thus, in current times, diseases of leucocytes are studied together with diseases of lymphoreticular tissues of the body.

LYMPH NODES: NORMAL AND REACTIVE *(p. 321)*

NORMAL STRUCTURE

The lymph nodes are bean-shaped or oval structures varying in length from 1 to 2 cm and form the part of lymphatic network distributed throughout the body. Each lymph node is covered by a connective tissue *capsule*. At the convex surface of the capsule several *afferent lymphatics* enter which drain into the peripheral *subcapsular sinus*, branch into the lymph node and terminate at the concavity (hilum) as a single *efferent lymphatic* vessel.

The inner structure of the lymph node is divided into a peripheral cortex and central medulla. The *cortex* consists of several rounded aggregates of lymphocytes called *lymphoid follicles*. The deeper region of the cortex or *paracortex* is the zone between the peripheral cortex and the inner medulla. The *medulla* is predominantly composed of cords of plasma cells and some lymphocytes.

Functionally, the lymph node is divided into T and B lymphocyte zones:
◈ *B-cell zone* lies in the follicles in the cortex, the mantle zone and the interfollicular space, while *plasma cells* are also present in the interfollicular zone.
◈ *T-cell zone* is predominantly present in the medulla.

There are two main functions of the lymph node—to mount immune response in the body, and to perform the function of active phagocytosis for particulate material.

REACTIVE LYMPHADENITIS *(p. 322)*

Lymph nodes undergo reactive changes in response to a wide variety of stimuli which include microbial infections, drugs, environmental pollutants, tissue injury, immune-complexes and malignant neoplasms.

ACUTE NONSPECIFIC LYMPHADENITIS

All kinds of acute inflammations may cause acute nonspecific lymphadenitis in the nodes draining the area of inflamed tissue. Most common causes are microbiologic infections or their breakdown products, and foreign bodies in the wound or into the circulation etc. Most frequently involved lymph nodes are: *cervical* (due to infections in the oral cavity), *axillary* (due to infection in the arm), *inguinal* (due to infection in the lower extremities), and *mesenteric* (due to acute appendicitis, acute enteritis etc).

CHRONIC NONSPECIFIC LYMPHADENITIS

Chronic nonspecific lymphadenitis, commonly called *reactive lymphoid hyperplasia,* is a common form of inflammatory reaction of draining lymph nodes as a response to antigenic stimuli.

G/A The affected lymph nodes are usually enlarged, firm and non-tender.

M/E The features of 3 patterns of reactive lymphoid hyperplasia are as under:

1. Follicular hyperplasia Besides nonspecific stimulation, a few specific causes are: rheumatoid arthritis, toxoplasmosis, syphilis and AIDS.
i)   There is marked enlargement and prominence of the germinal centres of lymphoid follicles (proliferation of B-cell areas).
ii)   Parafollicular and medullary regions are more cellular and contain plasma cells, histiocytes, and some neutrophils and eosinophils.
iii) There is hyperplasia of mononuclear phagocytic cells lining the lymphatic sinuses in the lymph node.
◈   *Angiofollicular lymphoid hyperplasia* or *Castleman's disease* is a clinicopathologic variant of follicular hyperplasia. Two histologic forms are distinguished: hyaline-vascular type, and plasma cell form.

2. Paracortical lymphoid hyperplasia This is due to hyperplasia of T-cell-dependent area of the lymph node.
◈   *Angioimmunoblastic lymphadenopathy* is characterised by diffuse hyperplasia of immunoblasts rather than paracortical hyperplasia only, and there is proliferation of blood vessels.
◈   *Dermatopathic lymphadenopathy* occurs in lymph node draining an area of skin lesion.

3. Sinus histiocytosis or sinus hyperplasia This is a very common type found in regional lymph nodes draining inflammatory lesions, or as an immune reaction of the host to a draining malignant tumour or its products. The hallmark of histologic diagnosis is the expansion of the sinuses by proliferating large histiocytes containing phagocytosed material.
◈   *Sinus histiocytosis with massive lymphadenopathy* is characterised by marked enlargement of lymph nodes, especially of the neck, in young adolescents.

HIV-RELATED LYMPHADENOPATHY

The presence of enlarged lymph nodes of more than 1 cm diameter at two or more extra-inguinal sites for more than 3 months without any other obvious cause is frequently the earliest symptom of primary HIV infection.

M/E The findings are as under:
1. *In the early stage* marked follicular hyperplasia is the dominant finding and reflects the polyclonal B-cell proliferation.
2. *In the intermediate stage,* there is a combination of follicular hyperplasia and follicular involution.
3. *In the last stage,* there is decrease in the lymph node size indicative of prognostic marker of disease progression. Microscopic findings of node at this stage reveal follicular involution and lymphocyte depletion.

WHITE BLOOD CELLS: NORMAL AND REACTIVE *(p. 324)*

The leucocytes of the peripheral blood are of 2 main varieties, distinguished by the presence or absence of granules: *granulocytes* and *nongranular leucocytes.* The granulocytes, according to the appearance of nuclei, are subdivided into polymorphonuclear leucocytes and monocytes. Further, depending upon the colour and content of granules, polymorphonuclear leucocytes are of 3 types: neutrophils, eosinophils and basophils. The nongranular leucocytes are 3 types of lymphocytes: T, B and natural killer (NK) cells.

GRANULOPOIESIS (p. 324)

SITE OF FORMATION AND KINETICS

All forms of granulocytes are produced in the bone marrow and are termed, 'myeloid series'. Myeloid series include maturing stages: myeloblast (most primitive precursor), promyelocyte, myelocyte, metamyelocyte, band forms and segmented granulocyte (mature form).

Normally the bone marrow contains more myeloid cells than the erythroid cells in the ratio of 2:1 to 15:1 (average 3:1), the largest proportion being that of metamyelocytes, band forms and segmented neutrophils.

MYELOID SERIES

1. MYELOBLAST The myeloblast is the earliest recognisable precursor of the granulocytes, normally comprising about 2% of the total marrow cells. The myeloblast varies considerably in size (10-18 μm in diameter), having a large round to oval nucleus nearly filling the cell, has fine nuclear chromatin and contains 2-5 well-defined pale nucleoli. The thin rim of cytoplasm is deeply basophilic and devoid of granules. The myeloblasts of acute myeloid leukaemia may, however, show the presence of rod-like cytoplasmic inclusions called *Auer's rods* which represent abnormal derivatives of primary azurophilic granules.

2. PROMYELOCYTE The promyelocyte is slightly larger than the myeloblast (12-18 μm diameter). It possesses a round to oval nucleus, having fine nuclear chromatin which is slightly condensed around the nuclear membrane. The nucleoli are present but are less prominent and fewer than those in the myeloblast. The main distinction of promyelocyte from myeloblast is in the cytoplasm which contains azurophilic (primary or non-specific) granules.

3. MYELOCYTE The myelocyte is the stage in which specific or secondary granules appear in the cytoplasm, and accordingly, the cell can be identified at this stage as belonging to the neutrophilic, eosinophilic or basophilic myelocyte. The myeloid cells up to the myelocyte stage continue to divide and, therefore, are included in *mitotic or proliferative pool*.

4. METAMYELOCYTE The metamyelocyte stage is 10-18 μm in diameter and is characterised by a clearly indented or horseshoe-shaped nucleus without nucleoli. The nuclear chromatin is dense and clumped. The cytoplasm contains both primary and secondary granules.

5. BAND FORMS Band form is juvenile granulocyte, 10-16 μm in diameter, characterised by further condensation of nuclear chromatin and transformation of nuclear shape into band configuration of uniform thickness.

6. SEGMENTED GRANULOCYTES The mature polymorphonuclear leucocytes, namely: the neutrophils, eosinophils and basophils, are described separately below.

MONOCYTE-MACROPHAGE SERIES

The monocyte-macrophage series of cells, comprise a part of myeloid series along with other granulocytic series.

1. MONOBLAST The monoblast is the least mature of the recognisable cell of monocyte-macrophage series. It is very similar in appearance to myeloblast except that it has ground-glass cytoplasm with irregular border and may show phagocytosis as indicated by the presence of engulfed red cells in the cytoplasm.

2. PROMONOCYTE The promonocyte is a young monocyte, about 20 μm in diameter and possesses a large indented nucleus containing a nucleolus. The cytoplasm is basophilic and contains no azurophilic granules but may have fine granules which are larger than those in the mature monocyte.

3. MONOCYTE The mature form of circulating monocytic series and in various tissues (i.e. macrophages) are a part of RE system.

LYMPHOPOIESIS (p. 326)

SITES OF FORMATION AND KINETICS

The lymphocytes and the plasma cells are immunocompetent cells of the body. In humans, the bone marrow and the thymus are the *primary lymphopoietic organs* where lymphoid stem cells undergo spontaneous division independent of antigenic stimulation. The *secondary or reactive lymphoid tissue* is comprised by the lymph nodes, spleen and gut-associated lymphoid tissue (GALT). These sites actively produce lymphocytes from the germinal centres of lymphoid follicles as a response to antigenic stimulation.

Functionally, the lymphocytes are divided into T, B and natural killer (NK) cells depending upon whether they are immunologically active in cell-mediated immunity (T cells), in humoral antibody response (B cells) or form part of the natural or innate immunity and act as killer of some viruses (NK cells).

LYMPHOID SERIES

1. LYMPHOBLAST The lymphoblast is the earliest identifiable precursor of lymphoid cells and is a rapidly dividing cell. It is a large cell, 10-18 μm in diameter, containing a large round to oval nucleus having slightly clumped or stippled nuclear chromatin. The nuclear membrane is denser and the number of nucleoli is fewer (1-2) as compared with those in myeloblast (2-5). The cytoplasm is scanty, basophilic and non-granular.

2. PROLYMPHOCYTE This stage is an intermediate stage between the lymphoblast and mature lymphocyte. These young lymphocytes are 9-18 μm in diameter, contain round to indented nucleus with slightly stippled or coarse chromatin and may have 0-1 nucleoli.

3. LYMPHOCYTE These are described below separately.

MATURE LEUCOCYTES IN HEALTH AND REACTIVE PROLIFERATION IN DISEASE (p. 326)

Normally, only mature leucocytes namely: polymorphs, lymphocytes, monocytes, eosinophils and basophils, are found in the peripheral blood. The normal range of total and differential leucocyte count (TLC and DLC expressed sequentially as P, L, M, E, B) in health in adults and children is given below:

	ABSOLUTE COUNT
TLC	
Adults	4,000–11,000/μl
Infants (Full term, at birth)	10,000–25,000/μl
Infants (1 year)	6,000–16,000/μl
Children (4–7 years)	5,000–15,000/μl
Children (8–12 years)	4,500–13,500/μl
DLC in adults	
Polymorphs (neutrophils) 40–75%	2,000–7,500/μl
Lymphocytes 20–50%	1,500–4,000/μl
Monocytes 2–10%	200–800/μl
Eosinophils 1–6%	40–400/μl
Basophils <l%	10–100/μl

POLYMORPHS (NEUTROPHILS)

MORPHOLOGY A polymorphonuclear neutrophil (PMN), commonly called polymorph or neutrophil, is 12-15 μm in diameter. It consists of a characteristic dense nucleus, having 2-5 lobes and pale cytoplasm containing numerous fine violet-pink granules. These lysosomal granules contain several enzymes and are of 2 types:

Primary or azurophilic granules are large and coarse and appear early at the promyelocyte stage.

Secondary or specific granules are smaller and more numerous.
The normal **functions** of neutrophils are:
1. *Chemotaxis* or cell mobilisation
2. *Phagocytosis*
3. *Killing* of the microorganism

VARIATION IN COUNT An increase in neutrophil count *(neutrophil leucocytosis or neutrophilia)* or a decrease in count *(neutropenia)* may occur in various diseases.

Neutrophil leucocytosis An increase in circulating neutrophils above 7,500/µl is the commonest type of leucocytosis.
1. *Acute infections, local or generalised.* For example: pneumonia, cholecystitis, salpingitis, meningitis, diphtheria, plague, peritonitis, appendicitis, actinomycosis, poliomyelitis, abscesses, furuncles, carbuncles, tonsillitis, otitis media, osteomyelitis etc.
2. *Other inflammations* e.g. tissue damage resulting from burns, operations, ischaemic necrosis (such as in MI), gout, collagen-vascular diseases, hypersensitivity reactions etc.
3. *Intoxication* e.g. uraemia, diabetic ketosis, eclampsia, poisonings by chemicals and drugs.
4. *Acute haemorrhage,* internal or external.
5. *Acute haemolysis.*
6. *Disseminated malignancies.*
7. *Myeloproliferative disorders* e.g. myeloid leukaemia, polycythaemia vera, myeloid metaplasia.
8. *Miscellaneous* e.g. following corticosteroid therapy, idiopathic neutrophilia.

Neutropenia When the absolute neutrophil count falls below 2,500/µl.
1. *Certain infections* e.g. typhoid, paratyphoid, brucellosis, influenza, measles, viral hepatitis, malaria, kala-azar etc.
2. *Overwhelming bacterial infections* especially in patients with poor resistance e.g. miliary tuberculosis, septicaemia.
3. *Drugs, chemicals and physical agents* which induce aplasia of the bone marrow cause neutropenia, e.g. antimetabolites, nitrogen mustards, benzene, ionising radiation. Occasionally, certain drugs produce neutropenia due to individual sensitivity such as: anti-inflammatory (amidopyrine, phenyl-butazone), antibacterial (chloramphenicol, cotrimoxazole), anticonvulsants, antithyroids, hypoglycaemics and antihistaminics.
4. *Certain haematological and other diseases* e.g. pernicious anaemia, aplastic anaemia, cirrhosis of the liver with splenomegaly, SLE, Gaucher's disease.
5. *Cachexia and debility.*
6. *Anaphylactoid shock.*
7. *Certain rare hereditary, congenital or familial disorders* e.g. cyclic neutropenia, primary splenic neutropenia, idiopathic benign neutropenia.

VARIATIONS IN MORPHOLOGY These are as under:

1. **Granules** Heavy, dark staining, coarse toxic granules are characteristic of bacterial infections.

2. **Vacuoles** In bacterial infections such as in septicaemia, cytoplasmic vacuolation may develop.

3. **Döhle bodies** These are small, round or oval patches, 2-3 µm in size, in the cytoplasm. They are mostly seen in bacterial infections.

4. **Nuclear abnormalities** These include the following:
i) *Sex chromatin* is a normal finding in 2-3% of neutrophils in female sex.
ii) A *'shift-to-left'* is the term used for appearance of neutrophils with decreased number of nuclear lobes in the peripheral blood.

iii) A *'shift-to-right'* is appearance of hypersegmented (more than 5 nuclear lobes) neutrophils in the peripheral blood such as in megaloblastic anaemia, uraemia, and sometimes in leukaemia.

iv) *Pelger-Huët anomaly* is an uncommon autosomal dominant inherited disorder in which nuclei in majority of neutrophils are distinctively bilobed (spectacle-shaped) and coarsely staining chromatin.

DEFECTIVE FUNCTIONS These are as follows:

1. Defective chemotaxis e.g. in a rare congenital abnormality called lazy-leucocyte syndrome.

2. Defective phagocytosis due to lack of opsonisation.

3. Defective killing e.g. in chronic granulomatous disease, Chédiak-Higashi syndrome, myeloid leukaemias.

LYMPHOCYTES

MORPHOLOGY Majority of lymphocytes in the peripheral blood are *small* (9-12 μm in diameter) but *large* lymphocytes (12-16 μm in diameter) are also found. Both small and large lymphocytes have round or slightly indented nucleus with coarsely-clumped chromatin and scanty basophilic cytoplasm. Plasma cells are derived from B lymphocytes under the influence of appropriate stimuli.

T lymphocytes i.e. thymus-dependent lymphocytes, which mature in the thymus and are also known as thymocytes. They are mainly involved in direct action on antigens and are therefore involved in *cell-mediated immune (CMI)* reaction by its subsets such as cytotoxic (killer) T cells (CD3+), CD8+ T cells, and *delayed hypersensitivity reaction* by CD4+ T cells.

B lymphocytes i.e. bone marrow-dependent or bursa-equivalent lymphocytes as well as their derivatives, plasma cells, are the source of specific immunoglobulin antibodies. They are, therefore, involved in *humoral immunity (HI) or circulating immune reactions.*

NK cells As the name indicates they are identified with *'natural'* or innate immunity and bring about direct *'killing'* of microorganisms (particularly certain viruses) or lysis of foreign body.

PATHOLOGIC VARIATIONS A rise in the absolute count of lymphocytes exceeding the upper limit of normal (above 4,000/μm) is termed *lymphocytosis,* while absolute lymphocyte count below 1,500/μm is referred to as *lymphopenia.*

Lymphocytosis

1. *Certain acute infections* e.g. pertussis, infectious mononucleosis, viral hepatitis, infectious lymphocytosis.
2. *Certain chronic infections* e.g. brucellosis, tuberculosis, secondary syphilis.
3. *Haematopoietic disorders* e.g. lymphocytic leukaemias, lymphoma, heavy chain disease.
4. *Relative lymphocytosis* is found in viral exanthemas, convalescence from acute infections, thyrotoxicosis, conditions causing neutropenia.

Lymphopenia

1. Most acute infections.
2. Severe bone marrow failure.
3. Corticosteroid and immunosuppressive therapy.
4. Widespread irradiation.

MONOCYTES

MORPHOLOGY The monocyte is the largest mature leucocyte in the peripheral blood measuring 12-20 μm in diameter. It possesses a large, central, oval, notched or indented or horseshoe-shaped nucleus which has characteristically fine reticulated chromatin network. The cytoplasm is abundant, pale blue and contains many fine dust-like granules and vacuoles.

The main **functions** of monocytes are:
1. *Phagocytosis*
2. Immunologic function as *antigen-presenting cells*
3. As *mediator of inflammation*.

PATHOLOGIC VARIATIONS A rise in the blood monocytes above 800/µl is termed *monocytosis*. These are:
1. *Certain bacterial infections* e.g. tuberculosis, subacute bacterial endocarditis, syphilis.
2. *Viral infections.*
3. *Protozoal and rickettsial infections* e.g. malaria, typhus, trypanosomiasis, kala-azar.
4. *Convalescence from acute infection.*
5. *Haematopoietic disorders* e.g. monocytic leukaemia, lymphomas, myeloproliferative disorders, multiple myeloma, lipid storage disease.
6. *Malignancies* e.g. cancer of the ovary, stomach, breast.
7. *Granulomatous diseases* e.g. sarcoidosis, inflammatory bowel disease.
8. *Collagen-vascular diseases.*

EOSINOPHILS

MORPHOLOGY Eosinophils are similar to segmented neutrophils in size (12-15 µm in diameter), and have coarse, deep red staining granules in the cytoplasm and have usually two nuclear lobes. Granules in eosinophils contain basic protein and stain more intensely for peroxidase than granules in the neutrophils.

Eosinophils are involved in reactions to foreign proteins and to antigen-antibody reactions.

PATHOLOGIC VARIATIONS An increase in the number of eosinophilic leucocytes above 400/µl is referred to as *eosinophilia* and below 40/µl is termed as *eosinopenia*.

Eosinophilia
1. *Allergic disorders* e.g. bronchial asthma, urticaria, angioneurotic oedema, hay fever, drug hypersensitivity.
2. *Parasitic infestations* e.g. trichinosis, echinococcosis, intestinal parasitism.
3. *Skin diseases* e.g. pemphigus, dermatitis herpetiformis, erythema multiforme.
4. *Löeffler's syndrome.*
5. *Pulmonary infiltration with eosinophilia* (PIE) syndrome.
6. *Tropical eosinophilia.*
7. *Haematopoietic diseases* e.g. CML, polycythaemia vera, pernicious anaemia, Hodgkin's disease, following splenectomy.
8. *Malignant diseases* with metastases.

Eosinopenia Adrenal steroids and ACTH induce eosinopenia in man.

BASOPHILS

MORPHOLOGY Basophils resemble the other mature granulocytes but are distinguished by coarse, intensely basophilic granules which usually fill the cytoplasm and often overlie and obscure the nucleus.

The granules of circulating basophils (as well as their tissue counterparts as mast cells) contain heparin, histamine and 5-HT. Mast cells or basophils on degranulation are associated with histamine release.

PATHOLOGIC VARIATIONS Basophil leucocytosis or *basophilia* refers to an increase in the number of basophilic leucocytes above 100/µl.
1. Chronic myeloid leukaemia
2. Polycythaemia vera
3. Myelosclerosis
4. Myxoedema
5. Ulcerative colitis
6. Following splenectomy

7. Hodgkin's disease
8. Urticaria pigmentosa.

INFECTIOUS MONONUCLEOSIS (p. 329)

Infectious mononucleosis (IM) or glandular fever is a benign, self-limited lymphoproliferative disease caused by Epstein-Barr virus (EBV), one of the herpesviruses. Infection may occur from childhood to old age but the classical acute infection is more common in teenagers and young adults. The infection is transmitted by person-to-person contact such as by kissing with transfer of virally-contaminated saliva.

PATHOGENESIS

EBV, the etiologic agent for IM, is a B lymphotropic herpesvirus. The disease is characterised by fever, generalised lymphadenopathy, hepatosplenomegaly, sore throat, and appearance in blood of atypical 'mononucleosis cells'.

1. In a susceptible sero-negative host who lacks antibodies, the virus in the contaminated saliva *invades and replicates within epithelial cells* of the salivary gland and then enters B cells in the lymphoid tissues.

2. Viraemia and death of infected B cells cause an acute febrile illness and appearance of specific humoral antibodies.

3. *EBV-infected B cells undergo polyclonal activation and proliferation.* These cells perform two important roles which are the characteristic diagnostic features of IM:

i) They secrete *antibodies*—initially IgM but later IgG class antibodies appear.

ii) They *activate CD8+ T lymphocytes*—also called cytotoxic T cells (or CTL) or suppressor T cells. CD8+ T cells bring about killing of B cells and are pathognomonic atypical lymphocytes seen in blood in IM.

4. The proliferation of these cells is responsible for *generalised lymphadenopathy and hepatosplenomegaly.*

5. The *sore throat* in IM may be caused by either necrosis of B cells or due to viral replication within the salivary epithelial cells in early stage.

CLINICAL FEATURES

The incubation period of IM is 30-50 days in young adults, while children have shorter incubation period.

1. **During prodromal period (first 3-5 days),** the symptoms are mild such as malaise, myalgia, headache and fatigue.

2. **Frank clinical features (next 7-21 days)** seen commonly are fever (90%), sore throat (80%) and bilateral cervical lymphadenopathy (95%).

3. **Complications** Although most cases of IM run a self-limited course, complications may develop in some cases.

LABORATORY FINDINGS

1. **HAEMATOLOGIC FINDINGS** These are as under:

i) TLC There is a moderate rise in total white cell count (10,000-20,000/µl) during 2nd to 3rd week after infection.

ii) DLC There is an absolute lymphocytosis. The lymphocytosis is due to rise in normal as well as atypical T lymphocytes. There is relative neutropenia.

iii) Atypical T cells Essential to the diagnosis of IM is the presence of at least 10-12% atypical T cells (or mononucleosis cells) lying in peripheral blood lymphocytosis. The mononucleosis cells are variable in appearance and are classed as Downey type I, II and III, of which Downey type I are found most frequently.

iv) CD4+ and CD8+ T cell counts There is reversal of CD4+/CD8+ T cell ratio. There is marked decrease in CD4+ T cells while there is substantial rise in CD8+ T cells.

v) Platelets There is generally thrombocytopenia in the first 4 weeks of illness.

2. SEROLOGIC DIAGNOSIS The second characteristic laboratory finding is the demonstration of antibodies in the serum of infected patient. These are
i) Heterophile antibody test (Paul-Bunnell test) is used for making the diagnosis of IM.
ii) Specific antibodies against the viral capsid and nucleus of EBV.
iii) Detection of EBV DNA or proteins can be done in blood or CSF by PCR method.

LEUKAEMOID REACTIONS (p. 331)

Leukaemoid reaction is defined as a reactive excessive leucocytosis in the peripheral blood resembling that of leukaemia in a subject who does not have leukaemia.

Leukaemoid reaction may be myeloid or lymphoid; the former is much more common.

MYELOID LEUKAEMOID REACTION

CAUSES Majority of leukaemoid reactions involve the granulocyte series. It may occur in association with a wide variety of diseases.
1. *Infections* e.g. staphylococcal pneumonia, disseminated tuberculosis, meningitis, diphtheria, sepsis, endocarditis, plague, infected abortions etc.
2. *Intoxication* e.g. eclampsia, mercury poisoning, severe burns.
3. *Malignant diseases* e.g. multiple myeloma, myelofibrosis, Hodgkin's disease, bone metastases.
4. *Severe haemorrhage and severe haemolysis.*

LABORATORY FINDINGS Major findings are:
1. *Leucocytosis,* usually moderate, not exceeding 100,000/μl.
2. Proportion of *immature cells* mild to moderate, comprised by metamyelocytes, myelocytes (5-15%), and blasts fewer than 5% i.e. the blood picture simulates somewhat with that of CML.
3. Infective cases may show *toxic granulation and Döhle bodies* in the cytoplasm of neutrophils.
4. *Neutrophil (or Leucocyte) alkaline phosphatase (NAP or LAP) score* in the cytoplasm of mature neutrophils in leukaemoid reaction is characteristically high and is very useful to distinguish it from chronic myeloid leukaemia in doubtful cases.
5. *Cytogenetic studies* may be helpful in exceptional cases which reveal negative Philadelphia chromosome i.e. t (9; 22) or BCR-ABL fusion gene in myeloid leukaemoid reaction but positive in cases of CML.

LYMPHOID LEUKAEMOID REACTION

CAUSES Lymphoid leukaemoid reaction may be found in the following conditions:
1. *Infections* e.g. infectious mononucleosis, cytomegalovirus infection, pertussis (whooping cough), chickenpox, measles, infectious lymphocytosis, tuberculosis.
2. *Malignant diseases* may rarely produce lymphoid leukaemoid reaction.

LABORATORY FINDINGS Main features are:
1. Leucocytosis not exceeding 100,000/μl.
2. The differential white cell count reveals mostly mature lymphocytes simulating the blood picture found in cases of CLL.

> **LYMPHOHAEMATOPOIETIC MALIGNANCIES**
> **(LEUKAEMIAS-LYMPHOMAS): GENERAL** (p. 333)

CLASSIFICATION: HISTORY AND CURRENT CONCEPTS

Neoplastic proliferations of white blood cells are termed leukaemias and lymphomas and are the most important group of leucocyte disorders.

Historically, **leukaemias** have been classified on the basis of cell types predominantly involved into *myeloid* and *lymphoid,* and on the basis of natural history of the disease, into *acute* and *chronic*. Thus, the main types of leukaemias have been: *acute myeloblastic leukaemia* and *acute lymphoblastic leukaemia* (AML and ALL), and *chronic myeloid leukaemia* and *chronic lymphocytic leukaemias* (CML and CLL). In general, acute leukaemias are characterised by predominance of undifferentiated leucocyte precursors or leukaemic blasts and have a rapidly downhill course. Chronic leukaemias, on the other hand, have easily recognisable late precursor series of leucocytes circulating in large number as the predominant leukaemic cell type and the patients tend to have more indolent behaviour. ALL is primarily a disease of children and young adults, whereas AML occurs at all ages. CLL tends to occur in the elderly, while CML is found in middle age.

Similarly, over the years, **lymphomas** which are malignant tumours of lymphoreticular tissues have been categorised into two distinct clinicopathologic groups: *Hodgkin's lymphoma* or *Hodgkin's disease (HD)* characterised by pathognomonic presence of Reed-Sternberg cells, and a heterogeneous group of *non-Hodgkin's lymphomas (NHL)*.

Over the last 50 years, several classification systems have been proposed for leukaemias and lymphomas. Newer classification schemes have been based on cytochemistry, immunophenotyping, cytogenetics and molecular markers which have become available to pathologists and haematologists. The last classification scheme proposed by the World Health Organization (WHO) in 2008 combines all tumours of haematopoietic and lymphoid tissues together. The basis of the WHO classification is the *cell type of the neoplasm* as identified by combined approach of clinical features and morphologic, cytogenetic and molecular characteristics, *rather than location of the neoplasm* (whether in blood or in tissues) because of the fact that haematopoietic cells are present in circulation as well as in tissues in general, and lymphoreticular tissues in particular.

As per WHO classification scheme, neoplasms of haematopoietic and lymphoid tissues are considered as a unified group and are divided into 3 broad categories:

I. Myeloid neoplasms
II. Lymphoid neoplasms
III. Histiocytic neoplasms

Besides the WHO classification, the FAB (French-American-British) Cooperative Group classification of lymphomas and leukaemias based on morphology and cytochemistry is also widely used.

ETIOLOGY OF LYMPHOHAEMATOPOIETIC MALIGNANCIES *(p. 334)*

The exact etiology of leukaemias and lymphomas is not known. However, a number of factors have been implicated:

1. HEREDITY There is evidence to suggest that there is role of family history, occurrence in identical twins and predisposition of these malignancies in certain genetic syndromes:

i) Identical twins There is high concordance rate among identical twins if acute leukaemia develops in the first year of life.

ii) Family history Families with excessive incidence of leukaemia have been identified.

iii) Genetic disease association Acute leukaemia occurs with increased frequency with a variety of congenital disorders such as Down's, Bloom's, Klinefelter's and Wiskott-Aldrich's syndromes.

2. INFECTIONS There is evidence to suggest that certain infections, particularly viruses, are involved in development of lymphomas and leukaemias:

i) *Human T cell leukaemia-lymphoma virus I (HTLV-I)* implicated in etiology of adult T cell leukaemia-lymphoma (ATLL).

ii) *HTLV II* for T cell variant of hairy cell leukaemia.

iii) *Epstein-Barr virus (EBV)* implicated in the etiology of Hodgkin's disease (mixed cellularity type and nodular sclerosis type), endemic variety of Burkitt's lymphoma, post-transplant lymphoma.

iv) HIV in diffuse large B-cell lymphoma and Burkitt's lymphoma.

v) Hepatitis C virus (HCV) in lymphoplasmacytic lymphoma.

vi) Human herpes virus 8 (HHV-8) in primary effusion lymphoma.

vii) Helicobacter pylori bacterial infection of gastric mucosa in MALT lymphoma of the stomach.

3. ENVIRONMENTAL FACTORS Certain environmental factors are known to play a role in the etiology of leukaemias and lymphomas e.g.

i) Ionising radiation

ii) Chemical carcinogens

iii) Certain drugs

4. ASSOCIATION WITH DISEASES OF IMMUNITY Since lymphoid cells are the immune cells of the body, diseases with derangements of the immune system have higher incidence of haematopoietic malignancies e.g.

i) Immunodeficiency diseases

ii) Autoimmune disease association

PATHOGENESIS *(p. 334)*

It needs to be emphasised that since haematopoietic cells have a rapid turnover, they are more vulnerable to chromosomal damages and cytogenetic changes under influence of various etiologic factors listed above.

1. Genetic damage to single clone of target cells Leukaemias and lymphomas arise following malignant transformation of a single clone of cells belonging to myeloid or lymphoid series, followed by proliferation of the transformed clone.

2. Chromosomal translocations A number of cytogenetic abnormalities have been detected in cases of leukaemias-lymphomas, most consistent of which are chromosomal translocations. In NHL, translocation involving antigen receptor genes, immunoglobulin genes, or overexpression of BCL-2 protein may be seen.

3. Maturation defect In acute leukaemia, the single most prominent characteristic of the leukaemic cells is a defect in maturation beyond the myeloblast or promyelocyte level in AML, and the lymphoblast level in ALL.

4. Myelosuppression As the leukaemic cells accumulate in the bone marrow, there is suppression of normal haematopoietic stem cells, partly by physically replacing the normal marrow precursors, and partly by inhibiting normal haematopoiesis.

5. Organ infiltration The leukaemic cells proliferate primarily in the bone marrow, circulate in the blood and infiltrate into other tissues such as lymph nodes, liver, spleen, skin, viscera and the central nervous system.

6. Cytokines Presence of reactive inflammatory cells in the Hodgkin's disease is due to secretion of cytokines from the Reed Sternberg cells e.g. IL-5, IL-13 and transforming growth factor-β.

MYELOID NEOPLASMS *(p. 335)*

Since myeloid trilineage stem cells differentiate into 3 series of progenitor cells: erythroid, granulocyte-monocyte, and megakaryocytic series, all examples of myeloid neoplasms fall into these three categories of cell-lines. Based on this concept, myeloid neoplasms has following 5 groups:

I. Myeloproliferative diseases

II. Myelodysplastic/myeloproliferative diseases

III. Myelodysplastic syndrome (MDS)

IV. Acute myeloid leukaemia (AML)

V. Acute biphenotypic leukaemia

MYELOPROLIFERATIVE DISEASES *(p. 335)*

The myeloproliferative disorders are a group of neoplastic proliferation of multipotent haematopoietic stem cells. Besides their common stem cell origin, these disorders are closely related, occasionally leading to evolution of one entity into another during the course of the disease.

Classic and common examples are chronic myeloid leukaemia (CML), polycythaemia vera (PV), and essential thrombocytosis (ET), each one representing corresponding excess of granulocytes, red blood cells, and platelets, respectively. The group as a whole has slow and insidious onset of clinical features and indolent clinical behaviour.

CHRONIC MYELOID LEUKAEMIA (CML)

DEFINITION AND PATHOPHYSIOLOGY

By WHO definition, CML is established by identification of the clone of haematopoietic stem cell that possesses the balanced reciprocal translocation between chromosomes 9 and 22, forming Philadelphia chromosome. The t(9;22) involves fusion of BCR (breakpoint cluster region) gene on chromosome 22q11 with ABL (named after Abelson murine leukaemia virus) gene located on chromosome 9q34. The fusion product so formed is termed "Ph chromosome t(9;22) (q34;11), BCR/ABL" which should be positive for making the diagnosis of CML. This identification may be done by PCR or by FISH.

CLINICAL FEATURES

Chronic myeloid (myelogenous, granulocytic) leukaemia comprises about 20% of all leukaemias and its peak incidence is seen in 3rd and 4th decades of life. A distinctive variant of CML seen in children is called *juvenile CML*. Both sexes are affected equally. The onset of CML is generally insidious. Some of the common presenting manifestations are:
1. Anaemia
2. Hypermetabolism
3. Splenomegaly
4. Bleeding tendencies

LABORATORY FINDINGS

I. **BLOOD PICTURE** The findings are as under:

1. Anaemia Anaemia is usually of moderate degree and is normocytic normochromic in type.

2. White blood cells Characteristically, there is marked leucocytosis (approximately 200,000/μl or more at the time of presentation). The natural history of CML consists of 3 phases—chronic, accelerated, and blastic.

❖ *Chronic phase of CML* begins as a myeloproliferative disorder and consists of excessive proliferation of myeloid cells of intermediate grade (i.e. myelocytes and metamyelocytes) and mature segmented neutrophils. Myeloblasts usually do not exceed 10% of cells in the peripheral blood and bone marrow.

❖ An *accelerated phase of CML* is also described in which there is progressively rising leucocytosis associated with thrombocytosis or thrombocytopenia and splenomegaly.

❖ *Blastic phase or blast crisis in CML* fulfills the definition of acute leukaemia in having blood or marrow blasts ≥20%. These blast cells may be myeloid, lymphoid, erythroid or undifferentiated and are established by morphology, cytochemistry, or immunophenotyping. Myeloid blast crisis in CML is more common and resembles AML.

3. Platelets Platelet count may be normal but is raised in about half the cases.

II. **BONE MARROW EXAMINATION** The findings are as under:

1. Cellularity Generally, there is hypercellularity with total or partial replacement of fat spaces by proliferating myeloid cells.

2. Myeloid cells The myeloid cells predominate in the bone marrow with increased myeloid-erythroid ratio.

3. Erythropoiesis Erythropoiesis is normoblastic but there is reduction in erythropoietic cells.

4. Megakaryocytes Megakaryocytes are conspicuous.

5. Cytogenetics Cytogenetic studies on blood and bone marrow cells show the characteristic chromosomal abnormality called Philadelphia (Ph) chromosome seen in 90-95% cases of CML.

II. CYTOCHEMISTRY The only significant finding on cytochemical stains is reduced scores of *neutrophil alkaline phosphatase (NAP)* which helps to distinguish CML from myeloid leukaemoid reaction in which case NAP scores are elevated.

IV. OTHER INVESTIGATIONS
1. Elevated serum B_{12} and vitamin B_{12} binding capacity.
2. Elevated serum uric acid (hyperuricaemia).

GENERAL PRINCIPLES OF TREATMENT AND PROGNOSIS

Insight into molecular mechanism of CML has brought about major changes in its therapy.
1. Imatinib oral therapy   Imatinib Induces apoptosis in BCR/ABL-positive cells and thus eliminates them.
2. Allogenic bone marrow (stem cell) transplantation
3. Interferon-α
4. Chemotherapy

POLYCYTHAEMIA VERA

DEFINITION AND PATHOPHYSIOLOGY

Polycythaemia vera (PV) is a clonal disorder characterised by increased production of all myeloid elements resulting in pancytosis (i.e increased red cells, granulocytes, platelets) in the absence of any recognisable cause.
❖ The term 'polycythaemia vera' or 'polycythaemia rubra vera' is used for *primary or idiopathic polycythaemia* only and is the most common of all the myeloproliferative disorders.
❖ *Secondary polycythaemia or erythrocytosis,* on the other hand, may occur secondary to several causes e.g.
i) High altitude.
ii) Cardiovascular disease.
iii) Pulmonary disease with alveolar hypoventilation.
iv) Heavy smoking.
v) Inappropriate increase in erythropoietin (renal cell carcinoma, hydronephrosis, hepatocellular carcinoma, cerebellar haemangioblastoma, massive uterine leiomyoma).

CLINICAL FEATURES

Clinical features are the result of hyperviscosity, hypervolaemia, hypermetabolism and decreased cerebral perfusion. These are as under:
1. Headache, vertigo, tinnitus, visual alterations syncope or even coma.
2. Increased risk of thrombosis.
3. Increased risk of haemorrhages.
4. Splenomegaly
5. Pruritus
6. Increased risk of urate stones and gout.

LABORATORY FINDINGS

1. *Raised haemoglobin* concentration (above 17.5 g/dl in males and 15.5 g/dl in females).
2. *Erythrocytosis* (above 6 million/μl in males and 5.5 million/μl in females).
3. Haematocrit (PCV) above 55% in males and above 47% in females.
4. Mild to moderate *leucocytosis* (15,000-25,000/μl) with basophilia and raised neutrophil alkaline phosphatase scores.
5. *Thrombocytosis* with defective platelet function.
6. Bone marrow examination reveals *panhyperplasia*.
7. *Cytogenetic abnormalities*
8. *Erythropoietin* levels in serum and urine are reduced.

1. *Phlebotomy* (venesection) by blood letting
2. *Anticoagulant therapy*
3. *Chemotherapy*
4. *Uricosuric drugs*
5. *Interferon-α*

ESSENTIAL THROMBOCYTHAEMIA

DEFINITION AND PATHOPHYSIOLOGY

Essential thrombocythaemia (ET), also termed essential thrombocytosis or primary (idiopathic) thrombocythaemia is a clonal disorder characterised by markedly elevated platelet count in the absence of any recognisable stimulus. *Secondary or reactive thrombocytosis,* on the other hand, occurs in response to known stimuli such as: chronic infection, haemorrhage, postoperative state, chronic iron deficiency, malignancy, rheumatoid arthritis and postsplenectomy.

CLINICAL FEATURES

1. Arterial or venous thrombosis.
2. Easy bruisability following minor trauma.
3. Spontaneous bleeding.
4. Transient ischaemic attack or frank stroke.

LABORATORY FINDINGS

1. Sustained elevation in platelet count (above 400,000 µl).
2. Blood film shows many large platelets, megakaryocyte fragments and hypogranular forms.
3. Consistently abnormal platelet functions, especially abnormality in platelet aggregation.
4. Bone marrow examination reveals a large number of hyperdiploid megakaryocytes and variable amount of increased fibrosis.

GENERAL PRINCIPLES OF TREATMENT AND PROGNOSIS

ET runs a benign course and may not require any therapy. Treatment is given only if platelet count is higher than one million.

CHRONIC IDIOPATHIC MYELOFIBROSIS

DEFINITION AND PATHOPHYSIOLOGY

Chronic idiopathic myelofibrosis (IMF), also called agnogenic (of unknown origin) myeloid metaplasia, primary myelofibrosis and myelosclerosis, is a clonal disorder characterised by proliferation of neoplastic stem cells at multiple sites outside the bone marrow (i.e. extramedullary haematopoiesis), especially in the liver and spleen, without an underlying etiology. Secondary myelofibrosis, on the other hand, develops in association with certain well-defined marrow disorders, or it is the result of toxic action of chemical agents or irradiation.

CLINICAL FEATURES

1. Anaemia
2. Massive splenomegaly
3. Hepatomegaly
4. Petechial and other bleeding problems
5. Less common findings are lymphadenopathy, jaundice, ascites, bone pain and hyperuricaemia.

LABORATORY FINDINGS

1. *Mild anaemia* is usual except in cases where features of polycythaemia vera are coexistent.

2. *Leucocytosis* at the time of presentation but later there may be leucopenia.

3. *Thrombocytosis* initially but advanced cases show thrombocytopenia.

4. *Peripheral blood smear* shows bizarre red cell shapes, tear drop poikilocytes, basophilic stippling, nucleated red cells, immature leucocytes (i.e. leucoerythroblastic reaction), basophilia and giant platelet forms.

5. *Bone marrow aspiration* is generally unsuccessful and yields 'dry tap'. Examination of trephine biopsy shows focal areas of hypercellularity and increased reticulin network and variable amount of collagen.

6. *Extramedullary haematopoiesis* can be documented by liver biopsy or splenic aspiration.

GENERAL PRINCIPLES OF TREATMENT AND PROGNOSIS

Chronic idiopathic myelofibrosis does not require any specific therapy. In general, chronic idiopathic myelofibrosis has poorer outcome compared with PV and ET.

ACUTE MYELOID LEUKAEMIA *(p. 340)*

DEFINITION AND PATHOPHYSIOLOGY

Acute myeloid leukaemia (AML) is a heterogeneous disease characterised by infiltration of malignant myeloid cells into the blood, bone marrow and other tissues. AML is mainly a disease of adults (median age 50 years), while children and older individuals may also develop it sometimes.

A few important examples of chromosomal mutations in AML are translocations {t(8;21)(q22q22)} and {t(15;17)(q22;q12)} and inversions {inv(16)(p13;q22)}.

CLASSIFICATION

Currently, two main classification schemes for AML are followed:

FAB CLASSIFICATION According to revised FAB classification system, a leukaemia is acute if the bone marrow consists of more than 30% blasts. Based on morphology and cytochemistry, FAB classification divides AML into 8 subtypes (M0 to M7).

WHO CLASSIFICATION WHO classification for AML differs from revised FAB classification in the following 2 ways:
◈ **Firstly**, it places limited reliance on blast morphology and cytochemistry for making the diagnosis of subtype of AML but instead takes into consideration *clinical, cytogenetic and molecular abnormalities* in different types.
◈ **Secondly**, WHO classification for AML has revised and lowered the cut off percentage of *marrow blasts to 20%* from 30% in the FAB classification for making the diagnosis of AML.

CLINICAL FEATURES

Clinical manifestations of AML are divided into 2 groups:

I.   DUE TO BONE MARROW FAILURE   The features are:
1.   Anaemia
2.   Bleeding manifestations
3.   Infections
4.   Fever

II.   DUE TO ORGAN INFILTRATION   These features are as under:
1.   Pain and tenderness of bones
2.   Lymphadenopathy
3.   Splenomegaly
4.   Hepatomegaly
5.   Leukaemic infiltration of the kidney
6.   Gum hypertrophy
7.   Chloroma or granulocytic sarcoma

8. Meningeal involvement
9. Other organ infiltrations include testicular swelling and mediastinal compression.

LABORATORY FINDINGS

I. BLOOD PICTURE The findings are as under:

1. Anaemia It is generally severe, progressive and normochromic.

2. Thrombocytopenia The platelet count is usually moderately to severely reduced (below 50,000/μl).

3. White blood cells The total WBC count ranges from subnormal-to-markedly elevated values. Typical characteristics of different forms of AML (M0 to M7) are given below:

FAB CLASS	MORPHOLOGY
M0:	Blasts lack definite cytologic and cytochemical features but have myeloid lineage antigens
M1:	Myeloblasts predominate; few if any granules or Auer rods
M2:	Myeloblasts with promyelocytes predominate; Auer rods may be present
M3:	Hypergranular promyelocytes; often with multiple Auer rods per cell
M4:	Mature cells of both myeloid and monocytic series in peripheral blood; myeloid cells resemble M2
M5:	Two subtypes: M5a shows poorly-differentiated monoblasts, M5b shows differentiated promonocytes and monocytes
M6:	Erythroblasts predominate (>50%); myeloblasts and promyelocytes also increased
M7:	Pleomorphic undifferentiated blasts predominate; react with antiplatelet antibodies

II. BONE MARROW EXAMINATION The findings are as follows:

1. Cellularity Typically, the marrow is hypercellular but sometimes a 'blood tap' or 'dry tap' occurs.

2. Leukaemic cells The bone marrow is generally tightly packed with leukaemic blast cells. As per WHO classification, these criteria have been revised and lowered to 20% blasts in the marrow for labelling and treating a case as AML.

3. Erythropoiesis Erythropoietic cells are reduced.

4. Megakaryocytes They are usually reduced or absent.

5. Cytogenetics Two of the most consistent cytogenetic abnormalities in specific FAB groups are as under:
i) M3 cases have $t(15;17)(q22;q12)$.
ii) M4E0 (E for abnormal eosinophils in the bone marrow) cases have $inv(16)(p13q22)$.

III. CYTOCHEMISTRY Some of the commonly employed cytochemical stains, as an aid to classify the type of AML are as:
1. Myeloperoxidase
2. Sudan Black
3. Periodic acid-Schiff (PAS)
4. Non-specific esterase (NSE)
5. Acid phosphatase

IV. BIOCHEMICAL INVESTIGATIONS These are:
1. Serum muramidase elevated
2. Serum uric acid increased

I.   TREATMENT OF ANAEMIA AND HAEMORRHAGE Anaemia and haemorrhage are managed by fresh blood transfusions and platelet concentrates.

II.   TREATMENT AND PROPHYLAXIS OF INFECTION   Neutropenia due to bone marrow replacement by leukaemic blasts and as a result of intensive cytotoxic therapy renders these patients highly susceptible to infection.

III.   CYTOTOXIC DRUG THERAPY   The aims of cytotoxic therapy are firstly to induce remission, and secondly to continue therapy to reduce the hidden leukaemic cell population by repeated courses of therapy.

IV.   BONE MARROW TRANSPLANTATION   Bone marrow (or stem cell) transplantation from suitable allogenic or autologous donor (HLA and mixed lymphocytes culture-matched) is increasingly being used for treating young adults with AML in first remission.

MYELODYSPLASTIC SYNDROMES *(p. 343)*

DEFINITION AND CLASSIFICATION

Myelodysplastic syndromes (MDS) are a heterogeneous group of haematopoietic clonal stem cell disorders having abnormal development of different marrow elements (i.e. dysmyelopoiesis), usually characterised by cytopenias, associated with cellular marrow and ineffective blood cell formation. These conditions are, therefore, also termed as preleukaemic syndromes or dysmyelopoietic syndromes.

FAB CLASSIFICATION OF MDS   FAB classified MDS into the following 5 groups:
1.   *Refractory anaemia (RA)*   Blood blasts <1%, marrow blasts <5%.
2.   *Refractory anaemia with ringed sideroblasts (RARS) (primary acquired sideroblastic anaemia)* Blood blast <1%, marrow blasts <5%; ring sideroblsts ≥15%.
3.   *Refractory anaemia with excess blasts (RAEB)*   Blood blasts 5%, marrow blasts 5-20%.
4.   *Refractory anaemia with excess of blasts in transformation (RAEB-t)* Blood blasts 5%, marrow blasts 21-30%.
5.   *Chronic myelomonocytic leukaemia (CMML)*   Blood blasts, 5%, monocytosis.

WHO CLASSIFICATION OF MDS   WHO classification differs from FAB classification in following ways:
i)   Marrow blast count for making the diagnosis of AML has been revised and brought down to 20%.
ii)   FAB category of RAEB-t (group 4 above) cases have prognosis similar to patients of AML and thus included in AML.
iii)   CMML category of FAB (category 4) has been excluded from WHO classification of MDS since these cases behave like a myeloproliferative disorder and thus CMML has been put in the hybrid category of myelodysplastic/myeloproliferative disorder.
     Thus, the WHO classification of MDS consists of following 8 categories:
1.   Refractory anaemia (RA)
2.   Refractory anaemia with ringed sideroblasts (RARS)
3.   Refractory cytopenia with multilineage dysplasia (RCMD)
4.   RCMD with ringed sideroblasts (RCMD-RS)
5.   Refractory anaemia with excess blasts (RAEB-1)
6.   RAEB-2
7.   Myelodysplastic syndrome unclassified (MDS-U)
8.   MDS with isolated del (5q)

PATHOPHYSIOLOGY

i)   *Primary MDS* is idiopathic but factors implicated in etiology are radiation exposure and benzene carcinogen.

ii) *Secondary (therapy-related) MDS* may occur following earlier anti-cancer treatment, aplastic anaemia treated with immunosuppressive therapy and in Fanconi's anaemia.

iii) *Several cytogenetic abnormalities* are seen in about 50% of MDS which include trisomy, translocations and deletions.

iv) *At molecular level*, mutations are seen in *N-RAS* oncogene and *p53* anti-oncogene.

CLINICAL FEATURES

In general, MDS is found more frequently in older people past 6th decade of life, with slight male preponderance. Clinical features are quite non-specific and MDS may be discovered during routine CBC examination done for some other cause.

LABORATORY FINDINGS

BLOOD FINDINGS There is cytopenia affecting two (bi-) or all the three blood cell lines (pancytopenia):

1. *Anaemia*
2. *TLC:* Usually normal
3. *DLC:* Neutrophils are hyposegmented and hypogranulated.
4. *Platelets:* Thrombocytopenia

BONE MARROW FINDINGS These are as under:

1. *Cellularity:* Normal to hypercellular to hypocellular.
2. *Erythroid series:* Dyserythropoiesis.
3. *Myeloid series:* Hypogranular and hyposegmented myeloid precursor cells.
4. *Megakaryocyte series:* Reduced in number.

LYMPHOID NEOPLASMS: GENERAL *(p. 344)*

HISTORY AND CLASSIFICATION

Conventionally, malignancies of lymphoid cells in blood have been termed as lymphatic leukaemias and those of lymphoid tissues as lymphomas. Discussed earlier, lymphoid leukaemias have been classified on the basis of survival and biologic course, into chronic and acute *(CLL and ALL)*. Similarly, two clinicopathologically distinct groups of lymphomas are distinguished: *Hodgkin's lymphoma* or *Hodgkin's disease (HD)* and *non-Hodgkin's lymphomas (NHL)*.

However, while HD can be identified by the pathognomonic presence of Reed-Sternberg cells, there have been controversies and confusion in classification of other lymphoid cancers (i.e. NHL and lymphoid leukaemias). In order to resolve the issue, over the years several classification schemes have emerged for lymphoid cancers due to following two main reasons:

1. **Biologic course of lymphoma-leukaemia** While some of the lymphoid malignancies initially present as leukaemias (i.e. in the blood and bone marrow), many others present as solid masses in the lymphoid tissues or in various other tissues, especially in the spleen, liver, bone marrow and other tissues.

2. **Technological advances** The additional tools include immuno-phenotyping, cytogenetics and molecular markers for the stage of differentiation of the cell of origin rather than location of the cell alone.

These aspects form the basis of current concept for WHO classification of malignancies of lymphoid cells of blood and lymphoreticular tissues as 'lymphoid neoplasms' as a unified group.

I. HISTORICAL CLASSIFICATIONS These classifications can be traced as under:

Morphologic classification *Rappaport classification (1966)* proposed a clinically relevant morphologic classification.

NHL was further classified according to the degree of differentiation of neoplastic cells into: *well-differentiated, poorly-differentiated,* and *histiocytic (large cells) types* of both nodular and diffuse lymphomas.

Immunologic classifications *Lukes-Collins classification (1974)* and *Kiel classification (1981)* employed immunologic markers for tumour cells, and divided all malignant lymphomas into either B-cell or T-cell origin, and rarely of macrophages.

II. OLD CLINICOPATHOLOGIC CLASSIFICATIONS

FAB classification of lymphoid leukaemia Although old FAB classification for lymphoid leukaemia based on morphology and cytochemistry divided ALL into 3 types (L1 to L3), but it was subsequently revised to include cytogenetic and immunologic features as well.

Working Formulations for Clinical Usage (1982) This classification proposed by a panel of experts from National Cancer Institute of the US incorporates the best features of all previous classification systems, and as the name implies, has strong clinical relevance. Based on the natural history of disease and long-term survival studies, Working Formulations divides all NHLs into following 3 prognostic groups:

◈ *Low-grade NHL:* 5-year survival 50-70%
◈ *Intermediate-grade NHL:* 5-year survival 35-45%
◈ *High-grade NHL:* 5-year survival 25-35%.

REAL classification (1994) International Lymphoma Study Group (Harris et al) proposed another classification called *r*evised *E*uropean-*A*merican classification of *l*ymphoid neoplasms abbreviated as REAL classification. This classification was based on the hypothesis that all forms of lymphoid malignancies (NHLs as well as lymphoblastic leukaemias) represent malignant counterparts of normal population of immune cells (B-cells, T-cells and histiocytes) present in the lymph node and bone marrow.

REAL classification subsequently merged into WHO classification described below.

III. WHO CLASSIFICATION OF LYMPHOID NEOPLASMS (2008) Although this classification has many similarities with REAL classification as regards identification of B and T cell types, WHO classification has more classes. WHO classification takes into account morphology, clinical features, immunophenotyping, and cytogenetic of the tumour cells.

As per current WHO classification, all lymphoid neoplasms (i.e. lymphoid leukaemias and lymphomas) fall into following 5 categories:

I.   Hodgkin's disease
II. B-cell malignancies: Precursor (or immature), and peripheral (or mature)
III. T-cell/NK cell malignancies: Precursor (or immature), and peripheral (or mature)
IV. Histiocytic and dendritic cell neoplasms
V.   Post-transplant lymphoproliferative disorders (PTLDs).

COMMON TO ALL LYMPHOID MALIGNANCIES *(p. 347)*

1.   Overall frequency Five major forms of lymphoid malignancies and their relative frequency are as under:
i)   NHL= 62%, *most common lymphoma*
ii) HD= 8%
iii) Plasma cell disorders = 16%
iv) CLL= 9%, *most common lymphoid leukaemia*
v)   ALL= 4%

2. Incidence of B, T, NK cell malignancies Majority of lymphoid malignancies are of B cell origin (75% of lymphoid leukaemias and 90% of lymphomas) while remaining are T cell malignancies; NK-cell lymphomas-leukaemias are rare.

3.   Diagnosis The diagnosis of lymphoma (both Hodgkin's and non-Hodgkin's) can only be reliably made on examination of lymph node biopsy.

While the initial diagnosis of ALL and CLL can be made on CBC examination, bone marrow biopsy is done for genetic and immunologic studies.

4.   Staging   In both HD and NHL, Ann Arbor staging is done for proper evaluation and planning treatment.

5.   Ancillary studies   CT scan, PET scan and gallium scan are additional imaging modalities which can be used in staging HD and NHL cases.

6.   Immune abnormalities   Since lymphoid neoplasms arise from immune cells of the body, immune derangements pertaining to the cell of origin may accompany these cancers.

HODGKIN'S DISEASE *(p. 348)*

Hodgkin's disease (HD) primarily arises within the lymph nodes and involves the extranodal sites secondarily. This group comprises about 8% of all cases of lymphoid neoplasms. The incidence of the disease has bimodal peaks—one in young adults between the age of 15 and 35 years and the other peak after 5th decade of life.

CLASSIFICATION

Unlike NHL, there is only one universally accepted classification of HD i.e. *Rye classification* adopted since 1966. Rye classification divides HD into the following 4 subtypes:
1.   Lymphocyte-predominance type
2.   Nodular-sclerosis type
3.   Mixed-cellularity type
4.   Lymphocyte-depletion type.

However, the WHO classification of lymphoid neoplasms divides HD into 2 main groups:
I.   Nodular lymphocyte-predominant HD (a new type).
II.   Classic HD (includes all the 4 above subtypes in the Rye classification).

Central to the diagnosis of HD is the essential identification of *Reed-Sternberg cell* though this is not the sole criteria (see below).

REED-STERNBERG CELL

The diagnosis of Hodgkin's disease rests on identification of RS cells, though uncommonly similar cells can occur in infectious mononucleosis and other forms of lymphomas.

1.   Classic RS cell   This is a large cell which has characteristically a bilobed nucleus appearing as mirror image of each other but occasionally the nucleus may be multilobed. Each lobe of the nucleus contains a prominent, eosinophilic, inclusion-like nucleolus with a clear halo around it, giving an owl-eye appearance. The cytoplasm of cell is abundant and amphophilic.

2.   Lacunar type RS cell   It is smaller and in addition to above features has a pericellular space or lacuna in which it lies, which is due to artefactual shrinkage of the cell cytoplasm. It is characteristically found in nodular sclerosis variety of HD.

3.   Polyploid type (or popcorn or lymphocytic-histiocytic i.e. L and H) RS cells   These are seen in lymphocyte predominance type of HD. This type of RS cell is larger with lobulated nucleus in the shape of popcorn.

4.   Pleomorphic RS cells   These are a feature of lymphocyte depletion type. These cells have pleomorphic and atypical nuclei.

Immunophenotyping of RS cells reveals monoclonal lymphoid cell origin of RS cell from B-cells of the germinal centre in most subtypes of Hodgkin's disease. RS cells in all types of Hodgkin's diseases, except in lymphocyte predominance type, express immunoreactivity for CD15 and CD30. RS cells in lymphocyte predominance type, however, are negative for both CD15 and CD30, but positive for CD20.

RS cells are invariably accompanied by variable number of *atypical Hodgkin cells* which are believed to be precursor RS cells.

G/A Initially, the lymph nodes are discrete and separate from one another but later the lymph nodes form a large matted mass due to infiltration into the surrounding connective tissue. The sectioned surface of the involved lymph nodes or extranodal organ involved appears grey-white and fishflesh-like.

M/E The findings are as under:

I. CLASSIC HD As per WHO classification, classic group of HD includes 4 types of HD of older Rye classification:

1. Lymphocyte-predominance type The lymphocyte-predominance type of HD is characterised by proliferation of small lymphocytes admixed with a varying number of histiocytes forming nodular or diffuse pattern.

For making the diagnosis, definite demonstration of RS cells is essential which are few in number, requiring a thorough search. In addition to typical RS cells, *polyploid variant* having polyploid, and twisted nucleus (popcorn-like) may be found in some cases.

2. Nodular-sclerosis type It is characterised by two essential features:

i) *Bands of collagen:* Variable amount of fibrous tissue is characteristically present in the involved lymph nodes.

ii) *Lacunar type RS cells:* Characteristic lacunar type of RS cells with distinctive pericellular halo are present.

3. Mixed-cellularity type This form of HD generally replaces the entire affected lymph nodes by heterogeneous mixture of various types of apparently normal cells. These include proliferating lymphocytes, histiocytes, eosinophils, neutrophils and plasma cells. Typical RS cells are frequent.

4. Lymphocyte-depletion type In this type of HD, the lymph node is depleted of lymphocytes. There are two variants of lymphocyte-depletion HD:

i) *Diffuse fibrotic variant* is hypocellular and the entire lymph node is replaced by diffuse fibrosis and infiltration by atypical histiocytes (Hodgkin cells), and numerous typical and atypical (pleomorphic) RS cells.

ii) *Reticular variant* is much more cellular and consists of large number of atypical pleomorphic histiocytes.

II. NODULAR LYMPHOCYTE-PREDOMINANT HD This is a newly described entity:

i) These cases of HD have a nodular growth pattern (similar to nodular sclerosis type).

ii) Like lymphocyte-predominant pattern of classic type, there is predominance of small lymphocytes with sparse number of RS cells.

iii) These cases of HD are CD45 positive, epithelial membrane antigen (EMA) positive but negative for the usual markers for RS cells (CD15 and CD30 negative).

CLINICAL FEATURES

Hodgkin's disease is particularly frequent among young and middle-aged adults. All histologic subtypes of HD, except the nodular sclerosis variety, are more common in males.

1. Most commonly, patients present with painless, movable and firm *lymphadenopathy.*

2. Approximately half the patients develop *splenomegaly* during the course of the disease. *Liver enlargement* too may occur.

3. *Constitutional symptoms* (type B symptoms) are present in 25-40% of patients.

OTHER LABORATORY FINDINGS

Haematologic abnormalities

1. Moderate, normocytic and normochromic *anaemia.*

2. *Serum iron and TIBC* are low.

3. *Marrow infiltration* by the disease.

4. *Routine blood counts* reveal moderate leukaemoid reaction.

5 *Platelet count* is normal or increased.

6. *ESR* is invariably elevated.

Immunologic abnormalities
1. There is progressive fall in immunocompetent T-cells with *defective cellular immunity.*
2. *Humoral antibody production* is normal.

STAGING

Ann Arbor staging classification takes into account both clinical and pathologic stage of the disease.

The suffix *A* or *B* are added to the above stages depending upon whether the three constitutional symptoms (fever, night sweats and unexplained weight loss exceeding 10% of normal) are absent (A) or present (B). The suffix *E* or *S* are used for extranodal involvement and splenomegaly respectively.

PROGNOSIS

With use of aggressive radiotherapy and chemotherapy, the outlook for Hodgkin's disease has improved significantly.

With appropriate treatment, the overall 5 years survival rate for *stage I and II A* is as high as about 100%, while the advanced stage of the disease may have upto 50% 5-year survival rate.

◈ Patients with *lymphocyte-predominance type* of HD tend to have localised form of the disease and have excellent prognosis.

◈ *Nodular sclerosis* variety too has very good prognosis.

◈ *Mixed cellularity type* occupies intermediate clinical position between the lymphocyte predominance and the lymphocyte-depletion type.

◈ *Lymphocyte-depletion type* is usually disseminated at the time of diagnosis. These patients usually have the most aggressive form of the disease.

NON-HODGKIN'S LYMPHOMAS-LEUKAEMIAS *(p. 352)*

Non-Hodgkin's lymphomas (NHLs) and lymphoid leukaemias comprise a large group of heterogeneous of neoplasms of lymphoid tissues and blood. NHLs have several types and are far more common (62%) than HD (8%).

PRECURSOR (IMMATURE) B- AND T-CELL LEUKAEMIA/LYMPHOMA
(*SYNONYM:* ACUTE LYMPHOBLASTIC LEUKAEMIA) *(p. 353)*

Lymphoid malignancy originating from precursor series of B or T cell (i.e. pre-B and pre-T) is the most common form of cancer of children under 4 years of age, together constituting 4% of all lymphoid malignancies. Pre-B cell ALL constitutes 90% cases while pre-T cell lymphoid malignancies comprise the remaining 10%.

CLINICAL FEATURES

PRECURSOR B-CELL LYMPHOBLASTIC LEUKAEMIA/LYMPHOMA Most often, it presents as ALL in children; rarely presentation may be in the form of lymphoma in children or adults and it rapidly transforms into leukaemia.

PRECURSOR T-CELL LYMPHOBLASTIC LEUKAEMIA/LYMPHOMA As the name implies, these cases may present as ALL or as lymphoma. Since the precursor T-cells differentiate in the thymus, this tumour often presents as mediastinal mass and pleural effusion and progresses rapidly to develop leukaemia in the blood and bone marrow.

Precursor T-cell lymphoma-leukaemia is, however, more aggressive than its B-cell counterpart.

MORPHOLOGIC FEATURES

Precursor B and T-cell ALL/lymphoma are indistinguishable on routine morphology. The diagnosis is made by following investigations:

1. Blood examination Peripheral blood generally shows anaemia and thrombocytopenia, and may show leucopenia-to-normal TLC to leucocytosis. DLC shows large number of circulating lymphoblasts (generally in excess of 20%) having round to convoluted nuclei, high nucleo-cytoplasmic ratio and absence of cytoplasmic granularity.

2. Bone marrow examination Marrow examination shows 20-95% malignant undifferentiated cells of precursor B or T cell origin. Mega-karyocytes are usually reduced or absent.

3. Cytochemistry
i) Periodic acid-Schiff (PAS): Positive in immature lymphoid cells in ALL.
ii) Acid phosphatase: Focal positivity in leukaemic blasts in ALL.
iii) Myeloperoxidase: Negative in immature cells in ALL.
iv) Sudan Black: Negative in immature cells in ALL.
v) Non-specific esterase (NSE): Negative in ALL.

Immunophenotyping TdT (terminal deoxynucleotidyl transferase) is expressed by the nuclei of both pre-B and pre-T stages of differentiation of lymphoid cells. Specific diagnosis is eastablished by following immunopheno-typing:
Pre-B-cell type: Typically positive for pan-B cell markers CD19, CD10, CD9a.
Pre-T-cell type: Typically positive for CD1, CD2, CD3, CD5, CD7.

PRINCIPLES OF TREATMENT AND PROGNOSIS

Treatment plan for children with pre-B or pre-T cell ALL is intensive remission induction with combination therapy. Patients presenting with pre-B or pre-T cell lymphoma are treated as a case of ALL.

Prognosis and disease-free survival of children with both pre-B cell and pre-T cell ALL is better than in adults.

PERIPHERAL(MATURE) B-CELL MALIGNANCIES *(p. 355)*

Peripheral or mature B-cell cancers are the most common lymphoid malignancies.

CHRONIC LYMPHOCYTIC LEUKAEMIA/ SMALL LYMPHOCYTIC LYMPHOMA (B-CELL CLL/SLL)

As the name implies, this subtype may present as leukaemia or lymphoma constituting 9% of all lymphoid neoplasms. As lymphoid leukaemia (CLL), this is the most common form while as SLL it constitutes 7% of all NHLs. B-cell CLL/SLL occurs more commonly in middle and older age groups (over 50 years of age) with a male preponderance (male-female ratio 2:1).

CLINICAL FEATURES

1. Features of anaemia
2. Enlargement of superficial lymph nodes
3. Splenomegaly and hepatomegaly are usual.
4. Haemorrhagic manifestations
5. Susceptibility to infections

MORPHOLOGIC FEATURES

I. BLOOD PICTURE The findings are as under:

1. Anaemia Anaemia is usually mild to moderate and normocytic normochromic in type.

2. White blood cells Typically, there is marked leucocytosis but less than that seen in CML (50,000-200,000/µl). Usually, more than 90% of leucocytes are mature small lymphocytes. Smudge or basket cells (degenerated forms) are present.

3. Platelets The platelet count is normal or moderately reduced.

II. BONE MARROW EXAMINATION Main findings are:

1. Increased lymphocyte count (25-95%). .
2. Reduced myeloid precursors.
3. Reduced erythroid precursors.

III. LYMPH NODE BIOPSY Cases with lymphadenopathy at presentation show replacement of the lymph node by diffuse proliferation of well-differentiated, mature, small and uniform lymphocytes without any cytologic atypia or significant mitoses.

IV. OTHER INVESTIGATIONS These are:

1. Positive for B-cell markers
2. Serum immunoglobulin levels are generally reduced.
3. Coombs' test is positive in 20% cases.

TREATMENT PLAN AND PROGNOSIS

Treatment is palliative and symptomatic. Prognosis of CLL/SLL is generally better than CML since *blastic transformation seldom occurs*. Generally, the course is indolent. However, some cases of SLL may transform into more aggressive diffuse large B-cell lymphoma.

FOLLICULAR LYMPHOMA

Follicular lymphomas occur in older individuals, most frequently presenting with painless peripheral lymphadenopathy.

MORPHOLOGIC FEATURES Following features are seen:

Lymph node biopsy As the name suggests, follicular lymphoma is characterised by follicular or nodular pattern of growth. The nuclei of tumour cells may vary from predominantly small cleaved (or indented) to predominantly large cleaved variety.

Blood and bone marrow Peripheral blood involvement as occurs in SLL is uncommon in this variety. Infiltration in the bone marrow is typically paratrabecular.

DIFFUSE LARGE B-CELL LYMPHOMA (DLBCL)

Diffuse large B-cell lymphoma (DLBCL), earlier termed as diffuse poorly-differentiated lymphocytic lymphoma is the most common comprising about 31% of all NHLs. It occurs in older patients with mean age of 60 years.

A few subtypes of diffuse large B-cell lymphoma are described with distinct clinicopathologic settings:

i) *Epstein-Barr virus (EBV)* infection has been etiologically implicated in diffuse large B-cell lymphoma in *immunosuppressed patients* of AIDS and organ transplant cases.

ii) *Human herpes virus type 8 (HHV-8)* infection along with presence of immunosuppression is associated with a subtype of diffuse large B-cell lymphoma presenting with effusion, termed *primary effusion lymphoma.*

iii) *Mediastinal large B-cell lymphoma* is diagnosed in patients with prominent involvement of mediastinum, occurs in young females and frequently spreads to CNS and abdominal viscera.

MORPHOLOGIC FEATURES DLBCL is the diffuse counterpart of follicular large cleaved cell lymphoma. In general, DLBCL is aggressive tumour and disseminates widely.

BURKITT'S LYMPHOMA/LEUKAEMIA

Burkitt's lymphoma/leukaemia is an uncommon tumour in adults but comprises about 30% of childhood NHLs. Burkitt's leukaemia corresponds to L3 ALL of FAB grouping and is uncommon. Three subgroups of Burkitt's lymphoma are recognised: *African endemic, sporadic and immuno-deficiency-associated.*

M/E All three types of Burkitt's lymphoma are similar. Tumour cells are intermediate in size, non-cleaved, and homogeneous in size and shape. The nuclei are round to oval and contain 2-5 nucleoli. The cytoplasm is basophilic and contains lipid vacuolation. The tumour cells have a very high mitotic rate, and therefore high cell death. This feature accounts for presence of numerous macrophages in the background of this tumour containing phago-cytosed tumour debris giving it a 'starry sky' appearance.

Burkitt's lymphoma is a high-grade tumour and is a very rapidly progressive human tumour.

EXTRANODAL MARGINAL ZONE B-CELL LYMPHOMA OF MALT TYPE (*SYNONYM: MALTOMA*)

MALT refers to mucosa-associated lymphoid tissue. This type comprises about 8% of all NHLs.

i)   *Etiologic association with H. pylori infection:* Most frequent is gastric lymphoma of MALT type with its characteristic etiologic association with *H. pylori*.

ii)   *Occurrence at extranodal sites:* Besides stomach, other extranodal sites for this subtype of NHL are intestine, orbit, lung, thyroid, salivary glands and CNS.

MORPHOLOGIC FEATURES It is characterised by diffuse infiltration by monoclonal small B lymphocytes which are negative for CD5.

MALT lymphoma has a good prognosis.

MANTLE CELL LYMPHOMA

It was earlier included in SLL but has been identified as a separate subtype due to characteristic chromosomal translocation, t(11;14) and overexpression of *BCL-1*. Patients of mantle cell lymphoma are generally older males. The disease involves bone marrow, spleen, liver and bowel.

HAIRY CELL LEUKAEMIA (HCL)

Hairy cell leukaemia (HCL) is an unusual and uncommon form of B-cell malignancy characterised by presence of hairy cells in the blood and bone marrow and splenomegaly. It occurs in the older males. HCL is characterised clinically by the manifestations due to infiltration of reticuloendothelial organs (bone marrow, liver and spleen).

MORPHOLOGIC FEATURES Laboratory diagnosis is made by the presence of pancytopenia due to marrow failure and splenic sequestration, and identification of characteristic hairy cells in the blood and bone marrow. These leukaemic 'hairy cells' have characteristically positive cytochemical staining for *tartrate-resistant acid phosphatase (TRAP)*.

PERIPHERAL(MATURE) T-CELL MALIGNANCIES (*p. 359*)

Peripheral or mature T-cell lymphoid malignancies are relatively less common compared to mature B cell cancers.

MYCOSIS FUNGOIDES/SÉZARY SYNDROME

Mycosis fungoides is a slowly evolving cutaneous T-cell lymphoma occurring in middle-aged adult males.

MORPHOLOGICAL FEATURES The condition is often preceded by eczema or dermatitis for several years (*premycotic stage*). This is followed by infiltration by CD4+T-cells in the epidermis and dermis as a plaque (*plaque stage*) and eventually as *tumour stage*. The disease may spread to viscera and to peripheral blood as a leukaemia characterised by Sézary cells having cerebriform nuclei termed as Sézary syndrome.

ADULT T-CELL LYMPHOMA/LEUKAEMIA (ATLL)

This is an uncommon T-cell malignancy but has gained much prominence due to association with retrovirus, human T-cell lymphotropic virus-I (HTLV-I).

ALCL is the T-cell counterpart of diffuse large B-cell lymphoma (DLBCL) and was previously included under malignant histiocytosis or diagnosed as anaplastic carcinoma. ALCL is defined by:
i)   documentation of t(2;5);
ii)   overexpression of ALK (anaplastic lymphoma kinase) protein.

LYMPH NODE METASTATIC TUMOURS (p. 360)

1.   Benign reactive hyperplasia, as already discussed is due to immunologic reaction by the lymph node in response to tumour-associated antigens. It may be expressed as sinus histiocytosis, follicular hyperplasia, plasmacytosis and occasionally may show non-caseating granulomas.

2.   Metastatic deposits in regional lymph nodes occur most commonly from carcinomas and malignant melanoma. Sarcomas often disseminate via haematogenous route but uncommonly may metastasise to the regional lymph nodes. The morphologic features of primary malignant tumour are recapitulated in metastatic tumour in lymph nodes.

PLASMA CELL DISORDERS (p. 360)

The plasma cell disorders are characterised by abnormal proliferation of immunoglobulin-producing cells and result in accumulation of monoclonal immunoglobulin in serum and urine. The group as a whole is known by various synonyms such as *plasma cell dyscrasias, paraproteinaemias, dysproteinaemias and monoclonal gammopathies*. The group comprises the following six disease entities:
1.   Multiple myeloma
2.   Localised plasmacytoma
3.   Lymphoplasmacytic lymphoma (discussed above)
4.   Waldenström's macroglobulinaemia
5.   Heavy chain disease
6.   Primary amyloidosis
7.   Monoclonal gammopathy of undetermined significance (MGUS).
      The feature common to all plasma cell disorders is the neoplastic proliferation of cells derived from B-lymphocyte lineage.

MULTIPLE MYELOMA

Multiple myeloma is a multifocal malignant proliferation of plasma cells derived from a single clone of cells (i.e. monoclonal). The terms multiple myeloma is used interchangeably with myeloma. Multiple myeloma primarily affects the elderly (peak incidence in 5th-6th decades) and increases in incidence with age. It is rare under the age of 40.

ETIOLOGY AND PATHOGENESIS

Myeloma is a monoclonal proliferation of B-cells. The etiology of myeloma remains unknown. However, following factors and abnormalities have been implicated:

1.   Radiation exposure Large dose exposure to radiation with a long latent period has been seen in myeloma.

2.   Epidemiologic factors Myeloma has higher incidence in blacks. Occupational exposure to petroleum products has been associated with higher incidence.

3.   Karyotypic abnormalities Several chromosomal alterations have been observed in cases of myeloma:

4.   Oncogenes-antioncogenes These are:
i) Overexpression of *MYC* and *RAS* growth promoting oncogenes in some cases.
ii) Mutation in *p53* and *RB* growth-suppressing antioncogene in some cases.

Based on above, **molecular pathogenesis** of multiple myeloma and its major manifestations can be summed up as under:

1. Cell-surface *adhesion molecules* bind myeloma cells to bone marrow stromal cells and extracellular matrix proteins.

2. This binding triggers *adhesion-mediated signaling* and mediates *production of several cytokines* by fibroblasts and macrophages of the marrow.

3. Adhesion-mediated signaling affects the cell cycle via cyclin-D and p21 causing abnormal production of *myeloma (M) proteins*.

4. *IL-6 cytokine* plays a central role in cytokine-mediated signaling and causes proliferation as well as cell survival of tumour cells via its antiapoptotic effects on tumour cells.

5. Certain cytokines produced by myeloma cells bring about bony destruction by acting as *osteoclast-activating factor (OAF)*.

MORPHOLOGIC FEATURES

The pathologic findings are described below under two headings—*osseous (bone marrow) lesions* and *extraosseous lesions*.

A. OSSEOUS (BONE MARROW) LESIONS In more than 95% of cases, multiple myeloma begins in the bone marrow. In majority of cases, the disease involves multiple bones. By the time the diagnosis is made, most of the bone marrow is involved. Most commonly affected bones are those with red marrow i.e. skull, spine, ribs and pelvis, but later long bones of the limbs are also involved.

G/A The normal bone marrow is replaced by soft, gelatinous, reddish-grey tumours.

M/E The diagnosis of multiple myeloma can be usually established by examining bone marrow aspiration from an area of bony rarefaction.

i) Cellularity There is usually hypercellularity of the bone marrow.

ii) Myeloma cells Myeloma cells constitute $\geq$10% of the marrow cellularity. These cells may form clumps or sheets, or may be scattered among the normal haematopoietic cells. Myeloma cells may vary in size from small, differentiated cells resembling normal plasma cells to large, immature and undifferentiated cells. Binucleate and multinucleate cells are sometimes present. The nucleus of myeloma cell is commonly eccentric similar to plasma cells but usually lacks the cart-wheel chromatin pattern seen in classical plasma cells. Nucleoli are frequently present. The cytoplasm of these cells is abundant and basophilic with perinuclear halo, vacuolisation and contains Russell bodies consisting of hyaline globules composed of synthesised immunoglobulin.

In addition to neoplastic proliferation of plasma cells in multiple myeloma, *reactive plasmacytosis* in the bone marrow can occur in some other disorders; these include: aplastic anaemia, rheumatoid arthritis, SLE, cirrhosis of liver, metastatic cancer and chronic inflammation and infections such as tuberculosis. However, in all these conditions the plasma cells are mature and they do not exceed 10% of the total marrow cells.

B. EXTRAOSSEOUS LESIONS Late in the course of disease, lesions at several extraosseous sites become evident.

1. Blood Approximately 50% of patients with multiple myeloma have a few atypical plasma cells in the blood. Other changes in the blood in myeloma are the presence of anaemia (usually normocytic normochromic type), marked red cell rouleaux formation and an elevated ESR.

2. Myeloma kidney Renal involvement in myeloma called myeloma nephrosis occurs in many cases.

3. Myeloma neuropathy Infiltration of the nerve trunk roots by tumour cells produces nonspecific polyneuropathy.

4. Systemic amyloidosis Systemic primary generalised amyloidosis (AL amyloid) may occur in 10% cases of multiple myeloma.

5. Liver, spleen involvement Organomegaly is seen in some cases.

1. *Bone pain* is the most common symptom.
2. *Susceptibility to infections*
3. *Renal failure*
4. *Anaemia* occurs in about 80% of patients
5. *Bleeding tendencies*
6. *Hyperviscosity syndrome* may produce headache, fatigue, visual disturbances and haemorrhages.
7. *Neurologic symptoms.*
8. *Biochemical abnormalities.* These include the following:
i) hypercalcaemia due to destruction of bone;
ii) hyperuricaemia from necrosis of tumour mass and from uraemia related to renal failure; and
iii) increased β-2 microglobulins and other globulins in urine and serum.
9. *POEMS syndrome* is seen in about 1% cases of myeloma and includes simultaneous manifestations of *p*olyneuropathy, *o*rganomegaly, *e*ndocrinopathy, *m*ultiple myeloma and *s*kin changes.

DIAGNOSIS

The diagnosis of myeloma is made by classic *triad* of features:
1. *Marrow plasmacytosis* of more than 10%
2. *Radiologic evidence* of *lytic bony lesions*
3. *Demonstration of serum and/or urine M component.*

There is rise in the total serum protein concentration due to *paraproteinaemia* but normal serum immunoglobulins (IgG, IgA and IgM) and albumin are depressed. Paraproteins are abnormal immunoglobulins or their parts circulating in plasma and excreted in urine. About two-third cases of myeloma excrete Bence Jones (light chain) proteins in the urine, consisting of either kappa (κ) or lambda (λ) light chains, along with presence of Bence Jones paraproteins in the serum. On serum electrophoresis, the paraprotein usually appears as a single narrow homogeneous *M-band* component, most commonly in the region of γ-globulin. Most frequent paraprotein is *IgG* seen in about 50% cases of myeloma, *IgA* in 25%, and IgD in 1%, while about 20% patients have only light chains in serum and urine (*light chain myeloma*).

TREATMENT PLAN AND PROGNOSIS

Treatment of multiple myeloma consists of systemic chemotherapy in the form of alkylating agents and symptomatic supportive care. The terminal phase is marked by the development of pancytopenia, severe anaemia and sepsis.

LOCALISED PLASMACYTOMA

Two variants of myeloma which do not fulfil the criteria of classical triad are the localised form of *solitary bone plasmacytoma* and *extramedullary plasmacytoma*. Both these are associated with M component in about a third of cases and occur in young individuals. Solitary bone plasmacytoma is a lytic bony lesion without marrow plasmacytosis.

WALDENSTRÖM'S MACROGLOBULINAEMIA

Waldenström's macroglobulinaemia is an uncommon malignant proliferation of monoclonal B lymphocytes which secrete IgM paraproteins called macroglobulins as they have high molecular weight. The condition is more common in men over 50 years of age and behaves clinically like a slowly progressive lymphoma.

MORPHOLOGIC FEATURES   Pathologically, the disease can be regarded as the hybrid between myeloma and small lymphocytic lymphoma.

CLINICAL FEATURES These are:
1. Hyperviscosity syndrome
2. Moderate organomegaly
3. Anaemia
4. Bleeding tendencies

HEAVY CHAIN DISEASES

Heavy chain diseases are rare malignant proliferations of B-cells accompanied by monoclonal excess of one of the heavy chains. Depending upon the type of excessive heavy chain, three types—γ, α and μ, of heavy chain diseases are distinguished:

MONOCLONAL GAMMOPATHY OF UNDETERMINED SIGNIFICANCE (MGUS)

Due to longevity, monoclonal gammopathy of undetermined significance (MGUS) is now increasingly diagnosed in asymptomatic healthy ageing population—1% at 50 years of age and in 10% individuals older than 75 years. This makes it the most common form of plasma cell dyscrasia. The defining criteria for MGUS are as under:
i) M-protein in serum <3 gm/dl
ii) Marrow plasmacytosis <10%
iii) No evidence of other B-cell proliferative disorder
iv) Absence of myeloma-related end-organ tissue damage (i.e. absence of lytic bone lesions, high calcium level, anaemia).

HISTIOCYTIC NEOPLASMS: LANGERHANS CELL HISTIOCYTOSIS (p. 365)

The term histiocytosis is used for a group of proliferations of dendritic cells, Langerhans cells or macrophages and includes both benign and malignant examples. Monoclonal proliferation of Langerhans cells are grouped under Langerhans cell histiocytosis (LCH) and are somewhat more common. LCH includes three clinicopathologically related conditions ocurring in children.

EOSINOPHILIC GRANULOMA

Unifocal eosinophilic granuloma is more common (60%) than the multifocal variety which is often a component of Hand-Schüller-Christian disease. Most of the patients are children and young adults, predominantly males. The condition commonly presents as a solitary osteolytic lesion in the femur, skull, vertebrae, ribs and pelvis. The diagnosis requires biopsy of the lytic bone lesion.

M/E The lesion consists largely of closely-packed aggregates of macrophages admixed with variable number of eosinophils. The macrophages contain droplets of fat or a few granules of brown pigment indicative of phagocytic activity. A few multinucleate macrophages may also be seen. The cytoplasm of these macrophages may contain rod-shaped inclusions called *histiocytosis-X bodies* or Birbeck granules, best seen by electron microscopy. Eosinophilic granuloma is clinically a benign disorder.

HAND-SCHÜLLER-CHRISTIAN DISEASE

A triad of features consisting of *multifocal bony defects, diabetes insipidus* and *exophthalmos* is termed Hand-Schüller-Christian disease. The disease develops in children under 5 years of age.

M/E The lesions are indistinguishable from those of unifocal eosinophilic granuloma.

Though the condition is benign, it is more disabling than the unifocal eosinophilic granuloma.

LETTERER-SIWE DISEASE

Letterer-Siwe disease is an acute disseminated form of LCH occurring in infants and children under 2 years of age. The disease is characterised by hepatosplenomegaly, lymphadenopathy, thrombocytopenia, anaemia and leucopenia.

M/E The involved organs contain aggregates of macrophages which are pleomorphic and show nuclear atypia. The cytoplasm of these cells contains vacuoles and rod-shaped *histiocytosis-X bodies*.

The condition is currently regarded as an unusual form of malignant lymphoma.

SPLEEN (p. 366)

NORMAL STRUCTURE

The spleen is the largest lymphoid organ of the body. Under normal conditions, the average weight of the spleen is about 150 gm in the adult. From the capsule extend connective tissue *trabeculae* into the pulp of the organ and serve as supportive network.

G/A The spleen consists of homogeneous, soft, dark red mass called the *red pulp* and long oval grey-white nodules called the *white pulp (malpighian bodies)*.

M/E The red pulp consists of a network of thin-walled venous sinuses and adjacent blood spaces. The blood spaces contain blood cells, lymphocytes and macrophages and appear to be arranged in cords called *splenic cords* or *cords of Billroth*. The white pulp is made up of lymphocytes surrounding an eccentrically placed arteriole.

SPLENIC ENLARGEMENT AND EFFECTS ON FUNCTION (p. 367)

SPLENOMEGALY

Enlargement of the spleen termed splenomegaly, occurs in a wide variety of disorders which increase the cellularity and vascularity of the organ. Many of the causes are exaggerated forms of normal splenic function. Splenic enlargement may occur as a result of one of the following pathophysiologic mechanisms:

I.   Infections
II. Disordered immunoregulation
III. Altered splenic blood flow
IV. Lymphohaematogenous malignancies
V.   Diseases with abnormal erythrocytes
VI. Storage diseases
VII. Miscellaneous causes.

The **degree of splenomegaly** varies with the disease entity:

◈ *Mild enlargement (upto 5 cm)* occurs in CVC of spleen in CHF, acute malaria, typhoid fever, bacterial endocarditis, SLE, rheumatoid arthritis and thalassaemia minor.

◈ *Moderate enlargement (upto umbilicus)* occurs in hepatitis, cirrhosis, lymphomas, infectious mononucleosis, haemolytic anaemia, splenic abscesses and amyloidosis.

◈ *Massive enlargement (below umbilicus)* occurs in CML, myeloid metaplasia with myelofibrosis, storage diseases, thalassaemia major, chronic malaria, leishmaniasis and portal vein obstruction.

G/A An enlarged spleen is heavy and firm. The capsule is tense and thickened. The sectioned surface of the organ is firm with prominent trabeculae.

M/E There is dilatation of sinusoids with prominence of splenic cords. The white pulp is atrophic while the trabeculae are thickened. Long-standing congestion may produce haemorrhages and *Gamna-Gandy bodies* resulting in *fibrocongestive splenomegaly*, also called *Banti's spleen*.

HYPERSPLENISM

The term hypersplenism is used for conditions which cause excessive removal of erythrocytes, granulocytes or platelets from the circulation. The mechanism for excessive removal could be due to increased sequestration of cells in the spleen by altered splenic blood flow or by production of antibodies against respective blood cells. The criteria for hypersplenism are as under:

1. Splenomegaly.
2. Splenic destruction of one or more of the cell types in the peripheral blood causing anaemia, leucopenia, thrombocytopenia, or pancytopenia.
3. Bone marrow cellularity is normal or hyperplastic.
4. Splenectomy is followed by improvement in the severity of blood cytopenia.

EFFECTS OF SPLENECTOMY

The blood changes following splenectomy are as under:

1. Red cells There is appearance of target cells in the blood film. Howell-Jolly bodies are present in the red cells as they are no longer cleared by the spleen.

2. White cells There is leucocytosis reaching its peak in 1-2 days after splenectomy.

3. Platelets Within hours after splenectomy, there is rise in platelet count upto 3-4 times normal.

SPLENIC RUPTURE

The most common cause of splenic rupture or laceration is blunt trauma. The trauma may be direct or indirect. Non-traumatic or spontaneous rupture occurs in an enlarged spleen but almost never in a normal spleen. In acute infections, the spleen can enlarge rapidly to 2 to 3 times its normal size causing acute splenic enlargement termed *acute splenic tumour*. Some of the other common causes of spontaneous splenic rupture are splenomegaly due to chronic malaria, infectious mononucleosis, typhoid fever, splenic abscess, thalassaemia and leukaemias.

TUMOURS

◆ **Primary tumours** of the spleen are extremely rare. The only notable benign tumours are haemangiomas and lymphangioma, while examples of primary malignant neoplasms of haematopoietic system i.e. Hodgkin's disease and non-Hodgkin's lymphomas.

◆ **Secondary tumours** occur late in the course of disease and represent haematogenous dissemination of the malignant tumour. Splenic metastases appear as multiple nodules.

THYMUS *(p. 368)*

NORMAL STRUCTURE

The thymus gland is a complex lymphoreticular organ lying buried within the mediastinum. At birth, the gland weighs 10-35 gm and grows in size upto puberty, following which there is progressive involution in the elderly. In the adult, thymus weighs 5-10 gm.

◆ **Epithelial cells** are similar throughout the thymus gland. *Hassall's corpuscles* are distinctive structures within the medulla.

◆ **Thymocytes** are predominantly present in the cortex. These cells include immature T lymphocytes in the cortex and mature T lymphocytes in the medulla.

The main **function** of the thymus is in the cell-mediated immunity by T-cells and by secretion of thymic hormones such as *thymopoietin* and *thymosin-α1*.

STRUCTURAL AND FUNCTIONAL CHANGES IN THYMUS *(p. 369)*

THYMIC HYPOPLASIA AND AGENESIS

Thymic hypoplasia and agenesis are acquired and congenital disorders respectively in which the gland is either unusually small or absent.

Enlargement of the thymus or failure to involute produces thymic hyperplasia. Hyperplasia is usually associated with appearance of lymphoid follicles in the medulla of the thymus and is called *thymic follicular hyperplasia*. Most common cause of follicular hyperplasia of the thymus is myasthenia gravis.

THYMOMA

Most common primary tumour present in the anterosuperior mediastinum is thymoma. Although thymus is a lymphoepithelial organ, the term thymoma is used for the tumour of epithelial origin.

G/A The tumour is spherical, measuring 5-10 cm in diameter with an average weight of 150 gm.

M/E Thymoma may be of following types:

Benign thymoma is more common. It consists of epithelial cells which are similar to the epithelial cells in the medulla of thymus and hence also called as medullary thymoma.

Malignant thymoma is less common and is further of 2 types:
Type 1 is cytologically benign looking but aggressive.
Type 2 is also called thymic carcinoma and has cytologic features of cancer.

SELF ASSESSMENT

1. The following myeloid cells partake in mitosis <u>except</u>:
   A. Myelocytes
   B. Metamyelocytes
   C. Promyelocytes
   D. Myeloblast
2. Basophils are increased in:
   A. Bronchial asthma
   B. CML
   C. Angioneurotic oedema
   D. Corticosteroid therapy
3. Heterophile antibody used to detect EBV infection in infectious mononucleosis is:
   A. IgA
   B. IgD
   C. IgG
   D. IgM
4. Atypical lymphoid cells (mononucleosis cells) in infectious mononucleosis are:
   A. Monocytes
   B. CD8 + T lymphocytes
   C. Killer T cells
   D. B-lymphocytes
5. Leucocyte alkaline phosphatase (LAP) scores are elevated in:
   A. AML
   B. CML
   C. Myeloid metaplasia
   D. Myeloid leukaemoid reaction
6. Radiation exposure is related to the following types of leukaemias <u>except</u>:
   A. AML
   B. CML
   C. ALL
   D. CLL
7. Gum hypertrophy is a feature of the following FAB type of AML:
   A. FAB type M1
   B. FAB type M2
   C. FAB type M3
   D. FAB type M4
8. Which of the following is not a type of paracortical lymphoid hyperplasia:
   A. Castleman's disease
   B. Angioimmunoblastic lymphadenopathy
   C. Dermatopathic lymphadenopathy
   D. Dilantin lymphadenopathy
9. Auer rods are derived from:
   A. RNA
   B. DNA
   C. Primary granules
   D. Secondary granules

10. **What is _not_ true about Pelger-Huet anomaly:**
    A. Autosomal dominant
    B. May be acquired
    C. Is characterised by bilobed neutrophils
    D. Causes severe impairment of neutrophil function

11. **Philadelphia chromosome is characterised by:**
    A. t(8;14)   B. t(9;22)
    C. t(22;9)   D. t(14;8)

12. **Tumours causing secondary polycythaemia include all _except_:**
    A. Renal cell carcinoma   B. Hepatocellular carcinoma
    C. Oat cell carcinoma   D. Uterine leiomyoma

13. **Mutation characteristic for polycythaemia vera is:**
    A. JAK2 mutation   B. Bcr-abl mutation
    C. p53 mutation   D. RAS mutation

14. **Difference between RAEB-1 and RAEB-2 is:**
    A. Blood cytopenia in RAEB-2
    B. Marrow blasts 5-9% in RAEB-2
    C. Marrow blasts 10-19% in RAEB-2
    D. Presence of ringed sideroblasts in RAEB-2

15. **Isotretinoin treatment is effective in which acute leukemia:**
    A. ALL   B. AML-M2
    C. AML-M6   D. AML-M3

16. **Which of the following is not included in classic Hodgkin's disease:**
    A. Nodular lymphocyte predominant HD
    B. Lymphocyte depletion HD
    C. Mixed cellularity HD
    D. Nodular sclerosis HD

17. **Which of the following is a specific marker for hairy cell?**
    A. CD22   B. CD5
    C. CD103   D. CD8

18. **Leukemic stage of cutaneous T cell lymphoma is called:**
    A. Hairy cell leukemia   B. Adult T cell leukemia
    C. Mycosis fungoides   D. Sezary syndrome

19. **A 40-year-old woman presents with increasing weakness and lethargy. Her peripheral white cell count is markedly elevated, and her leukocyte alkaline phosphatase score is markedly decreased. Which of the following chromosomal translocations is most likely in such a case?**
    A. t(9;22)   B. t(11;14)
    C. t(14;18)   D. t(15;17)

20. **A 16 years old boy has sore throat, enlarged tender cervical lymphadenopathy, and low-grade fever for one week. On examination, he has splenomegaly. His CBC shows TLC 20,000/μl and DLC 14, 80, 5, 1, 0. What is the possible diagnosis?**
    A. Acute lymphocytic leukaemia   B. Hodgkin's disease
    C. Non-Hodgkin's lymphoma   D. Infectious mononucleosis

KEY

1 = B	2 = B	3 = D	4 = C	5 = D
6 = D	7 = D	8 = A	9 = C	10 = D
11 = B	12 = C	13 = A	14 = C	15 = D
16 = A	17 = C	18 = D	19 = A	20 = D

13 The Blood Vessels and Lymphatics

NORMAL STRUCTURE *(p. 370)*

ARTERIES

Depending upon the calibre and certain histologic features, arteries are divided into 3 types: large (elastic) arteries, medium-sized (muscular) arteries and the smallest arterioles.

M/E All major arteries of the body have 3 layers in their walls: the tunica intima, the tunica media and the tunica adventitia. These layers progressively decrease with diminution in the size of the vessels.

1. Tunica intima This is the inner coat of the artery. It is composed of the lining endothelium, subendothelial connective tissue and bounded externally by internal elastic lamina.

2. Tunica media Tunica media is the middle coat of the arterial wall, bounded internally by internal elastic lamina and externally by external elastic lamina.

3. Tunica adventitia The outer coat of arteries is the tunica adventitia. It consists of loose mesh of connective tissue and some elastic fibres that merge with the adjacent tissues.

The layers of arterial wall receive nutrition and oxygen from 2 sources:

1. Tunica intima and inner third of the media are nourished by *direct diffusion* from the blood present in the lumen.

2. Outer two-thirds of the media and the adventitia are supplied by *vasa vasora (i.e. vessels of vessels)*, the nutrient vessels arising from the parent artery.

There are structural variations in three types of arteries:

◆ *Large, elastic arteries* such as the aorta, innominate, common carotid, major pulmonary, and common iliac arteries have very high content of elastic tissue in the media and thick elastic laminae and hence the name.

◆ *Medium-sized, muscular arteries* are the branches of elastic arteries. All the three layers of arterial wall are thinner than in the elastic arteries.

◆ *Arterioles* are the smallest branches with internal diameter 20-100 µm. Structurally, they consist of three layers as in muscular arteries but are much thinner and cannot be distinguished.

VEINS

The structure of normal veins is basically similar to that of arteries. The walls of the veins are thinner, the three tunicae (intima, media and adventitia) are less clearly demarcated, elastic tissue is scanty and not clearly organised into internal and external elastic laminae. The media contains very small amount of smooth muscle cells with abundant collagen. All veins, except vena cavae and common iliac veins, have valves best developed in veins of the lower limbs.

CAPILLARIES

Capillaries are about the size of an RBC (7-8 µm) and have 1-2 endothelial cells but no media. Blood from capillaries returns to the heart via *post-capillary venules* and from there into venules and then drained into veins.

LYMPHATICS

Lymphatic capillaries, lymphatic vessels and lymph nodes comprise the lymphatic system. Lymphatic capillaries resemble blood capillaries, and larger lymphatics are identical to veins. However, lymphatics lined by a single layer of endothelium have thin muscle in their walls than in veins of the same size and the valves are more numerous.

ARTERIOSCLEROSIS (p. 371)

Arteriosclerosis is a general term used to include all conditions with thickening and hardening of the arterial walls. The following morphologic entities are included under arteriosclerosis:

I. Senile arteriosclerosis (affects arteries)
II. Hypertensive arteriolosclerosis (affects arterioles)
III. Mönckeberg's arteriosclerosis (Medial calcific sclerosis) (affects arteries)
IV. Atherosclerosis (affects arteries)

SENILE ARTERIOSCLEROSIS (p. 371)

Senile arteriosclerosis is the thickening of media and intima of the arteries seen due to ageing.

M/E Findings are as under:
1. *Fibroelastosis:* The intima and media are thickened.
2. *Elastic reduplication:* The internal elastic lamina is split or reduplicated.

HYPERTENSIVE ARTERIOLOSCLEROSIS (p. 371)

Arteriolosclerosis is the term used to describe 3 morphologic forms of vascular disease affecting arterioles and small muscular arteries.

HYALINE ARTERIOLOSCLEROSIS

Hyaline sclerosis is a common arteriolar lesion that may be seen *physiologically* due to ageing, or may occur *pathologically* in benign nephrosclerosis in hypertensives.

M/E The thickened vessel wall shows structureless, eosinophilic, hyaline material in the intima and media.

HYPERPLASTIC ARTERIOLOSCLEROSIS

The hyperplastic or proliferative type of arteriolosclerosis is a characteristic lesion of malignant hypertension; other causes include haemolytic-uraemic syndrome, scleroderma and toxaemia of pregnancy.

M/E Main factors are as under:
i) *Onion-skin lesion* consists of loosely-placed concentric layers of hyperplastic intimal smooth muscle cells like the bulb of an onion.
ii) *Mucinous intimal thickening* is the deposition of amorphous ground substance, probably proteoglycans, with scanty cells.
iii) *Fibrous intimal thickening* is less common and consists of bundles of collagen, elastic fibres and hyaline deposits in the intima.

NECROTISING ARTERIOLITIS

In cases of severe hypertension and malignant hypertension, parts of small arteries and arterioles show changes of hyaline sclerosis and parts of these show necrosis, or necrosis may be superimposed on hyaline sclerosis.

M/E Besides the changes of hyaline sclerosis, the changes of necrotising arteriolitis include fibrinoid necrosis of vessel wall, acute inflammatory infiltrate of neutrophils in the adventitia.

MÖNCKEBERG'S ARTERIOSCLEROSIS (MEDIAL CALCIFIC SCLEROSIS) (p. 372)

Mönckeberg's arteriosclerosis is calcification of the media of large and medium-sized muscular arteries, especially of the extremities and of the genital tract, in persons past the age of 50.

M/E Mönckeberg's arteriosclerosis is characterised by deposits of calcium salts in the media without associated inflammatory reaction while the intima and the adventitia are spared. Often, coexistent changes of atherosclerosis are present altering the histologic appearance.

ATHEROSCLEROSIS *(p. 373)*

DEFINITION

Atherosclerosis is a thickening and hardening of large and medium-sized muscular arteries, primarily due to involvement of tunica intima and is characterised by fibrofatty plaques or atheromas.

The term atherosclerosis is derived from *athero-*(meaning porridge) referring to the soft lipid-rich material in the centre of atheroma, and *sclerosis* (scarring) referring to connective tissue in the plaques.

Atherosclerosis is the commonest and the most important of the arterial diseases. Though any large and medium-sized artery may be involved in atherosclerosis, the most commonly affected are the aorta, the coronaries and the cerebral arterial systems. Therefore, the major clinical syndromes resulting from ischaemia due to atherosclerosis are as under:
1. Heart (angina and myocardial infarcts or *heart attacks*)
2. Brain (transient cerebral ischaemia and cerebral infarcts or *strokes*)
3. Other sequelae are: peripheral vascular disease, aneurysmal dilatation due to weakened arterial wall, chronic ischaemic heart disease, ischaemic encephalopathy and mesenteric arterial occlusion.

ETIOLOGY

Cardiovascular disease, mostly related to atherosclerotic coronary heart disease or ischaemic heart disease (IHD) is the most common cause of premature death in the developed countries of the world. It is estimated that by the year 2020, cardiovascular disease, mainly atherosclerosis, will become the leading cause of total global disease burden.

Systematic large-scale studies of investigations on living populations have revealed a number of *risk factors* which are associated with increased risk of developing clinical atherosclerosis. These risk factors are divided into two groups as under:

I. MAJOR RISK FACTORS	II. EMERGING RISK FACTORS
A) Modifiable	1. Environmental influences
1. Dyslipidaemia	2. Obesity
2. Hypertension	3. Hormones: oestrogen deficiency,
3. Diabetes mellitus	oral contraceptives
4. Smoking	4. Physical inactivity
	5. Stressful life
B) Constitutional	6. Homocystinuria
1. Age	7. Role of alcohol
2. Sex	8. Prothrombotic factors
3. Genetic factors	9. Infections (*C. pneumoniae*,
4. Familial and racial factors	Herpesvirus, CMV)
	10. High CRP

MAJOR RISK FACTORS MODIFIABLE BY LIFE STYLE AND/OR THERAPY

1. DYSLIPIDAEMIAS Abnormalities in plasma lipoproteins have been firmly established as the most important major risk factor for atherosclerosis. It has been firmly established that hypercholesterolaemia has directly proportionate relationship with atherosclerosis and IHD. The following evidences are cited in support of this:

i) The atherosclerotic plaques contain cholesterol and cholesterol esters.

ii) The lesions of atherosclerosis can be induced in experimental animals.

iii) Individuals with hypercholesterolaemia due to various causes such as in diabetes mellitus, myxoedema, nephrotic syndrome, von Gierke's disease, xanthomatosis and familial hypercholesterolaemia have increased risk of developing atherosclerosis and IHD.

iv) Populations having hypercholesterolaemia have higher mortality from IHD.

The major classes of lipoprotein particles are *chylomicrons, very-low density lipoproteins (VLDL), low-density lipoproteins (LDL),* and *high-density lipoproteins (HDL).*

The major fractions of lipoproteins tested in blood lipid profile and their varying effects on atherosclerosis and IHD are as under:

i) **Total cholesterol** Desirable normal serum level is 140-200 mg/dl, while levels of borderline high are considered between 200-240 mg/dl. An elevation of total serum cholesterol levels above 260 mg/dl in men and women between 30 and 50 years of age has three times higher risk of developing IHD as compared with people with total serum cholesterol levels within normal limits.

ii) **Triglycerides** Normal serum level is below 150 mg/dl.

iii) **Low-density lipoproteins (LDL) cholesterol** Optimal serum level of LDL is <100 mg/dl. LDL is richest in cholesterol and has the *maximum association* with atherosclerosis.

iv) **Very-low-density lipoprotein (VLDL)** VLDL carries much of the triglycerides and its blood levels therefore parallel with that of triglycerides; VLDL has *less marked* effect than LDL.

v) **High-density lipoproteins (HDL) cholesterol** Normal desirable serum level is <50 mg/dl. HDL is *protective* ('good cholesterol') against atherosclerosis.

Many studies have demonstrated the harmful effect of diet containing larger quantities of saturated fats (e.g. in eggs, meat, milk, butter etc) and trans fats (i.e. unsaturated fats produced by artificial hydrogenation of polyunsaturated fats) which raise the plasma cholesterol level.

Familial hypercholesterolaemia, an autosomal codominant disorder, is characterised by elevated LDL cholesterol and normal triglycerides and occurrence of xanthomas and premature coronary artery disease.

Currently, management of dyslipidaemia is directed at *lowering LDL* in particular, and total cholesterol in general, by use of statins, and for *raising HDL* by weight loss, exercise and use of nicotinic acid.

2. HYPERTENSION Hypertension is a risk factor for all clinical manifestations of atherosclerosis. Hypertension doubles the risk of all forms of cardiovascular disease. It acts probably by mechanical injury to the arterial wall due to increased blood pressure.

3. SMOKING Men who smoke a pack of cigarettes a day are 3-5 times more likely to die of IHD than non-smokers. The increased risk and severity of atherosclerosis in smokers is due to reduced level of HDL, deranged coagulation system and accumulation of carbon monoxide.

4. DIABETES MELLITUS Clinical manifestations of atherosclerosis are far more common and develop at an early age in people with both type 1 and type 2 diabetes mellitus. In particular, association of type 2 diabetes mellitus characterised by metabolic (insulin resistance) syndrome and abnormal lipid profile termed 'diabetic dyslipidaemia' is common and heightens the risk of cardiovascular disease.

CONSTITUTIONAL RISK FACTORS

1. AGE Atherosclerosis is an age-related disease. Fully-developed atheromatous plaques usually appear in the 4th decade and beyond.

2. SEX The incidence and severity of atherosclerosis are more in men than in women and the changes appear a decade earlier in men (≥45 years) than in women (≥55 years).

3. GENETIC FACTORS Hereditary derangements of lipoprotein metabolism predispose the individual to high blood lipid level and familial hypercholesterolaemia.

4. FAMILIAL AND RACIAL FACTORS The familial predisposition to atherosclerosis may be related to other risk factors like diabetes, hypertension and hyperlipoproteinaemia. Racial differences too exist; Blacks have generally less severe atherosclerosis than Whites.

EMERGING RISK FACTORS

1. Higher incidence of atherosclerosis in developed countries and low prevalence in underdeveloped countries, suggesting the role of *environmental influences.*
2. *Metabolic syndrome* characterised by abdominal obesity along with glucose intolerance, insulin resistance and dyslipidaemia and hypertension.
3. Use of *exogenous hormones* (e.g. oral contraceptives) by women or *endogenous oestrogen deficiency* (e.g. in post-menopausal women).
4. *Physical inactivity* and lack of exercise.
5. *Stressful life style,* termed as 'type A' behaviour pattern.
6. *Hypercystinaemia* due to elevated serum homocysteine level from low folate and vitamin B_{12}.
7. Patients with *homocystinuria.*
8. *Prothrombotic factors* and elevated fibrinogen levels.
9. Role of *infections,* particularly of *Chlamydia pneumoniae* and viruses.
10. Markers of inflammation such as *elevated C reactive protein,* an acute phase reactant.

However, there are some reports in the literature which suggest that moderate consumption of *alcohol* has slightly beneficial effect by raising the level of HDL cholesterol.

PATHOGENESIS

As stated above, atherosclerosis is not caused by a single etiologic factor but is a multifactorial process whose exact pathogenesis is still not known.

Though, there is no consensus regarding the origin and progression of lesion of atherosclerosis, the role of four key factors—arterial smooth muscle cells, endothelial cells, blood monocytes and dyslipidaemia, is accepted by all. Currently, pathogenesis of atherosclerosis is explained on the basis of the following two theories:

1. *Reaction-to-injury hypothesis,* first described in 1973, and modified in 1986 and 1993 by Ross.
2. *Monoclonal theory,* based on neoplastic proliferation of smooth muscle cells, postulated by Benditt and Benditt in 1973.

1. REACTION-TO-INJURY HYPOTHESIS

This theory is most widely accepted and incorporates aspects of two older historical theories of atherosclerosis—the lipid theory of Virchow and thrombogenic (encrustation) theory of Rokitansky.

Following is the generally accepted role of key components involved in atherogenesis:

i) Endothelial injury It has been known for many years that endothelial injury is the initial triggering event in the development of lesions of atherosclerosis. Numerous causes ascribed to endothelial injury in experimental animals are: mechanical trauma, haemodynamic forces, immunological and chemical mechanisms, metabolic agent as chronic dyslipidaemia, homocysteine, circulating toxins from systemic infections, viruses, hypoxia, radiation, carbon monoxide and tobacco products.

In humans, two of the major risk factors which act together to produce endothelial injury are: *haemodynamic stress from hypertension and chronic dyslipidaemia.*

ii) Intimal smooth muscle cell proliferation Endothelial injury causes adherence, aggregation and platelet release reaction at the site of exposed subendothelial connective tissue and infiltration by inflammatory cells.

Proliferation of intimal smooth muscle cells and production of extracellular matrix are stimulated by various cytokines such as IL-1 and TNF-α released from invading monocyte-macrophages and by activated platelets at the site of endothelial injury.

◈ Platelet-derived growth factor *(PDGF)* and fibroblast growth factor *(FGF)*.

◈ Transforming growth factor-β *(TGF-β)* and interferon (IFN)-γ.

iii) Role of blood monocytes Though blood monocytes do not possess receptors for normal LDL, LDL does appear in the monocyte cytoplasm to form foam cell. Plasma LDL on entry into the intima undergoes oxidation. The 'oxidised LDL' formed in the intima performs the following all-important functions on monocytes and endothelium:

a) For monocytes: Oxidised LDL acts to attract, proliferate, immobilise and activate them as well as is readily taken up by scavenger receptor on the monocyte to transform it to a lipid-laden foam cell.

b) For endothelium: Oxidised LDL is cytotoxic.

iv) Role of dyslipidaemia As stated already, chronic dyslipidaemia in itself may initiate endothelial injury and dysfunction by causing increased permeability.

v) Thrombosis As apparent from the foregoing, endothelial injury exposes subendothelial connective tissue resulting in formation of small platelet aggregates at the site and causing proliferation of smooth muscle cells. This causes mild inflammatory reaction which together with foam cells is incorporated into the atheromatous plaque.

2. MONOCLONAL HYPOTHESIS

This hypothesis is based on the postulate that proliferation of smooth muscle cells is the primary event and that this proliferation is monoclonal in origin similar to cellular proliferation in neoplasms.

MORPHOLOGIC FEATURES

1. FATTY STREAKS AND DOTS Fatty streaks and dots on the intima by themselves are harmless but may be the precursor lesions of atheromatous plaques.

M/E Fatty streaks lying under the endothelium are composed of closely-packed foam cells, lipid-containing elongated smooth muscle cells and a few lymphoid cells.

2. GELATINOUS LESIONS Like fatty streaks, they may also be precursors of plaques. They are round or oval, circumscribed grey elevations, about 1 cm in diameter.

M/E Gelatinous lesions are foci of increased ground substance in the intima with thinned overlying endothelium.

3. ATHEROMATOUS PLAQUES A fully developed atherosclerotic lesion is called atheromatous plaque, also called *fibrous plaque, fibrofatty plaque or atheroma.* Most often and most severely affected is the abdominal aorta, though smaller lesions may be seen in descending thoracic aorta and aortic arch. The major branches of the aorta around the ostia are often severely involved, especially the iliac, femoral, carotid, coronary, and cerebral arteries.

G/A Atheromatous plaques are white to yellowish-white lesions, varying in diameter from 1-2 cm and raised on the surface by a few millimetres to a centimetre in thickness. Cut section of the plaque reveals the luminal surface as a firm, white *fibrous cap* and a *central core* composed of yellow to yellow-white, soft, porridge-like material and hence the name atheroma.

M/E Salient features are as under:

i) Superficial luminal part of the *fibrous cap* is covered by endothelium, and is composed of smooth muscle cells, dense connective tissue and extra-cellular matrix containing proteoglycans and collagen.

ii) Cellular area under the fibrous cap is comprised by a mixture of macrophages, foam cells, lymphocytes and a few smooth muscle cells which may contain lipid.

iii) Deeper *central soft core* consists of extracellular lipid material, cholesterol clefts, fibrin, necrotic debris and lipid-laden foam cells.

iv) In older and *more advanced lesions,* the collagen in the fibrous cap may be dense and hyalinised.

4. COMPLICATED PLAQUES These changes include calcification, ulceration, thrombosis, haemorrhage and aneurysmal dilatation. It is not uncommon to see more than one form of complication in a plaque.

CLINICAL EFFECTS

The clinical effects of atherosclerosis depend upon the size and type of arteries affected.

Large arteries affected most often are the aorta, renal, mesenteric and carotids, whereas the medium- and small-sized arteries frequently involved are the coronaries, cerebrals and arteries of the lower limbs. Accordingly, the symptomatic atherosclerotic disease involves most often the following:

i) *Heart*—Myocardial infarction, ischaemic heart disease.
ii) *Brain*—Chronic ischaemic brain damage, cerebral infarction and stroke.
iii) *Aorta*—Aneurysm formation, thrombosis and embolisation to other organs.
iv) *Small intestine*—Ischaemic bowel disease, infarction.
v) *Lower extremities*—Intermittent claudication, gangrene.

VASCULITIS *(p. 381)*

Arteritis, angiitis and vasculitis are the common terms used for inflammatory involvement of an artery, arterioles, venules and capillaries. It may occur following invasion of the vessel by infectious agents, or may be induced by non-infectious injuries such as chemical, mechanical, immunologic and radiation injury.

I. INFECTIOUS ARTERITIS *(p. 381)*

Direct invasion of the artery by infectious agents, especially bacteria and fungi, causes infectious arteritis.

ENDARTERITIS OBLITERANS

It is commonly seen close to the lesions of peptic ulcers of the stomach and duodenum, tuberculous and chronic abscesses in the lungs, chronic cutaneous ulcers, chronic meningitis, and in post-partum and post-menopausal uterine arteries.

M/E The obliteration of the lumen is due to concentric and symmetric proliferation of cellular fibrous tissue in the intima.

SYPHILITIC ARTERITIS

Syphilitic or luetic vascular involvement occurs in all stages of syphilis but is more prominent in the tertiary stage. Manifestations of the disease are particularly prominent at two sites—the aorta and the cerebral arteries.

SYPHILITIC AORTITIS Syphilitic involvement of the ascending aorta and the aortic arch is the commonest manifestation of cardiovascular syphilis. It occurs in about 80% cases of tertiary syphilis.

G/A The affected part of the aorta may be dilated, and its wall somewhat thickened and adherent to the neighbouring mediastinal structures. Longitudinally opened vessels show intimal surface studded with pearly-white thickenings, varying from a few millimeters to a centimeter in diameter. These lesions are separated by wrinkled normal intima, giving it characteristic *tree-bark appearance.*

M/E Salient features are:
i) Endarteritis and periarteritis of the vasa vasorum located in the media and adventitia.

ii) Perivascular accumulation of plasma cells, lymphocytes and macrophages that may form miliary gummas which undergo necrosis and are replaced by scar tissue.

iii) Intimal thickenings consist of dense avascular collagen that may undergo hyalinisation and calcification.

The *effects* of syphilitic aortitis may vary from trivial to catastrophic. These are:
a) Aortic aneurysm
b) Aortic valvular incompetence
c) Stenosis of coronary ostia

CEREBRAL SYPHILITIC ARTERITIS (HEUBNER'S ARTERITIS) Syphilitic involvement of small and medium-sized cerebral arteries occurs during the tertiary syphilis.

M/E Changes of endarteritis and periarteritis similar to those seen in syphilitic aortitis are found.

NON-SPECIFIC INFECTIVE ARTERITIS

Various forms of invasions of the artery by bacteria, fungi, parasites or viruses, either directly or by haematogenous route, cause non-syphilitic infective arteritis.

II. NON-INFECTIOUS ARTERITIS *(p. 382)*

This group consists of most of the important forms of vasculitis, more often affecting arterioles, venules and capillaries, and hence also termed as *small vessel vasculitis*. Their exact etiology is not known but available evidence suggests that many of them have immunologic origin. Serum from many of patients with vasculitis of immunologic origin show the presence of following immunologic features:
1. Anti-neutrophil cytoplasmic antibodies (ANCAs)
i) Cytoplasmic ANCA (c-ANCA) pattern
ii) Perinuclear ANCA (p-ANCA) pattern
2. Anti-endothelial cell antibodies (AECAs)
3. Pauci-immune vasculitis

POLYARTERITIS NODOSA

Polyarteritis nodosa (PAN) is a necrotising vasculitis involving small and medium-sized muscular arteries of multiple organs and tissues.

The disease occurs more commonly in adult males than females. Most commonly affected organs, in descending order of frequency of involvement, are the kidneys, heart, liver, gastrointestinal tract, muscle, pancreas, testes, nervous system and skin.

G/A The lesions of PAN involve segments of vessels, especially at the bifurcations and branchings, as tiny beaded nodules.

M/E There are 3 sequential stages in the evolution of lesions in PAN:
i) *Acute stage*—There is fibrinoid necrosis in the centre of the nodule located in the media.
ii) *Healing stage*—This is characterised by marked fibroblastic proliferation producing firm nodularity.
iii) *Healed stage*—In this stage, the affected arterial wall is markedly thickened due to dense fibrosis.

HYPERSENSITIVITY VASCULITIS

Hypersensitivity vasculitis, also called as allergic or leucocytoclastic vasculitis or microscopic polyarteritis, is a group of clinical syndromes with involvement of venules, capillaries and arterioles. The tissues and organs most commonly involved are the skin, mucous membranes, lungs, brain, heart, gastrointestinal tract, kidneys and muscle. The condition results from immunologic response to an identifiable antigen that may be bacteria (e.g. streptococci, staphylococci, mycobacteria), viruses (e.g. hepatitis B virus, influenza virus, CMV), malarial parasite, certain drugs and chemicals.

M/E

i) *Leucocytoclastic vasculitis,* characterised by fibrinoid necrosis with neutrophilic infiltrate in the vessel wall. Many of the neutrophils are fragmented. This form is found in vasculitis caused by deposits of immune complexes.

ii) *Lymphocytic vasculitis,* in which the involved vessel shows predominant infiltration by lymphocytes. This type is seen in vascular injury due to delayed hypersensitivity or cellular immune reactions.

WEGENER'S GRANULOMATOSIS

Wegener's granulomatosis is another form of necrotising vasculitis characterised by a *clinicopathologic triad* consisting of the following:

i)   Acute necrotising granulomas of the upper and lower respiratory tracts involving nose, sinuses and lungs;

ii)   focal necrotising vasculitis, particularly of the lungs and upper airways; and

iii)   focal or diffuse necrotising glomerulonephritis.

A *limited form* of Wegener's granulomatosis is the same condition without renal involvement.

M/E   Following features are seen:

i) The granulomas consist of fibrinoid necrosis with extensive infiltration by neutrophils, mononuclear cells, epithelioid cells, multinucleate giant cells and fibroblastic proliferation.

ii) The necrotising vasculitis may be segmental or circumferential.

iii) The renal lesions are those of focal or diffuse necrotising glomerulo-nephritis.

TEMPORAL (GIANT CELL) ARTERITIS

This is a form of granulomatous inflammation of medium-sized and large arteries. Preferential sites of involvement are the cranial arteries, especially the temporal, and hence the name. However, the aorta and other major arteries like common carotid, axillary, brachial, femoral and mesenteric arteries are also involved, and therefore, it is preferable to call the entity as *'giant cell arteritis'*. The patients are generally over the age of 70 years with slight female preponderance.

G/A   The affected artery is thickened, cord-like and the lumen is usually reduced to a narrow slit.

M/E   It shows following features:

i) There is chronic granulomatous reaction, usually around the internal elastic lamina and typically involves the entire circumference of the vessel.

ii) Giant cells of foreign body or Langhans' type are found in two-third of cases.

iii) The internal elastic lamina is often fragmented.

iv) There is eccentric or concentric intimal cellular proliferation causing marked narrowing of the lumen.

TAKAYASU'S ARTERITIS (PULSELESS DISEASE)

This is a form of granulomatous vasculitis affecting chiefly the aorta and its major branches and hence is also referred to as *aortic arch syndrome.* The disease affects chiefly young women and is typically characterised by absence of pulse in both arms and presence of ocular manifestations.

M/E   Following features are seen:

i) There is severe mononuclear inflammatory infiltrate involving the full thickness of the affected vessel wall.

ii) The inflammatory changes are more severe in the adventitia and media and there is perivascular infiltration of the vasa vasorum.

iii) Granulomatous changes in the media with central necrosis and Langhans' giant cells are found in many cases.

KAWASAKI'S DISEASE

Also known by more descriptive name of '*mucocutaneous lymph node syndrome*', it is an acute and subacute illness affecting mainly young children and infants. Kawasaki's disease is a febrile illness with mucocutaneous symptoms like erosions of oral mucosa and conjunctiva, skin rash and lymphadenopathy.

M/E The picture is of panarteritis resembling PAN, characterised by necrosis and inflammation of the entire thickness of the vessel wall. Therefore, some consider Kawasaki's disease as an infantile form of PAN.

BUERGER'S DISEASE (THROMBOANGIITIS OBLITERANS)

Buerger's disease is a specific disease entity affecting chiefly small and medium-sized arteries and veins of the extremities and characterised by acute and chronic occlusive inflammatory involvement. The disease affects chiefly men under the age of 35 years who are heavy cigarette smokers.

ETIOPATHOGENESIS Following possible mechanisms have been proposed:
i) There is consistent association with heavy cigarette smoking. This has led to the hypothesis that *tobacco products* cause either direct endothelial damage leading to hypercoagulability and thrombosis.
ii) *Genetic factors* play a role as the disease has familial occurrence and has HLA association.

G/A The lesions are typically segmental affecting small and medium-sized arteries, especially of the lower extremities. Involvement of the arteries is often accompanied with involvement of adjacent veins and nerves.

M/E Salient features are as follows:
i) In *early stage,* there is infiltration by polymorphs in all the layers of vessels and there is invariable presence of mural or occlusive thrombosis of the lumen.
ii) In *advanced stage,* the cellular infiltrate is predominantly mononuclear and may contain an occasional epithelioid cell granuloma with Langhans' giant cells. The thrombi undergo organisation and recanalisation.

RAYNAUD'S DISEASE AND RAYNAUD'S PHENOMENON

Raynaud's disease is not a vasculitis but is a functional vasospastic disorder affecting chiefly small arteries and arterioles of the extremities, occurring in otherwise young healthy females. The disease affects most commonly the fingers and hands. The ischaemic effect is provoked primarily by cold but other stimuli such as emotions, trauma, hormones and drugs also play a role. Clinically, the affected digits show *pallor,* followed by *cyanosis,* and then *redness,* corresponding to *arterial ischaemia, venostasis* and *hyperaemia* respectively.

Raynaud's phenomenon differs from Raynaud's disease in having an underlying cause e.g. secondary to artherosclerosis, connective tissue diseases like scleroderma and SLE, Buerger's disease, multiple myeloma, pulmonary hypertension and ingestion of ergot group of drugs. Raynaud's phenomenon like Raynaud's disease, also shows cold sensitivity but differs from the latter in having structural abnormalities in the affected vessels. These changes include segmental inflammation and fibrinoid change in the walls of capillaries.

ANEURYSMS *(p. 386)*

DEFINITION AND CLASSIFICATION

An aneurysm is defined as a permanent abnormal dilatation of a blood vessel occurring due to congenital or acquired weakening or destruction of the vessel wall. Most commonly, aneurysms involve large elastic arteries, especially the aorta and its major branches. Aneurysms can cause various ill-effects such as thrombosis and thromboembolism, alteration in the flow of blood, rupture of the vessel and compression of neighbouring structures.

Aneurysms can be classified on the basis of various features:

A. Depending upon the composition of the wall

1. *True aneurysm* composed of all the layers of a normal vessel wall.
2. *False aneurysm* having fibrous wall and occurring often from trauma to the vessel.

B. Depending upon the shape These are as under:
1. *Saccular* having large spherical outpouching.
2. *Fusiform* having slow spindle-shaped dilatation.
3. *Cylindrical* with a continuous parallel dilatation.
4. *Serpentine or varicose* which has tortuous dilatation of the vessel.
5. *Racemose or circoid* having mass of intercommunicating small arteries and veins.

C. Based on pathogenetic mechanisms
1. Atherosclerotic (arteriosclerotic) aneurysms
2. Syphilitic (luetic) aneurysms
3. Dissecting aneurysms (Dissecting haematoma)
4. Mycotic aneurysms
5. Berry aneurysms

ATHEROSCLEROTIC ANEURYSMS

Atherosclerotic aneurysms are the most common form of aortic aneurysms. They are seen more commonly in males and the frequency increases after the age of 50 years when the incidence of complicated lesions of advanced atherosclerosis is higher. They are most common in the abdominal aorta.

PATHOGENESIS Obviously, severe atherosclerotic lesions are the basic problem which cause thinning and destruction of the medial elastic tissue resulting in atrophy and weakening of the wall.

G/A Atherosclerotic aneurysms of the abdominal aorta are most frequently infra-renal, above the bifurcation of the aorta. They may be of variable size but are often larger than 5-6 cm in diameter. Atherosclerotic aneurysm is most frequently fusiform in shape and the lumen of aneurysm often contains mural thrombus.

M/E There is predominance of fibrous tissue in the media and adventitia with mild chronic inflammatory reaction. The intima and inner part of the media show remnants of atheromatous plaques and mural thrombus.

EFFECTS The clinical effects of atherosclerotic aneurysms are due to complications:
1. Rupture
2. Compression
3. Arterial occlusion

SYPHILITIC (LUETIC) ANEURYSMS

Cardiovascular syphilis occurs in about 10% cases of syphilis. It causes arteritis—syphilitic aortitis and cerebral arteritis, both of which are already described in this chapter. One of the major complications of syphilitic aortitis is syphilitic or luetic aneurysm that develops in the tertiary stage of syphilis.

PATHOGENESIS About 40% cases of syphilitic aortitis develop syphilitic aneurysms. The process begins from inflammatory infiltrate around the vasa vasorum of the adventitia, followed by endarteritis obliterans.

G/A Syphilitic aneurysms occurring most often in the ascending part and the arch of aorta are saccular in shape and usually 3-5 cm in diameter. Less often, they are fusiform or cylindrical. The intimal surface is wrinkled and shows *tree-bark appearance.*

M/E The features of healed syphilitic aortitis are seen. The adventitia shows fibrous thickening with endarteritis obliterans of vasa vasorum.

EFFECTS The clinical effects are due to:
1. Rupture

DISSECTING ANEURYSMS AND CYSTIC MEDIAL NECROSIS

The term dissecting aneurysm is applied for a dissecting haematoma in which the blood enters the separated (dissected) wall of the vessel and spreads for varying distance longitudinally. The most common site is the aorta and is an acute catastrophic aortic disease. The condition occurs most commonly in men in the age range of 50 to 70 years. In women, dissecting aneurysms may occur during pregnancy.

PATHOGENESIS The pathogenesis of dissecting aneurysm is explained on the basis of weakened aortic media. Various conditions causing weakening in the aortic wall resulting in dissection are as under:

i) Hypertensive state About 90% cases of dissecting aneurysm have hypertension.

ii) Non-hypertensive cases These are cases due to some local or systemic connective tissue disorder:
a) Marfan's syndrome
b) Cystic medial necrosis of Erdheim
c) Iatrogenic trauma
d) Pregnancy

G/A Dissecting aneurysm differs from atherosclerotic and syphilitic aneurysms in having no significant dilatation. Therefore, it is currently referred to as *'dissecting haematoma'*. Dissecting aneurysm classically begins in the arch of aorta. In 95% of cases, there is a sharply-incised, transverse or oblique intimal tear, 3-4 cm long, most often located in the ascending part of the aorta. The dissection is seen most characteristically between the outer and middle third of the aortic media so that the column of blood in the dissection separates the *intima and inner two-third of the media* on one side from the *outer one-third of the media and the adventitia* on the other.

If the patient survives, the false lumen may develop endothelial lining and *'double-barrel aorta'* is formed.

M/E Salient features are:
i) Focal separation of the fibromuscular and elastic tissue of the media.
ii) Numerous cystic spaces in the media containing basophilic ground substance.
iii) Fragmentation of the elastic tissue.
iv) Increased fibrosis of the media.

EFFECTS The complications arise from:
1. Rupture
2. Cardiac disease
3. Ischaemia

FIBROMUSCULAR DYSPLASIA

Fibromuscular dysplasia is a non-atherosclerotic and non-inflammatory disease affecting arterial wall, most often renal artery. Though the process may involve intima, media or adventitia, medial fibroplasia is the most common.

The main **effects** of renal fibromuscular dysplasia, depending upon the region of involvement, are renovascular hypertension and changes of renal atrophy.

COMMON DISEASES OF VEINS *(p. 389)*

VARICOSITIES

Varicosities are abnormally dilated and tortuous veins. The veins of lower extremities are involved most frequently, called *varicose veins*. The veins of other parts of the body which are affected are the lower oesophagus (*oeso-*

phageal varices), the anal region (haemorrhoids) and the spermatic cord (varicocele).

VARICOSE VEINS

Varicose veins are permanently dilated and tortuous superficial veins of the lower extremities, especially the long saphenous vein and its tributaries. About 10-12% of the general population develops varicose veins of lower legs, with the peak incidence in 4th and 5th decades of life. Adult females are affected more commonly than the males, especially during pregnancy. This is attributed to venous stasis in the lower legs because of compression on the iliac veins by pregnant uterus.

ETIOPATHOGENESIS A number of etiologic factors are involved in causation of varicose veins:

i)   Familial weakness of vein walls and valves is the most common cause.

ii)   Increased intraluminal pressure due to prolonged upright posture e.g. in nurses, policemen, surgeons etc.

iii)   Compression of iliac veins e.g. during pregnancy, intravascular thrombosis, growing tumour etc.

iv)   Hormonal effects on smooth muscle.

v)   Obesity.

vi)   Chronic constipation.

G/A The affected veins, especially of the lower extremities, are dilated, tortuous, elongated and nodular. Intraluminal thrombosis and valvular deformities are often found.

M/E There is variable fibromuscular thickening of the wall of the veins due to alternate dilatation and hypertrophy. Degeneration of the medial elastic tissue may occur which may be followed by calcific foci.

EFFECTS Varicose veins of the legs result in venous stasis which is followed by congestion, oedema, thrombosis, stasis, dermatitis, cellulitis and ulceration. Secondary infection results in chronic varicose ulcers.

PHLEBOTHROMBOSIS AND THROMBOPHLEBITIS

The terms 'phlebothrombosis' or thrombus formation in veins, and 'thrombophlebitis' or inflammatory changes within the vein wall, are currently used synonymously.

ETIOPATHOGENESIS Venous thrombosis that precedes thrombophlebitis is initiated by *triad* of changes: endothelial damage, alteration in the composition of blood and venous stasis.

MORPHOLOGIC FEATURES The most common locations for phlebothrombosis and thrombophlebitis are the deep veins of legs accounting for 90% of cases; it is commonly termed as *deep vein thrombosis (DVT)*.

G/A The affected veins may appear normal or may be distended and firm.

M/E The thrombus that is attached to the vein wall induces inflammatory-reparative response beginning from the intima and infiltrating into the thrombi.

EFFECTS The clinical effects may be local or systemic.

Local effects are oedema distal to occlusion, heat, swelling, tenderness, redness and pain.

Systemic effects are more severe and occur due to embolic phenomena, pulmonary thromboembolism being the most common and most important.

SPECIAL TYPES OF PHLEBOTHROMBOSIS

1.   Thrombophlebitis migrans Thrombophlebitis migrans or migratory thrombophlebitis or Trousseau's syndrome is the term used for multiple venous thrombi that disappear from one site so as to appear at another site.

2. **Phlegmasia alba dolens** This term meaning 'painful white leg' refers to extensive swelling of the leg, occurring most frequently due to iliofemoral venous thrombosis.

3. **Phlegmasia cerulea dolens** This term meaning 'painful blue leg' refers to markedly swollen bluish skin with superficial gangrene.

4. **Superior vena caval syndrome** Superior vena caval syndrome refers to obstruction of the superior vena cava.

5. **Inferior vena caval syndrome** Inferior vena caval syndrome is the obstruction of the inferior vena cava.

DISEASES OF LYMPHATICS (p. 390)

LYMPHANGITIS

Inflammation of the lymphatics or lymphangitis may be acute or chronic.

Acute lymphangitis occurs in the course of many bacterial infections. The most common organisms are β-haemolytic streptococci and staphylococci.

Chronic lymphangitis occurs due to persistent and recurrent acute lymphangitis or from chronic infections like tuberculosis, syphilis and actinomycosis.

LYMPHOEDEMA

Lymphoedema is swelling of soft tissues due to localised increase in the quantity of lymph. It may be primary (idiopathic) or secondary (obstructive).

I. PRIMARY (IDIOPATHIC) LYMPHOEDEMA Lymphoedema occurring without underlying secondary cause is called primary or idiopathic lymphoedema. Its various types are as under:

1. Congenital lymphoedema Congenital lymphoedema has further 2 subtypes—familial hereditary form (Milroy's disease) and non-familial (simple) form.

i) Milroy's disease is a form of congenital and familial oedema generally affecting one limb but at times may be more extensive and involve the eyelids and lips.

ii) Simple congenital lymphoedema is non-familial form with unknown etiology.

2. Lymphoedema praecox This is a rare form of lymphoedema affecting chiefly young females.

II. SECONDARY (OBSTRUCTIVE) LYMPHOEDEMA This is more common form of lymphoedema. Various causes of lymphatic obstruction causing lymphoedema are as under:

i) Lymphatic invasion by malignant tumour.

ii) Surgical removal of lymphatics e.g. in radical mastectomy.

iii) Post-irradiation fibrosis.

iv) Parasitic infestations e.g. in filariasis of lymphatics producing elephantiasis.

v) Lymphangitis causing scarring and obstruction.

Rupture of dilated large lymphatics may result in escape of milky chyle into the peritoneum (*chyloperitoneum*), into the pleural cavity (*chylothorax*), into pericardial cavity (*chylopericardium*) and into the urinary tract (*chyluria*).

TUMOURS AND TUMOUR-LIKE LESIONS (p. 391)

Majority of benign vascular tumours are malformations or hamartomas. On the other hand, there are true vascular tumours which are of intermediate grade and there are frank malignant tumours.

A. BENIGN TUMOURS AND HAMARTOMAS (p. 391)

HAEMANGIOMA

Haemangiomas are quite common lesions, especially in infancy and child-hood. The most common site is the skin of the face and mucosal surfaces.

CAPILLARY HAEMANGIOMA These are the most common type. Clinically, they appear as small or large, flat or slightly elevated, red to purple, soft and lobulated lesions, varying in size from a few millimeters to a few centimeters in diameter. They may be present at birth or appear in early childhood. Strawberry birthmarks and 'port-wine mark' are some good examples. The common sites are the skin, subcutaneous tissue and mucous membranes of oral cavity and lips.

M/E Capillary haemangiomas are well-defined but unencapsulated lobules. These lobules are composed of capillary-sized, thin-walled, blood-filled vessels. These vessels are lined by single layer of plump endothelial cells surrounded by a layer of pericytes.

CAVERNOUS HAEMANGIOMA Cavernous haemangiomas are single or multiple, discrete or diffuse, red to blue, soft and spongy masses. They are often 1 to 2 cm in diameter. They are most common in the skin (especially of the face and neck); other sites are mucosa of the oral cavity, stomach and small intestine, and internal visceral organs like the liver and spleen.

M/E Cavernous haemangiomas are composed of thin-walled cavernous vascular spaces, filled partly or completely with blood. The vascular spaces are lined by flattened endothelial cells.

GRANULOMA PYOGENICUM Granuloma pyogenicum is also referred to as *haemangioma of granulation tissue type*. True to its name, it appears as exophytic, red granulation tissue just like a nodule, commonly on the skin and mucosa of gingiva or oral cavity. *Pregnancy tumour* or *granuloma gravidarum* is a variant occurring on the gingiva during pregnancy and regresses after delivery.

M/E It shows proliferating capillaries similar to capillary haemangioma but the capillaries are separated by abundant oedema and inflammatory infiltrate, thus resembling inflammatory granulation tissue.

LYMPHANGIOMA

CAPILLARY LYMPHANGIOMA It is also called as lymphangioma simplex. It is a small, circumscribed, slightly elevated lesion measuring 1 to 2 cm in diameter. The common locations are the skin of head and neck, axilla and mucous membranes. Rarely, these may be found in the internal organs.

M/E Capillary lymphangioma is composed of a network of endothelium-lined, capillary-sized spaces containing lymph and often separated by lymphoid aggregates.

CAVERNOUS LYMPHANGIOMA It is more common than the capillary type. The common sites are in the region of head and neck or axilla. A large cystic variety called *cystic hygroma* occurs in the neck producing gross deformity in the neck.

M/E Cavernous lymphangioma consists of large dilated lymphatic spaces lined by flattened endothelial cells and containing lymph.

GLOMUS TUMOUR (GLOMANGIOMA)

Glomus tumour is an uncommon true benign tumour arising from contractile glomus cells that are present in the arteriovenous shunts (Sucquet-Hoyer anastomosis). These tumours are found most often in the dermis of the fingers or toes under a nail. These lesions are characterised by extreme pain.

M/E The tumours are composed of small blood vessels lined by endothelium and surrounded by aggregates, nests and masses of glomus cells. The glomus cells are round to cuboidal cells with scanty cytoplasm.

ARTERIOVENOUS MALFORMATIONS

An arteriovenous (AV) malformation is a communication between an artery and vein without an intervening capillary bed. It may be congenital or acquired type. Congenital AV malformations have thick-walled vessels with hyalinisation and calcification.

BACILLARY ANGIOMATOSIS AND PELIOSIS HEPATIS

Bacillary angiomatosis is a tumour-like lesion reported in association with HIV-AIDS with CD4+ T cell counts below 100/μl. In fact, it is an opportunistic infection with gram-negative bacilli of *Bartonella* genus.

M/E Lobules of proliferating blood vessels are seen lined by epithelioid endothelial cells having mild atypia. Mixed inflammatory cell infiltrate with nuclear debris of neutrophils is present in these areas.

The condition is treated with antibiotics.

B. INTERMEDIATE GRADE TUMOURS (p. 394)

HAEMANGIOENDOTHELIOMA

Haemangioendothelioma is a true tumour of endothelial cells, the behaviour of which is intermediate between a haemangioma and haemangiosarcoma. It is found most often in the skin and subcutaneous tissue in relation to medium-sized and large veins.

G/A The tumour is usually well-defined, grey-red, polypoid mass.

M/E There is an active proliferation of endothelial cells forming several layers around the blood vessels so that vascular lumina are difficult to identify. These cells may have variable mitotic activity. Reticulin stain delineates the pattern of cell proliferation inner to the basement membrane.

C. MALIGNANT TUMOURS (p. 394)

HAEMANGIOPERICYTOMA

Haemangiopericytoma is an uncommon tumour arising from pericytes. Pericytes are cells present external to the endothelial cells of capillaries and venules. This is a rare tumour that can occur at any site but is more common in lower extremities and the retroperitoneum. It may occur at any age and may vary in size from 1 to 8 cm.

M/E The tumour is composed of capillaries surrounded by spindle-shaped pericytes outside the vascular basement membrane forming whorled arrangement. These tumour cells may have high mitotic rate and areas of necrosis. Silver impregnation stain (i.e. reticulin stain) is employed to confirm the presence of pericytes outside the basement membrane of capillaries and to distinguish it from haemangioendothelioma.

ANGIOSARCOMA

Also known as haemangiosarcoma and malignant haemangioendothelioma, it is a malignant vascular tumour occurring most frequently in the skin, subcutaneous tissue, liver, spleen, bone, lung and retroperitoneal tissues. It can occur in both sexes and at any age. *Hepatic angiosarcomas* are of special interest in view of their association with carcinogens like polyvinyl chloride, arsenical pesticides and radioactive contrast medium, thorotrast, used in the past.

G/A The tumours are usually bulky, pale grey-white, firm masses with poorly-defined margins. Areas of haemorrhage, necrosis and central softening are frequently present.

M/E The tumours may be well-differentiated masses of proliferating endothelial cells around well-formed vascular channels, to poorly-differentiated lesions composed of plump, anaplastic and pleomorphic cells in solid clusters with poorly identifiable vascular channels.

KAPOSI'S SARCOMA

Kaposi's sarcoma is a malignant angiomatous tumour, first described by Kaposi, Hungarian dermatologist, in 1872. However, the tumour has attracted greater attention in the last two decades due to its frequent occurrence in patients with HIV/AIDS.

CLASSIFICATION Presently, four forms of Kaposi's sarcoma are described:

1. Classic (European) Kaposi's sarcoma This is the form which was first described by Kaposi. It is more common in men over 60 years of age of Eastern European descent.

2. African (Endemic) Kaposi's sarcoma This form is common in equatorial Africa. It is so common in Uganda that it comprises 9% of all malignant tumours in men.

3. Epidemic (AIDS-associated) Kaposi's sarcoma This form is seen in about 30% cases of AIDS, especially in young male homosexuals than the other high-risk groups.

4. Kaposi's sarcoma in renal transplant cases This form is associated with recipients of renal transplants who have been administered immunosuppressive therapy for a long time.

PATHOGENESIS Pathogenesis of Kaposi's sarcoma is complex. It is an opportunistic neoplasm in immunosupressed patients which has excessive proliferation of spindle cells of vascular origin having features of both endothelium and smooth muscle cells:

i) Epidemiological studies have suggested a *viral association* implicating HIV and human herpesvirus 8 (HSV 8, also called Kaposi's sarcoma-associated herpesvirus or KSHV).

ii) Occurrence of Kaposi's sarcoma involves interplay of HIV-1 infection, HHV-8 infection, activation of the immune system and secretion of cytokines (IL-6, TNF-α, GM-CSF, basic fibroblast factor, and oncostain M).

iii) Defective immunoregulation plays a role in its pathogenesis is further substantiated by observation of *second malignancy* (e.g. leukaemia, lymphoma and myeloma) in about one-third of patients with Kaposi's sarcoma.

G/A The lesions in the skin, gut and other organs form prominent, irregular, purple, dome-shaped plaques or nodules.

M/E The changes are nonspecific in early stage and more characteristic in late nodular stage.

◈ **Early patch stage** There are irregular vascular spaces separated by interstitial inflammatory cells and extravasated blood and haemosiderin.

◈ **Late nodular stage** There are slit-like vascular spaces containing red blood cells and separated by spindle-shaped, plump tumour cells.

CLINICAL COURSE The clinical course and biologic behaviour of Kaposi's sarcoma is quite variable. The classic form of Kaposi's sarcoma is largely confined to skin and the course is generally slow and insidious with long survival. The endemic (African) and epidemic (AIDS-associated) Kaposi's sarcoma, on the other hand, has a rapidly progressive course, often with widespread cutaneous as well as visceral involvement, and high mortality.

SELF ASSESSMENT

1. **Vasa vasora perfuse the vessel wall as follows:**
   - A. Whole thickness of vessel wall
   - B. Whole of adventitia and media
   - C. Adventitia and outer half of media
   - D. Adventitia and outer two-third of media

2. **Medial calcification of arteries is seen in the following except:**
   - A. Mönckeberg's arteriosclerosis
   - B. Atherosclerosis
   - C. Pseudoxanthoma elasticum
   - D. Idiopathic calcification of infancy

3. **Atherosclerosis is predominantly a disease of:**
   - A. Intima
   - B. Media
   - C. Adventitia
   - D. Entire vessel wall

4. **The following lipid has highest association with atherosclerosis:**
   A. Triglycerides
   B. Low-density lipoproteins
   C. Very-low density lipoproteins
   D. High density lipoproteins

5. **Hypertension with systolic pressure of 160 mmHg has greater risk of causing atherosclerosis as under:**
   A. 2-times
   B. 3-times
   C. 4-times
   D. 5-times

6. **The most important mitogen for smooth muscle proliferation in atherosclerosis is:**
   A. Platelet-derived growth factor
   B. Fibroblast growth factor
   C. Epidermal growth factor
   D. Transforming growth factor-α

7. **Cytoplasmic anti-neutrophil cytoplasmic antibodies (C-ANCA) is seen in:**
   A. Polyarteritis nodosa
   B. Wegener's granulomatosis
   C. Leucocytoclastic vasculitis
   D. Giant cell arteritis

8. **Biopsy of affected artery in the following condition is not only of diagnostic valve but also cures the main symptom of the patient:**
   A. Giant cell arteritis
   B. Takayasu's arteritis
   C. Kawasaki disease
   D. Raynaud's disease

9. **The most common site of involvement of atherosclerotic aneurysm is:**
   A. Arch of aorta
   B. Thoracic aorta
   C. Suprarenal abdominal aorta
   D. Infrarenal abdominal aorta

10. **The most common cause of dissecting haematoma is:**
    A. Cystic medial necrosis of Erdheim
    B. Trauma during cardiac catheterisation
    C. Systemic hypertension
    D. Marfan syndrome

11. **Dissecting haematoma causes separation of aortic wall as under:**
    A. Between intima and media
    B. Between inner third of media and outer two-third of media
    C. Between inner two-third of media and outer one-third
    D. Between media and adventitia

12. **In Kaposi's sarcoma, the lesions are more extensively distributed at different body sites and visceral organs in:**
    A. Classic (European) type
    B. African (Endemic) type
    C. AIDS-associated
    D. Renal transplant-associated

13. **Hyperplastic arteriosclerosis is seen in all except:**
    A. Haemolytic uraemic syndrome
    B. Benign nephrosclerosis
    C. Toxaemia of pregnancy
    D. Scleroderma

14. **Medial calcific sclerosis is a type of:**
    A. Dystrophic calcification
    B. Metastatic calcification
    C. Both metastatic and dystrophic calcification
    D. Neither metastatic nor dystrophic calcification

15. **Familial Hypercholesterolaemia is:**
    A. Autosomal recessive
    B. X-linked recessive
    C. Autosomal co-dominant
    D. Non-Mendelian disorder

16. **According to monoclonal hypothesis, the primary event in atherosclerosis is:**
    A. Monoclonal proliferation of endothelial cells

B. Monoclonal proliferation of smooth muscle cells
C. Monoclonal proliferation of monocytes
D. Monoclonal proliferation of foam cells

17. **All of the following may act as precursor of atheromatous plaque except:**
    A. Fatty streak   B. Fatty dots
    C. Gelatinous lesions   D. Fibrous plaque

18. **Huebner's arteritis is:**
    A. Endarteritis obliterans   B. Cerebral syphilitic arteritis
    C. Hypersensitivity vasculitis   D. Giant cell arteritis

19. **Pulseless disease is:**
    A. Temporal arteritis   B. Kawasaki's disease
    C. Takayasu arteritis   D. Buerger's disease

20. **DeBakey and Stanford classification systems are used for the categorisation of:**
    A. Arteritis   B. Dissecting aneurysm
    C. Vascular tumours   D. Arteriosclerosis

KEY

1 = D	2 = B	3 = A	4 = B	5 = D
6 = A	7 = B	8 = A	9 = D	10 = C
11 = C	12 = C	13 = B	14 = A	15 = C
16 = B	17 = D	18 = B	19 = C	20 = B

14 The Heart

ANATOMY AND PHYSIOLOGY

Average weight of the heart in an adult male is 300-350 gm while that of an adult female is 250-300 gm. Heart is divided into four chambers: a right and a left atrium both lying superiorly, and a right and a left ventricle both lying inferiorly and are larger. The atria are separated by a thin interatrial partition called *interatrial septum*, while the ventricles are separated by thick muscular partition called *interventricular septum*. The thickness of the right ventricular wall is 0.3 to 0.5 cm while that of the left ventricular wall is 1.3 to 1.5 cm. The blood in the heart chambers moves in a carefully prescribed pathway: venous blood from systemic circulation → right atrium → right ventricle → pulmonary arteries → lungs → pulmonary veins → left atrium → left ventricle → aorta → systemic arterial supply.

The transport of blood is regulated by cardiac valves: two loose flap-like atrioventricular valves, tricuspid on the right and mitral (bicuspid) on the left; and two semilunar valves with three leaflets each, the pulmonary and aortic valves, guarding the outflow tracts. The normal circumference of the valvular openings measures about 12 cm in tricuspid, 8.5 cm in pulmonary, 10 cm in mitral and 7.5 cm in aortic valve.

Wall of the heart consists mainly of the *myocardium* which is covered externally by thin membrane, the *epicardium* or visceral pericardium, and lined internally by another thin layer, the *endocardium*.

MYOCARDIAL BLOOD SUPPLY

The cardiac muscle, in order to function properly, must receive adequate supply of oxygen and nutrients. Blood is transported to myocardial cells by the coronary arteries which originate immediately above the aortic semilunar valve. Most of blood flow to the myocardium occurs during diastole. There are three major coronary trunks, each supplying blood to specific segments of the heart:

1. The **anterior descending branch of the left coronary artery,** commonly called **LAD** (left anterior descending coronary) supplies most of the apex of the heart, the anterior surface of the left ventricle, the adjacent third of the anterior wall of the right ventricle, and the anterior two-third of the interventricular septum.

2. The **circumflex branch of the left coronary artery,** commonly called **LCX** (left circumflex coronary) supplies the left atrium and a small portion of the lateral aspect of the left ventricle.

3. The **right coronary artery,** abbreviated as **RCA** supplies the right atrium, the remainder of the anterior surface of the right ventricle, the adjacent half of the posterior wall of the left ventricle and the posterior third of the interventricular septum.

There are 3 anatomic patterns of distribution of the coronary blood supply, depending upon which coronary artery crosses the crux. *Crux* is the region on the posterior surface of the heart where all the four cardiac chambers and the interatrial and interventricular septa meet. These patterns are as under:

◈ Right coronary artery preponderance
◈ Balanced cardiac circulation
◈ Left coronary preponderance

Coronary veins run parallel to the major coronary arteries to collect blood after the cellular needs of the heart are met. Subsequently, these veins drain into the *coronary sinus*.

HEART FAILURE *(p. 399)*

DEFINITION

Heart failure is defined as the pathophysiologic state in which impaired cardiac function is unable to maintain an adequate circulation for the metabolic needs of the tissues of the body. It may be *acute* or *chronic*. The term congestive heart failure (CHF) is used for the chronic form of heart failure in which the patient has evidence of congestion of peripheral circulation and of lungs.

ETIOLOGY *(p. 399)*

1. INTRINSIC PUMP FAILURE The most common and most important cause of heart failure is weakening of the ventricular muscle due to disease so that the heart fails to act as an efficient pump.
i)   Ischaemic heart disease
ii) Myocarditis
iii) Cardiomyopathies
iv) Metabolic disorders e.g. beriberi
v)   Disorders of the rhythm e.g. atrial fibrillation and flutter.

2. INCREASED WORKLOAD ON THE HEART Increased mechanical load on the heart results in increased myocardial demand resulting in myocardial failure.

i) Increased pressure load:
a) Systemic and pulmonary arterial hypertension.
b) Valvular disease e.g. mitral stenosis, aortic stenosis, pulmonary stenosis.
c) Chronic lung diseases.

ii) Increased volume load:
a) Valvular insufficiency
b) Severe anaemia
c) Thyrotoxicosis
d) Arteriovenous shunts
e) Hypoxia due to lung diseases.

3. IMPAIRED FILLING OF CARDIAC CHAMBERS Decreased cardiac output and cardiac failure may result from extra-cardiac causes or defect in filling of the heart:
a) Cardiac tamponade e.g. haemopericardium, hydropericardium
b) Constrictive pericarditis.

TYPES OF HEART FAILURE *(p. 399)*

Heart failure may be acute or chronic, right-sided or left-sided, and forward or backward failure.

ACUTE AND CHRONIC HEART FAILURE

Depending upon whether the heart failure develops rapidly or slowly, it may be acute or chronic.

Acute heart failure Sudden and rapid development of heart failure occurs in the following conditions:
i)   Larger myocardial infarction
ii) Valve rupture

iii) Cardiac tamponade
iv) Massive pulmonary embolism
v) Acute viral myocarditis
vi) Acute bacterial toxaemia.

Chronic heart failure More often, heart failure develops slowly as observed in the following states:
i) Myocardial ischaemia from atherosclerotic coronary artery disease
ii) Multivalvular heart disease
iii) Systemic arterial hypertension
iv) Chronic lung diseases resulting in hypoxia and pulmonary arterial hypertension
v) Progression of acute into chronic failure.

LEFT-SIDED AND RIGHT-SIDED HEART FAILURE

Though heart as an organ eventually fails as a whole, but functionally, the left and right heart act as independent units.

Left-sided heart failure:
i) Systemic hypertension
ii) Mitral or aortic valve disease (stenosis)
iii) Ischaemic heart disease
iv) Myocardial diseases e.g. cardiomyopathies, myocarditis.
v) Restrictive pericarditis.
   The clinical manifestations of left-sided heart failure result from decreased left ventricular output and hence there is accumulation of fluid *upstream* in the lungs. Accordingly, the major pathologic changes are as under:
i) Pulmonary congestion and oedema causes dyspnoea and orthopnoea.
ii) Decreased left ventricular output causing hypoperfusion and diminished oxygenation of tissues e.g. in kidneys causing ischaemic acute tubular necrosis, in brain causing hypoxic encephalopathy, and in skeletal muscles causing muscular weakness and fatigue.

Right-sided heart failure:
i) As a consequence of left ventricular failure.
ii) Cor pulmonale in which right heart failure occurs due to intrinsic lung diseases.
iii) Pulmonary or tricuspid valvular disease.
iv) Pulmonary hypertension secondary to pulmonary thromboembolism.
v) Myocardial disease affecting right heart.
vi) Congenital heart disease with left-to-right shunt.
   Whatever be the underlying cause, the clinical manifestations of right-sided heart failure are *upstream* of the right heart such as systemic (due to caval blood) and portal venous congestion, and reduced cardiac output. Accordingly, the pathologic changes are as under:
i) Systemic venous congestion in different tissues and organs e.g. subcutaneous oedema on dependent parts, passive congestion of the liver, spleen, and kidneys, ascites, hydrothorax, congestion of leg veins and neck veins.
ii) Reduced cardiac output resulting in circulatory stagnation causing anoxia, cyanosis and coldness of extremities.

BACKWARD AND FORWARD HEART FAILURE

Backward heart failure According to this concept, either of the ventricles fails to eject blood normally, resulting in rise of end-diastolic volume in the ventricle and increase in volume and pressure in the atrium which is transmitted *backward* producing elevated pressure in the veins.

Forward heart failure According to this hypothesis, clinical manifestations result directly from failure of the heart to pump blood causing diminished flow of blood to the tissues, especially diminished renal perfusion and activation of renin-angiotensin-aldosterone system.

In order to maintain normal cardiac output, several compensatory mechanisms play a role as under:

◈ Compensatory enlargement in the form of *cardiac hypertrophy, cardiac dilatation, or both.*

◈ *Tachycardia* (i.e. increased heart rate) due to activation of neurohumoral system e.g: release of norepinephrine and atrial natrouretic peptide, activation of renin-angiotensin-aldosterone mechanism.

CARDIAC HYPERTROPHY

Hypertrophy of the heart is defined as an increase in size and weight of the myocardium. It generally results from increased pressure load while increased volume load (e.g. valvular incompetence) results in hypertrophy with dilatation of the affected chamber due to regurgitation of the blood through incompetent valve.

CAUSES

Left ventricular hypertrophy:
i)   Systemic hypertension
ii)   Aortic stenosis and insufficiency
iii) Mitral insufficiency
iv)   Coarctation of the aorta
v)   Occlusive coronary artery disease
vi)   Congenital anomalies like septal defects and patent ductus arteriosus
vii) Conditions with increased cardiac output e.g. thyrotoxicosis, anaemia, arteriovenous fistulae.

Right ventricular hypertrophy:
i)   Pulmonary stenosis and insufficiency
ii)   Tricuspid insufficiency
iii) Mitral stenosis and/or insufficiency
iv)   Chronic lung diseases e.g. chronic emphysema, bronchiectasis, pneumoconiosis, pulmonary vascular disease etc.
v)   Left ventricular hypertrophy and failure of the left ventricle.

CARDIAC DILATATION

Quite often, hypertrophy of the heart is accompanied by cardiac dilatation. Stress leading to accumulation of excessive volume of blood in a chamber of the heart causes increase in length of myocardial fibres and hence cardiac dilatation as a compensatory mechanism.

CAUSES

i)   Valvular insufficiency (mitral and/or aortic insufficiency in left ventricular dilatation, tricuspid and/or pulmonary insufficiency in right ventricular dilatation)
ii)   Left-to-right shunts e.g. in VSD
iii) Conditions with high cardiac output e.g. thyrotoxicosis, arteriovenous shunt
iv)   Myocardial diseases e.g. cardiomyopathies, myocarditis
v)   Systemic hypertension.

MORPHOLOGIC FEATURES

Hypertrophy of the myocardium without dilatation is referred to as *concentric*, and when associated with dilatation is called *eccentric*. The weight of the heart is increased above normal, often over 500 gm. However, excessive epicardial fat is not indicative of true hypertrophy.

G/A Thickness of the left ventricular wall (excluding trabeculae carneae and papillary muscles) above 15 mm is indicative of significant hypertrophy. In concentric hypertrophy, the lumen of the chamber is smaller than usual, while in eccentric hypertrophy the lumen is dilated.

M/E There is increase in size of individual muscle fibres. There may be multiple minute foci of degenerative changes and necrosis in the hyper-trophied myocardium.

CONGENITAL HEART DISEASE *(p. 402)*

Congenital heart disease is the abnormality of the heart present from birth. It is the most common and important form of heart disease in the early years of life and is present in about 0.5% of newborn children. The incidence is higher in premature infants.

CLASSIFICATION Congenital anomalies of the heart may be either *shunts* (left-to-right or right-to-left), or defects causing *obstructions* to flow. However, complex anomalies involving *combinations* of shunts and obstructions are also often present.

I. MALPOSITIONS OF THE HEART *(p. 403)*

Dextrocardia is the condition when the apex of the heart points to the right side of the chest.

II. SHUNTS (CYANOTIC CONGENITAL HEART DISEASE) *(p. 403)*

A. LEFT-TO-RIGHT SHUNTS (ACYANOTIC OR LATE CYANOTIC GROUP)

In conditions where there is shunting of blood from left-to-right side of the heart, there is volume overload on the right heart producing pulmonary hypertension and right ventricular hypertrophy.

VENTRICULAR SEPTAL DEFECT (VSD) VSD is the most common congenital anomaly of the heart and comprises about 30% of all congenital heart diseases.

Depending upon the location of the defect, VSD may be of the following types:
1. In 90% of cases, the defect involves *membranous septum* and is very close to the bundle of His.
2. The remaining 10% cases have VSD immediately below the pulmonary valve (*subpulmonic*), below the aortic valve (*subaortic*).

MORPHOLOGIC FEATURES The *effects* of VSD are as under:
i) Volume hypertrophy of the right ventricle.
ii) Enlargement and haemodynamic changes in the tricuspid and pulmonary valves.
iii) Endocardial hypertrophy of the right ventricle.
iv) Pressure hypertrophy of the right atrium.
v) Volume hypertrophy of the left atrium and left ventricle.
vi) Enlargement and haemodynamic changes in the mitral and aortic valves.

ATRIAL SEPTAL DEFECT (ASD) Isolated ASD comprises about 10% of congenital heart diseases.

Depending upon the location of the defect, there are 3 types of ASD:

i) **Fossa ovalis type or ostium secundum type** is the most common form comprising about 90% cases of ASD.

ii) **Ostium primum type** comprises about 5% cases of ASD. The defect lies low in the interatrial septum adjacent to atrioventricular valves.

iii) **Sinus venosus type** accounts for about 5% cases of ASD. The defect is located high in the interatrial septum near the entry of the superior vena cava.

MORPHOLOGIC FEATURES The *effects* of ASD are as follows:
i) Volume hypertrophy of the right atrium and right ventricle.
ii) Enlargement and haemodynamic changes of tricuspid and pulmonary valves.
iii) Focal or diffuse endocardial hypertrophy of the right atrium and right ventricle.

iv) Volume atrophy of the left atrium and left ventricle.
v) Small-sized mitral and aortic orifices.

PATENT DUCTUS ARTERIOSUS (PDA) Normally, the ductus closes functionally within the first or second day of life. Its persistence after 3 months of age is considered abnormal. In about 90% of cases, it occurs as an isolated defect, while in the remaining cases it may be associated with other anomalies like VSD, coarctation of aorta and pulmonary or aortic stenosis.

MORPHOLOGIC FEATURES The *effects* of PDA on heart are as follows:
i) Volume hypertrophy of the left atrium and left ventricle.
ii) Enlargement and haemodynamic changes of the mitral and pulmonary valves.
iii) Enlargement of the ascending aorta.

B. RIGHT-TO-LEFT SHUNTS (CYANOTIC GROUP)

In conditions where there is shunting of blood from right side to the left side of the heart, there is entry of poorly-oxygenated blood into systemic circulation resulting in early cyanosis.

TETRALOGY OF FALLOT Tetralogy of Fallot is the most common cyanotic congenital heart disease, found in about 10% of children with anomalies of the heart.

MORPHOLOGIC FEATURES The four features of tetralogy are as under:
i) Ventricular septal defect (VSD) *('shunt')*.
ii) Displacement of the aorta to right so that it overrides the VSD.
iii) Pulmonary stenosis *('obstruction')*.
iv) Right ventricular hypertrophy.

There are two forms of tetralogy:

a) Cyanotic tetralogy The *effects* on the heart are as follows:
i) Pressure hypertrophy of the right atrium and right ventricle.
ii) Smaller and abnormal tricuspid valve.
iii) Smaller left atrium and left ventricle.
iv) Enlarged aortic orifice.

b) Acyanotic tetralogy The *effects* on the heart are as under:
i) Pressure hypertrophy of the left ventricle and right atrium.
ii) Volume hypertrophy of the left atrium and left ventricle.
iii) Enlargement of mitral and aortic orifices.

TRANSPOSITION OF GREAT ARTERIES The term transposition is used for complex malformations as regards position of the aorta, pulmonary trunk, atrioventricular orifices and the position of atria in relation to ventricles.

MORPHOLOGIC FEATURES These are as under:

i) Regular transposition is the most common type. In this, the aorta which is normally situated to the right and posterior with respect to the pulmonary trunk, is instead displaced anteriorly and to right.

ii) Corrected transposition is an uncommon anomaly. There is complete transposition of the great arteries with aorta arising from the right ventricle and the pulmonary trunk from the left ventricle.

III. OBSTRUCTIONS (OBSTRUCTIVE CONGENITAL HEART DISEASE) *(p. 406)*

Congenital obstruction to blood flow may result from obstruction in the aorta due to narrowing (*coarctation of aorta*), obstruction to outflow from the left ventricle (*aortic stenosis and atresia*), and obstruction to outflow from the right ventricle (*pulmonary stenosis and atresia*).

COARCTATION OF AORTA The word 'coarctation' means contracted or compressed. Coarctation of aorta is localised narrowing in any part of aorta, but the constriction is more often just distal to ductus arteriosus (*postductal or adult*), or occasionally proximal to the ductus arteriosus (*preductal or infantile type*) in the region of transverse aorta.

MORPHOLOGIC FEATURES The two common forms of coarctation of the aorta are as under:

i) Postductal or adult type The obstruction is just distal to the point of entry of ductus arteriosus which is often closed. In the stenotic segment, the aorta is drawn in as if a suture has been tied around it.

ii) Preductal or infantile type The narrowing is proximal to the ductus arteriosus which usually remains patent.

AORTIC STENOSIS AND ATRESIA The most common congenital anomaly of the aorta is bicuspid aortic valve which does not have much functional significance but predisposes it to calcification.

MORPHOLOGIC FEATURES Congenital aortic stenosis may be of three types:

i) Valvular stenosis The aortic valve cusps are malformed and are irregularly thickened.

ii) Subvalvular stenosis There is thick fibrous ring under the aortic valve causing subaortic stenosis.

iii) Supravalvular stenosis The most uncommon type, there is fibrous constriction above the sinuses of Valsalva.

PULMONARY STENOSIS AND ATRESIA Isolated pulmonary stenosis and atresia do not cause cyanosis and hence are included under acyanotic heart diseases.

MORPHOLOGIC FEATURES These are as under:

Pulmonary stenosis It may occur as a component of tetralogy of Fallot or as an isolated defect. Pulmonary stenosis is caused by fusion of cusps of the pulmonary valve forming a diaphragm-like obstruction.

Pulmonary atresia There is no communication between the right ventricle and lungs so that the blood bypasses the right ventricle through an interatrial septal defect.

ISCHAEMIC HEART DISEASE *(p. 407)*

Ischaemic heart disease (IHD) is defined as acute or chronic form of cardiac disability arising from imbalance between the myocardial supply and demand for oxygenated blood. Alternate term *'coronary artery disease (CAD)'* is used synonymously with IHD. As per rising trends of IHD worldwide, it is estimated that by the year 2020 it would become the most common cause of death throughout world.

ETIOPATHOGENESIS *(p. 407)*

IHD is invariably caused by disease affecting the coronary arteries, the most prevalent being atherosclerosis accounting for more than 90% cases, while other causes are responsible for less than 10% cases of IHD.

I. CORONARY ATHEROSCLEROSIS

Coronary atherosclerosis resulting in 'fixed' obstruction is the major cause of IHD in more than 90% cases.

1. Distribution Atherosclerotic lesions in coronary arteries are distributed in one or more of the three major coronary arterial trunks, the highest incidence being in the anterior descending branch of the left coronary (LAD), followed in decreasing frequency, by the right coronary artery (RCA) and still less in circumflex branch of the left coronary (CXA).

2. Location Almost all adults show atherosclerotic plaques scattered throughout the coronary arterial system. However, significant stenotic lesions that may produce chronic myocardial ischaemia show more than

75% (three-fourth) reduction in the cross-sectional area of a coronary artery or its branch.

3. **Fixed atherosclerotic plaques** The atherosclerotic plaques in the coronaries are more often eccentrically located bulging into the lumen from one side. Occasionally, there may be concentric thickening of the wall of the artery. Atherosclerosis produces gradual luminal narrowing that may eventually lead to 'fixed' coronary obstruction.

II. SUPERADDED CHANGES IN CORONARY ATHEROSCLEROSIS

The attacks of *acute coronary syndromes,* which include acute myocardial infarction, unstable angina and sudden ischaemic death, are precipitated by certain changes superimposed on a pre-existing fixed coronary athero-matous plaque.

1. **Acute changes in chronic atheromatous plaque** Though chronic fixed obstructions are the most frequent cause of IHD, acute coronary episodes are often precipitated by sudden changes in chronic plaques such as plaque haemorrhage, fissuring, or ulceration that results in thrombosis and embolisation of atheromatous debris.

2. **Coronary artery thrombosis** Transmural acute myocardial infarction is often precipitated by partial or complete coronary thrombosis. The initiation of thrombus occurs due to surface ulceration of fixed chronic atheromatous plaque, ultimately causing complete luminal occlusion.

3. **Local platelet aggregation and coronary artery spasm** Some cases of acute coronary episodes are caused by local aggregates of platelets on the atheromatous plaque, short of forming a thrombus.

III. NON-ATHEROSCLEROTIC CAUSES

Several other coronary lesions may cause IHD in less than 10% of cases.
1. Vasospasm
2. Stenosis of coronary ostia
3. Arteritis
4. Embolism
5. Thrombotic diseases
6. Trauma
7. Aneurysms
8. Compression

EFFECTS OF MYOCARDIAL ISCHAEMIA *(p. 408)*

Depending upon the suddenness of onset, duration, degree, location and extent of the area affected by myocardial ischaemia, the range of changes and clinical features may range from an asymptomatic state at one extreme to immediate mortality at another:
A. Asymptomatic state
B. Angina pectoris (AP)
C. Acute myocardial infarction (MI)
D. Chronic ischaemic heart disease (CIHD)/Ischaemic cardiomyopathy/ Myocardial fibrosis
E. Sudden cardiac death
    The term *acute coronary syndromes* include a triad of acute myocardial infarction, unstable angina and sudden cardiac death.

ANGINA PECTORIS

Angina pectoris is a clinical syndrome of IHD resulting from transient myocardial ischaemia. It is characterised by paroxysmal pain in the substernal or precordial region of the chest which is aggravated by an increase in the demand of the heart and relieved by a decrease in the work of the heart. Often, the pain radiates to the left arm, neck, jaw or right arm. It is more common in men past 5th decade of life.

There are 3 overlapping clinical patterns of angina pectoris with some differences in their pathogenesis:

STABLE OR TYPICAL ANGINA This is the most common pattern. Stable or typical angina is characterised by attacks of pain following physical exertion or emotional excitement and is relieved by rest. The pathogenesis of condition lies in *chronic stenosing coronary atherosclerosis* that cannot perfuse the myocardium adequately when the workload on the heart increases.

PRINZMETAL'S VARIANT ANGINA This pattern of angina is characterised by pain at rest and has no relationship with physical activity. The exact pathogenesis of Prinzmetal's angina is not known. It may occur due to *sudden vasospasm* of a coronary trunk induced by coronary atherosclerosis, or may be due to release of humoral vasoconstrictors.

UNSTABLE OR CRESCENDO ANGINA Also referred to as 'pre-infarction angina' or 'acute coronary insufficiency', this is the most serious pattern of angina. It is characterised by more frequent onset of pain of prolonged duration and occurring often at rest. It is thus indicative of an impending acute myocardial infarction.

ACUTE MYOCARDIAL INFARCTION

Acute myocardial infarction (MI) is the most important and feared consequence of coronary artery disease. A significant factor that may prevent or diminish the myocardial damage is the development of collateral circulation through anastomotic channels over a period of time. A regular and well-planned exercise programme encourages good collateral circulation and improved cardiac performance.

INCIDENCE In developed countries, acute MI accounts for 10-25% of all deaths. Due to the dominant etiologic role of coronary atherosclerosis in acute MI, the incidence of acute MI correlates well with the incidence of atherosclerosis in a geographic area.

Age Acute MI may virtually occur at all ages, though the incidence is higher in the elderly.

Sex Males throughout their life are at a significantly higher risk of developing acute MI as compared to females. Women during reproductive period have remarkably low incidence of acute MI, probably due to the protective influence of oestrogen.

ETIOPATHOGENESIS The etiologic role of severe coronary atherosclerosis (more than 75% compromise of lumen) of one or more of the three major coronary arterial trunks in the pathogenesis of about 90% cases of acute MI is well documented by autopsy studies as well as by coronary angiographic studies.

1. **Myocardial ischaemia** Myocardial ischaemia is brought about by one or more of the following mechanisms:
i) Diminished coronary blood flow e.g. in coronary artery disease, shock.
ii) Increased myocardial demand e.g. in exercise, emotions.
iii) Hypertrophy of the heart without simultaneous increase of coronary blood flow e.g. in hypertension, valvular heart disease.

2. **Role of platelets** Rupture of an atherosclerotic plaque exposes the subendothelial collagen to platelets which undergo aggregation, activation and release reaction.

3. **Acute plaque rupture** But acute complications in coronary atherosclerotic plaques in the form of superimposed coronary thrombosis due to plaque rupture and plaque haemorrhage is frequently encountered in cases of acute MI:
i) *Superimposed coronary thrombosis* due to disruption of plaque is seen in about half the cases of acute MI. Infusion of intracoronary fibrinolysins in the first half an hour of development of acute MI in such cases restores blood flow in the blocked vessel in majority of cases.
ii) *Intramural haemorrhage* is found in about one-third cases of acute MI.

4. Non-atherosclerotic causes About 10% cases of acute MI are caused by non-atherosclerotic factors such as coronary vasospasm, arteritis, coronary ostial stenosis, embolism, thrombotic diseases, trauma and outside compression as already described.

5. Transmural *versus* subendocardial infarcts There are some differences in the pathogenesis of the *transmural infarcts* involving the full thickness of ventricular wall and the *subendocardial (laminar) infarcts* affecting the inner subendocardial one-third to half. These are as under:

i) *Transmural (full thickness) infarcts* are the most common type seen in 95% cases. Critical coronary narrowing (more than 75% compromised lumen) is of great significance in the causation of such infarcts.

ii) *Subendocardial (laminar) infarcts* have their genesis in reduced coronary perfusion due to coronary atherosclerosis but without critical stenosis (not necessarily 75% compromised lumen), aortic stenosis or haemorrhagic shock.

TYPES OF INFARCTS Infarcts have been classified in a number of ways by the physicians and the pathologists:

1. *According to the anatomic region of the left ventricle involved,* they are called anterior, posterior (inferior), lateral, septal and circumferential, and their combinations like anterolateral, posterolateral (or inferolateral) and anteroseptal.

2. *According to the degree of thickness of the ventricular wall involved,* infarcts are of two types:

i) Full-thickness or transmural, when they involve the entire thickness of the ventricular wall.

ii) Subendocardial or laminar, when they occupy the inner subendocardial half of the myocardium.

3. *According to the age of infarcts,* they are of two types:

i) Newly-formed infarcts called as acute, recent or fresh.

ii) Advanced infarcts called as old, healed or organised.

LOCATION OF INFARCTS Infarcts are most frequently located in the left ventricle. Right ventricle is less susceptible to infarction due to its thin wall, having less metabolic requirements and is thus adequately nourished by the thebesian vessels. Atrial infarcts, whenever present, are more often in the right atrium, usually accompanying the infarct of the left ventricle. Left atrium is relatively protected from infarction because it is supplied by the oxygenated blood in the left atrial chamber.

The region of infarction depends upon the area of obstructed blood supply by one or more of the three coronary arterial trunks. Accordingly, there are three regions of myocardial infarction:

1. *Stenosis of the left anterior descending coronary artery* is the most common (40-50%). The region of infarction is the anterior part of the left ventricle including the apex and the anterior two-thirds of the interventricular septum.

2. *Stenosis of the right coronary artery* is the next most frequent (30-40%). It involves the posterior part of the left ventricle and the posterior one-third of the interventricular septum.

3. *Stenosis of the left circumflex coronary artery* is seen least frequently (15-20%). Its area of involvement is the lateral wall of the left ventricle.

G/A As explained above, they are found most often in the left ventricle. The transmural infarcts, which by definition involve the entire thickness of the ventricular wall, usually have a thin rim of preserved subendocardial myocardium which is perfused directly by the blood in the ventricular chamber. The subendocardial infarcts which affect the inner subendocardial half of the myocardium produce less well-defined gross changes than the transmural infarcts.

1. *In 6 to 12 hours old infarcts,* no striking gross changes are discernible except that the affected myocardium is slightly paler and drier than normal. However, the early infarcts (3 to 6 hours old) can be detected by histo-chemical staining for *dehydrogenases* on unfixed slice of the heart. This consists of immersing a slice of unfixed heart in the solution of triphe-

nyltetrazolium chloride (TTC) which imparts red brown colour to the normal heart muscle, while the area of infarcted muscle fails to stain due to lack of dehydrogenases.

2. *By about 24 hours,* the infarct develops cyanotic, red-purple, blotchy areas of haemorrhage.

3. *During the next 48 to 72 hours,* the infarct develops a yellow border.

4. *In 3-7 days,* the infarct has hyperaemic border while the centre is yellow and soft.

5. *By 10 days,* the periphery of the infarct appears reddish-purple due to growth of granulation tissue. With the passage of time, further healing takes place; the necrotic muscle is resorbed and the infarct shrinks and becomes pale grey.

6. *By the end of 6 weeks,* the infarcted area is replaced by a thin, grey-white, hard, shrunken fibrous scar which is well developed in about 2 to 3 months.

M/E Sequential time-lined changes are as under:

1. First week

i) In the *first 6 hours* after infarction, usually no detectable histologic change is observed in routine light microscopy. However, some investigators have described stretching and waviness of the myocardial fibres within one hour of the onset of ischaemia.

ii) *After 6 hours,* there is appearance of some oedema fluid between the myocardial fibres.

iii) By *12 hours,* coagulative necrosis of the myocardial fibres sets in and neutrophils begin to appear at the margin of the infarct.

iv) During *first 24 hours,* coagulative necrosis progresses further as evidenced by shrunken eosinophilic cytoplasm and pyknosis of the nuclei.

v) During *first 48 to 72 hours,* coagulative necrosis is complete with loss of nuclei. The neutrophilic infiltrate is well developed and extends centrally into the interstitium.

vi) *In 3-7 days,* neutrophils are necrosed and gradually disappear. The process of resorption of necrosed muscle fibres by macrophages begins. Simultaneously, there is onset of proliferation of capillaries and fibroblasts from the margins of the infarct.

2. Second week

i) By *10th day,* most of the necrosed muscle at the periphery of infarct is removed. The fibrovascular reaction at the margin of infarct is more prominent.

ii) By the *end of the 2nd week,* most of the necrosed muscle in small infarcts is removed, neutrophils have almost disappeared, and newly laid collagen fibres replace the periphery of the infarct.

3. Third week
Necrosed muscle fibres from larger infarcts continue to be removed and replaced by ingrowth of newly formed collagen fibres.

4. Fourth to sixth week
With further removal of necrotic tissue, there is increase in collagenous connective tissue, decreased vascularity and fewer pigmented macrophages, lymphocytes and plasma cells.

SALVAGE IN EARLY INFARCTS AND REPERFUSION INJURY
In vast majority of cases of acute MI, occlusive coronary artery thrombosis has been demonstrated superimposed on fibrofatty plaque. The ischaemic injury to myocardium is reversible if perfusion is restored within the first 30 minutes of onset of infarction failing which irreversible ischaemic necrosis of myocardium sets in. The salvage in early infarcts can be achieved by the following interventions:

1. Institution of *thrombolytic therapy* with thrombolytic agents.
2. *Percutaneous transluminal coronary angioplasty (PTCA).*
3. *Coronary artery stenting.*
4. *Coronary artery bypass surgery.*

However, late attempt at reperfusion is fraught with the risk of ischaemic reperfusion injury. Further myonecrosis during reperfusion occurs due to rapid influx of calcium ions and generation of toxic oxygen free radicals.

CHANGES IN EARLY INFARCTS These are as under:

1. Electron microscopic changes

i) Disappearance of perinuclear glycogen granules within 5 minutes of ischaemia.

ii) Swelling of mitochondria in 20 to 30 minutes.

iii) Disruption of sarcolemma.

iv) Nuclear alterations like peripheral clumping of nuclear chromatin.

2. Chemical and histochemical changes

i) Glycogen depletion in myocardial fibres within 30 to 60 minutes of infarction.

ii) Increase in lactic acid in the myocardial fibres.

iii) Loss of K^+ from the ischaemic fibres.

iv) Increase of Na^+ in the ischaemic cells.

v) Influx of Ca^{++} into the cells causing irreversible cell injury.

DIAGNOSIS The diagnosis of acute MI is made on the observations of 3 types of features:

1. Clinical features Typically, acute MI has a sudden onset.

i) Pain

ii) Indigestion

iii) Apprehension

iv) Shock

v) Oliguria

vi) Low grade fever

vii) Acute pulmonary oedema.

2. ECG changes The ECG changes are one of the most important parameters. Most characteristic ECG change is ST segment elevation in acute MI (termed as STEMI); other changes inlcude T wave inversion and appearance of wide deep Q waves.

3. Serum cardiac markers Certain proteins and enzymes are released into the blood from necrotic heart muscle after acute MI. Measurement of their levels in serum is helpful in making a diagnosis and plan management.

i) *Creatine phosphokinase (CK) and CK-MB* CK has three forms—

a) CK-MM derived from skeletal muscle;

b) CK-BB derived from brain and lungs; and

c) CK-MB, mainly from cardiac muscles and insignificant amount from extracardiac tissue.

Thus, total CK estimation lacks specificity while elevation of CK-MB isoenzyme is considerably specific for myocardial damage. CK-MB has further 2 forms—CK-MB2 is the myocardial form while CK-MB1 is extracardiac form. A ratio of CK-MB2: CK-MB1 above 1.5 is highly sensitive for the diagnosis of acute MI after 4-6 hours of onset of myocardial ischaemia. CK-MB disappears from blood by 48 hours.

ii) *Lactate dehydrogenase (LDH)* Total LDH estimation also lacks specificity since this enzyme is present in various tissues besides myocardium such as in skeletal muscle, kidneys, liver, lungs and red blood cells. However, like CK, LDH too has two isoforms of which LDH-1 is myocardial-specific. Estimation of ratio of LDH-1: LDH-2 above 1 is reasonably helpful in making a diagnosis. LDH levels begin to rise after 24 hours, reach peak in 3 to 6 days and return to normal in 14 days.

iii) *Cardiac-specific troponins (cTn)* Troponins are contractile muscle proteins present in human cardiac and skeletal muscle but cardiac troponins are specific for myocardium. There are two types of cTn:

a) cardiac troponin T (cTnT); and

b) cardiac troponin I (cTnI).

Both cTnT and cTnI are not found in the blood normally, but after myocardial injury their levels rise very high around the same time when CK-MB is elevated (i.e. after 4-6 hours). Both troponin levels remain high for much longer duration; cTnI for 7-10 days and cTnT for 10-14 days.

iv) *Myoglobin* Though myoglobin is the first cardiac marker to become elevated after myocardial infarction, it lacks cardiac specificity and is excreted in the urine rapidly. Its levels, thus, return to normal within 24 hours of attack of acute MI.

COMPLICATIONS Following an attack of acute MI, only 10-20% cases do not develop major complications and recover.
1. Arrhythmias
2. Congestive heart failure
3. Cardiogenic shock
4. Mural thrombosis and thromboembolism
5. Rupture
6. Cardiac aneurysm
7. Pericarditis
8. Postmyocardial infarction syndrome

CHRONIC ISCHAEMIC HEART DISEASE

Chronic ischaemic heart disease, ischaemic cardiomyopathy or myocardial fibrosis, are the terms used for focal or diffuse fibrosis in the myocardium characteristically found in elderly patients of progressive IHD. The patients generally have gradually developing CHF due to decompensation over a period of years.

ETIOPATHOGENESIS In majority of cases, coronary atherosclerosis causes progressive ischaemic myocardial damage and replacement by myocardial fibrosis. A small percentage of cases may result from other causes such as emboli, coronary arteritis and myocarditis.

G/A The heart may be normal in size or hypertrophied. The left ventricular wall generally shows foci of grey-white fibrosis in brown myocardium.

M/E Salient features are as under:
i) There are scattered areas of diffuse myocardial fibrosis, especially around the small blood vessels in the interstitial tissue of the myocardium.
ii) Intervening single fibres and groups of myocardial fibres show variation in fibre size and foci of myocytolysis.
iii) Areas of brown atrophy of the myocardium may also be present.
iv) Coronary arteries show atherosclerotic plaques and may have complicated lesions in the form of superimposed thrombosis.

SUDDEN CARDIAC DEATH

Sudden cardiac death is defined as sudden death within 24 hours of the onset of cardiac symptoms. The most important cause is coronary atherosclerosis; less commonly it may be due to coronary vasospasm and other non-ischaemic causes. The mechanism of sudden death by myocardial ischaemia is almost always by fatal arrhythmias, chiefly ventricular asystole or fibrillation.

G/A At autopsy, such cases reveal most commonly critical atherosclerotic coronary narrowing (more than 75% compromised lumen) in one or more of the three major coronary arterial trunks with superimposed thrombosis or plaque-haemorrhage.

HYPERTENSIVE HEART DISEASE *(p. 417)*

Hypertensive heart disease or hypertensive cardiomyopathy is the disease of the heart resulting from systemic hypertension of prolonged duration and manifesting by left ventricular hypertrophy. Even mild hypertension (blood pressure higher than 140/90 mmHg) of sufficient duration may induce hypertensive heart disease. It is the second most common form of heart disease after IHD. As already pointed out, hypertension predisposes to atherosclerosis.

PATHOGENESIS Stimulus to LVH is pressure overload in systemic hypertension. Both genetic and haemodynamic factors contribute to LVH. The stress of pressure on the ventricular wall causes increased production of myofilaments, myofibrils, other cell organelles and nuclear enlargement. Since the adult myocardial fibres do not divide, the fibres are hypertrophied.

G/A The most significant finding is marked hypertrophy of the heart, chiefly of the left ventricle. The weight of the heart increases to 500 gm or more (normal weight about 300 gm). The thickness of the left ventricular wall increases from its normal 13 to 15 mm up to 20 mm or more. The papillary muscles and trabeculae carneae are rounded and prominent. Initially, there is *concentric hypertrophy* of the left ventricle (without dilatation). But when decompensation and cardiac failure supervene, there is *eccentric hypertrophy* (with dilatation) with thinning of the ventricular wall and there may be dilatation and hypertrophy of right heart as well.

M/E The changes include enlargement and degeneration of myocardial fibres with focal areas of myocardial fibrosis.

COR PULMONALE *(p. 418)*

Cor pulmonale (*cor* = heart; *pulmonale* = lung) or pulmonary heart disease is the disease of right side of the heart resulting from disorders of the lungs. It is characterised by right ventricular dilatation or hypertrophy, or both. Thus, cor pulmonale is the right-sided counterpart of the hypertensive heart disease just described.

Depending upon the rapidity of development, cor pulmonale may be acute or chronic:

◈ *Acute cor pulmonale* occurs following massive pulmonary embolism resulting in sudden dilatation of the pulmonary trunk, conus and right ventricle.

◈ *Chronic cor pulmonale* is more common and is often preceded by chronic pulmonary hypertension. Following chronic lung diseases can cause chronic pulmonary hypertension and subsequent cor pulmonale:
   i)   Chronic emphysema
   ii) Chronic bronchitis
   iii) Pulmonary tuberculosis
   iv) Pneumoconiosis
   v)   Cystic fibrosis
   vi) Hyperventilation in marked obesity (Pickwickian syndrome)
   vii) Multiple organised pulmonary emboli.

PATHOGENESIS Chronic lung diseases as well as diseases of the pulmonary vessels cause increased pulmonary vascular resistance. The most common underlying mechanism causing increased pulmonary blood pressure (pulmonary hypertension) is by pulmonary vasoconstriction, activation of coagulation pathway and obliteration of pulmonary arterial vessels. Pulmonary hypertension causes pressure overload on the right ventricle and hence right ventricular enlargement.

G/A In *acute cor pulmonale,* there is characteristic ovoid dilatation of the right ventricle, and sometimes of the right atrium. In *chronic cor pulmonale,* there is increase in thickness of the right ventricular wall from its normal 3 to 5 mm up to 10 mm or more.

RHEUMATIC FEVER AND RHEUMATIC HEART DISEASE *(p. 418)*

DEFINITION

Rheumatic fever (RF) is a systemic, post-streptococcal, non-suppurative inflammatory disease, principally affecting the heart, joints, central nervous system, skin and subcutaneous tissues. The chronic stage of RF involves all the layers of the heart (pancarditis) causing major cardiac sequelae referred to as rheumatic heart disease (RHD). In spite of its name suggesting an acute arthritis migrating from joint to joint, it is the heart rather than the joints which is first and major organ affected. Decades ago, William Boyd gave the dictum *'rheumatism licks the joint, but bites the whole heart'.*

INCIDENCE

The disease appears most commonly in children between the age of 5 to 15 years when the streptococcal infection is most frequent and intense. Both the sexes are affected equally, though some investigators have noted a slight female preponderance.

The disease is seen more commonly in poor socioeconomic strata of the society living in damp and overcrowded places which promote interpersonal spread of the streptococcal infection. It is still common in the developing countries of the world, particularly prevalent in Indian subcontinent (India, Pakistan, Bangladesh, Nepal, Afghanistan), some Arab countries, sub-Saharan Africa and some South American countries. In India, RHD and RF continue to be a major public health problem.

ETIOPATHOGENESIS

After a long controversy, the etiologic role of preceding throat infection with β-haemolytic streptococci of group A in RF is now well accepted. However, the mechanism of lesions in the heart, joints and other tissues is not by direct infection but by induction of hypersensitivity or autoimmunity in a susceptible host. Thus, there are 3 types of factors in the etiology and pathogenesis of RF and RHD: *environmental factors, host susceptibility* and *immunologic evidences.*

A. ENVIRONMENTAL FACTORS Evidences in support are as under:
1. There is often a *history* of infection of the pharynx, upper respiratory tract with this microorganism about 2 to 3 weeks prior to the attack of RF.
2. *Subsequent or ongoing attacks* of streptococcal infection are generally associated with recurrent episodes of acute RF.
3. A higher incidence of RF has been observed after outbreaks and *epidemics* of streptococcal infection of throat in children.
4. Administration of *antibiotics* leads to lowering of the incidence.
5. Cardiac lesions similar to those seen in RHD have been produced in experimental animals by *induction* of repeated infection with β-haemolytic streptococci of group A.
6. *Socioeconomic factors* like poverty, poor nutrition, density of population, overcrowding in quarters for sleeping etc are associated with spread of infection.
7. The *geographic distribution* of the disease, as already pointed out, shows higher frequency and severity of the disease in the developing countries of the world where the living conditions in underprivileged populations are substandard and medical facilities are insufficient.
8. The incidence of the disease is higher in subtropical and tropical regions with cold, damp *climate* near the rivers and waterways which favour the spread of infection.

B. HOST SUSCEPTIBILITY Since all individuals with streptococcal infections do not develop RF, role of inherited characteristic for the disease has been reported:
1. Clustering of disease in *families.*
2. Occurrence in *identical twins.*
3. Individuals with *HLA class II* alleles have strong association with RF.
4. First-degree relatives of patients with RF and RHD have increased expression of a particular alloantigen.

C. IMMUNOLOGIC EVIDENCE Following evidences support immunologic injury:
1. Patients with RF have *elevated titres* of antibodies to the antigens of β-haemolytic streptococci of group A such as anti-streptolysin O (ASO) and S, anti-streptokinase, anti-streptohyaluronidase and anti-DNAase B.
2. *Cell wall polysaccharide* of group A *Streptococcus* forms antibodies which are reactive against cardiac valves.
3. *Hyaluronate capsule* of group A *Streptococcus* is identical to human hyaluronate present in joint tissues and thus these tissues are the target of attack.
4. *Membrane antigens* of group A *Streptococcus* react with sarcolemma of smooth and cardiac muscle, dermal fibroblasts and neurons of caudate nucleus.

A. CARDIAC LESIONS

The cardiac manifestations of RF are in the form of focal inflammatory involvement of the interstitial tissue of all the three layers of the heart, the so-called *pancarditis.* The pathognomonic feature of pancarditis in RF is the presence of distinctive *Aschoff nodules* or *Aschoff bodies.*

THE ASCHOFF NODULES OR BODIES The Aschoff nodules or the Aschoff bodies are spheroidal or fusiform distinct tiny structures, 1-2 mm in size, occurring in the interstitium of the heart in RF and may be visible to naked eye. Lesions similar to the Aschoff nodules may be found in the extracardiac tissues.

Evolution of fully-developed Aschoff bodies occurs through 3 stages:

1.   Early (exudative or degenerative) stage   The earliest sign of injury in the heart in RF is apparent by *about 4th week* of illness. Initially, there is oedema of the connective tissue and increase in acid mucopolysaccharide in the ground substance. Eventually, the collagen fibres are fragmented and disintegrated. This change is referred to as *fibrinoid degeneration.*

2. Intermediate (proliferative or granulomatous) stage   It is this stage of the Aschoff body which is pathognomonic of rheumatic conditions. This stage is apparent in 4th to 13th week of illness. The early stage of fibrinoid change is followed by proliferation of cells that includes infiltration by lymphocytes (mostly T cells), plasma cells, a few neutrophils and the characteristic *cardiac histiocytes (Anitschkow cells)* at the margin of the lesion. Some of these modified cardiac histiocytes become multinucleate cells containing 1 to 4 nuclei and are called *Aschoff cells* and are pathognomonic of RHD.

3. Late (healing or fibrous) stage   The stage of healing by fibrosis of the Aschoff nodule occurs in about *12 to 16 weeks* after the illness. The nodule becomes oval or fusiform in shape, about 200 µm wide and 600 µm long. These cells tend to be arranged in a palisaded manner. Eventually, it is replaced by a small fibrocollagenous scar with little cellularity, frequently in perivascular location.

1.   RHEUMATIC ENDOCARDITIS   Endocardial lesions of RF may involve the valvular and mural endocardium, causing *rheumatic valvulitis* and *mural endocarditis,* respectively.

RHEUMATIC VALVULITIS   *G/A* The valves in **acute RF** show thickening and loss of translucency of the valve leaflets or cusps. This is followed by the formation of characteristic, small (1 to 3 mm in diameter), multiple, warty *vegetations* or *verrucae,* chiefly along the line of closure of the leaflets and cusps.

Though all the four heart valves are affected, their frequency and severity of involvement varies: mitral valve alone being the most common site, followed in decreasing order of frequency, by combined mitral and aortic valve. The higher incidence of vegetations on left side of the heart is possibly because of the greater mechanical stresses on the valves of the left heart, especially along the line of closure of the valve cusps.

The **chronic stage of RHD** is characterised by permanent deformity of one or more valves, especially the mitral (in 98% cases alone or along with other valves) and aortic.

Gross appearance of chronic healed mitral valve in RHD is characteristically *'fish mouth'* or *'button hole'* stenosis. Mitral stenosis and insufficiency are commonly combined in chronic RHD; calcific aortic stenosis may also be found.

M/E The inflammatory changes begin in the region of the valve rings (where the leaflets are attached to the fibrous annulus) and then extend throughout the entire leaflet, whereas vegetations are usually located on the free margin of the leaflets and cusps.

i)   In the **early (acute) stage,** the histological changes are oedema of the valve leaflet, presence of increased number of capillaries and infiltration with lymphocytes, plasma cells, histiocytes with many Anitschkow cells and a few polymorphs.

ii) In the **healed (chronic) stage,** the vegetations have undergone organisation. The valves show diffuse thickening as a result of fibrous tissue with hyalinisation, and often calcification.

RHEUMATIC MURAL ENDOCARDITIS Mural endocardium may also show features of rheumatic carditis though the changes are less conspicuous as compared to valvular changes.

G/A The lesions are seen most commonly as *MacCallum's patch* which is the region of endocardial surface in the posterior wall of the left atrium just above the posterior leaflet of the mitral valve.

M/E The affected area shows oedema, fibrinoid change in the collagen, and cellular infiltrate of lymphocytes, plasma cells and macrophages with many Anitschkow cells.

2. RHEUMATIC MYOCARDITIS **G/A** In the *early (acute) stage,* the myocardium, especially of the left ventricle, is soft and flabby. In the *intermediate stage,* the interstitial tissue of the myocardium shows small foci of necrosis. Later, tiny pale foci of the Aschoff bodies may be visible throughout the myocardium.

M/E The most characteristic feature of rheumatic myocarditis is the presence of distinctive Aschoff bodies. These diagnostic nodules are scattered throughout the interstitial tissue of the myocardium and are most frequent in the interventricular septum, left ventricle and left atrium.

3. RHEUMATIC PERICARDITIS It commonly accompanies RHD.

G/A If the parietal pericardium is pulled off from the visceral pericardium, the two separated surfaces are shaggy due to thick fibrin covering them. This appearance is often likened to *'bread and butter appearance'*.

M/E Fibrin is identified on the surfaces. The subserosal connective tissue is infiltrated by lymphocytes, plasma cells, histiocytes and a few neutrophils. Characteristic Aschoff bodies may be seen which later undergo organisation and fibrosis.

B. EXTRACARDIAC LESIONS

1. POLYARTHRITIS Acute and painful inflammation of the synovial membranes of some of the joints, especially the larger joints of the limbs, is seen in about 90% cases of RF in adults and less often in children. As pain and swelling subside in one joint, others tend to get involved, producing the characteristic *'migratory polyarthritis'* involving two or more joints at a time.

2. SUBCUTANEOUS NODULES The subcutaneous nodules of RF occur more often in children than in adult. These nodules are small (0.5 to 2 cm in diameter), spherical or ovoid and painless. They are attached to deeper structures like tendons, ligaments, fascia or periosteum and therefore often remain unnoticed by the patient.

3. ERYTHEMA MARGINATUM This non-pruritic erythematous rash is characteristic of RF. The lesions occur mainly on the trunk and proximal parts of the extremities.

4. RHEUMATIC ARTERITIS Arteritis in RF involves not only the coronary arteries and the aorta but also occurs in arteries of various other organs such as renal, mesenteric and cerebral arteries.

5. CHOREA MINOR Chorea minor or Sydenham's chorea or Saint Vitus' dance is a delayed manifestation of RF as a result of involvement of the central nervous system.

6. RHEUMATIC PNEUMONITIS AND PLEURITIS Involvement of the lungs and pleura occurs rarely in RF. Pleuritis is often accompanied with serofibrinous pleural effusion.

CLINICAL FEATURES AND PROGNOSIS

The first attack of acute RF generally appears 2 to 3 weeks after streptococcal pharyngitis, most often in children between the age of 5 to 15 years. With subsequent streptococcal pharyngitis, there is reactivation of the disease and similar clinical manifestations appear with each recurrent attack. The disease generally presents with migratory polyarthritis and fever.

Clinical **diagnosis of RF** and RHD is made in a case with antecedent laboratory evidence of streptococcal throat infection in the presence of *any two of the major criteria, or occurrence of one major and two minor criteria.*

The long-term sequelae or **stigmata** are the chronic valvular deformities, especially the mitral stenosis, as already just explained.

The major **causes of death** in RHD are cardiac failure, bacterial endocarditis and embolism:

NON-RHEUMATIC ENDOCARDITIS (p. 424)

Several workers designate endocarditis on the basis of anatomic area of the involved endocardium such as: *valvular* for valvular endocardium, *mural* for inner lining of the lumina of cardiac chambers, *chordal* for the endocardium of the chordae tendineae. Endocarditis can be broadly grouped into *non-infective* and *infective* types. Most types of endocarditis are characterised by the presence of 'vegetations' or 'verrucae' which have distinct features.

ATYPICAL VERRUCOUS (LIBMAN-SACKS) ENDOCARDITIS (p. 424)

Libman and Sacks, two American physicians, described a form of endocarditis in 1924 that is characterised by sterile endocardial vegetations which are distinguishable from the vegetations of RHD and bacterial endocarditis.

ETIOPATHOGENESIS Atypical verrucous endocarditis is one of the manifestations of 'collagen diseases'. Characteristic lesions of Libman-Sacks endocarditis are seen in *50% cases* of *acute systemic lupus erythematosus (SLE);* other diseases associated with this form of endocarditis are systemic sclerosis, thrombotic thrombocytopenic purpura (TTP) and other collagen diseases.

G/A Characteristic vegetations occur most frequently on the mitral and tricuspid valves. The vegetations of atypical verrucous endocarditis are small (1 to 4 mm in diameter), granular, multiple and tend to occur on both surfaces of affected valves. The vegetations are sterile unless superimposed by bacterial endocarditis.

M/E The verrucae of Libman-Sacks endocarditis are composed of fibrinoid material with superimposed fibrin and platelet thrombi. The endocardium underlying the verrucae shows characteristic histological changes which include fibrinoid necrosis, proliferation of capillaries and infiltration by histiocytes, plasma cells, lymphocytes, neutrophils and the pathognomonic *haematoxylin bodies of Gross* which are counterparts of LE cells of the blood.

NON-BACTERIAL THROMBOTIC (CACHECTIC, MARANTIC) ENDOCARDITIS (p. 425)

Non-bacterial thrombotic, cachectic, marantic or terminal endocarditis or endocarditis simplex is an involvement of the heart valves by sterile thrombotic vegetations.

ETIOPATHOGENESIS The exact pathogenesis of lesions in non-bacterial thrombotic endocarditis (NBTE) is not clear. Following diseases and conditions are frequently associated with their presence:
1. In patients having *hypercoagulable state* from various etiologies.
2. Occurrence of these lesions in young and well-nourished patients is explained on the basis of *alternative hypothesis* such as allergy, vitamin C deficiency, deep vein thrombosis, and endocardial trauma.

G/A The verrucae of NBTE are located on cardiac valves, chiefly mitral, and less often aortic and tricuspid valve. These verrucae are usually small (1 to 5 mm in diameter), single or multiple, brownish and occur along the line of closure of the leaflets but are more friable than the vegetations of RHD.

M/E The vegetations in NBTE are composed of fibrin along with entangled RBCs, WBCs and platelets. Vegetations in NBTE are sterile, bland and do not cause tissue destruction.

INFECTIVE (BACTERIAL) ENDOCARDITIS *(p. 425)*

DEFINITION Infective or bacterial endocarditis (IE or BE) is serious infection of the valvular and mural endocardium caused by different forms of microorganisms and is characterised by typical infected and friable vegetations. Depending upon the severity of infection, BE is subdivided into 2 clinical forms:

1. Acute bacterial endocarditis (ABE) is fulminant and destructive acute infection of the endocardium by highly virulent bacteria in a previously normal heart and almost invariably runs a rapidly fatal course in a period of 2-6 weeks.

2. Subacute bacterial endocarditis (SABE) or endocarditis lenta (*lenta* = slow) is caused by less virulent bacteria in a previously diseased heart and has a gradual downhill course in a period of 6 weeks to a few months and sometimes years.

INCIDENCE Introduction of antibiotic drugs has helped greatly in lowering the incidence of BE as compared with its incidence in the pre-antibiotic era. Though BE may occur at any age, most cases of ABE as well as SABE occur over 50 years of age. Males are affected more often than females.

ETIOLOGY All cases of BE are caused by *infection with microorganisms* in patients having certain *predisposing factors*.

A. Infective agents About 90% cases of BE are caused by streptococci and staphylococci.

◈ *In ABE,* the most common causative organisms are virulent strains of staphylococci, chiefly *Staphylococcus aureus*. Others are pneumococci, gonococci, β-streptococci and enterococci.

◈ *In SABE,* the commonest causative organisms are the streptococci with low virulence, predominantly *Streptococcus viridans,* which forms part of normal flora of the mouth and pharynx. Other less common etiologic agents include other strains of streptococci and staphylococci.

B. Predisposing factors There are 3 main types of factors which predispose to the development of both forms of BE:

1. *Bacteraemia, septicaemia and pyaemia:* Bacteria gain entry to the blood stream causing transient and clinically silent bacteraemia in a variety of day-to-day procedures as well as from other sources of infection. Some of the common examples are:
i) Periodontal infections
ii) Infections of the genitourinary tract
iii) Infections of gastrointestinal and biliary tract
iv) Surgery of the bowel, biliary tract and genitourinary tracts
v) Skin infections
vi) Upper and lower respiratory tract infections
vii) Intravenous drug abuse.
viii) Cardiac catheterisation and cardiac surgery.

2. *Underlying heart disease:* SABE occurs much more frequently in previously diseased heart valves, whereas the ABE is common in previously normal heart. Amongst the commonly associated underlying heart diseases are the following:
i) Chronic rheumatic valvular disease in about 50% cases.
ii) Congenital heart diseases in about 20% cases.
iii) Other causes are syphilitic aortic valve disease, atherosclerotic valvular disease, floppy mitral valve, and prosthetic heart valves.

3. *Impaired host defenses:* All conditions in which there is depression of specific immunity, deficiency of complement and defective phagocytic function, predispose to BE.

MORPHOLOGIC FEATURES The characteristic pathologic feature in both ABE and SABE is the presence of typical vegetations or verrucae on the valve cusps or leaflets. A summary of the distinguishing features of vegetations of BE and RHD is given below:

	FEATURE	RHEUMATIC	BACTERIAL (INFECTIVE)
1.	*Valves commonly affected*	Mitral alone; mitral and aortic combined	Mitral; aortic; combined mitral and aortic
2.	*Location on valve cusps or leaflets*	Occur along the line of closure, atrial surface of atrioventricular valves and ventricular surface of semilunar valves	SABE more often on diseased valves: ABE on previously normal valves; location same as in RHD
3.	*Macroscopy*	Small, multiple, warty, grey brown, translucent, firmly attached, generally produce permanent valvular deformity	Often large, grey-tawny to greenish, irregular, single or multiple, typically friable
4.	*Microscopy*	Composed of fibrin with superimposed platelet thrombi and no bacteria, Adjacent and underlying endocardium shows oedema, proliferation of capillaries, mononuclear inflammatory infiltrate and occasional Aschoff bodies.	Composed of outer eosinophilic zone of fibrin and platelets, covering colonies of bacteria and deeper zone of non-specific acute and chronic inflammatory cells. The underlying endocardium may show abscesses in ABE and inflammatory granulation tissue in the SABE.

G/A The lesions are found commonly on the valves of the left heart, most frequently on the mitral, followed in descending frequency, by the aortic, simultaneous involvement of both mitral and aortic valves. The vegetations in SABE are more often seen on previously diseased valves, whereas the vegetations of ABE are often found on previously normal valves. Like in RHD, the vegetations are often located on the atrial surface of atrioventricular valves and ventricular surface of the semilunar valves.

The *vegetations* of BE vary in size from a few millimeters to several centimeters, grey-tawny to greenish, irregular, single or multiple, and typically *friable*. They may appear flat, filiform, fungating or polypoid.

M/E The vegetations of BE consist of 3 zones:

i) The *outer layer or cap* consists of eosinophilic material composed of fibrin and platelets.

ii) Underneath this layer is the *basophilic zone* containing colonies of bacteria.

iii) The *deeper zone* consists of non-specific inflammatory reaction in the cusp itself.

COMPLICATIONS AND SEQUELAE Most cases of BE present with fever. The acute form of BE is characterised by high grade fever, chills, weakness and malaise while the subacute form of the disease has non-specific manifestations like slight fever, fatigue, loss of weight and flu-like symptoms. In the early stage, the lesions are confined to the heart. Complications and sequelae of BE are divided into cardiac and extracardiac:

A. Cardiac complications These include the following:

i) Valvular stenosis or insufficiency

ii) Perforation, rupture, and aneurysm of valve leaflets

iii) Abscesses in the valve ring

iv) Myocardial abscesses

v) Suppurative pericarditis

vi) Cardiac failure from one or more of the foregoing complications.

B. Extracardiac complications Since the vegetations in BE are typically friable, they tend to get dislodged due to rapid stream of blood and give rise to embolism which is responsible for very common and serious extra-cardiac complications. These are as follows:

i) Emboli originating from the *left side of the heart* and entering the systemic circulation affect organs like the spleen, kidneys, and brain causing infarcts, abscesses and mycotic aneurisms.

ii) Emboli arising from *right side of the heart* enter the pulmonary circulation and produce pulmonary abscesses.

iii) *Petechiae* may be seen in the skin and conjunctiva due to either emboli or toxic damage to the capillaries.

iv) In SABE, there are painful, tender nodules on the finger tips of hands and feet called *Osler's nodes,* while in ABE there is appearance of painless, non-tender subcutaneous maculapapular lesions on the pulp of the fingers called *Janeway's spots.*

v) *Focal necrotising glomerulonephritis* is seen more commonly in SABE than in ABE.

SPECIFIC TYPES OF INFECTIVE ENDOCARDITIS Based on etiologic agent, following specific types of IE are described:

1. Tuberculous endocarditis Though tubercle bacilli are bacteria, tuberculous endocarditis is described separate from the bacterial endocarditis due to specific granulomatous inflammation found in tuberculosis. It is characterised by presence of typical tubercles on the valvular as well as mural endocardium and may form tuberculous thromboemboli.

2. Syphilitic endocarditis The endocardial lesions in syphilis are seen. The severest manifestation of cardiovascular syphilis is aortic valvular incompetence.

3. Fungal endocarditis Rarely, endocardium may be infected such as from *Candida albicans, Histoplasma capsulatum, Aspergillus, Mucor,* coccidioidomycosis, cryptococcosis, blastomycosis and actinomycosis. Opportunistic fungal infections like candidiasis and aspergillosis are seen more commonly in patients receiving long-term antibiotic therapy, intravenous drug abusers and after prosthetic valve replacement.

VALVULAR DISEASES AND DEFORMITIES *(p. 429)*

Valvular diseases are various forms of congenital and acquired diseases which cause valvular deformities. Many of them result in cardiac failure. Rheumatic heart disease is the most common form of acquired valvular disease. Valves of the left side of the heart are involved much more frequently than those of the right side of the heart. The mitral valve is affected most often, followed in descending frequency, by the aortic valve, and combined mitral and aortic valves. The valvular deformities may be of 2 types: stenosis and insufficiency:

◆ *Stenosis* is the term used for failure of a valve to open completely during diastole resulting in obstruction to the forward flow of the blood.

◆ *Insufficiency or incompetence or regurgitation* is the failure of a valve to close completely during systole resulting in back flow or regurgitation of the blood.

Various acquired valvular diseases that may deform the heart valves are listed below:

1. RHD, the commonest cause
2. Infective endocarditis
3. Non-bacterial thrombotic endocarditis
4. Libman-Sacks endocarditis
5. Syphilitic valvulitis
6. Calcific aortic valve stenosis
7. Calcification of mitral annulus
8. Myxomatous degeneration (floppy valve syndrome)
9. Carcinoid heart disease.

Mitral stenosis occurs in approximately 40% of all patients with RHD. About 70% of the patients are women. The latent period between the rheumatic carditis and development of symptomatic mitral stenosis is about two decades.

G/A Generally, the valve leaflets are diffusely thickened by fibrous tissue and/or calcific deposits, especially towards the closing margin. In less extensive involvement, the bases of the leaflets of mitral valve are mobile while the free margins have puckered and thickened tissue with narrowed orifice; this is called as *'purse-string puckering'*. The more advanced cases have rigid, fixed and immobile diaphragm-like valve leaflets with narrow, slit-like or oval mitral opening, commonly referred to as *'button-hole'* or *'fish-mouth'* mitral orifice.

EFFECTS These are as under:
1. Dilatation and hypertrophy of the left atrium.
2. Normal-sized or atrophic left ventricle due to reduced inflow of blood.
3. Pulmonary hypertension resulting from passive backward transmission of elevated left artial pressure which causes:
    i) chronic passive congestion of the lungs;
    ii) hypertrophy and dilatation of the right ventricle; and
    iii) dilatation of the right atrium when right heart failure supervenes.

MITRAL INSUFFICIENCY

Mitral insufficiency is caused by RHD in about 50% of patients but in contrast to mitral stenosis, pure mitral insufficiency occurs more often in men (75%). Subsequently, mitral insufficiency is associated with some degree of mitral stenosis.

MORPHOLOGIC FEATURES The appearance of the mitral valve in insufficiency varies according to the underlying cause.
◆ In *myxomatous degeneration* of the mitral valve leaflets (floppy valve syndrome), there is prolapse of one or both leaflets into the left atrium during systole.
◆ In *non-inflammatory calcification* of mitral annulus seen in the aged, there is irregular, stony-hard, bead-like thickening.

EFFECTS These are summarised below:
1. Dilatation and hypertrophy of the left ventricle.
2. Marked dilatation of the left atrium.
3. Features of pulmonary hypertension such as:
    i) chronic passive congestion of the lungs;
    ii) hypertrophy and dilatation of the right ventricle; and
    iii) dilatation of the right atrium when right heart failure supervenes.

AORTIC STENOSIS

Aortic stenosis comprises about one-fourth of all patients with chronic valvular heart disease.

1. **Non-calcific aortic stenosis** The most common cause of non-calcific aortic stenosis is chronic RHD.

2. **Calcific aortic stenosis** Various causes include healing by scarring followed by calcification of aortic valve such as in RHD, bacterial endocarditis, *Brucella* endocarditis, Mönckeberg's calcific aortic stenosis.

EFFECTS The *three cardinal symptoms* of aortic stenosis are: exertional dyspnoea, angina pectoris and syncope.
◆ Exertional dyspnoea results from elevation of pulmonary capillary pressure.
◆ Angina pectoris usually results from elevation of pulmonary capillary pressure and usually develops due to increased demand of hypertrophied myocardial mass.

AORTIC INSUFFICIENCY

About three-fourth of all patients with aortic insufficiency are males with some having family history of Marfan's syndrome.

G/A The aortic valve cusps are thickened, deformed and shortened and fail to close. There is generally distension and distortion of the ring.

EFFECTS As a result of regurgitant aortic orifice, there is increase of the left ventricular end-diastolic volume. This leads to hypertrophy and dilatation of the left ventricle producing massive cardiac enlargement so that the heart may weigh as much as 1000 gm. Failure of the left ventricle increases the pressure in the left atrium and eventually pulmonary hypertension and right heart failure occurs.

CARCINOID HEART DISEASE

ETIOLOGY Carcinoid syndrome developing in patients with extensive hepatic metastases from a carcinoid tumour is characterised by cardiac manifestations in about half the cases. The lesions are characteristically located in the valves and endocardium of the right side of the heart. The pathogenesis of the cardiac lesions is not certain. But in carcinoid tumour with hepatic metastasis, there is increased blood level of serotonin secreted by the tumour.

G/A In majority of cases, the lesions are limited to the right side of the heart. Both pulmonary and tricuspid valves as well as the endocardium of the right chambers show characteristic cartilage-like fibrous plaques.

EFFECTS The thickening and contraction of the cusps and leaflets of the valves of the outflow tracts of the right heart result mainly in pulmonary stenosis and tricuspid regurgitation.

MYXOMATOUS DEGENERATION OF MITRAL VALVE
(MITRAL VALVE PROLAPSE)

Myxomatous or mucoid degeneration of the valves of the heart is a peculiar condition occurring in young patients between the age of 20 and 40 years and is more common in women. The condition is common and seen in 5% of general adult population. The condition is also known by other synonyms like 'floppy valve syndrome' or 'mitral valve prolapse'.

ETIOLOGY The cause of the condition is not known but in some cases it may be genetically determined collagen disorder. Association with Marfan's syndrome has been observed in 90% of patients. Others have noted myxomatous degeneration in cases of Ehlers-Danlos syndrome and in myotonic dystrophy.

G/A Any cardiac valve may be involved but mitral valve is affected most frequently. A significant feature is the ballooning or aneurysmal protrusion of the affected leaflet and hence the name 'mitral valve prolapse' and 'floppy valve syndrome'.

M/E The enlarged cusp shows loose connective tissue with abundant mucoid or myxoid material due to abundance of mucopolysaccharide.

MYOCARDIAL DISEASES (p. 432)

Involvement of the myocardium occurs in three major forms of diseases already discussed—ischaemic heart disease, hypertensive heart disease and rheumatic heart disease. In addition, there are two other broad groups of isolated myocardial diseases:

I. *Myocarditis* i.e. inflammatory involvement of the myocardium
II. *Cardiomyopathy* i.e. a non-inflammatory myocardial involvement.

Inflammation of the heart muscle is called myocarditis. It is a rather common form of heart disease that can occur at any age. Its exact incidence is difficult to ascertain as the histological examination has been largely confined to autopsy material.

Currently most commonly used is *etiologic classification*.

I. INFECTIVE MYOCARDITIS

1. VIRAL MYOCARDITIS A number of viral infections are associated with myocarditis. Some of the common examples are influenza, poliomyelitis, infectious mononucleosis, hepatitis, smallpox, chickenpox, measles, mumps, rubella, viral pneumonias, coxsackievirus and HIV infections.

G/A The myocardium is pale and flabby with dilatation of the chambers. There may be focal or patchy areas of necrosis.

M/E There are changes of acute myocarditis.

2. SUPPURATIVE MYOCARDITIS Pyogenic bacteria, chiefly *Staphylococcus aureus* or *Streptococcus pyogenes*, which cause septicaemia and pyaemia may produce suppurative myocarditis.

G/A There are either abscesses in the myocardium or there is diffuse myocardial involvement.

M/E The exudate chiefly consists of neutrophils, admixed with lymphocytes, plasma cells and macrophages.

3. TOXIC MYOCARDITIS A number of acute bacterial infections produce myocarditis by toxins e.g. in diphtheria, typhoid fever and pneumococcal pneumonia.

4. GRANULOMATOUS MYOCARDITIS Tuberculosis, brucellosis and tularaemia are some examples of bacterial infections characterised by granulomatous inflammation in the myocardium. Sarcoidosis, though not a bacterial infection, has histological resemblance to other granulomatous myocarditis.

5. SYPHILITIC MYOCARDITIS Syphilitic involvement of the myocardium may occur in 2 forms—a *gummatous lesion* consisting of granulomatous inflammation which is more common, and a *primary non-specific myocarditis* which is rare.

6. PROTOZOAL MYOCARDITIS Chagas' disease and toxoplasmosis are the two protozoal diseases causing myocarditis. Chagas' disease caused by *Trypanosoma cruzi* frequently attacks myocardium besides involving the skeletal muscle and the central nervous system. Toxoplasmosis caused by intracellular protozoan, *Toxoplasma gondii,* sometimes causes myocarditis in children and adults.

7. HELMINTHIC MYOCARDITIS *Echinococcus granulosus* and *Trichinella spiralis* are the two intestinal helminths which may cause myocarditis. *Echinococcus* rarely produces hydatid cyst in the myocardium while the larvae of *Trichinella* in trichinosis cause heavy inflammation in the myocardium as well as in the interstitial tissue.

8. FUNGAL MYOCARDITIS Patients with immunodeficiency, cancer and other chronic debilitating diseases are more prone to develop fungal myocarditis. These include: candidiasis, aspergillosis, blastomycosis, actinomyosis, cryptococcosis, coccidioidomycosis and histoplasmosis.

II. IDIOPATHIC (FIEDLER'S) MYOCARDITIS

Idiopathic or Fiedler's myocarditis is an isolated myocarditis unaccompanied by inflammatory changes in the endocardium or pericardium and occurs without the usual apparent causes. The condition is rapidly progressive and causes sudden severe cardiac failure or sudden death.

M/E Two forms of idiopathic myocarditis are described: diffuse type and giant cell (idiopathic granulomatous) type.

III. MYOCARDITIS IN CONNECTIVE TISSUE DISEASES

Inflammatory involvement of the myocardium occurs in a number of connective tissue diseases such as rheumatoid arthritis, lupus erythematosus, polyarteritis nodosa, dermatomyositis and scleroderma.

CARDIOMYOPATHY (p. 434)

Cardiomyopathy literally means disease of the heart muscle but the term was originally coined to restrict its usage to *myocardial disease of unknown cause,* commonly called primary cardiomyopathy. The WHO definition of cardiomyopathy also excludes heart muscle diseases of known etiologies which are termed secondary cardiomyopathies.

A. PRIMARY CARDIOMYOPATHY

This is a group of myocardial diseases of unknown cause. It is subdivided into the following 3 pathophysiologic categories:

IDIOPATHIC DILATED (CONGESTIVE) CARDIOMYOPATHY

This type of cardiomyopathy is characterised by gradually progressive cardiac failure along with dilatation of all the four chambers of the heart. The condition occurs more often in adults and the average survival from onset to death is less than 5 years.

ETIOLOGY A few hypothesis have been proposed:
i) Possible association of viral myocarditis.
ii) Association with toxic damage from cobalt and chemotherapy.
iii) Inherited mutations.
iv) Chronic alcoholism.
v) Peripartum association.

G/A The heart is enlarged and increased in weight (up to 1000 gm). The most characteristic feature is prominent dilatation of all the four chambers giving the heart typical globular appearance.

M/E The endomyocardial biopsies or autopsy examination of the heart reveal non-specific and variable changes. There may be hypertrophy of some myocardial fibres and atrophy of others.

IDIOPATHIC HYPERTROPHIC CARDIOMYOPATHY

This form of cardiomyopathy is known by various synonyms like asymmetrical hypertrophy, hypertrophic subaortic stenosis and Teare's disease. The disease occurs more frequently between the age of 25 and 50 years.

ETIOLOGY Following factors have been implicated:
i) Autosomal dominant inheritance
ii) Inherited mutations

G/A The characteristic features are cardiac enlargement, increase in weight, normal or small ventricular cavities and myocardial hypertrophy. The hypertrophy of the myocardium is typically asymmetrical and affects the interventricular septum more than the free walls of the ventricles. The designation of *rhabdomyoma of the septum* was applied to this form of cardiomyopathy.

M/E The classical feature is the myocardial cell disorganisation in the ventricular septum.

IDIOPATHIC RESTRICTIVE (OBLITERATIVE OR INFILTRATIVE) CARDIOMYOPATHY

This form of cardiomyopathy is characterised by restriction in ventricular filling due to reduction in the volume of the ventricles. The common feature in this heterogeneous group of conditions producing restrictive cardiomyopathy is abnormal diastolic function. Restrictive cardiomyopathy includes the following entities:

I) CARDIAC AMYLOIDOSIS Amyloidosis of the heart may occur in any form of systemic amyloidosis or may occur as isolated organ amyloidosis in amyloid of ageing and result in subendocardial deposits.

II) ENDOCARDIAL FIBROELASTOSIS This is an unusual and uncommon form of heart disease occurring predominantly in infants and children under 2 years of age and less often in adults. The *infantile form* is clinically characterised by sudden breathlessness, cyanosis, cardiac failure and death whereas the symptoms in the *adult form* last for longer duration.

G/A The characteristic feature is the diffuse or patchy, rigid, pearly-white thickening of the mural endocardium. Left ventricle is predominantly involved.

M/E Typical finding is the proliferation of the collagen and elastic tissue (fibroelastosis) comprising the thickened endocardium.

III) ENDOMYOCARDIAL FIBROSIS It is seen in children and young adults. The clinical manifestations consist of congestive heart failure of unknown cause just as in adult variety of endocardial fibroelastosis.

G/A Endomyocardial fibrosis is characterised by fibrous scarring of the ventricular endocardium that extends to involve the inner third of the myocardium.

M/E The endocardium and parts of inner third of the myocardium show destruction of normal tissue and replacement by fibrous tissue.

IV) LÖEFFLER'S ENDOCARDITIS Also known by the more descriptive term of 'fibroplastic parietal endocarditis with peripheral blood eosinophilia', the condition is considered by some as a variant of the entity described above, endomyocardial fibrosis. However, it differs from the latter in following respects:
a)   There is generally a peripheral blood eosinophilic leucocytosis.
b)   The inflammatory infiltrate in the endocardium and in the part of affected myocardium chiefly consists of eosinophils.

B. SECONDARY CARDIOMYOPATHY

This is a group of myocardial diseases of known etiologies or having clinical associations. This, however, excludes well-defined entities such as ischaemic, hypertensive, valvular, pericardial, congenital and inflammatory involvements of the heart. The main entities included in this group are:
1.   Nutritional disorders
2.   Toxic chemicals
3.   Drugs
4.   Metabolic diseases
5.   Neuromuscular diseases
6.   Infiltrations
7.   Connective tissue diseases.

PERICARDIAL DISEASES (p. 437)

PERICARDIAL FLUID ACCUMULATIONS (p. 437)

A. HYDROPERICARDIUM (PERICARDIAL EFFUSION) Accumulation of fluid in the pericardial cavity due to non-inflammatory causes is called hydropericardium or pericardial effusion. Normally, the pericardial cavity contains 30 to 50 ml of clear watery fluid. Considerable quantities of fluid (up to 1000 ml) can be accommodated in the pericardial cavity without seriously affecting the cardiac function if the accumulation is slow.

1.   Serous effusions This is the most common type occurring in conditions in which there is generalised oedema.

2.   Serosanguineous effusion This type is found following blunt trauma to chest and cardiopulmonary resuscitation.

3.   Chylous effusion Milky or chylous fluid accumulates in conditions causing lymphatic obstruction.

4. Cholesterol effusion This is a rare type of fluid accumulation characterised by the presence of cholesterol crystals such as in myxoedema.

B. HAEMOPERICARDIUM Accumulation of pure blood in the pericardial sac is termed haemopericardium. Massive and sudden bleeding into the sac causes compression of the heart leading to cardiac tamponade. The causes of haemopericardium are as under:

i)   Rupture of the heart through a myocardial infarct.
ii) Rupture of dissecting aneurysm.
iii) Bleeding diathesis such as in scurvy, acute leukaemias, thrombocytopenia.
iv) Trauma following cardiopulmonary resuscitation or by laceration of a coronary artery.

PERICARDITIS (p. 437)

Pericarditis is the inflammation of the pericardial layers and is generally secondary to diseases in the heart or caused by systemic diseases. Based on the morphologic appearance, pericarditis is classified into acute and chronic types.

A.   ACUTE PERICARDITIS

Acute bacterial and non-bacterial pericarditis are the most frequently encountered forms of pericarditis. These may have the following subtypes:

1.   SEROUS PERICARDITIS   Its various causes are:
i)   Viral infection
ii) Rheumatic fever.
iii) Rheumatoid arthritis.
iv) Systemic lupus erythematosus.
v)   Involvement of the pericardium by malignant tumour in the vicinity e.g. carcinoma lung, mesothelioma and mediastinal tumours.
vi) Tuberculous pericarditis in the early stage.

2.   FIBRINOUS AND SEROFIBRINOUS PERICARDITIS   The response of the pericardium by fibrinous exudate is the most common type of pericarditis. The various causes of this type of pericarditis are as follows:
i)   Uraemia
ii) Myocardial infarction
iii) Rheumatic fever
iv) Trauma such as in cardiac surgery
v)   Acute bacterial infections.

3.   PURULENT OR FIBRINOPURULENT PERICARDITIS   Purulent or fibrinopurulent pericarditis is mainly caused by pyogenic bacteria (e.g. staphylococci, streptococci and pneumococci) and less frequently by fungi and parasites. The infection may spread to the pericardium by the following routes:
i)   By direct extension
ii) By haematogenous spread.
iii) By lymphatic permeation.
iv) Direct implantation during cardiac surgery.

4.   HAEMORRHAGIC PERICARDITIS   Its causes are:
i)   Neoplastic involvement of the pericardium
ii) Haemorrhagic diathesis with effusion
iii) Tuberculosis
iv) Severe acute infections

B.   CHRONIC PERICARDITIS

1.   TUBERCULOUS PERICARDITIS   Tuberculous pericarditis is the most frequent form of granulomatous inflammation of the pericardium. The lesions may occur by one of the following mechanisms:
i)   Direct extension from an adjacent focus of tuberculosis.
ii) By lymphatic spread e.g. from tracheobronchial lymph nodes, chronic pulmonary tuberculosis or infected pleura.

The exudate is slightly turbid, caseous or blood-stained with sufficient fibrin. Tubercles are generally visible on the pericardial surfaces and sometimes caseous areas are also visible to the naked eye.

M/E Typical tuberculous granulomas with caseation necrosis are seen in the pericardial wall.

2. CHRONIC ADHESIVE PERICARDITIS Chronic adhesive pericarditis is the stage of organisation and healing by formation of fibrous adhesions in the pericardium following preceding fibrinous, suppurative or haemorrhagic pericarditis. The process begins by formation of granulation tissue and neovascularisation. Subsequently, fibrous adhesions develop between the parietal and the visceral layers of the pericardium and obliterate the pericardial space.

3. CHRONIC CONSTRICTIVE PERICARDITIS This is a rare condition characterised by dense fibrous or fibrocalcific thickening of the pericardium resulting in mechanical interference with the function of the heart and reduced cardiac output. The condition usually results from long-standing preceding causes, e.g.
i)   Tuberculous pericarditis
ii)   Purulent pericarditis
iii) Haemopericardium
iv)   Concato's disease (polyserositis)
v)   Rarely, acute non-specific and viral pericarditis.
      The heart is encased in 0.5 to 1 cm thick and dense collagenous scar which may be calcified. As a result, the heart fails to dilate during diastole.

4. PERICARDIAL PLAQUES (MILK SPOTS, SOLDIERS' SPOTS) These are opaque, white, shining and well-circumscribed areas of organisation with fibrosis in the pericardium measuring 1 to 3 cm in diameter. The exact cause is not known but they are generally believed to arise from healing of preceding pericarditis.

TUMOURS OF THE HEART *(p. 439)*

PRIMARY TUMOURS

Primary tumours of the heart are quite rare, found in 0.04% of autopsies. In decreasing order of frequency, the benign tumours encountered in the heart are: myxoma, lipoma, fibroelastoma, rhabdomyoma, haemangioma and lymphangioma. The malignant tumours are still rarer.

MYXOMA This is the most common primary tumour of the heart comprising about 50% of all primary cardiac tumours. Majority of them occur in the age range of 30 to 60 years. Myxomas may be located in any cardiac chamber or the valves, but 90% of them are situated in the left atrium.

G/A They are often single but may be multiple. They range in size from less than 1 to 10 cm, polypoid, pedunculated, spherical, soft and haemorrhagic masses resembling an organising mural thrombus.

M/E The tumour shows following features:
i)   There is abundant myxoid or mucoid intercellular stroma positive for mucin.
ii)   The cellularity is sparse. The tumour cells are generally stellate-shaped, spindled and polyhedral, scattered in the stroma. Occasional multinucleate tumour giant cells are present.

SECONDARY TUMOURS

Metastatic tumours of the heart are more common than the primary tumours. About 10% cases with disseminated cancer have metastases in the heart. Most of these result from haematogenous or lymphatic spread.

ENDOMYOCARDIAL BIOPSY

Endomyocardial biopsy (EMB) is done for making a final histopathologic diagnosis in certain cardiac diseases. The main *indications* for EMB are: myocarditis, cardiac transplant cases, restrictive heart disease, infiltrative heart diseases such as in amyloidosis, storage disorders etc.

BALLOON ANGIOPLASTY

Balloon angioplasty or percutaneous coronary intervention (PCI) is a non-surgical procedure that employs percutaneous insertion and manipulation of a balloon catheter into the occluded coronary artery. The balloon is inflated to dilate the stenotic artery which causes endothelial damage, plaque fracture, medial dissection and haemorrhage in the affected arterial wall. PCI is accompanied with insertion of coronary stents in the blocked coronaries with a success rate of symptoms in over 95% cases.

CORONARY ARTERY BYPASS GRAFTING

Coronary artery bypass grafting (CABG) employs the use of autologous grafts to replace or bypass the blocked coronary arteries. Most frequently used is autologous graft of saphenous vein which is reversed (due to valves in the vein) and transplanted, or left internal mammary artery may be used being in the operative area of the heart.

CARDIAC TRANSPLANTATION

Since the first human-to-human cardiac transplant was carried out successfully by South African surgeon Dr Christian Barnard in 1967, cardiac transplantation and prolonged assisted circulation is being done in many countries in end-stage cardiac diseases, most often in idiopathic dilated cardiomyopathy, heart failure and IHD. Worldwide, about 3,000 cardiac transplants are performed annually. The survival following heart transplants is reported as: 1 year in 85%, 5 years in 65% and 10 years in 45% cases. Major complications are: transplant rejection reaction, infections (particularly with *Toxoplasma gondii* and cytomegaloviruses), graft coronary atherosclerosis and higher incidence of malignancy due to long-term administration of immunosuppressive therapy.

SELF ASSESSMENT

1. **The most common anatomic pattern of distribution of coronary blood supply is:**
   A. Left coronary preponderance
   B. Right coronary preponderance
   C. Circumflex preponderance
   D. Balanced circulation

2. **Right heart failure is predominantly characterised by the following <u>except</u>:**
   A. Chronic venous congestion liver
   B. Chronic venous congestion spleen
   C. Chronic venous congestion kidney
   D. Pulmonary congestion

3. **The thickness of left ventricular wall in left ventricular hyper-trophy is at least:**
   A. 13 mm
   B. 15 mm
   C. 17 mm
   D. 19 mm

4. **The features of tetralogy of Fallot are as under <u>except</u>:**
   A. VSD
   B. Displacement of aorta to right to override the VSD

C. Pulmonary stenosis
D. Left ventricular hypertrophy

5. **Post-ductal coarctation of aorta has following features <u>except</u>:**
   A. Hypertension in upper extremities
   B. Weak pulses
   C. High blood pressure in lower extremities
   D. Claudication in lower legs

6. **Non-infarct effects of myocardial ischaemia are as under <u>except</u>:**
   A. Sudden cardiac death
   B. Angina pectoris
   C. Subendocardial infarcts
   D. Chronic ischaemic heart disease

7. **The most thrombogenic constituent of atheroma is:**
   A. Fibrous cap   B. Lipid core
   C. Foam cells   D. Smooth muscle cells

8. **The most important and common complicated atheromatous lesion in coronary artery in acute myocardial infarction is:**
   A. Calcification   B. Coronary thrombosis
   C. Aneurysm   D. Ulceration

9. **Infarcts are least common in:**
   A. Left ventricle   B. Right ventricle
   C. Left atrium   D. Right atrium

10. **CKMB2:CKMB1 ratio sensitive for the diagnosis of acute MI is:**
    A. >0.5   B. >1.0
    C. 1.5   D. >2.0

11. **Chronic ischaemic heart disease is most often due to:**
    A. Coronary atherosclerosis
    B. Repetitive coronary vasospasm
    C. Embolisation to coronary branches
    D. Stenosis of coronary ostia

12. **In hypertensive heart disease left ventricular hypertrophy is correlated with:**
    A. Duration of hypertension
    B. Severity of hypertension
    C. Cause of hypertension
    D. Severity of coronary atherosclerosis

13. **In rheumatic heart disease, antibodies against the following streptococcal products are seen in the serum <u>except</u>:**
    A. DNAase B   B. Streptokinase
    C. Streptolysin S   D. Streptohyaluronidase

14. **Anitschkow cells are believed to be derivative of:**
    A. Cardiac myocyte
    B. Cardiac histiocyte
    C. Endocardial smooth muscle cells
    D. Endothelial cells of lymphatics

15. **In chronic RHD, the most common valvular deformities are:**
    A. Mitral stenosis and insufficiency
    B. Mitral stenosis alone
    C. Mitral insufficiency alone
    D. Mitral and aortic stenosis combined

16. **MacCallum's patch appears in the region of:**
    A. Pericardial surface in the posterior wall of left atrium
    B. Pericardial surface in the posterior wall of left ventricle
    C. Endocardial surface in the posterior wall of left atrium
    D. Endocardial surface in the posterior wall of left ventricle

17. Major criteria in the modified Jones' criteria include the following <u>except</u>:
    A. Carditis
    B. Polyarthritis
    C. Raised C-reactive proteins
    D. Subcutaneous nodules

18. Haematoxylin bodies of Gross may be seen in vegetations of:
    A. Rheumatic valvulitis
    B. Libman-Sacks endocarditis
    C. Non-bacterial thrombotic endocarditis
    D. Subacute bacterial valvulitis

19. Most frequent underlying heart disease in causation of SABE is:
    A. Ventricular septal defect
    B. Chronic rheumatic valvular disease
    C. Floppy mitral valve
    D. Atherosclerotic valvular disease

20. Vegetations of the following types of endocarditis are generally not friable <u>except</u> that of:
    A. Rheumatic endocarditis
    B. Libman-Sacks endocarditis
    C. Subacute bacterial endocarditis
    D. Non-bacterial thrombotic endocarditis

21. Mitral stenosis causes the following effects on the heart <u>except</u>:
    A. Dilatation and hypertrophy of left atrium
    B. Dilatation and hypertrophy of left ventricle
    C. Dilatation and hypertrophy of right ventricle
    D. Dilatation of right atrium

22. In the following heart disease, there is generally involvement of valves of right heart:
    A. Heart disease in SLE
    B. Carcinoid heart disease
    C. Non-bacterial thrombotic endocarditis
    D. Subacute bacterial endocarditis

23. The following type of cardiomyopathy is classically characterised by four chamber dilatation:
    A. Idiopathic congestive cardiomyopathy
    B. Idiopathic hypertrophic cardiomyopathy
    C. Endomyocardial fibrosis
    D. Loeffler's endocarditis

24. All of the following cause left-sided heart failure <u>except</u>:
    A. Cor pulmonale
    B. Systemic hypertension
    C. Mitral stenosis
    D. Aortic stenosis

25. The most common location for myxoma of heart is:
    A. Left ventricle
    B. Right ventricle
    C. Left atrium
    D. Interventricular septum

26. An important protein from bacterial cell surface implicated in pathogenesis of RHD is:
    A. G-protein
    B. M-protein
    C. L-protein
    D. X-protein

27. For endomyocardial biopsy, the safest site for biopsy is:
    A. Left ventricle
    B. Left atrium
    C. Right ventricle
    D. Right atrium

28. Which of the following produces right ventricular hypertrophy:
    A. Coarctation of aorta
    B. Aortic stenosis
    C. Pulmonary insufficiency
    D. Systemic hypertension

29. Most common congenital anomaly of the heart is:
    A. VSD
    B. ASD
    C. PDA
    D. Tetralogy of Fallot

30. Acronym "STEMI" stands for:
    A. Standard Treatment and Evaluation in MI
    B. Serial Testing of Enzyme levels in MI
    C. ST segment Elevation in acute MI
    D. Steps Taken in Emergency in case of Multiple Infarcts
31. Reported incidence of RHD in school going children by the Indian Council of Medical Research is:
    A. 1 to 5.5 per 100 children
    B. 5.5 to 10 per 100 children
    C. 10 to 15.5 per 100 children
    D. 15.5 to 20 per 100 children
32. MacCallum's patch is seen in:
    A. Right atrium   B. Right ventricle
    C. Left atrium   D. Left ventricle
33. Chronic alcoholism is associated with:
    A. Hypertrophic cardiomyopathy
    B. Dilated cardiomyopathy
    C. Restrictive cardiomyopathy
    D. Infiltrative cardiomyopathy
34. Most common location for performing endomyocardial biopsy is:
    A. Right atrium   B. Right ventricle
    C. Left atrium   D. Left ventricle
35. A one month old male baby is brought to paediatric emergency due to difficulty in feeding and lethargy. On auscultation, a loud murmur is heard. Which of the following is the most likely congenital heart disease in this baby?
    A. Tetralogy of Fallot's   B. VSD
    C. ASD   D. Aortic atresia

KEY

1 = B	2 = D	3 = B	4 = D	5 = C
6 = C	7 = B	8 = B	9 = C	10 = C
11 = A	12 = A	13 = C	14 = B	15 = A
16 = C	17 = C	18 = B	19 = B	20 = C
21 = B	22 = B	23 = A	24 = A	25 = C
26 = B	27 = C	28 = C	29 = A	30 = C
31 = A	32 = C	33 = B	34 = B	35 = B

15   The Respiratory System

ANATOMY The normal *adult right lung* weighs 375 to 550 gm (average 450 gm) and is divided by two fissures into three lobes—the upper, middle and lower lobes. The weight of the normal *adult left lung* is 325 to 450 gm (average 400 gm) and has one fissure dividing it into two lobes—the upper and lower lobes, while the middle lobe is represented by the lingula.

The trachea, major bronchi and their branchings possess cartilage, smooth muscle and mucous glands in their walls, while the bronchioles have smooth muscle but lack cartilage as well as the mucous glands. Between the tracheal bifurcation and the smallest bronchi, about 8 divisions take place. The *bronchioles* so formed further undergo 3 to 4 divisions leading to the *terminal bronchioles* which are less than 2 mm in diameter. The part of the lung tissue distal to a terminal bronchiole is called an *acinus*. An acinus consists of 3 parts:

1. Several (usually 3 to 5 generations) *respiratory bronchioles* originate from a terminal bronchiole.
2. Each respiratory bronchiole divides into several *alveolar ducts.*
3. Each alveolar duct opens into many *alveolar sacs (alveoli)* which are blind ends of the respiratory passages.

The lungs have double blood supply—oxygenated blood from the bronchial arteries and venous blood from the pulmonary arteries, and there is mixing of the blood to some extent.

HISTOLOGY The bronchi and their subdivisions up to bronchioles are lined by pseudostratified columnar ciliated epithelial cells, also called *respiratory epithelium.*

The **alveolar walls or alveolar septa** are the sites of exchange between the blood and air and have the following microscopic features:

1. The *capillary endothelium* lines the anastomotic capillaries in the alveolar walls.
2. The capillary endothelium and the, alveolar lining epithelial cells are separated by the *capillary basement membrane and some interstitial tissue.*
3. The *alveolar epithelium* consists of 2 types of cells: *type I* or *membranous pneumocytes* are the most numerous covering about 95% of alveolar surface, while *type II* or *granular pneumocytes* project into the alveoli and are covered by microvilli.
4. The *alveolar macrophages* belonging to mononuclear-phagocyte system are present either free in the alveolar spaces or are attached to the alveolar cells.
5. The *pores of Kohn* are the sites of alveolar connections between the adjacent alveoli and allow the passage of bacteria and exudate.

FUNCTIONS The primary functions of lungs are oxygenation of the blood and removal of carbon dioxide. The respiratory tract is particularly exposed to infection as well as to the hazards of inhalation of pollutants from the inhaled air and cigarette smoke.

CONGENITAL CYSTS

Developmental defects involving deficiency of bronchial or bronchiolar cartilage, elastic tissue and muscle result in congenital cystic disease of lungs. A single large cyst of this type occupying almost a lobe is called *pneumatocele*. Multiple small cysts are more common and give sponge-like appearance to the lung.

BRONCHOPULMONARY SEQUESTRATION

Sequestration is the presence of lobes or segments of lung tissue which are not connected to the airway system.

◈ **Intralobar sequestration** is the sequestered bronchopulmonary mass within the pleural covering of the affected lung.

◈ **Extralobar sequestration** is the sequestered mass of lung tissue lying outside the pleural investing layer such as in the base of left lung or below the diaphragm.

ACUTE RESPIRATORY DISTRESS SYNDROME (HYALINE MEMBRANE DISEASE)

Acute respiratory distress syndrome (ARDS) is a severe, at times life-threatening, form of progressive respiratory insufficiency which involves pulmonary tissues diffusely i.e. involvement of the alveolar epithelium, alveolar lumina and interstitial tissue. ARDS exists in 2 forms: neonatal and adult type. Both have the common morphological feature of formation of hyaline membrane in the alveoli and hence is also termed as hyaline membrane disease (HMD).

CLINICAL FEATURES AND CONSEQUENCES These are different in children and adults:

◈ **Neonatal ARDS** occurring in newborn infants begins with dyspnoea within a few hours after birth with tachypnoea, hypoxia and cyanosis; in severe cases death may occur within a few hours.

◈ **Adult ARDS** is known by various synonyms such as shock-lung syndrome, diffuse alveolar damage (DAD), acute alveolar injury, traumatic wet lungs and post-traumatic respiratory insufficiency. Adult ARDS also presents clinically by sudden and severe respiratory distress, tachypnoea, tachycardia, cyanosis and severe hypoxaemia.

ETIOLOGY The two forms of ARDS have distinct etiology:

◈ **Neonatal ARDS** is primarily initiated by hypoxia, either shortly before birth or immediately afterward.
1. Preterm infants
2. Infants born to diabetic mothers
3. Delivery by caesarean section
4. Infants born to mothers with previous premature infants
5. Excessive sedation of the mother causing depression in respiration of the infant
6. Birth asphyxia from various causes such as coils of umbilical cord around the neck
7. Male preponderance (1.5 to 2 times) over female babies due to early maturation of female lungs
8. Finally, many cases of neonatal ARDS remain idiopathic.

◈ **Adult ARDS**

a) Direct lung injury:
1. Diffuse pulmonary infections, chiefly viral pneumonia
2. Oxygen toxicity
3. Inhalation of toxins and irritants e.g. smoke, war gases, nitrogen dioxide, metal fumes etc.
4. Aspiration of gastric contents
5. Near drowning

b) Indirect lung injury:
1. Shock due to sepsis, trauma, burns
2. Narcotic overdose
3. Pancreatitis
4. Drugs e.g. salicylates, colchicines
5. Fat embolism
6. Radiation .
7. Multiple transfusions

PATHOGENESIS In both neonatal and adult type ARDS, there is damage to alveolocapillary wall triggered by etiologic factors listed above, and the final pathologic consequence of formation of hyaline membrane is also similar.

❖ **Neonatal ARDS** *Entry of air into alveoli is essential for formation of hyaline membrane i.e. still born infants do not develop HMD.*

i) The basic defect in neonatal ARDS is a *deficiency of pulmonary surfactant*, normally synthesised by type II alveolar cells. The main function of alveolar surfactant being lowering of alveolar surface tension, its deficiency leads to increased alveolar surface tension which in turn causes *atelectasis*.

ii) Atelectasis of the lungs results in hypoventilation, pulmonary hypoperfusion and ischaemic damage to capillary endothelium.

iii) This results in *ischaemic necrosis* of the alveolocapillary wall, exudation of plasma proteins including fibrinogen into the alveoli.

❖ **Adult ARDS** The mechanism of acute injury by etiologic agents listed earlier depends upon the *imbalance between pro-inflammatory and anti-inflammatory cytokines:*

i) Activated pulmonary macrophages release *proinflammatory cytokines* such as IL8, IL1, and tumour necrosis factor (TNF), while macrophage inhibitory factor (MIF) helps to sustain inflammation in the alveoli.

In either case, injury to the capillary endothelium leads to increased vascular permeability while injured pneumocytes, especially type 1, undergo necrosis. The net effect of injury to both capillary endothelium and alveolar epithelium is interstitial and intra-alveolar oedema, congestion, fibrin deposition and formation of hyaline membranes.

G/A The lungs are normal in size. They are characteristically stiff, congested, heavy and airless so that they sink in water.

M/E It shows following features:

1. There is presence of collapsed alveoli (atelectasis) alternating with dilated alveoli.

2. Necrosis of alveolar epithelial cells and formation of characteristic eosinophilic hyaline membranes lining the respiratory bronchioles, alveolar ducts and the proximal alveoli.

3. Changes of bronchopneumonia may supervene.

CONSEQUENCES ARDS may have following outcome:

1. **Death** The mortality rate in neonatal ARDS is high (20 to 30%) and is still higher in babies under 1 kg of body weight.

2. **Resolution** Milder cases of neonatal ARDS recover with adequate oxygen therapy by ventilator-assist methods in a few days, while in adult ARDS control of the trigger which initiated it may result in resolution.

BRONCHOPULMONARY DYSPLASIA

Bronchopulmonary dysplasia occurs as a complication in infants treated for neonatal ARDS with oxygen and assisted ventilation.

M/E There is organisation of hyaline membranes resulting in fibrous thickening of the alveolar walls, bronchiolitis, peribronchial fibrosis, and development of emphysema due to alveolar dilatation.

ATELECTASIS AND COLLAPSE

Atelectasis in the newborn or *primary atelectasis* is defined as incomplete expansion of a lung or part of a lung, while pulmonary collapse or *secondary atelectasis* is the term used for reduction in lung size of a previously expanded and well-aerated lung. Obviously, the former occurs in newborn whereas the latter may occur at any age.

ATELECTASIS Stillborn infants have total atelectasis, while the newborn infants with weak respiratory action develop incomplete expansion of the lungs and clinical atelectasis. The common causes are prematurity, cerebral birth injury, CNS malformations and intrauterine hypoxia.

COLLAPSE Pulmonary collapse or secondary atelectasis in children and adults may occur from various causes such as compression, obstruction, contraction and lack of pulmonary surfactant.

Sudden infant death syndrome (SIDS) or crib death is an uncommon condition seen more often in the developed countries. It affects infants in the age group of 2 to 6 months. The condition is seen in premature babies born to mothers who have been smokers and indulged in drug abuse.

PULMONARY VASCULAR DISEASE *(p. 446)*

PULMONARY HYPERTENSION

Pulmonary hypertension is defined as a systolic blood pressure in the pulmonary arterial circulation above 30 mmHg. Pulmonary hypertension is broadly classified into 2 groups: primary (idiopathic) and secondary; the latter being more common.

PRIMARY (IDIOPATHIC) PULMONARY HYPERTENSION

Primary or idiopathic pulmonary hypertension is an uncommon condition of unknown cause. The diagnosis can be established only after a thorough search for the usual causes of secondary pulmonary hypertension. The patients are usually young females between the age of 20 and 40 years, or children around 5 years of age.

ETIOPATHOGENESIS Though the etiology of primary pulmonary hypertension is unknown, a number of etiologic factors have been suggested to explain its pathogenesis:
1. A *neurohumoral vasoconstrictor mechanism*
2. *Unrecognised thromboemboli* or *amniotic fluid emboli* during pregnancy may play a role.
3. There is a suggestion that primary pulmonary hypertension may be a form of *collagen vascular disease.*
4. *Pulmonary veno-occlusive disease* characterised by fibrous obliteration of small pulmonary veins is believed to be responsible for some cases of primary pulmonary hypertension.
5. *Ingestion of substances* like 'bush tea', oral contraceptives and appetite depressant agents like aminorex are believed to be related to primary pulmonary hypertension.
6. *Familial occurrence* has been reported in a number of cases.

SECONDARY PULMONARY HYPERTENSION

It is the more common type and may be encountered at any age, but is seen more frequently over the age of 50 years.

ETIOPATHOGENESIS Based on the underlying mechanism, it is divided into the following 3 groups:

A. Passive pulmonary hypertension e.g.
1. Mitral stenosis.
2. Chronic left ventricular failure (e.g. in severe systemic hypertension, aortic stenosis, myocardial fibrosis).

B. Hyperkinetic (Reactive) pulmonary hypertension e.g.
1. Patent ductus arteriosus.
2. Atrial or ventricular septal defects.

C. Vaso-occlusive pulmonary hypertension

1. *Obstructive type* e.g.
i) Multiple emboli or thrombi
ii) Sickle cell disease
iii) Schistosomiasis

2. *Obliterative type* e.g.
i) Chronic emphysema
ii) Chronic bronchitis
iii) Bronchiectasis
iv) Pulmonary tuberculosis
v) Pneumoconiosis

3. *Vasoconstrictive type* e.g.
i) In those residing at high altitude
ii) Pathologic obesity (Pickwickian disease)
iii) Upper airway disease such as tonsillar hypertrophy
iv) Neuromuscular diseases such as poliomyelitis
v) Severe kyphoscoliosis.

MORPHOLOGIC FEATURES Irrespective of the type of pulmonary hypertension (primary or secondary), chronic cases invariably lead to cor pulmonale. There is hypertrophy of the right ventricle and dilatation of the right atrium. The vascular changes are similar in primary and secondary types and involve the entire arterial tree from the main pulmonary arteries down to the arterioles.

1. Arterioles and small pulmonary arteries
i) Medial hypertrophy.
ii) Thickening and reduplication of elastic laminae.
iii) Plexiform pulmonary arteriopathy

2. Medium-sized pulmonary arteries
i) Medial hypertrophy.
ii) Concentric intimal thickening.
iii) Adventitial fibrosis.
iv) Thickening and reduplication of elastic laminae.

3. Large pulmonary arteries
i) Atheromatous deposits.

PULMONARY INFECTIONS *(p. 448)*

PNEUMONIAS *(p. 448)*

Pneumonia is defined as acute inflammation of the lung parenchyma distal to the terminal bronchioles (consisting of the respiratory bronchiole, alveolar ducts, alveolar sacs and alveoli). The terms 'pneumonia' and 'pneumonitis' are often used synonymously for inflammation of the lungs, while 'consolidation' (meaning solidification) is the term used for gross and radiologic appearance of the lungs in pneumonia.

PATHOGENESIS

The microorganisms gain entry into the lungs by one of the following four routes:
1. *Inhalation* of the microbes present in the air.
2. *Aspiration* of organisms from the nasopharynx or oropharynx.
3. *Haematogenous spread* from a distant focus of infection.
4. *Direct spread* from an adjoining site of infection.
   Failure of defense mechanisms and presence of certain predisposing factors result in pneumonias. These conditions are as under:
1. Altered consciousness
2. Depressed cough and glottic reflexes
3. Impaired mucociliary transport
4. Impaired alveolar macrophage function
5. Endobronchial obstruction
6. Immunocompromised states

CLASSIFICATION

I. On the basis of the *anatomic region* of the lung parenchyma involved, pneumonias are traditionally classified into 3 main types:
1. Lobar pneumonia
2. Bronchopneumonia (or Lobular pneumonia)
3. Interstitial pneumonia.

II. Based on the *clinical settings* in which infection occurred, pneumonias are classified as under:
1. Community-acquire pneumonia
2. Health care-associated pneumonia (including hospital-acquired pneumonia)
3. Ventilator-associated pneumonia

III. Based on *etiology and pathogenesis*, pneumonias are classified as under:

A. Bacterial pneumonia

B. Viral pneumonia

C. Pneumonias from other etiologies.

A. BACTERIAL PNEUMONIA

Bacterial infection of the lung parenchyma is the most common cause of pneumonia or consolidation of one or both the lungs. Two types of acute bacterial pneumonias are distinguished—lobar pneumonia and broncho-(lobular-) pneumonia, each with distinct etiologic agent and morphologic changes.

LOBAR PNEUMONIA

Lobar pneumonia is an acute bacterial infection of a part of a lobe, the entire lobe, or even two lobes of one or both the lungs.

ETIOLOGY Based on the etiologic microbial agent causing lobar pneumonia, following types are described:

1. Pneumococcal pneumonia More than 90% of all lobar pneumonias are caused by *Streptococcus pneumoniae,* a lancet-shaped diplococcus. Out of various types, type *3 S. pneumoniae* causes particularly virulent form of lobar pneumonia. Pneumococcal pneumonia in majority of cases is community-acquired infection.

2. Staphylococcal pneumonia *Staphylococcus aureus* causes pneumonia by haematogenous spread of infection from another focus or after viral infections.

3. Streptococcal pneumonia β-haemolytic streptococci may rarely cause pneumonia such as in children after measles or influenza, in severely debilitated elderly patients and in diabetics.

4. Pneumonia by gram-negative aerobic bacteria Less common causes of lobar pneumonia are gram-negative bacteria like *Haemophilus influenzae, Klebsiella pneumoniae (Friedlander's bacillus), Pseudomonas, Proteus* and *Escherichia coli, H. influenzae* commonly causes pneumonia in children below 3 years of age after a preceding viral infection.

MORPHOLOGIC FEATURES Laennec's original description divides lobar pneumonia into 4 sequential pathologic phases: *stage of congestion* (initial phase), *red hepatisation* (early consolidation), *grey hepatisation* (late consolidation) and *resolution*. However, these classic stages seen in untreated cases are found much less often nowadays due to early institution of antibiotic therapy and improved medical care.

1 STAGE OF CONGESTION: INITIAL PHASE The initial phase represents the early acute inflammatory response to bacterial infection that lasts for 1 to 2 days.

G/A The affected lobe is enlarged, heavy, dark red and congested. Cut surface exudes blood-stained frothy fluid.

M/E Salient features are:

i) Dilatation and congestion of the capillaries in the alveolar walls.

ii) Pale eosinophilic oedema fluid in the air spaces.

iii) A few red cells and neutrophils in the intra-alveolar fluid.

iv) Numerous bacteria demonstrated in the alveolar fluid by Gram's staining.

2. RED HEPATISATION: EARLY CONSOLIDATION This phase lasts for 2 to 4 days. The term hepatisation in pneumonia refers to liver-like consistency of the affected lobe on cut section.

G/A The affected lobe is red, firm and consolidated. The cut surface of the involved lobe is airless, red-pink, dry, granular and has liver-like consistency. The stage of red hepatisation is accompanied by serofibrinous pleurisy.

M/E Salient features are:

i) The oedema fluid of the preceding stage is replaced by strands of fibrin.

ii) There is marked cellular exudate of neutrophils and extravasation of red cells.

iii) Many neutrophils show ingested bacteria.

iv) The alveolar septa are less prominent than in the first stage due to cellular exudation.

3. GREY HEPATISATION: LATE CONSOLIDATION This phase lasts for 4 to 8 days.

G/A The affected lobe is firm and heavy. The cut surface is dry, granular and grey in appearance with liver-like consistency.

M/E Salient features are:

i) The fibrin strands are dense and more numerous.

ii) The cellular exudate of neutrophils is reduced due to disintegration of many inflammatory cells as evidenced by their pyknotic nuclei. The red cells are also fewer. The macrophages begin to appear in the exudate.

iii) The cellular exudate is often separated from the septal walls by a thin clear space.

iv) The organisms are less numerous and appear as degenerated forms.

4. RESOLUTION This stage begins by 8th to 9th day if no chemotherapy is administered and is completed in 1 to 3 weeks.

G/A The previously solid fibrinous constituent is liquefied by enzymatic action, eventually restoring the normal aeration in the affected lobe. The cut surface is grey-red or dirty brown and frothy, yellow, creamy fluid can be expressed on pressing.

M/E Salient features are:

i) Macrophages are the predominant cells in the alveolar spaces, while neutrophils diminish in number. Many of the macrophages contain engulfed neutrophils and debris.

ii) Granular and fragmented strands of fibrin in the alveolar spaces are seen due to progressive enzymatic digestion.

iii) Alveolar capillaries are engorged.

iv) There is progressive removal of fluid content as well as cellular exudate from the air spaces, partly by expectoration but mainly by lymphatics.

COMPLICATIONS Since the advent of antibiotics, serious complications of lobar pneumonia are uncommon. However, they may develop in neglected cases and in patients with impaired immunologic defenses. These are:

1. Organisation
2. Pleural effusion
3. Empyema
4. Lung abscess
5. Metastatic infection

CLINICAL FEATURES Classically, the onset of lobar pneumonia is sudden. The major symptoms are: shaking chills, fever, malaise with pleuritic chest pain, dyspnoea and cough with expectoration which may be mucoid, purulent or even bloody. The common physical findings are fever, tachycardia, and tachypnoea, and sometimes cyanosis if the patient is severely hypoxaemic. There is generally a marked neutrophilic leucocytosis. Blood cultures are positive in about 30% of cases. Chest radiograph may reveal consolidation.

BRONCHOPNEUMONIA (LOBULAR PNEUMONIA)

Bronchopneumonia or lobular pneumonia is infection of the terminal bronchioles that extends into the surrounding alveoli resulting in patchy consolidation of the lung. The condition is particularly frequent at the extremes of life (i.e. in infancy and old age), as a terminal event in chronic debilitating diseases and as a secondary infection following viral respiratory infections such as influenza, measles etc.

ETIOLOGY The common organisms responsible for bronchopneumonia are staphylococci, streptococci, pneumococci, *Klebsiella pneumoniae, Haemophilus influenzae,* and gram-negative bacilli like *Pseudomonas* and coliform bacteria.

G/A Bronchopneumonia is identified by patchy areas of red or grey consolidation affecting one or more lobes, frequently found bilaterally and more often involving the lower zones of the lungs due to gravitation of the secretions. On cut surface, these patchy consolidated lesions are dry, granular, firm, red or grey in colour, 3 to 4 cm in diameter, slightly elevated over the surface and are often centred around a bronchiole.

M/E Main findings are:
i) Acute bronchiolitis.
ii) Suppurative exudate, consisting chiefly of neutrophils, in the peribronchiolar alveoli.
iii) Thickening of the alveolar septa by congested capillaries and leucocytic infiltration.
iv) Less involved alveoli contain oedema fluid.

COMPLICATIONS The complications of lobar pneumonia may occur in bronchopneumonia as well.

CLINICAL FEATURES The patients of bronchopneumonia are generally infants or elderly individuals. There may be history of preceding bed-ridden illness, chronic debility, aspiration of gastric contents or upper respiratory infection. For initial 2 to 3 days, there are features of acute bronchitis but subsequently signs and symptoms similar to those of lobar pneumonia appear. Blood examination usually shows a neutrophilic leucocytosis. Chest radiograph shows mottled, focal opacities in both the lungs, chiefly in the lower zones.

LEGIONELLA PNEUMONIA

Legionella pneumonia or Legionnaire's disease is an epidemic illness caused by gram-negative bacilli, *Legionella pneumophila* that thrives in aquatic environment. The epidemic occurs in summer months by spread of organisms through contaminated drinking water or in air-conditioning cooling towers. Impaired host defenses in the form of immunodeficiency, corticosteroid therapy, old age and cigarette smoking play important roles.

CLINICAL FEATURES The disease begins with malaise, headache and muscle-aches followed by high fever, chills, cough and tachypnoea. Systemic manifestations unrelated to pathologic changes in the lungs are seen due to bacteraemia and include abdominal pain, watery diarrhoea, proteinuria and mild hepatic dysfunction.

B. VIRAL AND MYCOPLASMAL PNEUMONIA (PRIMARY ATYPICAL PNEUMONIA)

Viral and mycoplasmal pneumonia is characterised by patchy inflammatory changes, largely confined to interstitial tissue of the lungs, without any alveolar exudate. Other terms used for these respiratory tract infections are *interstitial pneumonitis,* reflecting the interstitial location of the inflammation, and *primary atypical pneumonia,* atypicality being the absence of alveolar exudate commonly present in other pneumonias.

ETIOLOGY Interstitial pneumonitis is caused by a wide variety of agents, the most common being *respiratory syncytial virus* (RSV). Others are *Mycoplasma pneumoniae* and many viruses such as influenza and para-influenza viruses, adenoviruses, rhinoviruses, coxsackieviruses and cyto-megaloviruses (CMV). Occasionally, psittacosis *(Chlamydia)* and Q fever *(Coxiella)* are associated with interstitial pneumonitis.

G/A Depending upon the severity of infection, the involvement may be patchy to massive and widespread consolidation of one or both the lungs. The lungs are heavy, congested and subcrepitant. Sectioned surface of the lung exudes small amount of frothy or bloody fluid. The pleural reaction is usually infrequent and mild.

M/E Main changes are as under:

i) Interstitial inflammation There is thickening of alveolar walls due to congestion, oedema and mononuclear inflammatory infiltrate.

ii) Necrotising bronchiolitis This is characterised by foci of necrosis of the bronchiolar epithelium, inspissated secretions in the lumina and mononuclear infiltrate in the walls and lumina.

iii) Reactive changes The lining epithelial cells of the bronchioles and alveoli proliferate in the presence of virus and may form multinucleate giant cells and syncytia in the bronchiolar and alveolar walls.

iv) Alveolar changes In severe cases, the alveolar lumina may contain oedema fluid, fibrin, scanty inflammatory exudate and coating of alveolar walls by pink, hyaline membrane.

COMPLICATIONS The major complication of interstitial pneumonitis is superimposed bacterial infection and its complications.

CLINICAL FEATURES Majority of cases of interstitial pneumonitis initially have upper respiratory symptoms with fever, headache and muscle-aches. A few days later, dry, hacking, non-productive cough with retrosternal burning appears due to tracheitis and bronchitis. Blood film shows characteristic neutrophilic leucocytosis. Chest radiograph may show patchy or diffuse consolidation.

C. FUNGAL INFECTIONS OF LUNG (FUNGAL PNEUMONIAS)

PNEUMOCYSTIS PNEUMONIA

Pneumocystis is an opportunistic fungal infection of the lungs. The original species *P. carinii* infects rats while *P. jirovecii* causes pneumonia by inhalation of the organisms in neonates and immunosuppressed people. Almost 100% cases of HIV/AIDS develop opportunistic infection during the course of disease, most commonly *Pneumocystis* pneumonia.

G/A The affected parts of the lung are consolidated, dry and grey.

M/E Salient features are:

i) Interstitial pneumonitis with thickening and mononuclear infiltration of the alveolar walls.

ii) Alveolar lumina contain pink frothy fluid having the organisms.

iii) By Grocott's methenamine-silver (GMS) stain, the characteristic oval or crescentic cysts, about 5 µm in diameter and surrounded by numerous tiny black dot-like organism *P. jirovecii* are demonstrable in the frothy fluid.

OTHER FUNGAL INFECTIONS OF LUNG

1. Aspergillosis Aspergillosis is the most common fungal infection of the lung caused by *Aspergillus fumigatus* that grows best in cool, wet climate. The infection may result in *allergic bronchopulmonary aspergillosis, aspergilloma* and *necrotising bronchitis.* Immunocompromised persons develop more serious manifestations of aspergillus infection, especially in leukaemic patients on cytotoxic drug therapy and HIV/AIDS.

G/A Pulmonary aspergillosis may occur within pre-existing pulmonary cavities or in bronchiectasis as fungal ball.

M/E The fungus may appear as a tangled mass within the cavity. The organisms are identified by their characteristic morphology—thin septate hyphae with dichotomous branching at acute angles which stain positive for fungal stains such as PAS and silver impregnation technique.

2. Mucormycosis Mucormycosis or phycomycosis is caused by *Mucor* and *Rhizopus*. The infection in the lung occurs in a similar way as in aspergillosis. Mucor is distinguished by its broad, non-parallel, nonseptate hyphae which branch at an obtuse angle. Mucormycosis is more often angioinvasive, and disseminates; hence it is more destructive than aspergillosis.

3.   **Candidiasis**   Candidiasis or moniliasis caused by *Candida albicans* is a normal commensal in oral cavity, gut and vagina but attains pathologic form in immunocompromised host.

4.   **Histoplasmosis**   It is caused by oval organism, *Histoplasma capsulatum,* by inhalation of infected dust or bird droppings.

5.   **Cryptococcosis**   It is caused by *Cryptococcus neoformans* which is round yeast having a halo around it due to shrinkage in tissue sections. The infection occurs from infection by inhalation of pigeon droppings.

6.   **Coccidioidomycosis**   Coccidioidomycosis is caused by *Coccidioides immitis* which are spherical spores.

7.   **Blastomycosis**   It is an uncommon condition caused by *Blastomyces dermatitidis.* The lesions result from inhalation of spores in the ground.

D. NON INFECTIVE PNEUMONIAS

ASPIRATION (INHALATION) PNEUMONIA

Aspiration or inhalation pneumonia results from inhalation of different agents into the lungs. These substances include food, gastric contents, foreign body and infected material from oral cavity. A number of factors predispose to inhalation pneumonia which include: unconsciousness, drunkenness, neurological disorders affecting swallowing, drowning, necrotic oropharyngeal tumours, in premature infants and congenital tracheo-oeso-phageal fistula.

M/E Main features are:
1. Aspiration of small amount of **sterile foreign matter** such as acidic gastric contents produces *chemical pneumonitis.*
2. **Non-sterile aspirate** causes widespread *bronchopneumonia* with multiple areas of necrosis and suppuration.

HYPOSTATIC PNEUMONIA

Hypostatic pneumonia is the term used for collection of oedema fluid and secretions in the dependent parts of the lungs in severely debilitated, bed-ridden patients.

LIPID PNEUMONIA

Another variety of non-infective pneumonia is lipid pneumonia which is of 2 types: exogenous and endogenous.

G/A The exogenous lipid pneumonia affects the right lung more frequently due to direct path from the main bronchus. Quite often, the lesions are bilateral.

M/E Main findings are:
i) Lipid is finely dispersed in the cytoplasm of macrophages forming foamy macrophages within the alveolar spaces.
ii) There may be formation of cholesterol clefts due to liberation of cholesterol and other lipids.
iii) Formation of granulomas with foreign body giant cells may be seen around the large lipid droplets.

LUNG ABSCESS *(p. 457)*

Lung abscess is a localised area of necrosis of lung tissue with suppuration. It is of 2 types:
◈   *Primary lung abscess* that develops in an otherwise normal lung. The commonest cause is aspiration of infected material.
◈   *Secondary lung abscess* that develops as a complication of some other disease of the lung or from another site.

ETIOPATHOGENESIS   The microorganisms are introduced into the lungs from one of the following mechanisms:

1. Aspiration of infected foreign material
2. Preceding bacterial infection
3. Bronchial obstruction
4. Septic embolism
5. Miscellaneous e.g. infection of lung infarct, amoebic abscess of lung, trauma to lungs and direct extension from a suppurative focus in the vicinity.

MORPHOLOGIC FEATURES Abscesses due to aspiration are more likely to be in right lung due to more vertical main bronchus and are frequently single. They are commonly located in the lower part of the right upper lobe or apex of right lower lobe. Abscesses developing from preceding pneumonia and septic or pyaemic abscesses are often multiple and scattered throughout the lung.

G/A Abscesses may be of variable size from a few millimeters to large cavities, 5 to 6 cm in diameter. The cavity often contains exudate.

M/E The characteristic feature is the destruction of lung parenchyma with suppurative exudate in the lung cavity. The cavity is initially surrounded by acute inflammation in the wall but later there is replacement by chronic inflammatory cell infiltrate composed of lymphocytes, plasma cells and macrophages.

CLINICAL FEATURES The clinical manifestations are fever, malaise, loss of weight, cough, purulent expectoration and haemoptysis in half the cases. Clubbing of the fingers and toes appears in about 20% of patients. Secondary amyloidosis may occur in chronic long-standing cases.

CHRONIC OBSTRUCTIVE PULMONARY DISEASE (p. 458)

Chronic obstructive pulmonary disease (COPD) or chronic obstructive airway disease (COAD) are commonly used clinical terms for a group of pathological conditions in which there is chronic, partial or complete, obstruction to the airflow at any level from trachea to the smallest airways resulting in functional disability of the lungs i.e. these are diffuse lung diseases. One etiologic factor which is a common denominator in all forms of COPD is smoking. The following entities are included in COPD:
I. Chronic bronchitis
II. Emphysema
III. Bronchial asthma
IV. Bronchiectasis
V. Small airways disease (bronchiolitis)

CHRONIC BRONCHITIS (p. 458)

Chronic bronchitis is a common condition defined *clinically* as persistent cough with expectoration on most days for at least three months of the year for two or more consecutive years. The cough is caused by oversecretion of mucus.

ETIOPATHOGENESIS The two most important etiologic factors responsible for majority of cases of chronic bronchitis are: cigarette smoking and atmospheric pollution. Other contributory factors are occupation, infection, familial and genetic factors.

G/A The bronchial wall is thickened, hyperaemic and oedematous. Lumina of the bronchi and bronchioles may contain mucus plugs and purulent exudate.

M/E Just as there is clinical definition, there is histologic definition of chronic bronchitis by increased Reid index. *Reid index* is the ratio between thickness of the submucosal mucus glands (i.e. hypertrophy and hyperplasia) in the cartilage-containing large airways to that of the total bronchial wall.

CLINICAL FEATURES Some important features of 'predominant bronchitis' are as under:
1. Persistent cough with copious expectoration of long duration; initially beginning in a heavy smoker with 'morning catarrh' or 'throat clearing' which worsens in winter.

2.   Recurrent respiratory infections are common.
3.   Dyspnoea is generally not prominent at rest but is more on exertion.

EMPHYSEMA (p. 459)

The WHO has defined pulmonary emphysema as combination of permanent dilatation of air spaces distal to the terminal bronchioles and the destruction of the walls of dilated air spaces. *Thus, emphysema is defined morphologically, while chronic bronchitis is defined clinically.*

CLASSIFICATION   As per WHO definition of pulmonary emphysema, it is classified according to the portion of the acinus involved, into 5 types: centriacinar, panacinar (panlobular), para-septal (distal acinar), irregular (para-cicatricial) and mixed (unclassified) emphysema. A number of other conditions to which the term 'emphysema' is loosely applied are, in fact, examples of 'overinflation'.

ETIOPATHOGENESIS   The commonest form of COPD is the combination of chronic bronchitis and pulmonary emphysema. The association of the two conditions is principally linked to the common etiologic factors—most importantly *tobacco smoke* and *air pollutants*. Other less significant contributory factors are occupational exposure, infection and somewhat poorly-understood familial and genetic influences. All these factors have already been discussed above.

However, pathogenesis of the most significant event in emphysema, the *destruction of the alveolar walls*, is not linked to bronchial changes but is closely related to deficiency of serum α-1-antitrypsin (α1-protease inhibitor) commonly termed *protease-antiprotease hypothesis.*

The α1-AT deficiency develops in adults and causes pulmonary emphysema in smokers as well as in non-smokers, though smokers become symptomatic about 15 years earlier than non-smokers. The other organ showing effects of α1-AT deficiency is the liver which may develop obstructive jaundice early in infancy, and cirrhosis and hepatoma late in adulthood.

The mechanism of alveolar wall destruction in emphysema by elastolytic action is based on the imbalance between proteases (chiefly *elastase)* and anti-proteases (chiefly *anti-elastase):*
i)   By decreased anti-elastase activity i.e. deficiency of α-1 antitrypsin.
ii)   By increased activity of elastase i.e. increased neutrophilic infiltration in the lungs causing excessive elaboration of neutrophil elastase.

G/A   The lungs are voluminous, pale with little blood. The edges of the lungs are rounded. Advanced cases show subpleural bullae and blebs bulging outwards from the surface of the lungs with rib markings between them. The *bullae* are air-filled cyst-like or bubble-like structures, larger than 1 cm in diameter.

M/E   Depending upon the type of emphysema, there is dilatation of air spaces and destruction of septal walls of part of acinus involved i.e. respiratory bronchioles, alveolar ducts and alveolar sacs. Changes of bronchitis may be present. Bullae and blebs when present show fibrosis and chronic inflammation of the walls.

CLINICAL FEATURES   Though there is considerable overlap between the clinical features of chronic bronchitis and emphysema. Following features generally characterise 'predominant emphysema':
1.   There is long history of slowly increasing severe exertional dyspnoea.
2.   Patient is quite distressed with obvious use of accessory muscles of respiration.
3.   Chest is barrel-shaped and hyperresonant.
4.   Cough occurs late after dyspnoea starts and is associated with scanty mucoid sputum.
5.   Recurrent respiratory infections are not frequent.

MORPHOLOGY OF INDIVIDUAL TYPES OF EMPHYSEMA

1.   CENTRIACINAR (CENTRILOBULAR) EMPHYSEMA   Centriacinar or centrilobular emphysema is one of the common types. It is characterised by initial involvement of respiratory bronchioles i.e. the central or proximal part of the acinus.

G/A The lesions are more common and more severe in the upper lobes of the lungs. The characteristic appearance is obvious in cut surface of the lung. It shows distended air spaces in the centre of the lobules surrounded by a rim of normal lung parenchyma in the same lobule.

M/E There is distension and destruction of the respiratory bronchiole in the centre of lobules, surrounded peripherally by normal uninvolved alveoli.

2. PANACINAR (PANLOBULAR) EMPHYSEMA Panacinar or panlobular emphysema is the other common type. In this type, all portions of the acinus are affected but not of the entire lung.

G/A In contrast to centriacinar emphysema, the panacinar emphysema involves lower zone of lungs more frequently and more severely than the upper zone.

M/E Usually all the alveoli within a lobule are affected to the same degree. All portions of acini are distended—respiratory bronchioles, alveolar ducts and alveoli, are all dilated and their walls stretched and thin. Ruptured alveolar walls and spurs of broken septa are seen between the adjacent alveoli.

3. PARASEPTAL (DISTAL ACINAR) EMPHYSEMA This type of emphysema involves distal part of acinus while the proximal part is normal. Paraseptal or distal acinar emphysema is localised along the pleura and along the perilobular septa.

4. IRREGULAR (PARA-CICATRICIAL) EMPHYSEMA This is the most common form of emphysema, seen surrounding scars from any cause.

5. MIXED (UNCLASSIFIED) EMPHYSEMA Quite often, the same lung may show more than one type of emphysema.

MORPHOLOGY OF TYPES OF OVERINFLATION

Under this heading are covered a group of lung conditions of heterogeneous etiology characterised by overinflation of the parts of acini but without significant destruction of the walls and are sometimes loosely termed emphysema.

1. COMPENSATORY OVERINFLATION (COMPENSATORY EMPHY-SEMA) When part of a lung or a lobe of lung is surgically removed, the residual lung parenchyma undergoes compensatory hyperinflation so as to fill the pleural cavity.

2. SENILE HYPERINFLATION (AGEING LUNG, SENILE EMPHYSEMA) In old people, the lungs become voluminous due to loss of elastic tissue, thinning and atrophy of the alveolar ducts and alveoli:

3. OBSTRUCTIVE OVERINFLATION (INFANTILE LOBAR EMPHYSEMA) Partial obstruction to the bronchial tree such as by a tumour or a foreign body causes overinflation of the region supplied by obstructed bronchus.

4. UNILATERAL TRANSLUCENT LUNG (UNILATERAL EMPHYSEMA) This is a form of overinflation in which one lung or one of its lobes or segments of a lobe are radiolucent.

5. INTERSTITIAL EMPHYSEMA (SURGICAL EMPHYSEMA) The entry of air into the connective tissue framework of the lung is called interstitial or surgical emphysema. The causes are as under:
i)   Violent coughing with bronchiolar obstruction.
ii)   Rupture of the oesophagus, trauma to the lung, or major bronchus and trachea.
iii) Entry of air through surgical incision.
iv)   Fractured rib puncturing the lung parenchyma.
v)   Sudden change in atmospheric pressure e.g. in decompression sickness.
      The condition may affect patients of all ages.

BRONCHIAL ASTHMA *(p. 463)*

Asthma is a disease of airways that is characterised by increased responsiveness of the tracheobronchial tree to a variety of stimuli resulting in widespread spasmodic narrowing of the air passages which may be relieved spontaneously or by therapy. Asthma is an episodic disease manifested clinically by paroxysms of dyspnoea, cough and wheezing. However, a severe and unremitting form of the disease termed *status asthmaticus* may prove fatal.

ETIOPATHOGENESIS AND TYPES Based on the stimuli initiating bronchial asthma, two broad etiologic types are traditionally described: *extrinsic (allergic, atopic)* and *intrinsic (idiosyncratic, non-atopic)* asthma. A third type is a *mixed pattern* in which the features do not fit clearly into either of the two main types.

1. Extrinsic (atopic, allergic) asthma This is the most common type of asthma. It usually begins in childhood or in early adult life. Most patients of this type of asthma have personal and/or family history of preceding allergic diseases such as rhinitis, urticaria or infantile eczema. Hypersensitivity to various extrinsic antigenic substances or 'allergens' is usually present in these cases. There is increased level of IgE in the serum and positive skin test with the specific offending inhaled antigen representing an IgE-mediated type I hypersensitivity reaction which includes an 'acute immediate response' and a 'late phase reaction'.

2. Intrinsic (idiosyncratic, non-atopic) asthma This type of asthma develops later in adult life with negative personal or family history of allergy, negative skin test and normal serum levels of IgE. Most of these patients develop typical symptom-complex after an upper respiratory tract infection by viruses.

3. Mixed type Many patients do not clearly fit into either of the above two categories and have mixed features of both. Those patients who develop asthma in early life have strong allergic component, while those who develop the disease late tend to be non-allergic.

G/A The lungs are overdistended due to over-inflation. The cut surface shows characteristic occlusion of the bronchi and bronchioles by viscid mucus plugs.

M/E
1. The mucus plugs contain normal or degenerated respiratory epithelium forming twisted strips called *Curschmann's spirals*.
2. The sputum usually contains numerous eosinophils and diamond-shaped crystals derived from eosinophils called *Charcot-Leyden crystals*.
3. The bronchial wall shows thickened basement membrane of the bronchial epithelium, submucosal oedema and inflammatory infiltrate consisting of lymphocytes and plasma cells with prominence of eosinophils.

BRONCHIECTASIS *(p. 465)*

Bronchiectasis is defined as abnormal and irreversible dilatation of the bronchi and bronchioles (greater than 2 mm in diameter) developing secondary to inflammatory weakening of the bronchial walls. The most characteristic clinical manifestation of bronchiectasis is persistent cough with expectoration of copious amounts of foul-smelling, purulent sputum.

ETIOPATHOGENESIS The origin of inflammatory destructive process of bronchial walls is nearly always a result of two basic mechanisms: endobronchial obstruction and infection.

These 2 mechanisms are seen in a number of clinical settings as under:

1. Hereditary and congenital factors e.g.
i) Congenital bronchiectasis
ii) Cystic fibrosis
iii) Hereditary immune deficiency diseases
iv) Immotile cilia syndrome
v) Atopic bronchial asthma.

2. Obstruction Post-obstructive bronchiectasis, unlike the congenital-hereditary forms, is of the localised variety, usually confined to one part of the bronchial system. The causes of endobronchial obstruction include foreign bodies, endobronchial tumours, compression by enlarged hilar lymph nodes and post-inflammatory scarring (e.g. in healed tuberculosis).

3. As secondary complication *Necrotising pneumonias* such as in staphylococcal suppurative pneumonia and *tuberculosis* may develop bronchiectasis as a complication.

G/A The lungs may be involved diffusely or segmentally. Bilateral involvement of lower lobes occurs most frequently. The pleura is usually fibrotic and thickened with adhesions to the chest wall. The dilated airways, depending upon their gross or bronchographic appearance, have been subclassified into the following different types:

i) Cylindrical
ii) Fusiform
iii) Saccular
iv) Varicose

Cut surface of the affected lobes, generally the lower zones, shows characteristic honey-combed appearance. The bronchi are extensively dilated nearly to the pleura, their walls are thickened and the lumina are filled with mucus or mucopus.

M/E Main findings are as under:

i) The bronchial epithelium may be normal, ulcerated or may show squamous metaplasia.
ii) The bronchial wall shows infiltration by acute and chronic inflammatory cells and destruction of normal muscle and elastic tissue with replacement by fibrosis.
iii) The intervening lung parenchyma shows fibrosis, while the surrounding lung tissue shows changes of interstitial pneumonia.

CLINICAL FEATURES The clinical manifestations of bronchiectasis typically consist of chronic cough with foul-smelling sputum production, haemoptysis and recurrent pneumonia. Sinusitis is a common accompaniment of diffuse bronchiectasis. Late complications occurring in cases uncontrolled for years include development of clubbing of the fingers, metastatic abscesses (often to the brain), amyloidosis and cor pulmonale.

SMALL AIRWAYS DISEASE *(p. 466)*

Bronchiolitis and bronchiolitis obliterans are the inflammatory conditions affecting the small airways occurring predominantly in older paediatric age group and in quite elderly persons. A number of etiologic factors have been stated to cause this condition. These include viral infection (frequently adenovirus and respiratory syncytial virus), bacterial infection, fungal infection, inhalation of toxic gases (e.g. in silo-fillers' disease) and aspiration of gastric contents.

M/E The lumina of affected bronchioles are narrow and occluded by fibrous plugs. The bronchiolar walls are inflamed and are infiltrated by lymphocytes and plasma cells. There are changes of interstitial pneumonitis and fibrosis in the alveoli around the affected bronchioles.

CHRONIC RESTRICTIVE PULMONARY DISEASE *(p. 467)*

The second large group of diffuse lung disease is 'chronic restrictive pulmonary disease' characterised by reduced expansion of lung parenchyma with decreased total lung capacity.

Restrictive lung disease includes 2 types of conditions:

A. Restriction due to chest wall disorder
1. Kyphoscoliosis
2. Poliomyelitis
3. Severe obesity
4. Pleural diseases.

B. Restriction due to interstitial and infiltrative diseases Commonly called as '*interstitial lung diseases (ILDs)*', these are diseases characterised by non-infectious diffuse parenchymal involvement of the lung i.e. the alveolar lumina and alveolar epithelium, capillary basement membrane, the intervening space, perivascular tissue and lymphatic tissue. The term 'infiltrative' is used here to denote the radiologic appearance of lungs in chest radiographs which show characteristic diffuse interstitial ground-glass opacities. Depending upon the underlying pathologic findings, ILDs have been broadly classified as under:

I. WITH PREDOMINANT FIBROSIS
   1. Pneumoconiosis with inorganic minerals: coal, asbestos, fumes, gases
   2. Idiopathic pulmonary fibrosis (Idiopathic interstitial pneumonias)
   3. Nonspecific interstitial pneumonia
   4. Acute interstitial pneumonia (Hamman-Rich syndrome)
   5. Cryptogenic organising pneumonia
   6. Therapy related-ILD (radiation, antibiotics, chemotherapy)
   7. Connective tissue diseases
   8. Residual effects of ARDS

II. WITH PREDOMINANT GRANULOMATOUS REACTION
   1. Sarcoidosis
   2. Pneumoconiosis with inorganic dusts: silica, beryllium
   3. Granulomatous vasculitis
   4. Wegener's granulomatosis

III. IMMUNOLOGIC LUNG DISEASES (EOSINOPHILIC PNEUMONIAS)
   1. Hypersensitivity pneumonitis: with organic dusts
   2. Pulmonary infiltrates with eosinophilia (PIE)
   3. Pulmonary haemorrhage syndromes (Goodpasture's syndrome)
   4. Pulmonary alveolar proteinosis

IV. SMOKING-ASSOCIATED ILDs
   1. Desquamative interstitial pneumonia (DIP)
   2. Respiratory bronchiolitis-associated ILD
   3. Pulmonary Langerhans cell histiocytosis (eosinophilic granuloma of the lung)

PNEUMOCONIOSES *(p. 467)*

Pneumoconiosis is the term used for lung diseases caused by inhalation of dust, mostly at work (*pneumo* = lung; *conis* = dust in Greek). These diseases are, therefore, also called 'dust diseases' or 'occupational lung diseases'.

The type of lung disease varies according to the nature of inhaled dust. Some dusts are inert and cause no reaction and no damage at all, while others cause immunologic damage and predispose to tuberculosis or to neoplasia. The factors which determine the extent of damage caused by inhaled dusts are as under:
1. size and shape of the particles;
2. their solubility and physicochemical composition;
3. the amount of dust retained in the lungs;
4. the additional effect of other irritants such as tobacco smoke; and
5. host factors such as efficiency of clearance mechanism and immune status of the host.

The tissue response to inhaled dust may be one of the following three types:
❖ *Fibrous nodules* e.g. in coal-workers' pneumoconiosis and silicosis.
❖ *Interstitial fibrosis* e.g. in asbestosis.
❖ *Hypersensitivity reaction* e.g. in berylliosis.

COAL-WORKERS' PNEUMOCONIOSIS

This is the commonest form of pneumoconiosis and is defined as the lung disease resulting from inhalation of coal dust particles, especially in coal-miners engaged in handling soft bituminous coal for a number of years, often 20 to 30 years.

PATHOGENESIS Anthracosis, simple coal-workers' pneumoconiosis and progressive massive fibrosis are different stages in the evolution of fully-developed coal-workers' pneumoconiosis. A number of predisposing factors have been implicated in this transformation as follows:

1. Older age of the miners.
2. Severity of coal dust burden engulfed by macrophages.
3. Prolonged exposure (20 to 30 years) to coal dust.
4. Concomitant tuberculosis.
5. Additional role of silica dust.

Activation of alveolar macrophage plays the most significant role in the pathogenesis of progressive massive fibrosis by release of various mediators e.g.

i) *Free radicals* which are reactive oxygen species which damage the lung parenchyma.

ii) *Chemotactic factors* for various leucocytes (leukotrienes, TNF, IL-8 and IL-6) resulting in infiltration into pulmonary tissues by these inflammatory cells which on activation cause further damage.

iii) *Fibrogenic cytokines* such as IL-1, TNF and platelet derived growth factor (PDGF).

MORPHOLOGIC FEATURES The pathologic findings at autopsy of lungs in the major forms of coal-workers' pneumoconiosis are given under 3 headings:

SIMPLE COAL-WORKERS' PNEUMOCONIOSIS *G/A* The lung parenchyma shows small, black focal lesions, measuring less than 5 mm in diameter and evenly distributed throughout the lung but have a tendency to be more numerous in the upper lobes. These are termed *coal macules,* and if palpable are called *nodules.*

M/E Main features are as under:

1. Coal macules are composed of aggregates of dust-laden macrophages. These are present in the alveoli and in the bronchiolar and alveolar walls.
2. There is some increase in the network of reticulin and collagen in the coal macules.
3. Respiratory bronchioles and alveoli surrounding the macules are distended.

PROGRESSIVE MASSIVE FIBROSIS *G/A* Besides the coal macules and nodules of simple pneumoconiosis, there are larger, hard, black scattered areas measuring more than 2 cm in diameter and sometimes massive. They are usually bilateral and located more often in the upper parts of the lungs posteriorly. Sometimes, these masses break down centrally due to ischaemic necrosis or due to tuberculosis forming cavities filled with black semifluid resembling India ink.

M/E Main findings are as under:

1. The fibrous lesions are composed almost entirely of dense collagen and carbon pigment.
2. The wall of respiratory bronchioles and pulmonary vessels included in the massive scars are thickened and their lumina obliterated.
3. There is scanty inflammatory infiltrate of lymphocytes and plasma cells around the areas of massive scars.
4. The alveoli surrounding the scars are markedly dilated.

RHEUMATOID PNEUMOCONIOSIS (CAPLAN'S SYNDROME) Development of rheumatoid arthritis in a few cases of pneumoconiosis is termed Caplan's syndrome.

G/A The lungs have rounded, firm nodules with central necrosis, cavitation or calcification.

M/E The lung lesions are modified rheumatoid nodules with central zone of dust-laden fibrinoid necrosis enclosed by palisading fibroblasts and mononuclear cells.

CLINICAL FEATURES Simple coal-workers' pneumoconiosis is the mild form of disease characterised by chronic cough with black expectoration. The radiological findings of nodularities in the lungs appear after working for several years in coal-mines. Progressive massive fibrosis is, however, a serious disabling condition manifested by progressive dyspnoea and chronic cough with jet-black sputum. More advanced cases develop pulmonary hypertension and right ventricular hypertrophy (cor pulmonale).

SILICOSIS

Historically, silicosis used to be called 'knife grinders' lung. Silicosis is caused by prolonged inhalation of silicon dioxide, commonly called silica. Silica constitutes about one-fourth of earth's crust. Therefore, a number of occupations engaged in silceous rocks or sand and products manufactured from them are at increased risk. These include miners (e.g. of granite, sandstone, slate, coal, gold, tin and copper), quarry workers, tunnellers, sandblasters, grinders, ceramic workers, foundry workers and those involved in the manufacture of abrasives containing silica. Peculiar to India are the occupational exposure to pencil, slate and agate-grinding industry carrying high risk of silicosis (agate = very hard stone containing silica).

PATHOGENESIS Silicosis appears after prolonged exposure to silica dust, often a few decades. Besides, it depends upon a number of other factors such as total dose, duration of exposure, the type of silica inhaled and individual host factors. The mechanisms involved in the formation of silicotic nodules are not clearly understood. The following sequence of events has been proposed:

1. Silica particles between 0.5 to 5 μm size on reaching the alveoli are taken by the macrophages which undergo necrosis. New macrophages engulf the debris and thus a repetitive cycle of *phagocytosis and necrosis* is set up.
2. Some silica-laden macrophages are carried to the respiratory bronchioles, alveoli and in the interstitial tissue. Some of the silica dust is transported to the subpleural and interlobar lymphatics and into the regional lymph nodes. The *cellular aggregates* containing silica become associated with lymphocytes, plasma cells, mast cells and fibroblasts.
3. Silica dust is *fibrogenic*. Crystalline form, particularly quartz, is more fibrogenic than non-crystalline form of silica.
4. Simultaneously, there is *activation of T and B lymphocytes*.
5. As noted above, silica is *cytotoxic* and kills the macrophages which engulf it.

G/A The chronic silicotic lung is studded with well-circumscribed, hard, fibrotic nodules, 1 to 5 mm in diameters. They are scattered throughout the lung parenchyma but are initially more often located in the upper zones of the lungs. The pleura is grossly thickened and adherent to the chest wall. The lesions may undergo ischaemic necrosis and develop cavitation, or be complicated by tuberculosis and rheumatoid pneumoconiosis.

M/E Main findings are as under:

1. The silicotic nodules are located in the region of respiratory bronchioles, adjacent alveoli, pulmonary arteries, in the pleura and the regional lymph nodes.
2. The *silicotic nodules* consist of central hyalinised material with scanty cellularity and some amount of dust. The hyalinised centre is surrounded by concentric laminations of collagen which is further enclosed by more cellular connective tissue, dust-filled macrophages and a few lymphocytes and plasma cells.
3. The collagenous nodules have cleft-like spaces between the lamellae of collagen which when examined polariscopically may demonstrate numerous birefringent particles of silica.
4. The severe and progressive form of the disease may result in coalescence of adjacent nodules.
5. The intervening lung parenchyma may show hyperinflation or emphysema.

CLINICAL FEATURES The main presenting complaint is dyspnoea. In time, the patient may develop features of obstructive or restrictive pattern of disease. Other complications such as pulmonary tuberculosis, rheumatoid arthritis (Caplan's syndrome) and cor pulmonale may occur.

Asbestos as a mineral is known to mankind for more than 4000 years but its harmful effects have come to light during the last few decades. In general, if *coal is lot of dust and little fibrosis, asbestos is little dust and a lot of fibrosis*. In nature, asbestos exists as long thin fibrils which are fire-resistant and can be spun into yarns and fabrics suitable for thermal and electrical insulation and has many applications in industries. Particularly at risk are workers engaged in mining, fabrication and manufacture of a number of products from asbestos such as asbestos pipes, tiles, roofs, textiles, insulating boards, sewer and water conduits, brake lining, clutch castings etc.

There are two major geometric forms of asbestos:

◈ *Serpentine* consisting of curly and flexible fibres. It includes the most common chemical form *chrysotile* (white asbestos) comprising more than 90% of commercially used asbestos.

◈ *Amphibole* consists of straight, stiff and rigid fibres. It includes the less common chemical forms *crocidolite* (blue asbestos), *amosite* (brown asbestos), *tremolite, anthophyllite* and *actinolite.*

PATHOGENESIS Overexposure to asbestos for more than a decade may produce asbestosis of the lung, pleural lesions and certain tumours. Following mechanisms have been suggested:

1. The inhaled asbestos fibres are *phagocytosed by alveolar macrophages* from where they reach the interstitium.
2. The asbestos-laden macrophages release *chemo-attractants* for neutrophils and for more macrophages.
3. Asbestos fibres are coated with glycoprotein and endogenous haemosiderin to produce characteristic beaded or dumbbell-shaped *asbestos bodies.*
4. All types of asbestos are *fibrogenic* and result in interstitial fibrosis.
5. A few *immunological abnormalities* such as antinuclear antibodies and rheumatoid factor have been found in cases of asbestosis.
6. Asbestos fibres are *carcinogenic,* the most carcinogenic being crocidolite. There is high incidence of bronchogenic carcinoma in asbestosis.

MORPHOLOGIC FEATURES Over-exposure to asbestos is associated with 3 types of lesions: asbestosis, pleural disease and certain tumours.

A. ASBESTOSIS Its features are as under:

G/A The affected lungs are small and firm with cartilage-like thickening of the pleura. The sectioned surface shows variable degree of pulmonary fibrosis, especially in the subpleural areas and in the bases of lungs.

M/E The features are as under:
1. There is non-specific interstitial fibrosis.
2. There is presence of characteristic *asbestos bodies* in the involved area.
3. There may be changes of emphysema in the pulmonary parenchyma between the areas of interstitial fibrosis.

B. PLEURAL DISEASE Pleural disease in asbestos exposure may produce one of the following 3 types of lesions:
1. Pleural effusion
2. Visceral pleural fibrosis
3. Pleural plaques

C. TUMOURS Asbestos exposure predisposes to a number of cancers, most importantly bronchogenic carcinoma and malignant mesothelioma. A few others are: carcinomas of the oesophagus, stomach, colon, kidneys and larynx and various lymphoid malignancies.

CLINICAL FEATURES Asbestosis is a slow and insidious illness. The patient may remain asymptomatic for a number of years in spite of radiological evidence of calcific pleural plaques and parenchymatous changes. However, onset of interstitial fibrosis brings about dyspnoea with dry or productive cough. More advanced cases show development of Caplan's syndrome, pulmonary hypertension, cor pulmonale and various forms of cancers.

Berylliosis is caused by heavy exposure to dust or fumes of metallic beryllium or its salts. Beryllium was used in the past in fluorescent tubes and light bulbs but currently it is principally used in nuclear and aerospace industries and in the manufacture of electrical and electronic equipment. Two forms of pulmonary berylliosis are recognised—*acute* and *chronic*.

ACUTE BERYLLIOSIS Acute berylliosis occurs in individuals who are unusually sensitive to it and are heavily exposed to it for 2 to 4 weeks. The pulmonary reaction is in the form of an exudative chemical pneumonitis in which the alveoli are filled with protein-rich fluid with formation of hyaline membrane.

CHRONIC BERYLLIOSIS Chronic berylliosis develops in individuals who are sensitised to it for a number of years, often after a delay of 20 or more years. The disease is a cell-mediated hypersensitivity reaction in which the metal beryllium acts as a hapten. The condition is characterised by development of non-caseating epithelioid granulomas like those of sarcoidosis. The granulomas have giant cells which frequently contain 3 types of inclusions:
1. Birefringent crystals.
2. Concentrically-laminated haematoxyphilic Schaumann or conchoid bodies.
3. Acidophilic stellate-shaped asteroid bodies.

These inclusions are described in giant cells of granulomas in sarcoidosis too. Similar sarcoid-like granulomas can occur in other organs such as in the liver, kidneys, spleen or lymph nodes in chronic berylliosis.

ILDs ASSOCIATED WITH IMMUNOLOGIC LUNG DISEASES *(p. 474)*

HYPERSENSITIVITY (ALLERGIC) PNEUMONITIS

Hypersensitivity pneumonitis is a group of immunologically-mediated ILDs occurring in workers inhaling a variety of organic (biologic) antigenic materials. The condition may have an *acute* onset due to isolated exposure or may be *chronic* due to repeated low-dose exposure.

ETIOPATHOGENESIS The immunologic mechanisms underlying hypersensitivity pneumonitis from any of causes appear to be either type III immune-complex disease or type IV delayed-hypersensitivity reaction.

1. **Farmers' lung** is the classic example resulting from exposure to thermophilic actinomycetes generated by humid and warm mouldy hay.

2. **Bagassosis** occurs in individuals engaged in manufacture of paper and cardboard from sugarcane bagasse.

3. **Byssinosis** is an occupational lung disease occurring in workers exposed to fibres of cotton, flex and hemp for a number of years.

4. **Bird-breeders' (Bird-fanciers') lung** occurs in pigeon breeders, parrot breeders, chicken farmers and bird-fanciers who are exposed to bird-droppings.

5. **Mushroom-workers' lung** is found in mushroom cultivators exposed to mushroom compost dust.

6. **Malt-workers' lung** is seen in distillery and brewery workers who are exposed to mouldy barley and malt dust.

7. **Maple-bark disease** occurs in those involved in stripping of maple bark and inhale mouldy maple bark.

8. **Silo-fillers' disease** occurs in individuals who enter the *silo* (silo is an airtight store-house of fodder for farm animals) in which toxic fumes of nitric oxide and nitrogen dioxide are formed due to fermentation of silage.
◈ *In early stage,* the alveolar walls are diffusely infiltrated with lymphocytes, plasma cells and macrophages.
◈ *In chronic cases,* the lungs show interstitial fibrosis with some inflammatory infiltrate.

PULMONARY INFILTRATES WITH EOSINOPHILIA

Pulmonary eosinophilia, eosinophilic pneumonias or pulmonary infiltration with eosinophilia (PIE) syndrome are a group of immunologically-mediated lung diseases characterised by combination of 2 features:

◈ Infiltration of the lungs in chest radiographs.

◈ Elevated eosinophil count in the peripheral blood.

ETIOPATHOGENESIS PIE syndrome has a number of diverse causes and pathogenesis.

1. **Löeffler's syndrome** is characterised by eosinophilia in the blood and typical wandering radiologic shadows, appearing in some part of the lung for a few days, and then disappearing to appear again somewhere else in the lung.

2. **Tropical pulmonary eosinophilia** is caused by the passage of larvae of worms through the lungs e.g. in filariasis, ascariasis, strongyloidosis, toxocariasis and ancylostomiasis.

3. **Secondary chronic pulmonary eosinophilia** occurs secondary to adverse drug reactions; infection with fungi, bacteria, and helminths; allergic bronchopulmonary aspergillosis and in association with asthma.

4. **Idiopathic chronic eosinophilic pneumonia** is characterised by prominent focal areas of consolidation of the lung.

5. **Hypereosinophilic syndrome** is occurrence of eosinophilia of over 1500/μl for more than 6 months without any identifiable cause and without eosinophilic infiltrates in the lungs and other organs.

GOODPASTURE'S SYNDROME

Goodpasture's syndrome or pulmonary haemorrhage syndrome is combination of necrotising haemorrhagic interstitial pneumonitis and rapidly progressive glomerulonephritis.

ETIOPATHOGENESIS The condition results from immunologic damage produced by anti-basement membrane antibodies formed against antigens common to the glomerular and pulmonary basement membranes.

G/A The lungs are heavy with red-brown areas of consolidation.

M/E The features are different in early and late stages:

◈ *In acute stage,* there are focal areas of haemorrhages in the alveoli and focal necrosis in the alveolar walls.

◈ *In more chronic cases,* there is organisation of the haemorrhage leading to interstitial fibrosis and filling of alveoli with haemosiderin-laden macrophages.

PULMONARY ALVEOLAR PROTEINOSIS

Pulmonary alveolar proteinosis is a rare chronic disease in which the distal airspaces of the lungs are filled with granular, PAS-positive, eosinophilic material with abundant lipid in it. The condition can occur at any age from infancy to old age.

ETIOPATHOGENESIS The etiology and pathogenesis of alveolar proteinosis are unknown.

1. Since the alveolar material is combination of lipid and protein, it is not simply an overproduction of surfactant.

2. Alveolar proteinosis may have an occupational etiology as seen in patients heavily exposed to silica.

3. It may have an etiologic association with haematologic malignancies.

4. There may be defective alveolar clearance of debris.

ILDs ASSOCIATED WITH CONNECTIVE TISSUE DISEASES *(p. 475)*

1.˙ **SCLERODERMA (PROGRESSIVE SYSTEMIC SCLEROSIS)** The lungs are involved in 80% cases of scleroderma. Interstitial pulmonary fibrosis is the most common form of pulmonary involvement. The disease usually involves the lower lobes and subpleural regions of the lungs and may lead to honeycombing of the lung.

2. RHEUMATOID ARTHRITIS Pulmonary involvement in rheumatoid arthritis may result in pleural effusion, interstitial pneumonitis, necrobiotic nodules and rheumatoid pneumoconiosis.

3. SYSTEMIC LUPUS ERYTHEMATOSUS Patients with systemic lupus erythematosus (SLE) commonly develop some form of lung disease during the course. The most common manifestation of SLE is pleurisy with small amount of pleural effusion that may contain LE cells.

4. SJÖGREN'S SYNDROME Patients with Sjögren's syndrome often have rheumatoid arthritis and associated pulmonary changes. Involvement of the bronchial mucous gland by a process similar to that in the salivary glands can lead to inadequate bronchial clearance and repeated infections.

5. DERMATOMYOSITIS AND POLYMYOSITIS Interstitial pneumonitis and interstitial fibrosis commonly accompany dermatomyositis and polymyositis.

6. WEGENER'S GRANULOMATOSIS Wegener's granulomatosis is an necro-inflammatory lesion having 4 components—granulomas of the upper respiratory tract, granulomas of the lungs, systemic vasculitis and focal necrotising glomerulonephritis. *Localised or limited form* of the disease occurs in the lungs without involvement of other organs.

M/E Granulomas have foci of fibrinoid necrosis and intense infiltrate of lymphocytes, plasma cells and macrophages with scattered multinucleate giant cells. Besides necrotising granulomas, there is associated vasculitis.

IDIOPATHIC PULMONARY FIBROSIS (p. 476)

Idiopathic pulmonary fibrosis is the most common form of diffuse interstitial pneumonia and has bad prognosis compared with other forms of lung fibrosis. Diffuse interstitial fibrosis can occur as a result of a number of pathologic entities such as pneumoconiosis, hypersensitivity pneumonitis and collagen-vascular disease. However, in half the cases of diffuse interstitial fibrosis, no apparent cause or underlying disease is identifiable.

PATHOGENESIS The pathogenesis of idiopathic pulmonary fibrosis is unknown and the condition is diagnosed by excluding all known causes of interstitial fibrosis. However, a few evidences point toward immunologic mechanism:
1. High levels of autoantibodies such as rheumatoid factor and antinuclear antibodies.
2. Elevated titres of circulating immune complexes.
3. Immunofluorescent demonstration of the deposits of immunoglobulins and complement on the alveolar walls in biopsy specimens.

G/A The lungs are firm, heavier with reduced volume. Honeycombing (i.e. enlarged, thick-walled air spaces) develops in parts of lung, particularly in the subpleural region.

M/E The features are different in early and advanced stage:
◈ **In early stage,** there is widening of the alveolar septa by oedema and cellular infiltrate by mononuclear inflammatory cells. Based on the obser-vation of desquamative component in the cellular exudate, some authors label the early stage of idiopathic pulmonary fibrosis as *'desquamative interstitial pneumonitis'*.
◈ **In advanced stage,** there is organisation of the alveolar exudate and replacement fibrosis in the alveoli as well as in the interstitial septal wall with variable amount of inflammation. Eventually, there are small cystic areas (honeycomb lung) with alternating areas of fibrosis containing thick-walled and narrowed vessels. This stage is often referred to as *'chronic interstitial pneumonitis'* or *'usual interstitial pneumonitis'*.

ILDs ASSOCIATED WITH SMOKING (p. 476)

Long-term consequence of smoking is associated with following non-neoplastic respiratory insufficiency:
◈ **Smoking-related COPD** These are chronic bronchitis and emphysema, which frequently coexist.

◈ **Smoking-related ILD** These are chronic restrictive pulmonary diseases due to desquamative interstitial pneumonia (DIP), respiratory bronchiolitis-associated ILD, and pulmonary Langerhans cell histiocytosis (eosinophilic granuloma of the lung).

DESQUAMATIVE INTERSTITIAL PNEUMONIA (DIP) It is an uncommon condition occurring exclusively in smokers in 4th to 5th decades of life and is more common in males. Most patients present with dyspnoea and cough. Chest X-ray shows peculiar diffuse hazy opacities which characterise all ILDs.

M/E Main findings are as under:

i) Hallmark finding is collections of large number of intra-alveolar macrophages having abundant cytoplasm and containing brown-black pigment and are termed as smokers' macrophages.

ii) The intervening septa contain a few lymphocytes, plasma cells and an occasional eosinophil.

RESPIRATORY BRONCHIOLITIS ASSOCIATED ILD Respiratory bronchiolitis is a far more common lesion in chronic smokers than DIP and is considered a milder form of DIP having similar clinical presentation. Respiratory bronchiolitis associated ILD is the term used for advanced cases who develop impaired pulmonary function and radiologic features.

M/E The features are as under:

i) Patchy and bronchiolocentric location of smokers' macrophages similar to those seen in DIP.

ii) Peribronchial infiltrate of lymphocytes and histiocytes.

iii) There may be mild peribronchial fibrosis.

iv) Centriacinar emphysema may coexist.

PULMONARY LANGERHANS CELL HISTIOCYTOSIS This is an uncommon smoking-related ILD occurring in younger men (20-40 years). Clinically, the features may vary from an asymptomatic state to a rapidly progressive course. Symptomatic cases present with cough, dyspnoea, weight loss and fever. CT scan shows presence of ill-defined stellate nodules and thin-walled cysts. Discontinuation of smoking leads to reversal of the condition.

M/E Main features are as under:

i) There is presence of poorly-defined nodules distributed in peribronchiolar location while intervening lung parenchyma is uninvolved.

ii) Characteristically, these nodules are sclerosing and contain Langerhans cells along with other inflammatory cells.

TUMOURS OF LUNGS *(P. 477)*

A number of benign and malignant tumours occur in the lungs but the primary lung cancer, commonly termed bronchogenic carcinoma, is the most common (95% of all primary lung tumours). The lung is also the commonest site for metastasis from carcinomas and sarcomas as follows:

    I. EPITHELIAL TUMOURS
        A. *Benign*
            1. Papilloma
            2. Adenoma
        B. *Dysplasia and carcinoma in situ*
        C. *Malignant*
            Bronchogenic carcinoma
            1. Squamous cell (epidermoid) carcinoma
            2. Small cell carcinoma
                i) Pure
                ii) Combined (with any other non-small cell carcinoma lung)
            3. Adenocarcinoma
                i) Acinar predominant
                ii) Papillary predominant
                iii) Lepidic predominant (formerly bronchiolo-alveolar carcinoma)

iv) Solid predominant with mucin formation
v) Micropapillary predominant
4. Large cell carcinoma
5. Adenosquamous carcinoma
Other carcinomas
1. Pulmonary neuroendocrine tumour (carcinoid tumour)
2. Bronchial gland carcinomas
   i) Adenoid cystic carcinoma
   ii) Mucoepidermoid carcinoma

II. SOFT TISSUE TUMOURS
(Fibroma, fibrosarcoma; leiomyoma, leiomyosarcoma; lipoma, chondroma, haemangioma, lymphangioma, granular cell myoblastoma)

III. PLEURAL TUMOURS
   A. Benign mesothelioma
   B. Malignant mesothelioma

IV. MISCELLANEOUS TUMOURS
   1. Carcinosarcoma
   2. Pulmonary blastoma
   3. Malignant melanoma
   4. Malignant lymphoma

V. SECONDARY TUMOURS

BRONCHOGENIC CARCINOMA *(p. 477)*

The term bronchogenic carcinoma is commonly used for cancer of the lungs which includes carcinomas arising from the respiratory epithelium lining the bronchi, bronchioles and alveoli.

INCIDENCE AND CLASSIFICATION

Lung cancer is the most common primary malignant tumour in men and accounts for nearly 30% of all cancer deaths in both sexes in developing countries. Currently, the incidence of lung cancer in females in the United States has already exceeded breast cancer as a cause of death in women. Of late, there has been slight decline in lung cancer deaths in males due to smoking cessation efforts which started in the West 4 decades back and has started yielding results.

For therapeutic purposes, bronchogenic carcinoma can be classified into 3 groups:
1. Small cell carcinomas, SCC (20-25%)
2. Non-small cell carcinomas, NSCC (70-75%) (includes squamous cell carcinoma, adenocarcinoma, and large cell carcinoma)
3. Combined/mixed patterns (5-10%).

As per reports on international data for the last 25 years, while there has been decline in the incidence of small cell carcinoma, incidence of adenocarcinoma of the lung has risen and is most frequent histologic subtype of lung cancer, accounting for almost half of all lung cancers.

ETIOLOGY

The high incidence of lung cancer is associated with a number of etiologic factors, notably *cigarette smoking*.

1. SMOKING The most important factor for high incidence of all forms of bronchogenic carcinoma is tobacco smoking. About 80% of the lung cancer occurs in active smokers.

i) Total dose There is a direct statistical correlation between death rate from lung cancer and the total amount of cigarettes smoked

ii) Histologic alterations The association of tobacco smoking is strongest for squamous cell carcinoma and small cell carcinoma of the lung. More than 90% of smokers have sequential epithelial changes in the respiratory tract in the form of squamous metaplasia, dysplasia and carcinoma *in situ*.

iii) Mechanism How tobacco smoking causes lung cancer is not quite clear. However, following facts have been observed:

a) Analysis of the tar from cigarette smoke has revealed a number of known carcinogens (e.g. polycyclic aromatic hydrocarbons, nitrosamines) and tumour promoters (e.g. phenol derivatives).

b) In experimental animal studies, it has been possible to induce cancer by skin painting experiments with smoke-tar.

2. OTHER FACTORS 15% cases of lung cancer occur in non-smokers, more so in women probably related to hormonal factors. A few other factors implicated in lung cancer are as follows:

i) Radiation exposure
ii) Atmospheric pollution
iii) Occupational causes
iv) Dietary factors
v) Chronic scarring

MOLECULAR PATHOGENESIS

Molecular studies have revealed that there are several genetic alterations in cancer stem cells which produce clones of malignant cells to form tumour mass. Following genetic changes have been found:

1. Activation of growth-promoting oncogenes Mutation in *K-RAS* oncogene has been seen as the dominant change in lung cancer. Besides, there is mutation in tyrosine kinase domain of *EGFR* oncogene in cases of adenocarcinoma lung in non-smokers.

2. Inactivation of tumour-suppressor genes Many tumour suppressor genes have been found on chromosome 3p in lung cancer cases. These include inactivation of *p53* and *Rb* gene.

3. Autocrine growth factors Studies have shown that lung cancer is a multistep process—initiator carcinogen causing mutation, followed by action of tumour promoters.

4. Inherited predisposition Although not common, there are a few examples of inheritance of lung cancer as under:

i) Patients of Li-Fraumeni syndrome
ii) Clinical cases of retinoblastoma
iii) First-degree relatives of lung cancer
iv) Mutations of cytochrome P450 system.

5. Molecular targets for therapy and survival prediction Knowledge on the insight into molecular biology and pathogenesis of lung cancer has applications in discovery of newer molecules for targeted therapy, predicting response to treatment and survival:

i) EGFR mutations and NSCC therapy: It has been reported that 70% cases of NSCC have overexpression of *EGFR* protein or amplification of the *EGFR* gene.

ii) VEGF and monoclonal therapy: Although not mutated, VEGF is excessively produced in lung cancer and contributes to tumour angiogenesis.

MORPHOLOGIC FEATURES

Bronchogenic carcinoma can occur anywhere in the lung but the most common location is *hilar*, followed in descending frequency by *peripheral* type.

G/A Two gross patterns are distinguished:

1. Hilar type Most commonly, the lung cancer arises in the main bronchus or one of its segmental branches in the hilar parts of the lung, more often on the right side. The tumour begins as a small roughened area on the bronchial mucosa at the bifurcation. As the tumour enlarges, it thickens the bronchial mucosa producing nodular or ulcerated surface. As the nodules coalesce, the carcinoma grows into a friable spherical mass, 1 to 5 cm in diameter, narrowing and occluding the lumen. The cut surface of the tumour is yellowish-white with foci of necrosis and haemorrhages which may produce cavitary lesions.

Systemic Pathology

2. Peripheral type A small proportion of lung cancers, chiefly adenocarcinomas including bronchioloalveolar carcinomas, originate from a small peripheral bronchiole but the exact site of origin may not be discernible.

M/E Five main histologic types of bronchogenic carcinoma are distinguished which is important because of prognostic and therapeutic considerations. However, from clinical point of view, distinction between small cell (SCC) and non-small cell carcinoma (NSCC) is important because the two not only differ in morphology, but there are major differences in immunophenotyping and response to treatment discussed above.

1. Squamous cell (epidermoid) carcinoma This has been the most common histologic subtype of bronchogenic carcinoma until recently and is found more commonly in men, often with history of tobacco smoking. The tumour is diagnosed microscopically by identification of either intercellular bridges or keratinisation. The tumour may show varying histologic grades of differentiation such as well-differentiated, moderately-differentiated and poorly-differentiated.

2. Small cell carcinoma Small cell carcinomas are frequently hilar or central in location, have strong relation-ship to cigarette smoking and are highly malignant tumours. They are most often associated with ectopic hormone production because of the presence of neurosecretory granules in majority of tumour cells. By immunohistochemistry, these tumour cells are positive for neuroendocrine markers: chromogranin, neuron-specific enolase (NSE) and synaptophysin. Small cell carcinomas have 2 subtypes:
i) *Pure small cell carcinoma* is composed of uniform, small (or oat-like) cells, larger than lymphocytes with dense, round or oval nuclei having diffuse chromatin, inconspicuous nucleoli and very sparse cytoplasm (*oat* = a form of grain).
ii) *Combined small cell carcinoma* is a tumour in which there is a definite component of small cell carcinoma with component of other non-small lung carcinoma such as squamous cell and/or adenocarcinoma.

3. Adenocarcinoma Adenocarcinoma, also called *peripheral carcinoma* due to its location and *scar carcinoma* due to its association with areas of chronic scarring, is the most common bronchogenic carcinoma in women and is slow-growing. Recent estimates on adenocarcinoma place this as the most frequent histologic subtype of lung cancer. *Invasive adenocarcinoma* is further subclassified into 5 types:
i) *Acinar predominant adenocarcinoma* which has predominance of glandular structure.
ii) *Papillary predominant adenocarcinoma* which has a pronounced macropapillary configuration.
iii) *Lepidic predominant (formerly bronchiolo-alveolar carcinoma)* is characterised by cuboidal to tall columnar and mucus-secreting epithelial cells growing along the existing alveoli.
iv) *Solid predominant carcinoma* is a poorly-differentiated adenocarcinoma lacking acini, tubules or papillae.
v) *Micropapillary predominant adenocarcinoma* has tumour cells growing in tiny papillary tufts lacking fibrovascular core.

4. Large cell carcinoma These are undifferentiated carcinomas which lack the specific features by which they could be assigned into squamous cell carcinoma or adenocarcinoma.

5. Adenosquamous carcinoma These are a small pro-portion of peripheral scar carcinomas having clear evidence of both keratinisation and glandular differentiation.

SPREAD

Bronchogenic carcinoma can invade the adjoining structures directly, or may spread by lymphatic and haematogenous routes.

1. Direct spread The tumour extends directly by invading through the wall of the bronchus and destroys and replaces the peribronchial lung tissue. As it grows further, it spreads to the opposite bronchus and lung, into the pleural cavity, the pericardium and the myocardium and along the great vessels of the heart causing their constriction.

2. **Lymphatic spread** Initially, hilar lymph nodes are affected. Later, lymphatic metastases occur to the other groups leading to spread to mediastinal, cervical, supraclavicular and para-aortic lymph nodes.

3. **Haematogenous spread** Distant metastases via blood stream are widespread and early. The sites affected, in descending order of involvement, are: the liver, adrenals, bones, pancreas, brain, opposite lung, kidneys and thyroid.

CLINICAL FEATURES

Symptoms of lung cancer are quite variable and result from local effects, effects due to occlusion of a bronchus, direct and distant metastases, and paraneoplastic syndromes. Diagnostic aids include radiologic examination and CT scan of the chest, cytologic examination of the sputum, bronchial washings and bronchioalveolar lavage.

STAGING AND PROGNOSIS

The widely accepted clinical staging of lung cancer is according to the TNM classification, combining features of primary *Tumours*, *Nodal* involvement and distant *Metastases*. TNM staging divides all lung cancers into the following 4 stages:

Occult: Malignant cells in the bronchopulmonary secretions but no evidence of primary tumour or metastasis.

Stage I: Tumour less than 3 cm, with or without ipsilateral nodal involvement, no distant metastasis.

Stage II: Tumour larger than 3 cm, with ipsilateral hilar lymph node involvement, no distant metastasis.

Stage III: Tumour of any size, involving adjacent structures, involving contralateral lymph nodes or distant metastasis.

In general, tumour size larger than 5 cm has worse prognosis. Symptomatic patients, particularly with systemic symptoms, fare far badly than the nonsymptomatic patients. The overall prognosis of bronchogenic carcinoma is dismal. *Small cell carcinoma has the worst prognosis* since surgical treatment is ineffective though the tumour is sensitive to radiotherapy and chemotherapy.

BRONCHIAL CARCINOID AND OTHER NEUROENDOCRINE TUMOURS *(p. 483)*

Neuroendocrine tumours of the lung represent a continuum spectrum of lung tumours with progressively increasing aggressiveness which include: typical carcinoid (*least aggressive*), atypical carcinoid, and large cell endocrine carcinoma, and also small cell carcinoma (*most aggressive*). Bronchial carcinoids tend to occur at a younger age than bronchogenic carcinoma, often appearing below the age of 40 years, and are not related to cigarette smoking.

G/A Bronchial carcinoids most commonly arise from a major bronchus and project into the bronchial lumen as a spherical polypoid mass, 3-4 cm in diameter.

M/E The tumour is composed of uniform cuboidal cells forming aggregates, trabeculae or ribbons separated by fine fibrous septa. The tumour cells have abundant, finely granular cytoplasm and oval central nuclei with clumped nuclear chromatin. The secretory granules of bronchial carcinoids resemble those of other foregut carcinoids and stain positively with argyrophilic stains in which exogenous reducing agent is added for the reaction. Immunohistochemically, markers for neuroendocrine are stained positive e.g. NSE, chromogranin, synaptophysin and neurofilaments.

CLINICAL FEATURES Bronchial carcinoids occur at a relatively early age and have equal sex incidence. Most of the symptoms in bronchial carcinoids occur as a result of bronchial obstruction such as cough, haemoptysis, atelectasis and secondary infection. About 5-10% of bronchial carcinoids metastasise to the liver and these cases are capable of producing carcinoid syndrome.

HAMARTOMA *(p. 484)*

Hamartoma is a tumour-like lesion composed of an abnormal admixture of pulmonary tissue components and is discovered incidentally as a coin-lesion in the chest-X-ray. Pulmonary hamartomas are of 2 types: chondromatous and leiomyomatous.

◈ **Chondromatous hamartoma** is more common and usually asymptomatic.

◈ **Leiomyomatous hamartoma** has a prominent smooth muscle component and bronchiolar structures.

METASTATIC LUNG TUMOURS *(p. 484)*

Secondary tumours of the lungs are more common than the primary pulmonary tumours. Metastases from carcinomas as well as sarcomas arising from anywhere in the body may spread to the lung by haematogenous or lymphatic routes, or by direct extension. Blood-borne metastases are the most common since emboli of tumour cells from any malignant tumour entering the systemic venous circulation are likely to be lodged in the lungs.

Most common sources of metastases in the lungs are: carcinomas of the bowel, breast, thyroid, kidney, pancreas, lung (ipsilateral or contralateral) and liver. Other tumours which frequently metastasise to the lungs are osteogenic sarcoma, neuroblastoma, Wilms' tumour, melanoma, lymphomas and leukaemias.

DISEASES OF PLEURA *(p. 485)*

NORMAL STRUCTURE Visceral pleura covers the lungs and extends into the fissures while the parietal pleura limits the mediastinum and covers the dome of the diaphragm and inner aspect of the chest wall. The two layers between them enclose pleural cavity which contains less than 15 ml of clear serous fluid.

M/E Both the pleural layers are lined by a single layer of flattened mesothelial cells facing each other.

INFLAMMATIONS *(p. 485)*

Inflammatory involvement of the pleura is commonly termed *pleuritis or pleurisy.*

1. SEROUS, FIBRINOUS AND SEROFIBRINOUS PLEURITIS Acute inflammation of the pleural sac (acute pleuritis) can result in serous, serofibrinous and fibrinous exudate. Most of the causes of such pleuritis are infective in origin, particularly within the lungs, such as tuberculosis, pneumonias, pulmonary infarcts, lung abscess and bronchiectasis. Other causes include a few collagen diseases.

2. SUPPURATIVE PLEURITIS (EMPYEMA THORACIS) Bacterial or mycotic infection of the pleural cavity that converts a serofibrinous effusion into purulent exudate is termed suppurative pleuritis or empyema thoracis. The most common cause is direct spread of pyogenic infection from the lung.

In empyema, the exudate is yellow-green, creamy pus that accumulates in large volumes. Empyema is eventually replaced by granulation tissue and fibrous tissue. In time, tough fibrocollagenic adhesions develop which obliterate the cavity, and with passage of years, calcification may occur.

3. HAEMORRHAGIC PLEURITIS Haemorrhagic pleuritis differs from haemothorax in having inflammatory cells or exfoliated tumour cells in the exudate. The causes of haemorrhagic pleuritis are metastatic involvement of the pleura, bleeding disorders and rickettsial diseases.

1. HYDROTHORAX Hydrothorax is non-inflammatory accumulation of serous fluid within the pleural cavities. Hydrothorax may be unilateral or bilateral depending upon the underlying cause. Occasionally, an effusion is limited to part of a pleural cavity by pre-existing pleural adhesions.

The most common cause of hydrothorax, often bilateral, is congestive heart failure. Other causes are renal failure, cirrhosis of liver, Meig's syndrome, pulmonary oedema and primary and secondary tumours of the lungs.

The non-inflammatory serous effusion in hydrothorax is clear and straw-coloured and has the characteristics of transudate with a specific gravity of under 1.012, protein content below 1 gm/dl and little cellular content.

2. HAEMOTHORAX Accumulation of pure blood in the pleural cavity is termed as haemothorax. The most common causes of haemothorax are trauma to the chest wall or to the thoracic viscera and rupture of aortic aneurysm.

3. CHYLOTHORAX Chylothorax is an uncommon condition in which there is accumulation of milky fluid of lymphatic origin into the pleural cavity. Chylothorax results most commonly from rupture of the thoracic duct by trauma or obstruction of the thoracic duct such as by malignant tumours, most often malignant lymphomas.

PNEUMOTHORAX (p. 485)

An accumulation of air in the pleural cavity is called pneumothorax. It may occur in one of the three circumstances: spontaneous, traumatic and therapeutic.

i) Spontaneous pneumothorax occurs due to spontaneous rupture of alveoli in any form of pulmonary disease. Most commonly, spontaneous pneumothorax occurs in association with emphysema, asthma and tuber-culosis.

ii) Traumatic pneumothorax is caused by trauma to the chest wall or lungs, ruptured oesophagus or stomach, and surgical operations of the thorax.

iii) Therapeutic (artificial) pneumothorax used to be employed formerly in the treatment of chronic pulmonary tuberculosis in which air was introduced into the pleural sac so as to collapse the lung and limit its respiratory movements.

TUMOURS OF PLEURA (p. 486)

Pleural tumours may be primary or secondary. In line with pulmonary tumours, the secondary tumours in the pleura are more common.

MESOTHELIOMA

Mesothelioma is an uncommon tumour arising from mesothelial lining of serous cavities, most often in pleural cavity, and rarely in peritoneal cavity and pericardial sac. Mesotheliomas are of 2 types—*benign (solitary) and malignant (diffuse)*.

BENIGN (SOLITARY) MESOTHELIOMA

Benign or solitary mesothelioma is also called as pleural fibroma. *Asbestos exposure plays no role in etiology of benign mesothelioma.*

G/A It consists of a solitary, circumscribed, small, firm mass, generally less than 3 cm in diameter. Cut surface shows whorls of dense fibrous tissue.

M/E The tumour is predominantly composed of whorls of collagen fibres and reticulin with interspersed fibroblasts.

MALIGNANT (DIFFUSE) MESOTHELIOMA

Malignant or diffuse mesothelioma is rare. It is a highly malignant tumour associated with high mortality. The tumour is significant in view of its recognised association with occupational exposure to asbestos (particularly crocidolite) for a number of years, usually 20 to 40 years. About 90% of malignant mesotheliomas are asbestos-related.

G/A The tumour is characteristically diffuse, forming a thick, white, fleshy coating over the parietal and visceral surfaces.

M/E Malignant mesothelioma may have epithelial, sarcomatoid or biphasic patterns.

i) **Epithelioid pattern** resembles an adenocarcinoma, consisting of tubular and tubulo-papillary formations. The tumour cells are usually well-differentiated, cuboidal, flattened or columnar cells.

ii) **Sarcomatoid pattern** consists of spindle cell sarcoma resembling fibrosarcoma.

iii) **Mixed pattern** shows mixed growth having epithelial as well as sarcomatoid pattern. Usually, there are slit-like or gland-like spaces lined by neoplastic mesothelial cells separated by proliferating spindle-shaped tumour cells.

SECONDARY PLEURAL TUMOURS (p. 487)

Metastatic malignancies in the pleura are more common than the primary tumours and appear as small nodules scattered over the lung surface. The most frequent primary malignant tumours metastasising to the pleura are of the lung and breast through lymphatics, and ovarian cancers via haematogenous route.

SELF ASSESSMENT

1. **Source of pulmonary surfactant is:**
   A. Alveolar macrophages
   B. Type I pneumocytes
   C. Type II pneumocytes
   D. Capillary basement membrane

2. **The basic defect in neonatal hyaline membrane disease is:**
   A. Shock due to sepsis
   B. Deficient production of surfactant
   C. Inhalation of toxins
   D. Aspiration pneumonitis

3. **Adult respiratory distress syndrome occurs from the following causes <u>except</u>:**
   A. Pancreatitis
   B. Oxygen toxicity
   C. Deficiency of surfactant
   D. Diffuse pulmonary infections

4. **Primary atelectasis is defined as:**
   A. Incomplete expansion of a previously unexpanded lung
   B. Reduction in size of a previously expanded lung due to compression
   C. Reduction in size of a lung due to obstruction
   D. Reduction in lung size due to contraction

5. **Pulmonary hypertension is defined as systolic blood pressure in the pulmonary arterial circulation above the following cut off figure:**
   A. 120 mmHg
   B. 90 mmHg
   C. 60 mmHg
   D. 30 mmHg

6. **Bronchopneumonia is grossly characterised by:**
   A. Diffuse consolidation of a lobe or lobes of one or both lungs
   B. Diffuse consolidation of a lobe of one lung
   C. Diffuse consolidation of a lobe of both lungs
   D. Patchy consolidation of a lobe or lobes of one or both lungs

7. **The most common causative organism for lobar pneumonia is:**
   A. Staphylococci
   B. Streptococci
   C. Pneumococci
   D. Haemophilus

8. **Viral pneumonias are characterised by the following features except:**
   A. Presence of interstitial inflammation
   B. Presence of alveolar exudate
   C. Necrotising bronchiolitis
   D. Multinucleate giant cells in the bronchiolar wall
9. **The organism in *Pneumocystis* pneumonia is:**
   A. Mycoplasma
   B. Fungus
   C. Protozoa
   D. Chlamydia
10. **Lung abscess secondary to aspiration pneumonia develops more often in:**
    A. Lower lobe of right lung
    B. Lower lobe of left lung
    C. Upper lobe of either lung
    D. Middle lobe of right lung
11. **Reid index used as a criteria of quantitation in chronic bronchitis is the ratio of thickness of:**
    A. Bronchial mucosa to that of bronchial wall
    B. Submucosal glands to that of bronchial wall
    C. Bronchial cartilage to that of bronchial wall
    D. Inflammatory infiltrate to that of bronchial wall
12. **The most fibrogenic dust in pneumoconiosis is:**
    A. Coal
    B. Asbestos
    C. Silica
    D. Beryllium
13. **Classic a-1 antitrypsin deficiency in emphysema has the following phenotype of protease inhibitor:**
    A. PiMM
    B. PiZZ
    C. PiMZ
    D. PiMO
14. **The extent of damage to pulmonary parenchyma is severest in the following type of emphysema:**
    A. Centriacinar
    B. Panacinar
    C. Distal acinar
    D. Irregular
15. **Emphysema associated most often with α1 antitrypsin deficiency is:**
    A. Panacinar
    B. Centriacinar
    C. Distal acinar
    D. Irregular
16. **Serum IgE levels are elevated in:**
    A. Intrinsic bronchial asthma
    B. Extrinsic bronchial asthma
    C. Predominant chronic bronchitis
    D. Predominant emphysema
17. **Bronchiectasis commonly develops in the following microanatomic zone of bronchial tree:**
    A. Acini beyond respiratory bronchioles
    B. Acini beyond terminal bronchioles
    C. Terminal bronchioles less than 2 mm diameter
    D. Bronchioles more than 2 mm diameter
18. **Restrictive lung disease is characterised by the following features except:**
    A. Dyspnoea
    B. Tachypnoea
    C. Cyanosis
    D. Wheezing
19. **Inhaled dust particles of the following size are generally eliminated by expectoration:**
    A. Smaller than 1 μm
    B. 1-3 μm
    C. 3-5 μm
    D. Larger than 5 μm
20. **Bronchogenic carcinoma has increased incidence in the following pneumoconiosis:**
    A. Coal workers' pneumoconiosis
    B. Silicosis
    C. Asbestosis
    D. Berylliosis

21. Silicosis occurs in following occupational exposure except:
    A. Ceramic workers
    B. Foundry workers
    C. Textile workers
    D. Construction workers

22. Out of various forms of asbestos, the following type is implicated in etiology of malignant pleural tumour:
    A. Chrysotite
    B. Crocidolite
    C. Amosite
    D. Anthophyllite

23. Caplan's syndrome may develop in the following types of pneumoconiosis except:
    A. Coal-workers' pneumoconiosis
    B. Asbestosis
    C. Berylliosis
    D. Silicosis

24. Non-caseating sarcoid-like epithelioid cell granulomas are seen in:
    A. Silicosis
    B. Asbestosis
    C. Coal-workers' pneumoconiosis
    D. Chronic berylliosis

25. The following histologic types of bronchogenic carcinoma have strong association with cigarette smoking except:
    A. Squamous cell carcinoma
    B. Small cell carcinoma
    C. Large cell carcinoma
    D. Adenocarcinoma

26. The following type of bronchogenic carcinoma has worst prognosis:
    A. Squamous cell carcinoma
    B. Small cell carcinoma
    C. Large cell carcinoma
    D. Adenocarcinoma

27. Bronchial carcinoid arises from:
    A. Columnar ciliated epithelium
    B. Goblet cells
    C. Kulchitsky cells
    D. Alveolar lining cells

28. The following tumour does not have association with occupational exposure to asbestosis:
    A. Benign mesothelioma
    B. Malignant mesothelioma
    C. Bronchogenic carcinoma
    D. Laryngeal carcinoma

29. Macrophage-derived fibrogenic cytokine is:
    A. IL-1
    B. IL-8
    C. TNF
    D. TGF α

30. The most important mutation in small cell carcinoma is in the following gene:
    A. *RB* gene
    B. *MYC* gene
    C. *CDK* gene
    D. *RAS* gene

31. Hamman-Rich syndrome is:
    A. Bronchopulmonary dysplasia
    B. Desquamative interstitial pneumonia
    C. Diffuse fibrosing alveolitis
    D. ARDS

32. Most common etiologic factor implicated in chronic bronchitis is:
    A. Atmospheric pollution
    B. Cotton mills
    C. Mycoplasma infection
    D. Cigarette smoking

33. Which type of asthma occurs in late adult life:
    A. Atopic asthma
    B. Intrinsic asthma
    C. Mixed asthma
    D. Allergic asthma

34. Asbestos exposure results in all of the following changes except:
    A. Interstitial pneumonia
    B. Pleural effusion
    C. Malignant mesothelioma
    D. Pleural fibrosis

35. All are types of allergic pneumonitis except:
    A. Bagassosis
    B. Byssinosis
    C. Berryliosis
    D. Farmer's lung

36. Which of the following mutation is being used to develop targeted molecular therapy in non-small cell cancer of lung?
    A. EGFR mutation
    B. p53 mutation
    C. K-RAS mutation
    D. p16 mutation

37. **Which of the following histologic types of carcinomas is most likely to be found at the periphery of the lung preceded by healed lung lesions?**
   A. Adenocarcinoma
   B. Large cell carcinoma
   C. Small cell carcinoma
   D. Squamous cell carcinoma

KEY

1 = C	2 = B	3 = C	4 = A	5 = D
6 = D	7 = C	8 = B	9 = B	10 = A
11 = B	12 = C	13 = B	14 = B	15 = A
16 = B	17 = D	18 = D	19 = D	20 = C
21 = C	22 = B	23 = C	24 = D	25 = D
26 = B	27 = C	28 = A	29 = D	30 = A
31 = C	32 = D	33 = B	34 = A	35 = C
36 = A	37 = A			

16 The Eye, ENT and Neck

EYE (p. 488)

NORMAL STRUCTURE

The *eyelids* are covered externally by the skin and internally by *conjunctiva* which is reflected over the globe of the eye. The *lacrimal glands* which are compound racemose glands are situated at the outer upper angle of the orbit. The *globe of the eye* is composed of 3 layers: the cornea-sclera, choroid-iris, and retina.

◈   The **cornea** is covered by stratified epithelium which may be regarded as continuation of the conjunctiva over the cornea.

◈   The **sclera** is composed of dense fibrous tissue which is thickest at the back of the eyeball.

◈   The **choroid** is the vascular membrane in contact with the sclera.

◈   The **iris** is the continuation of the choroid which extends in front of the lens.

◈   The **uveal tract** consists of 3 parts—the choroid and ciliary body posteriorly, and the iris anteriorly.

◈   The **retina** is part of the central nervous system and corresponds in extent to the choroid which it lines internally. The retina is composed of a number of layers of cells and their synapses which are of 3 types—external photoreceptor cells (rods and cones), intermediate relay layer of bipolar cells, and internal layer of ganglion cells with their axons running into the central nervous system.

◈   The **lens** is the biconvex mass of laminated transparent tissue with elastic capsule.

◈   The **anterior chamber** is the space filled with the aqueous humour, and is bounded by the cornea in front and the iris behind, with anterior surface of the lens exposed in the pupil.

◈   The **posterior chamber** containing aqueous humour is the triangular space between the back of the iris, the anterior surface of the lens and the ciliary body forming its apex at the pupillary margin.

◈   The **vitreous chamber** is the large space behind the lens containing gelatinous material, the vitreous humour.

The main *function* of the eye is visual acuity which depends upon a transparent focussing system comprised by the cornea, lens, transparent media consisting of aqueous and vitreous humours, and a normal retinal and neural conduction system.

CONGENITAL LESIONS (p. 488)

RETROLENTAL FIBROPLASIA (RETINOPATHY OF PREMATURITY)
This is a developmental disorder occurring in premature infants who have been given oxygen-therapy at birth. The basic defect lies in the developmental prematurity of the retinal blood vessels which are extremely sensitive to high dose of oxygen-therapy.

RETINITIS PIGMENTOSA   Retinitis pigmentosa is a group of systemic and ocular diseases of unknown etiology, characterised by degeneration of the retinal pigment epithelium. The condition can have various inheritance patterns—autosomal dominant, autosomal recessive trait, or sex-linked recessive trait. The earliest clinical finding is night blindness due to loss of rods and may progress to total blindness.

INFLAMMATORY CONDITIONS (p. 489)

Inflammatory conditions of the eye are designated according to the tissue affected. 'Uveitis' is the commonly used term for the ocular inflammation of the uveal tract which is the most vascular tissue of the eye.

STYE (HORDEOLUM) Stye or 'external hordeolum' is an acute suppurative inflammation of the sebaceous glands of Zeis, the apocrine glands of Moll and the eyelash follicles.

CHALAZION Chalazion is a very common lesion and is the chronic inflammatory process involving the meibomian glands. It occurs as a result of obstruction to the drainage of secretions.

M/E The chalazion gives the appearance of a chronic inflammatory granuloma located in the tarsus and contains fat globules in the centre of the granulomas i.e. appearance of a lipogranuloma.

ENDOPHTHALMITIS-PANOPHTHALMITIS Endophthalmitis is an acute suppurative intraocular inflammation. Panophthalmitis is the term used for inflammation involving retina, choroid and sclera and extending to the orbit. Infection may be of exogenous or endogenous origin. The exogenous agents may be bacteria, viruses or fungi introduced into the eye during an accidental or surgical perforating wound. The endogenous agents include opportunistic infections which may cause endophthalmitis via haematogenous route e.g. candidiasis, toxoplasmosis, nocardiosis, aspergillosis and cryptococcosis.

CONJUNCTIVITIS AND KERATOCONJUNCTIVITIS Conjunctiva and cornea are constantly exposed to various types of physical, chemical, microbial (bacteria, fungi, viruses) and allergic agents and hence prone to develop acute, subacute and chronic inflammations.

TRACHOMA AND INCLUSION CONJUNCTIVITIS Both these conditions are caused by *Chlamydia* or TRIC agents. Trachoma is caused by *C. trachomatis* while inclusion conjunctivitis is caused by *C. oculogenitalis*. Trachoma is widely prevalent in the developing countries of the world and is responsible for blindness on a large scale.

GRANULOMATOUS UVEITIS A number of chronic granulomatous conditions may cause granulomatous uveitis. These include bacteria (e.g. tuberculosis, leprosy, syphilis), viruses (e.g. CMV disease, herpes zoster), fungi (e.g. aspergillosis, blastomycosis, phycomycosis, histoplasmosis), and certain parasites (e.g. toxoplasmosis, onchocerciasis). Granulomatous uveitis is common in sarcoidosis as well.

SYMPATHETIC OPHTHALMIA (SYMPATHETIC UVEITIS) This is an uncommon condition in which there is bilateral diffuse granulomatous uveitis following penetrating injury to one eye. The condition probably results from an autosensitivity reaction to injured uveal tissue.

M/E There is granulomatous uveal inflammation consisting of epithelioid cells and lymphocytes affecting both the eyes.

VASCULAR LESIONS (p. 489)

DIABETIC RETINOPATHY Diabetic retinopathy is an important cause of blindness. It is related to the degree and duration of glycaemic control. The condition develops in more than 60% of diabetics 15-20 years after the onset of disease, and in about 2% of diabetics causes blindness. Other ocular complications of diabetes include glaucoma, cataract and corneal disease. Most cases of diabetic retinopathy occur over the age of 50 years. The risk is greater in type 1 diabetes mellitus than in type 2 diabetes mellitus, although in clinical practice there are more patients of diabetic retinopathy due to type 2 diabetes mellitus because of its higher prevalence.

M/E Two types of changes are described in diabetic retinopathy:

1. Background (non-proliferative) retinopathy This is the initial retinal capillary microangiopathy. The following changes are seen:
i)   Basement membrane shows varying thickness.
ii) Degeneration of pericytes and some loss of endothelial cells.
iii) Capillary microaneurysms.
iv) 'Waxy exudates'.
v)   'Dot and blot haemorrhages'.
vi) Soft 'cotton-wool spots'.

2. Proliferative retinopathy (retinitis proliferans) After many years, retinopathy becomes proliferative.
i)   Neovascularisation of the retina at the optic disc.
ii) Friability of newly-formed blood vessels causes them to bleed easily.
iii) Proliferation of astrocytes and fibrous tissue around the new blood vessels.
iv) Fibrovascular and gliotic tissue contracts to cause retinal detachment and blindness.

HYPERTENSIVE RETINOPATHY In hypertensive retinopathy, the retinal arterioles are reduced in their diameter leading to retinal ischaemia. In acute severe hypertension as happens at the onset of malignant hypertension and in toxaemia of pregnancy, the vascular changes are in the form of spasms, while in chronic hypertension the changes are diffuse in the form of onion-skin thickening of the arteriolar walls with narrowing of the lumina.

M/E Features of hypertensive retinopathy include the following:
i)   Variable degree of arteriolar narrowing.
ii)   'Flame-shaped' haemorrhages.
iii) Macular star.
iv)   Cotton-wool spots.
v)   Microaneurysms.
vi)   Arteriovenous nicking.
vii) Hard exudates.
     Hypertensive retinopathy is classified according to the severity of above lesions from grade I to IV.

RETINAL INFARCTS Infarcts of the retina may result from thrombosis or embolism in central artery of the retina, causing ischaemic necrosis of the inner two-third of the retina while occlusion of the posterior ciliary arteries causes ischaemia of the inner photoreceptor layer only.

MISCELLANEOUS CONDITIONS *(p. 491)*

PINGUECULA AND PTERYGIUM **Pinguecula** is a degenerative condition of the collagen of the bulbar conjunctiva. Clinically, the condition appears as raised yellowish lesions on the interpalpebral bulbar conjunctiva of both eyes in middle-aged and elderly patients.
     Pterygium is a lesion closely related to pinguecula but differs from the latter by being located at the limbus and often involves the cornea.

SENILE MACULAR DEGENERATION Age-related degeneration of the macular region of the retina is an important cause of bilateral central visual loss in the elderly people.

RETINAL DETACHMENT Retinal detachment is the separation of the neurosensory retina from the retinal pigment epithelium. It may occur spontaneously in older individuals past 50 years of age, or may be secondary to trauma in the region of head and neck. There are 3 pathogenetic mechanisms of retinal detachment:
i)   Pathologic processes in the vitreous or anterior segment, causing traction on the retina.
ii)   Collection of serous fluid in the sub-retinal space from inflammation or tumour in the choroid.
iii) Accumulation of vitreous under the retina through a hole or a tear in the retina.

PHTHISIS BULBI Phthisis bulbi is the end-stage of advanced degeneration and disorganisation of the entire eyeball in which the intraocular pressure is decreased and the eyeball shrinks. The causes of such end-stage blind eye are trauma, glaucoma and intraocular inflammations.

CATARACT The cataract is the opacification of the normally crystalline lens which leads to gradual painless blurring of vision. The various causes of cataract are: senility, congenital (e.g. Down syndrome, rubella, galactosaemia), traumatic (e.g. penetrating injury, electrical injury), metabolic (e.g. diabetes, hypoparathyroidism), association with drugs (e.g. long-term corticosteroid therapy), smoking and heavy alcohol consumption. The most common is, however, idiopathic senile cataract.

GLAUCOMA Glaucoma is a group of ocular disorders that have in common increased intraocular pressure. Glaucoma is one of the leading causes of blindness because of the ocular tissue damage produced by raised intraocular pressure. In all types of glaucoma, degenerative changes appear after some duration and eventually damage to the optic nerve and retina occurs.

PAPILLOEDEMA Papilloedema is oedema of the optic disc resulting from increased intracranial pressure. This is due to anatomic continuation of the subarachnoid space of the brain around the optic nerve so that raised intracranial pressure is passed onto the optic disc area.

SJÖGREN'S SYNDROME Sjögren's syndrome is characterised by triad of keratoconjunctivitis sicca, xerostomia (sicca syndrome) and rheumatoid arthritis. The condition occurs due to immunologically-mediated destruction of the lacrimal and salivary glands.

MIKULICZ'S SYNDROME This is characterised by inflammatory enlargement of lacrimal and salivary glands. The condition may occur with Sjögren's syndrome, or with some diseases.

TUMOURS AND TUMOUR-LIKE LESIONS (p. 492)

The eye and its adnexal structures are the site of a variety of benign and malignant tumours as well as tumour-like lesions.

INFLAMMATORY PSEUDOTUMOURS

These are a group of inflammatory enlargements, especially in the orbit, which clinically look like tumours but surgical exploration and pathologic examination fail to reveal any evidence of neoplasm.

G/A These lesions are circumscribed and sometimes have fibrous capsule.

M/E Many of the lesions can be placed in well-established categories such as tuberculous, syphilitic, mycotic, parasitic, foreign-body granuloma etc, while others show non-specific histologic appearance having abundant fibrous tissue, lymphoid follicles and inflammatory infiltrate with prominence of eosinophils.

SEBACEOUS CARCINOMA

This is the *most frequent tumour of the eyelid* next only to basal cell carcinoma, although it is very rare tumour elsewhere in the body. It arises either from the meibomian glands in the tarsus or from Zeis' glands of eyelash follicles. The tumour is seen mostly in the upper eyelid (basal cell carcinoma is seen more frequently in the lower eyelid).

G/A The tumour appears as a localised or diffuse swelling of the tarsus.

M/E The tumour may show well-differentiated lobules of tumour cells with sebaceous differentiation, or may be poorly-differentiated tumour requiring confirmation by fat stains.

UVEAL MALIGNANT MELANOMA

Malignant melanomas arising from neural crest-derived pigment epithelium of the uvea is the most common primary ocular malignancy in the white adults in North America and Europe.

G/A The malignant melanoma appears as a pigmented mass, most commonly in the posterior choroid, and less often in the ciliary body and iris.

M/E Types of melanomas are as under:

1. **Spindle A melanoma** is composed of uniform, spindle-shaped cells containing spindled nuclei. Nucleoli are indistinct and mitotic figures are rare.

2. **Spindle B melanoma** is composed of larger and plump spindle-shaped cells with ovoid nuclei. Nucleoli are conspicuous and a few mitotic figures are present.

3. **Epithelioid melanoma** consists of larger, irregular and pleomorphic cells with larger nuclei and abundant acidophilic cytoplasm. These tumours are the most malignant of the uveal melanomas and have poor prognosis.

4. **Mixed cell type melanomas** have features of spindle cell type as well as of epithelioid cell type.

In general, uveal malignant melanomas are usually slow-growing, late metastasising and have a better prognosis than malignant melanoma of the skin. Uveal melanomas spread via haematogenous route and the liver is eventually involved in 90% of cases.

RETINOBLASTOMA

This is the most common malignant ocular tumour in children. It may be present at birth or recognised in early childhood before the age of 4 years. Retinoblastoma has some peculiar features. About 60% cases of retinoblastoma are sporadic and the remaining 40% are familial. Familial tumours are often multiple and multifocal and transmitted as an autosomal dominant trait by retinoblastoma susceptibility gene *(RB)* located on chromosome 13. Such individuals have a higher incidence of bilateral tumours and have increased risk of developing second primary tumour, particularly osteogenic sarcoma.

G/A The tumour characteristically appears as a white mass within the retina which may be partly solid and partly necrotic. The tumour may be *endophytic* when it protrudes into the vitreous, or *exophytic* when it grows between the retina and the pigment epithelium.

M/E The tumour is composed of undifferentiated retinal cells with tendency towards formation of photo-receptor elements. In the better differentiated area, the tumour cells are characteristically arranged in rosettes. The rosettes may be of 2 types—*Flexner-Wintersteiner rosettes* characterised by small tumour cells arranged around a lumen with their nuclei away from the lumen, and *Homer-Wright rosettes* having radial arrangement of tumour cells around the central neurofibrillar structure.

Besides direct spread, the tumour can spread widely via haematogenous route as well.

METASTATIC TUMOURS

Ocular metastatic tumours are far more common than primary ocular malignant tumours, choroid and iris being the preferential site for metastasis. Common primary tumours that metastasise to the eye are cancers of the breast in women and lung in men. Leukaemia and malignant lymphoma also commonly invade ocular tissues.

EAR *(p. 495)*

NORMAL STRUCTURE

The ear is divided into 3 parts—the external, middle and inner ear.

◈ The **external ear** comprises the auricle or pinna composed of cartilage, the external cartilaginous meatus and the external bony meatus. The external meatus is lined by stratified epithelium which is continued on to the external layer of the tympanic membrane.

◈ The **middle ear** consists of 3 parts—the uppermost portion is the *attic*, the middle portion is *mesotympanum,* and the lowermost portion is the *hypotympanum*. Besides, the middle ear has an opening, eustachian tube, the mastoid antrum and cells, and the three ossicles (the malleus, incus and stapes).

◈   The **inner ear** or labyrinth consists of bony capsule embedded in the petrous bone and contains the membranous labyrinth.

INFLAMMATORY AND MISCELLANEOUS LESIONS *(p. 495)*

OTITIS MEDIA   This is the term used for inflammatory involvement of the middle ear. It may be acute or chronic. The usual source of infection is via the eustachian tube and the common causative organisms are *Streptococcus pneumoniae, Haemophilus influenzae* and β-*Streptococcus haemolyticus*. Otitis media may be suppurative, serous or mucoid. Acute suppurative otitis media (SOM) clinically presents as tense and hyperaemic tympanic membrane along with pain and tenderness and sometimes mastoiditis as well. Chronic SOM manifests clinically as draining ear with perforated tympanic membrane and partially impaired hearing.

RELAPSING POLYCHONDRITIS   This is an uncommon autoimmune disease characterised by complete loss of glycosaminoglycans resulting in destruction of cartilage of the ear, nose, eustachian tube, larynx and lower respiratory tract.

CHONDRODERMATITIS NODULARIS CHRONICA HELICIS   This condition involves the external ear superficially and presents as a 'painful nodule of the ear'. The skin in this location is in direct contact with the cartilage without protective subcutaneous layer.

CAULIFLOWER EAR   This is an acquired deformity of the external ear due to degeneration of cartilage as a result of repeated trauma as occurs in boxers and wrestlers.

OTOSCLEROSIS   This is a dystrophic disease of labyrinth of the temporal bone. The footplate of stapes first undergoes fibrous replacement and is subsequently replaced by sclerotic bone.

TUMOURS AND TUMOUR-LIKE LESIONS *(p. 495)*

Tumours and tumour-like lesions which are specific to the ear are as under:
◈   In the external ear—aural (otic) polyps and cerumen-gland tumours.
◈   In the middle ear—cholesteatoma (keratoma) and jugular paraganglioma (glomus jugulare tumour).
◈   In the inner ear—acoustic neuroma.

AURAL (OTIC) POLYPS   Aural or otic polyps are tumour-like lesions arising from the middle ear as a complication of the chronic otitis media and project into the external auditory canal.

CERUMEN-GLAND TUMOURS   Tumours arising from cerumen-secreting apocrine sweat glands of the external auditory canal are cerumen-gland adenomas or cerumen-gland adenocarcinomas and are counter-parts of sweat gland tumours (hideradenoma and adenocarcinoma) of the skin.

CHOLESTEATOMA (KERATOMA)   This is a post-inflammatory 'pseudo-tumour' found in the middle ear or mastoid air cells. There is invariable history of acute or chronic otitis media which the squamous epithelium enters the middle ear and results in exfoliation of squamous and formation of the keratin.

M/E   The lesion consists of cyst containing abundant keratin material admixed with cholesterol crystals and large number of histiocytes. In advanced cases, there may be pressure erosion of the bone.

JUGULAR PARAGANGLIOMA (GLOMUS JUGULARE TUMOUR, NON-CHROMAFFIN PARAGANGLIOMA)   Tumours originating from parasympathetic ganglia are called 'paraganglioma' and are named according to the location of the tissue of origin. The one arising from glomus jugulare bodies of the middle ear (jugulotympanic bodies) is called jugular paraganglioma or chemodectoma or non-chromaffin paraganglioma and is the most common benign tumour of the middle ear.

M/E The tumour cells containing neurosecretory granules are arranged in typical organoid pattern or nests.

ACOUSTIC NEUROMA (ACOUSTIC SCHWANNOMA) This is a tumour of Schwann cells of 8th cranial nerve. It is usually located in the internal auditory canal and cerebellopontine angle. It is a benign tumour similar to other schwannomas but by virtue of its location and large size, may produce compression of the important neighbouring tissues leading to deafness, tinnitus, paralysis of 5th and 7th nerves, compression of the brainstem and hydrocephalus.

NOSE AND PARANASAL SINUSES (p. 496)

NORMAL STRUCTURE

The external nose and the septum are composed of bone and cartilage. On the lateral wall of the nasal cavity, there is a system of 3 ridges on each side known as conchae or turbinates—the inferior, middle and superior. The nasal accessory sinuses are air spaces in the bones of the skull and communicate with the nasal cavity.

M/E Nasal mucous membranes as well as the lining of the nasal sinus are lined by respiratory epithelium (pseudostratified columnar ciliated cells). Mucous and serous glands lie under the mucous membrane.

INFLAMMATORY CONDITIONS (p. 496)

ACUTE RHINITIS (COMMON COLD) Acute rhinitis or common cold is the common inflammatory disorder of the nasal cavities that may extend into the nasal sinuses. It begins with rhinorrhoea, nasal obstruction and sneezing. Initially, the nasal discharge is watery, but later it becomes thick and purulent. The etiologic agents are generally adenoviruses that evoke catarrhal discharge. Chilling of the body is a contributory factor. Secondary bacterial invasion is common.

ALLERGIC RHINITIS (HAY FEVER) Allergic rhinitis occurs due to sensitivity to allergens such as pollens. It is an IgE-mediated immune response consisting of an early acute response due to degranulation of mast cells, and a delayed prolonged response.

SINUSITIS Acute sinusitis is generally a complication of acute or allergic rhinitis and rarely secondary to dental sepsis. The ostia are occluded due to inflammation and oedema and the sinuses are full. *'Mucocele'* is filling up of the sinus with mucus while *'empyema'* of the sinus occurs due to collection of pus.

NASAL POLYPS Nasal polyps are common and are pedunculated grape-like masses of tissue. They are the end-result of prolonged chronic inflammation causing polypoid thickening of the mucosa. They may be *allergic* or *inflammatory*.

G/A They are gelatinous masses with smooth and shining surface.

M/E They are composed of loose oedematous connective tissue containing some mucous glands and varying number of inflammatory cells like lymphocytes, plasma cells and eosinophils. Allergic polyps have plenty of eosinophils and hyperplasia of mucous glands.

RHINOSPORIDIOSIS Rhinosporidiosis is caused by a fungus, *Rhinosporidium seeberi*. Typically it occurs in a nasal polyp but may be found in other locations like nasopharynx, larynx and conjunctiva.

M/E Besides the structure of inflammatory or allergic polyp, large number of organisms of the size of erythrocytes with chitinous wall are seen in the thick-walled *sporangia*. Each sporangium may contain a few thousand spores.

RHINOSCLEROMA This is a chronic destructive inflammatory lesion of the nose and upper respiratory airways caused by diplobacilli, *Klebsiella rhinoscleromatis*.

M/E There is extensive infiltration by foamy histiocytes containing the organisms (Mikulicz cells) and other chronic inflammatory cells like lymphocytes and plasma cells.

GRANULOMAS Many types of granulomatous inflammations may involve the nose.

1. **Tuberculosis or lupus** of the nose is uncommon and occurs secondary to pulmonary tuberculosis and usually produces ulcerative lesions on the anterior part of the septum of the nose.

2. **Leprosy** begins as a nodule that may ulcerate and perforate the septum.

3. **Syphilis** may involve the nose in congenital form causing destruction of the septum, or in acquired tertiary syphilis in the form of gummas perforating the septum.

4. **Aspergillosis** may involve the paranasal sinuses where the septate hyphae grow to form a mass called *aspergilloma*.

5. **Mucormycosis** is an opportunistic infection caused by *Mucorales* which are non-septate hyphae and involve the nerves and blood vessels.

6. **Wegener's granulomatosis** is a form of necrotising vasculitis with granuloma formation affecting the upper respiratory tract, lungs and kidneys.

7. **Lethal midline granuloma or polymorphic reticulosis** is a rare and lethal lesion of the upper respiratory tract that causes extensive destruction of cartilage and necrosis of tissues. Currently, the condition is considered to be a nasal type extranodal T cell lymphoma.

TUMOURS *(p. 498)*

BENIGN TUMOURS

CAPILLARY HAEMANGIOMA Capillary haemangioma of the septum of nose is a common benign lesion and is similar to its counterparts elsewhere.

SINONASAL PAPILLOMAS Papillomas may occur in the nasal vestibule, nasal cavity and paranasal sinuses. They are mainly of 2 types—*fungiform papilloma* with exophytic growth, and *inverted papilloma* with everted growth, also called Schneiderian papilloma. Papillomas of either type may be lined with various combinations of epithelia: respiratory, squamous and mucous type.

MALIGNANT TUMOURS

OLFACTORY NEUROBLASTOMA OR ESTHESIONEUROBLASTOMA It occurs over the olfactory mucosa as a polypoid mass that may invade the paranasal sinuses or skull. It is a highly malignant small cell tumour of neural crest origin that may, at times, be indistinguishable from other small cell malignancies.

CARCINOMAS Carcinomas of the nasal cavity and paranasal sinuses are called *sinonasal carcinomas*. Most commonly, these are squamous cell carcinomas of varying grades of differentiation.

PHARYNX *(p. 499)*

NORMAL STRUCTURE

The pharynx has 3 parts—the nasopharynx, oropharynx (pharynx proper) and the laryngopharynx. The whole of pharynx is lined by stratified squamous epithelium. The lymphoid tissue of the pharynx is comprised by the tonsils and adenoids.

LUDWIG'S ANGINA This is a severe, acute streptococcal cellulitis involving the neck, tongue and back of the throat.

VINCENT'S ANGINA Vincent's angina is a painful condition of the throat characterised by local ulceration of the tonsils, mouth and pharynx. The causative organism is *Vincent's bacillus.*

DIPHTHERIA Diphtheria is an acute communicable disease caused by *Corynebacterium diphtheriae.* It usually occurs in children and results in the formation of a yellowish-grey *pseudomembrane* in the mucosa of nasopharynx, oropharynx, tonsils, larynx and trachea.

TONSILLITIS Tonsillitis caused by staphylococci or streptococci may be acute or chronic.
◈ *Acute tonsillitis* is characterised by enlargement, redness and inflammation.
◈ *Chronic tonsillitis* is caused by repeated attacks of acute tonsillitis in which case the tonsils are small and fibrosed.

PERITONSILLAR ABSCESS (QUINSY) Peritonsillar abscess or quinsy occurs as a complication of acute tonsillitis. The causative organisms are staphylococci or streptococci which are associated with infection of the tonsils.

RETROPHARYNGEAL ABSCESS Formation of abscess in the soft tissue between the posterior wall of the pharynx and the vertebral column is called retropharyngeal abscess.

TUMOURS *(p. 499)*

NASOPHARYNGEAL ANGIOFIBROMA This is a peculiar tumour that occurs exclusively in adolescent males (10-20 years of age) suggesting the role of testosterone hormone in its production. Though a benign tumour of the nasopharynx, it may grow into paranasal sinuses, cheek and orbit but does not metastasise.

M/E The tumour is composed of 2 components as the name suggests—numerous small endothelium-lined vascular spaces and the stromal cells which are myofibroblasts.

NASOPHARYNGEAL CARCINOMA Nasopharyngeal carcinoma is a common cancer in South-East Asia, especially prevalent in people of Chinese descent under 45 years of age. Genetic susceptibility and role of Epstein-Barr virus are considered important factors in its etiology. In fact, EBV-genome is found virtually in all cases of nasopharyngeal carcinoma.

M/E Nasopharyngeal carcinoma has 3 histologic variants:
i) Non-keratinising squamous cell carcinoma
ii) Keratinising squamous cell carcinoma
iii) Undifferentiated (transitional cell) carcinoma
    A variant of undifferentiated carcinoma is *'lymphoepithelioma'* in which undifferentiated carcinoma is infiltrated by abundant non-neoplastic mature lymphocytes.

EMBRYONAL RHABDOMYOSARCOMA Also termed as botyroid rhabdomyosarcoma, this is one of the common malignant tumours in children lesion is highly cellular and mitotically active. Other locations include vagina, orbit, middle ear, oral cavity, retroperitoneum and bile duct.

MALIGNANT LYMPHOMA The lymphoid tissue of the nasopharynx and tonsils may be the site for development of malignant lymphomas which resemble similar tumours elsewhere in the body.

NORMAL STRUCTURE

The larynx is composed of cartilages which are bound together by ligaments and muscles and is covered by mucous membrane. The cartilages of the larynx are of 2 types—unpaired and paired.

The larynx as well as trachea are lined by respiratory epithelium, except over the true vocal cords and the epiglottis, which are lined by stratified squamous epithelium.

INFLAMMATORY CONDITIONS (p. 500)

ACUTE LARYNGITIS This may occur as a part of the upper or lower respiratory tract infection. Atmospheric pollutants like cigarette smoke, exhaust fumes, industrial and domestic smoke etc predispose the larynx to acute bacterial and viral infections. *Streptococci* and *H. influenzae* cause acute epiglottitis which may be life-threatening.

CHRONIC LARYNGITIS Chronic laryngitis may occur from repeated attacks of acute inflammation, excessive smoking, chronic alcoholism or vocal abuse.

TUBERCULOUS LARYNGITIS Tuberculous laryngitis occurs secondary to pulmonary tuberculosis. Typical caseating tubercles are present on the surface of the larynx.

ACUTE OEDEMA OF THE LARYNX This hazardous condition is an acute inflammatory condition, causing swelling of the larynx that may lead to airway obstruction and death by suffocation.

TUMOURS (p. 500)

LARYNGEAL PAPILLOMA AND PAPILLOMATOSIS Juvenile laryngeal papillomas are found in children or adolescents and are often multiple, while the adults have usually a single lesion. Human papilloma virus (HPV type 11 and 6) has been implicated in the etiology of papillomas of the larynx.

G/A The lesions appear as warty growths on the true vocal cords, epiglottis and sometimes extend to the trachea and bronchi.

M/E Papillomas are composed of finger-like papillae, each papilla contains fibrovascular core covered by stratified squamous epithelium.

LARYNGEAL NODULES Laryngeal nodules or polyps are seen mainly in adults and are found more often in heavy smokers and in individuals subjected to vocal abuse. Therefore, they are known by various synonyms like singers' nodes, preachers' node, and screamers' nodes.

G/A It is a small lesion, less than 1 cm in diameter, rounded, smooth, usually sessile and polypoid swelling on the true vocal cords.

M/E The nodules have prominent oedema with sparse fibrous tissue and numerous irregular and dilated vascular channels.

LARYNGEAL CARCINOMA Cancer of the larynx in 99% of cases is squamous cell carcinoma. Rarely, adenocarcinoma and sarcoma are encountered. Squamous carcinoma of the larynx occurs in males beyond 4th decade of life. Important etiologic factor is heavy smoking of cigarettes, cigar or pipe; other factors include excessive alcohol consumption, radiation and asbestos exposure.

However, based on the anatomic location, laryngeal carcinoma is classified as under:
1. *Glottic* is the most common location, found in the region of true vocal cords and anterior and posterior commissures.
2. *Supraglottic* involving ventricles and arytenoids.
3. *Subglottic* in the walls of subglottis.

4. *Marginal zone* between the tip of epiglottis and ary-epiglottic folds.

5. *Laryngo-(hypo-) pharynx* in the pyriform fossa, postcricoid fossa and posterior pharyngeal wall.

G/A The glottic carcinoma is the most common form and appears as a small, pearly white, plaque-like thickening that may be ulcerated or fungated.

M/E Keratinising and non-keratinising squamous carcinomas of varying grades are found. Two special varieties of squamous carcinoma in the larynx are: *verrucous carcinoma* (or Ackerman's tumour) which is a variant of well-differentiated squamous carcinoma, and *spindle cell carcinoma* which has elongated tumour cells resembling sarcoma (pseudosarcoma) at the other extreme of prognosis.

NORMAL STRUCTURE

The neck is the region from where important structures like oesophagus, trachea, carotid arteries, great veins and nerve trunks pass through it. Besides, the neck has structures such as carotid body, sympathetic ganglia, larynx, thyroid, parathyroids and lymph nodes.

CYSTS OF NECK *(p. 502)*

The cysts of neck may be medial (midline) or lateral.

MEDIAL (MIDLINE) CERVICAL CYSTS

THYROGLOSSAL CYST Thyroglossal cyst arises from the vestiges of thyroglossal duct that connects the foramen caecum at the base of the tongue with the normally located thyroid gland.

M/E The cyst is lined by respiratory and/or stratified squamous epithelium.

MIDLINE DERMOID CYST Dermoid cyst located in the midline of the neck occurs due to sequestration of dermal cells along the lines of closure of embryonic clefts.

M/E It is lined by epidermis and contains skin adnexal structures.

LATERAL CERVICAL CYSTS

BRANCHIAL (LYMPHOEPITHELIAL) CYST Branchial or lymphoepithelial cyst arises from incomplete closure of 2nd or 3rd branchial clefts. The cyst is generally located anterior to the sternocleidomastoid muscle near the angle of the mandible.

M/E True to its name, the cyst has an *epithelial lining*, usually stratified squamous or respiratory epithelium, and *subepithelial lymphoid* tissue aggregates or follicles with germinal centres.

PARATHYROID CYST Parathyroid cyst is a lateral cyst of the neck usually located deep to the sternocleidomastoid muscle at the angle of the mandible.

M/E Parathyroid cyst is lined by flattened cuboidal to low columnar epithelium and the cyst wall may contain any type of parathyroid cells.

CERVICAL THYMIC CYST Cervical thymic cyst originates from cystic degeneration of Hassall's corpuscles.

M/E The cyst is lined by stratified squamous epithelium and the cyst wall may contain thymic structures.

CYSTIC HYGROMA Cystic hygroma is a lateral swelling at the root of the neck, usually located behind the sternocleidomastoid muscle. It may be present congenitally or may manifest in the first 2 years of life.

M/E Cystic hygroma is a diffuse lymphangioma containing large cavernous spaces lined by endothelium and containing lymph fluid.

Tumours of the neck may be primary or metastatic in cervical lymph nodes.

PRIMARY TUMOURS

CAROTID BODY TUMOUR (CHEMODECTOMA, CAROTID BODY PARAGANGLIOMA) Carotid body tumour arises in the carotid bodies which are situated at the bifurcation of the common carotid arteries. Histologically similar tumours are found in other parasympathetic ganglia represented by the vagus and glomus jugulare (jugulotympanic bodies).

G/A They are small, firm, dark tan, encapsulated nodules.

M/E Well-differentiated tumour cells form characteristic organoid or alveolar pattern, as is the case with all other neuroendocrine tumours. The tumour cells contain dark neurosecretory granules containing catecholamines.

TORTICOLLIS (FIBROMATOSIS COLLI, WRY NECK) This is a deformity in which the head is bent to one side while the chin points to the other side. The deformity may occur as congenital torticollis or may be an acquired form. The *acquired form* may occur secondary to fracture dislocation of the cervical spine, Pott's disease of the cervical spine, scoliosis, spasm of the muscles of neck, exposure to chill causing myositis, and contracture following burns or wound healing.

MALIGNANT LYMPHOMAS Various forms of non-Hodgkin's lymphomas and Hodgkin's disease occur in the cervical lymph nodes as discussed in Chapter 12.

SECONDARY TUMOURS

Cervical lymph nodes are common site for metastases of a large number of carcinomas. These include: squamous cell carcinoma of the lips, mouth, tongue, larynx and oesophagus; transitional cell carcinoma of the pharynx and nasopharynx; thoracic and abdominal cancers such as of the stomach, lungs, ovaries, uterus and testis.

SELF ASSESSMENT

1. **Chalazion is chronic inflammatory process involving:**
   - A. Sebaceous gland of Zeis
   - B. Apocrine gland of Moll
   - C. Meibomian glands
   - D. Eyelash follicle

2. **Proliferative retinopathy consists of the following lesions except:**
   - A. Capillary microaneurysms
   - B. Neovascularisation of the retina at optic disc
   - C. Vitreous haemorrhages
   - D. Proliferation of astrocytes and fibrous tissue around blood vessels

3. **Hypertensive retinopathy has the following features except:**
   - A. Flame-shaped haemorrhages in retinal nerve layer
   - B. Arteriolosclerosis
   - C. Vitreous haemorrhages
   - D. Microaneurysm

4. **Mikulicz's syndrome is inflammatory enlargement of lacrimal and salivary glands which may occur with following conditions except:**
   - A. Sjögren's syndrome
   - B. Sarcoidosis
   - C. Tuberculosis
   - D. Lymphoma

5. **Sebaceous carcinoma occurs most commonly at:**
   - A. Axilla
   - B. Groin
   - C. Upper eyelid
   - D. Lower eyelid

6. **Following histologic type of uveal malignant melanoma has the worst prognosis:**
   A. Spindle A
   B. Spindle B
   C. Epithelioid
   D. Mixed

7. **The most common ocular metastatic tumour is from the following primary cancer:**
   A. Melanoma
   B. Breast
   C. Epidermoid
   D. Neuroblastoma

8. **Sjögren's syndrome produces the following pathological change in the eye:**
   A. Uveitis
   B. Phthisis bulbi
   C. Keratoconjunctivitis
   D. Glaucoma

9. **Most common eyelid tumour is:**
   A. Sebaceous carcinoma
   B. Squamous cell carcinoma
   C. Malignant melanoma
   D. Basal cell carcinoma

10. **What is true about retinoblastoma:**
    A. 60% cases are sporadic and 40% are familial
    B. 40% cases are sporadic and 60% are familial
    C. 80% cases are sporadic and 20% are familial
    D. 20% cases are sporadic and 80% are familial

11. **Wegener's granulomatosis generally produces lesions in the following tissues <u>except</u>:**
    A. Nose
    B. Ears
    C. Lungs
    D. Kidneys

12. **Nasopharyngeal angiofibroma has the following features <u>except</u>:**
    A. It is endemic in people of South-East Asia
    B. It occurs exclusively in adolescent males
    C. It is a benign nasopharyngeal tumour
    D. Testosterone hormone plays a role in its etiology

13. **Nasopharyngeal carcinoma has the following features <u>except</u>:**
    A. It is common cancer in South-East Asia
    B. It occurs in males exclusively
    C. EB virus plays a role in its etiology
    D. The prognosis is usually fatal

14. **Sebaceous carcinoma is commonest tumour in the following location:**
    A. Upper eyelid
    B. Lower eyelid
    C. External auditory canal
    D. Lip

15. **Lateral cervical cysts of the neck include the following examples <u>except</u>:**
    A. Branchial cyst
    B. Thyroglossal cyst
    C. Cervical thymic cyst
    D. Parathyroid cyst

16. **Which of the following is post-inflammatory pseudotumour of ear:**
    A. Chondrodermatitis nodularis
    B. Cauliflower ear
    C. Otosclerosis
    D. Cholesteatoma

17. **Characteristic cells seen in rhinoscleroma are known as:**
    A. Mikulicz cells
    B. Dendritic cells
    C. Langerhans cells
    D. Touton cells

18. **Which HPV types are implicated in causation of laryngeal papilloma:**
    A. HPV type 6 and 11
    B. HPV type 8 and 16
    C. HPV type 33 and 36
    D. HPV type 46 and 52

19. **Ackerman's tumour is:**
    A. Spindle cell carcinoma of larynx
    B. Verrucous carcinoma of larynx

C. Adenocarcinoma of larynx
D. Sarcoma of larynx

20. Which one of the following viruses is a member of the herpes family, infects B cells and epithelial cells of the oropharynx, and causes a positive heterophil antibody test?
   A. CMV
   B. EBV
   C. HBV
   D. HIV

KEY

1 = C	2 = A	3 = C	4 = C	5 = C
6 = C	7 = B	8 = C	9 = A	10 = A
11 = B	12 = A	13 = B	14 = A	15 = B
16 = D	17 = B	18 = A	19 = B	20 = B

The Oral Cavity and Salivary Glands

ORAL SOFT TISSUES *(p. 504)*

NORMAL STRUCTURE

The oral cavity is the point of entry for digestive and respiratory tracts. The mucous membrane of the mouth consists of squamous epithelium covering vascularised connective tissue. The epithelium is keratinised over the hard palate, lips and gingiva, while elsewhere it is non-keratinised. Mucous glands (minor salivary glands) are scattered throughout the oral mucosa.

DEVELOPMENTAL ANOMALIES *(p. 504)*

1.   FACIAL CLEFTS   *Cleft upper lip (harelip) and cleft palate,* alone or in combination, are the commonest developmental anomalies of the face.

2.   FORDYCE'S GRANULES   Fordyce's granules are symmetric, small, light yellow macular spots on the lips and buccal mucosa and represent collections of sebaceous glands.

3.   LEUKOEDEMA   This is an asymptomatic condition occurring in children and is characterised by symmetric, grey-white areas on the buccal mucosa.

4.   DEVELOPMENTAL DEFECTS OF THE TONGUE   These are as under:

i)   Macroglossia is the enlargement of the tongue, usually due to lymphangioma or haemangioma, sometimes due to amyloid tumour.

ii)   Microglossia and aglossia are rare congenital anomalies representing small-sized and absence of tongue respectively.

iii)   Fissured tongue (scrotal, furrowed or grooved tongue) is a genetically-determined condition characterised by numerous small furrows or grooves on the dorsum of the tongue.

iv)   Bifid tongue is a rare condition occurring due to failure of the two lateral halves of the tongue to fuse in the midline.

v)   Tongue tie occurs when the lingual fraenum is quite short.

vi)   Hairy tongue is not a true developmental defect. The filiform papillae are hypertrophied and elongated. These 'hairs' (papillae) are stained black, brown or yellowish-white by food, tobacco, oxidising agents or by oral flora.

MUCOCUTANEOUS LESIONS *(p. 504)*

LICHEN PLANUS   Characteristically, oral lichen planus appears as interlacing network of whitening or keratosis on the buccal mucosa but other oral tissues such as gingiva, tongue and palate may also be involved.

VESICULAR LESIONS   A number of vesicular or bullous diseases of the skin have oral lesions.

i)   Pemphigus vulgaris   Vesicular oral lesions appear invariably in all cases at some time in the course of pemphigus vulgaris.

ii)   Pemphigoid   Vesicles or bullae appear on oral mucosa as well as on conjunctiva in pemphigoid.

iii)   Erythema multiforme   Subepithelial vesicles may occur on the skin as well as mucosae.

iv) Stevens-Johnson syndrome It is a rather fatal and severe form of erythema multiforme involving oral and other mucous membranes occurring following ingestion of sulfa drugs.

v) Epidermolysis bullosa It is a hereditary condition having subepidermal bullae on the skin as well as has oral lesions.

INFLAMMATORY AND PIGMENTARY DISEASES *(p. 504)*

STOMATITIS Inflammation of the mucous membrane of the mouth is called stomatitis. It can occur in the course of several different diseases.

i) Aphthous, ulcers (Canker sores) These are the commonest form of oral ulcerations. The etiology is unknown but may be precipitated by emotional factors, stress, allergy, hormonal imbalance, nutritional deficiencies, gastrointestinal disturbances, trauma etc.

ii) Herpetic stomatitis It is an acute disease occurring in infants and young children. It is the most common manifestation of primary infection with herpes simplex virus.

iii) Necrotising stomatitis (Noma or Cancrum oris) This occurs more commonly in poorly-nourished children like in kwashiorkor; infectious diseases such as measles, immunodeficiencies and emotional stress.

iv) Mycotic infections Common examples are as under:
◈ *Cervicofacial actinomycosis* is the commonest form of the disease developing at the angle of the mandible.
◈ *Candidiasis (moniliasis or thrush)* is caused by *Candida albicans* which is a commensal in the mouth.

GLOSSITIS **Acute glossitis** characterised by swollen papillae occurs in eruptions of measles and scarlet fever. In **chronic glossitis,** the tongue is raw and red without swollen papillae and is seen in malnutrition such as in pellagra, ariboflavinosis and niacin deficiency.

SYPHILITIC LESIONS Oral lesions may occur in primary, secondary, tertiary and congenital syphilis.
i) Extragenital chancre of *primary syphilis* occurs most commonly on the lips.
ii) Secondary *syphilis* shows maculopapular eruptions and mucous patches in the mouth.
iii) In the *tertiary syphilis*, gummas or diffuse fibrosis may be seen on the hard palate and tongue.
iv) Oral lesions of the *congenital syphilis* are fissures at the angles of mouth and characteristic peg-shaped notched Hutchinson's incisors.

TUBERCULOUS LESIONS Involvement of the mouth in tuberculosis is rare.

HIV INFECTION HIV infection of low grade as well as full-blown acquired immunodeficiency syndrome (AIDS) are associated with oral manifestations such as opportunistic infections, malignancy, hairy leukoplakia and others. About half the cases of Kaposi's sarcoma have intraoral lesions as part of systemic involvement.

PIGMENTARY LESIONS Oral and labial melanotic pigmentation may be observed in certain systemic and metabolic disorders such as Addison's disease, Albright syndrome, Peutz-Jeghers syndrome and haemochromatosis. All types of pigmented naevi as well as malignant melanoma can occur in oral cavity.

TUMOURS AND TUMOUR-LIKE LESIONS *(p. 505)*

A. TUMOUR-LIKE LESIONS

FIBROUS GROWTHS These are not true tumours (unlike intraoral fibroma and papilloma), but are instead inflammatory or irritative in origin. A few common varieties are as under:

i) Fibroepithelial polyps occur due to irritation or chronic trauma. These are composed of reparative fibrous tissue, covered by a thin layer of stratified squamous epithelium.

ii) Fibrous epulis is a lesion occurring on the gingiva and is localised hyperplasia of the connective tissue following trauma or inflammation in the area.

iii) Denture hyperplasia occurs in edentulous or partly edentulous patients. The lesion is an inflammatory hyperplasia in response to local irritation by ill-fitting denture or an elongated tooth.

PYOGENIC GRANULOMA This is an elevated, bright red swelling of variable size occurring on the lips, tongue, buccal mucosa and gingiva. *Pregnancy tumour* is a variant of pyogenic granuloma.

MUCOCELE Also called mucous cyst or retention cyst, it is a cystic dilatation of the mucous glands of the oral mucosa.

RANULA It is a large mucocele located on the floor of the mouth. The cyst is lined by true epithelial lining.

DERMOID CYST This tumour-like mass in the floor of the mouth represents a developmental malformation. The cyst is lined by stratified squamous epithelium. The cyst wall contains sebaceous glands, sweat glands, hair follicles and other mature tissues.

B. BENIGN TUMOURS

SQUAMOUS PAPILLOMA Papilloma can occur anywhere in the mouth and has the usual papillary or finger-like projections.

M/E Each papilla is composed of vascularised connective tissue covered by squamous epithelium.

HAEMANGIOMA Haemangioma can occur anywhere in the mouth; when it occurs on the tongue it may cause macroglossia. It is most commonly capillary type, although cavernous and mixed types may also occur.

LYMPHANGIOMA Lymphangioma may develop most commonly on the tongue producing macroglossia; on the lips producing macrocheilia, and on the cheek. *Cystic hygroma* is a special variety of lymphangioma occurring in children on the lateral side of neck.

FIBROMA Although most common benign oral mucous membrane mass is fibroma appearing as a discrete superficial pedunculated mass. It probably arises as a response to physical trauma.

FIBROMATOSIS GINGIVAE This is a fibrous overgrowth of unknown etiology involving the entire gingiva.

TUMOURS OF MINOR SALIVARY GLANDS Minor salivary glands present in the oral cavity may sometimes be the site of origin of salivary tumours similar to those seen in the major salivary glands. Pleomorphic adenoma is a common example.

GRANULAR CELL TUMOUR Earlier called as granular cell myoblastoma, it is benign tumour, which now by electron microscopic studies, is known to be mesenchymal in origin than odontogenic.

M/E The tumour is composed of large polyhedral cells with granular, acidophilic cytoplasm.

C. ORAL LEUKOPLAKIA (WHITE LESIONS)

DEFINITION Leukoplakia *(white plaque)* may be clinically defined as a white patch or plaque on the oral mucosa, exceeding 5 mm in diameter, which cannot be rubbed off nor can be classified into any other diagnosable disease. However, from the pathologist's point of view, the term 'leukoplakia' is reserved for epithelial thickening which may range from completely benign to atypical and to premalignant cellular changes.

INCIDENCE It occurs more frequently in males than females. The lesions may be of variable size and appearance. The sites of predilection, in descending order of frequency, are: cheek mucosa, angles of mouth, alveolar mucosa, tongue, lip, hard and soft palate, and floor of the mouth. In about 4-6% cases of leukoplakia, carcinomatous change is reported.

ETIOLOGY The etiological factors are similar to those suggested for carcinoma of the oral mucosa. *It has the strongest association with the use of tobacco in various forms,* e.g. in heavy smokers (especially in pipe and cigar smokers) and improves when smoking is discontinued, and in those who chew tobacco containing products e.g. *paan, paan masaala, zarda, gutka* etc. The condition is also known by other names such as *smokers' keratosis* and *stomatitis nicotina.*

G/A The lesions of leukoplakia may appear white, whitish-yellow, or red-velvety of more than 5 mm diameter and variable in appearance. They are usually circumscribed, slightly elevated, smooth or wrinkled, speckled or nodular.

M/E Leukoplakia is of 2 types:

1. Hyperkeratotic type This is characterised by an orderly and regular hyperplasia of squamous epithelium with hyperkeratosis on the surface.

2. Dysplastic type When the changes such as irregular stratification of the epithelium, focal areas of increased and abnormal mitotic figures, hyper-chromatism, pleomorphism, loss of polarity and individual cell keratinisation are present, the lesion is considered as epithelial dysplasia. The subepithelial tissues usually show an inflammatory infiltrate composed of lymphocytes and plasma cells. If the epithelial dysplasia is extensive so as to involve the entire thickness of the epithelium, the lesion is called carcinoma *in situ* which may progress to invasive carcinoma.

D. MALIGNANT TUMOURS

SQUAMOUS CELL (EPIDERMOID) CARCINOMA

Oral cancer is a disease with very poor prognosis because it is not recognised and treated when small and early.

INCIDENCE Squamous cell (epidermoid) carcinoma comprises 90% of all oral malignant tumours and 5% of all human malignancies. Oral cancer is a very frequent malignancy in India, Sri Lanka and some Eastern countries, probably related to habits of betel-nut chewing and reversed smoking. It can occur anywhere in the mouth but certain sites are more commonly involved. These sites, in descending order of frequency, are: the lips (more commonly lower), tongue, anterior floor of mouth, buccal mucosa in the region of alveolar lingual sulcus, and palate.

ETIOLOGY A number of etiological factors have been implicated:

Strong association is seen with following:
i) Tobacco smoking and tobacco chewing causing leukoplakia
ii) Chronic alcohol consumption.
iii) Human papilloma virus infection, particularly HPV 16, 18 and 33 types.

Weak association is observed with following:
i) Chronic irritation from ill-fitting denture or jagged teeth.
ii) Submucosal fibrosis
iii) Poor orodental hygiene.
iv) Nutritional deficiencies.
v) Exposure to sunlight (in relation to lip cancer).
vi) Exposure to radiation.
vii) Plummer-Vinson syndrome.

G/A Squamous cell carcinoma of oral cavity may have the following types:
i) Ulcerative type—is the most frequent type.
ii) Papillary or verrucous type—is soft and wart-like growth.
iii) Nodular type—appears as a firm, slow growing submucosal nodule.
iv) Scirrhous type—is characterised by infiltration into deeper structures.

M/E Squamous cell carcinoma ranges from well-differentiated keratinising carcinoma to highly-undifferentiated neoplasm.

    Verrucous carcinoma, on the other hand, is composed of very well-differentiated squamous epithelium with minimal atypia and hence has very good prognosis.

Other less common malignant neoplasms which may be encountered in the oral cavity are: malignant melanoma, lymphoepithelial carcinoma, malignant lymphoma, malignant tumours of minor salivary glands, and various sarcomas like rhabdomyosarcoma, liposarcoma, alveolar soft part sarcoma, Kaposi's sarcoma and fibrosarcoma.

TEETH AND PERIODONTAL TISSUES (p. 509)

NORMAL STRUCTURE

The teeth are normally composed of 3 calcified tissues, namely: *enamel*, *dentin* and *cementum*; and the *pulp* which is composed of connective tissue. The teeth are peculiar than other calcified tissues of the body by being surrounded by the portion of oral mucosa called the gingiva or gum, and that they are part of a highly specialised odontogenic apparatus; other parts of this apparatus being the mandible and maxilla.

❖ Inner epithelial layer of the dental lamina is ectoderm-derived columnar to cuboidal oral epithelium called **ameloblasts** which secrete enamel matrix, also called enamel organ.

❖ Mesoderm-derived connective tissue gives rise to structures in the **dental papilla** (i.e. dental pulp or core of loose connective tissue, blood vessels and nerves).

❖ Outer margin of the dental papilla differentiates into **odontoblasts**, which continue with ameloblastic epithelium; odontoblasts secrete dentin.

Dental pulp is inner to dentine and occupies the pulp cavity and root canal. It consists of connective tissue, blood vessels and nerves.

INFLAMMATORY DISEASES (p. 510)

DENTAL CARIES

Dental caries is the most common disease of dental tissues, causing destruction of the calcified tissues of the teeth.

ETIOPATHOGENESIS Dental caries is essentially a disease of modern society, associated with diet containing high proportion of refined carbohydrates. Diets rich in carbohydrates do not require much chewing and thus the soft and sticky food gets clung to the teeth rather than being cleared away, particularly in the areas of occlusal pits and fissures. '*Bacterial plaques*' are formed in such stagnation areas.

G/A The earliest change is the appearance of a small, chalky-white spot on the enamel which subsequently enlarges and often becomes yellow or brown and breaks down to form carious cavity.

M/E Inflammation (pulpitis) and necrosis of pulp take place. There is evidence of reaction of the tooth to the carious process in the form of *secondary dentin*, which is a layer of odontoblasts laid down under the original dentin.

SEQUELAE OF CARIES Carious destruction of dental hard tissues frequently produces pulpitis and other inflammatory lesions like apical granuloma and apical abscess. Less common causes of these lesions are fracture of tooth and accidental exposure of pulp by the dentist.

PERIODONTAL DISEASE

Chronic inflammation and degeneration of the supporting tissues of teeth resulting in teeth loss is a common condition. Besides inflammation, other diseases associated with gingival swelling are leukaemia, scurvy, fibrous hyperplasia and epulis.

The inflammatory periodontal disease affects adults more commonly. Pregnancy, puberty and use of drugs like dilantin are associated with periodontal disease more often. The disease begins as *chronic marginal gingivitis,* secondary to bacterial plaques around the teeth such as due to calculus (tartar) on the tooth surface, impacted food, uncontrolled diabetes, tooth-decay and ill-fitting dental appliances.

M/E Untreated chronic marginal gingivitis slowly progresses to *chronic periodontitis* or *pyorrhoea* in which there is inflammatory destruction of deeper tissues. At this stage, progressive resorption of alveolar bone occurs and the tooth ultimately gets detached.

EPITHELIAL CYSTS OF THE JAW *(p. 511)*

A. INFLAMMATORY CYSTS

RADICULAR CYST

Radicular cyst, also called as apical, periodontal or simply dental cyst, is the most common cyst originating from the dental tissues. It arises consequent to inflammation following destruction of dental pulp such as in dental caries, pulpitis, and apical granuloma. Most often, radicular cyst is observed at the apex of an erupted tooth and sometimes contains thick pultaceous material.

M/E The radicular cyst is lined by nonkeratinised squamous epithelium. Epithelial rete processes may penetrate the underlying connective tissues. Radicular cyst of the maxilla may be lined by respiratory epithelium. The cyst wall is fibrous and contains chronic inflammatory cells (lymphocytes, plasma cells with Russell bodies and macrophages).

B. DEVELOPMENTAL CYSTS

ODONTOGENIC CYSTS

DENTIGEROUS (FOLLICULAR) CYST Dentigerous cyst arises from enamel of an unerupted tooth. The mandibular third molars and the maxillary canines are most often involved. Dentigerous cysts are less common than radicular cysts and occur more commonly in children and young individuals.

M/E Dentigerous cyst is composed of a thin fibrous tissue wall lined by stratified squamous epithelium. Thus, the cyst may resemble radicular cyst, except that chronic inflammatory changes so characteristic of radicular cyst, are usually absent in dentigerous cyst.

NON-ODONTOGENIC AND FISSURAL CYSTS

NASOPALATINE DUCT (INCISIVE CANAL, MEDIAN, ANTERIOR MAXILLARY) CYST This is the most common non-odontogenic (fissural) cyst and arises from the epithelial remnants of the nasopalatine duct.

NASOLABIAL (NASOALVEOLAR) CYST This cyst is situated in the soft tissues at the junction of median nasal, lateral nasal and maxillary processes, at the ala of the nose, and sometimes extending into the nostril.

DERMOID CYST The dermoid cyst is common in the region of head and neck, especially in the floor of the mouth. The cyst arises from remains in the midline during closure of mandibular and branchial arches.

ODONTOGENIC TUMOURS *(p. 513)*

Odontogenic tumours are a group of uncommon lesions of the jaw derived from the odontogenic apparatus. These tumours are usually benign but some have malignant counterparts.

A. BENIGN ODONTOGENIC TUMOURS

AMELOBLASTOMA

Ameloblastoma is the most common benign but locally invasive epithelial odontogenic tumour. It is most frequent in the 3rd to 5th decades of life. Preferential sites are the mandible in the molar-ramus area and the maxilla.

The tumour originates from dental epithelium of the enamel itself or its epithelial residues.

G/A The tumour is greyish-white, usually solid, sometimes cystic, replacing and expanding the affected bone.

M/E Ameloblastoma can show different patterns as follows:

i) Follicular pattern is the most common. The tumour consists of follicles of variable size and shape and separated from each other by fibrous tissue.

ii) Plexiform pattern is the next common pattern after follicular pattern. The tumour epithelium is seen to form irregular plexiform masses or network of strands.

iii) Acanthomatous pattern is squamous metaplasia within the islands of tumour cells.

iv) Basal cell pattern of ameloblastoma is similar to basal cell carcinoma of the skin.

v) Granular cell pattern is characterised by appearance of acidophilic granularity in the cytoplasm of tumour cells.

ODONTOGENIC ADENOMATOID TUMOUR (ADENO-AMELOBLASTOMA)

This is a benign tumour seen more often in females in their 2nd decade of life. The tumour is commonly associated with an unerupted tooth and thus closely resembles dentigerous cyst radiologically.

M/E The lesion has extensive cyst formations. The wall of cyst contains scanty fibrous connective tissue in which are present characteristic tubule-like structures composed of epithelial cells.

CALCIFYING EPITHELIAL ODONTOGENIC TUMOUR

This is a rare lesion which is locally invasive and recurrent like ameloblastoma. It is seen commonly in 4th and 5th decades and occurs more commonly in the region of mandible.

M/E The tumour consists of closely packed polyhedral epithelial cells having features of nuclear pleomorphism, giant nuclei and rare mitotic figures. The stroma is often scanty and appears homogeneous and hyalinised in which small calcified deposits are seen which are a striking feature of this tumour.

ODONTOGENIC MYXOMA (MYXOFIBROMA)

Odontogenic myxoma is a locally invasive and recurring tumour.

AMELOBLASTIC FIBROMA

This is a benign tumour consisting of epithelial and connective tissues derived from odontogenic apparatus. It resembles ameloblastoma but can be distinguished from it because ameloblastic fibroma occurs in younger age group (below 20 years).

ODONTOMAS

Odontomas are hamartomas that contain both epithelial and mesodermal dental tissue components. There are 3 subtypes:

i) **Complex odontoma** is always benign and consists of enamel, dentin and cementum which are not differentiated.

ii) **Compound odontoma** is also benign and is comprised of differentiated dental tissue elements forming a number of denticles in fibrous tissue.

iii) **Ameloblastic fibro-odontoma** is a lesion that resembles ameloblastic fibroma with odontoma formation.

CEMENTOMAS

Cementomas are a variety of benign lesions which are characterised by the presence of cementum or cementum-like tissue. Five types of cementomas are described:

i) Benign cementoblastoma (true cementoma)
ii) Cementifying fibroma
iii) Periapical cemental dysplasia (Periapical fibrous dysplasia)
iv) Multiple apical cementomas
v) Gigantiform cementoma

B. MALIGNANT ODONTOGENIC TUMOURS

ODONTOGENIC CARCINOMA

i) *Malignant ameloblastoma* is the term used for the uncommon metastasising ameloblastoma.
ii) *Ameloblastic carcinoma* is the term employed for the ameloblastic tumour having cytologic features of malignancy in the primary tumour.
iii) *Primary intraosseous carcinoma* may develop within the jaw from the rests of odontogenic epithelium.
iv) Rarely, carcinomas may arise from the odontogenic epithelium lining the *odontogenic cysts*.

ODONTOGENIC SARCOMAS

The only example of odontogenic sarcoma is a rare ameloblastic fibrosarcoma.

SALIVARY GLANDS (p. 515)

NORMAL STRUCTURE

There are two main groups of salivary glands—major and minor. The major salivary glands are the three paired glands: parotid, submandibular and sublingual. The minor salivary glands are numerous and are widely distributed in the mucosa of oral cavity.

M/E The salivary glands are tubuloalveolar glands and may contain mucous cells, serous cells, or both.
    The secretory acini of the major salivary glands are drained by ducts lined by:
◈ low cuboidal epithelium in the intercalated portion,
◈ tall columnar epithelium in the intralobular ducts, and
◈ simpler epithelium in the secretory ducts.

INFLAMMATORY AND SALIVARY FLOW DISEASES (p. 515)

SIALORRHOEA (PTYALISM)

Increased flow of saliva is termed sialorrhoea or ptyalism. It occurs commonly due to: stomatitis, teething, mentally retarded state, schizophrenia, neurological disturbances, increased gastric secretion and sialosis (i.e. uniform, symmetric, painless hypertrophy of salivary glands).

XEROSTOMIA

Decreased salivary flow is termed xerostomia. It is associated with the following conditions: Sjögren's syndrome, sarcoidosis, mumps parotitis, Mikulicz's syndrome, megaloblastic anaemia, dehydration, drug intake (e.g. antihistamines, antihypertensives, antidepressants).

SIALADENITIS

Inflammation of salivary glands, sialadenitis, may be acute or chronic; the latter being more common.

ETIOLOGY It may occur from following causes:

1. Viral infections The most common inflammatory lesion of the salivary glands particularly of the parotid glands, is mumps occurring in children of school-age. It is characterised by triad of pathological involvement—*epidemic parotitis (mumps), orchitis-oophoritis, and pancreatitis.*

2. Bacterial and mycotic infections Bacterial infections may cause acute sialadenitis more often.

i) *Acute sialadenitis* The causes are:
a) Acute infectious fevers
b) Acute postoperative parotitis (ascent of microorganisms up the parotid duct from the mouth)
c) General debility
d) Old age
e) Dehydration.

ii) *Chronic sialadenitis* This may result from the following causes:
a) *Recurrent obstructive type* Recurrent obstruction due to calculi (sialolithiasis), stricture, surgery, injury etc.
b) *Recurrent non-obstructive type* Recurrent mild ascending infection of the parotid gland due to intake of drugs causing hyposalivation (e.g. antihistamines, antihypertensives, antidepressants), effect of irradiation and congenital malformations of the duct system.
c) *Chronic inflammatory diseases* Tuberculosis, actinomycosis and other mycoses.

3. Autoimmune disease These are:
i) Sjögren's syndrome
ii) Mikulicz's syndrome.

G/A Irrespective of the underlying etiology of sialadenitis, there is swelling of the affected salivary gland, usually restricted by the fibrous capsule.

M/E *Acute viral sialadenitis* in mumps shows swelling and cytoplasmic vacuolation of the acinar epithelial cells and degenerative changes in the ductal epithelium. *Chronic and recurrent sialadenitis* is characterised by increased lymphoid tissue in the interstitium, progressive loss of secretory tissue and replacement by fibrosis.

TUMOURS OF SALIVARY GLANDS (p. 516)

The major glands, particularly the parotid glands (85%), are the most common sites. Majority of parotid gland tumour (65-85%) are benign, while in the other major and minor salivary glands 35-50% of the tumours are malignant. Most of the salivary gland tumours originate from the ductal lining epithelium and the underlying myoepithelial cells; a few arise from acini.

A. BENIGN SALIVARY GLAND TUMOURS

ADENOMAS

The adenomas of the salivary glands are benign epithelial tumours. They are broadly classified into 2 major groups—pleomorphic and monomorphic adenomas.

PLEOMORPHIC ADENOMA (MIXED SALIVARY TUMOUR)

This is the most common tumour of major (60-75%) and minor (50%) salivary glands. Pleomorphic adenoma is the commonest tumour in the parotid gland and occurs less often in other major and minor salivary glands. The tumour is commoner in women and is seen more frequently in 3rd to 5th decades of life.

G/A Pleomorphic adenoma is a circumscribed, pseudoencapsulated, rounded, at times multilobulated, firm mass, 2-5 cm in diameter, with bosselated surface. The cut surface is grey-white and bluish, variegated, semitranslucent.

M/E The pleomorphic adenoma is characterised by pleomorphic or 'mixed' appearance.

◈ **Epithelial component** may form various patterns like ducts, acini, tubules, sheets and strands of cells of ductal or myoepithelial origin. The ductal cells are cuboidal or columnar, while the underlying myoepithelial cells may be polygonal or spindle-shaped resembling smooth muscle cells.

◈ **Stromal elements** are present as loose connective tissue, and as myxoid, mucoid and chondroid matrix, which simulates cartilage (*pseudocartilage*). However, true cartilage and even bone may also be observed in a small proportion of these tumours.

PROGNOSIS Pleomorphic adenoma is notorious for recurrences, sometimes after many years. The main factors responsible for the tendency to recur are incomplete surgical removal due to proximity to the facial nerve, multiple foci of tumour, pseudoencapsulation, and implantation in the surgical field.

MONOMORPHIC ADENOMAS

These are benign epithelial tumours of salivary glands without any evidence of mesenchyme-like tissues. Their various forms are as under:

WARTHIN'S TUMOUR (PAPILLARY CYSTADENOMA LYMPHOMATO-SUM, ADENOLYMPHOMA) It is a benign tumour of the parotid gland comprising about 8% of all parotid neoplasms, seen more commonly in men from 4th to 7th decades of life.

G/A The tumour is encapsulated, round or oval with smooth surface. The cut surface shows characteristic slit-like or cystic spaces, containing milky fluid and having papillary projections.

M/E The tumour shows 2 components:
◈ **Epithelial parenchyma** is composed of glandular and cystic structures having papillary arrangement and is lined by characteristic eosinophilic epithelium.
◈ **Lymphoid stroma** is present under the epithelium in the form of prominent lymphoid tissue, often with germinal centres.

OXYPHIL ADENOMA (ONCOCYTOMA) It is a benign slow-growing tumour of the major salivary glands. The tumour consists of parallel sheets, acini or tubules of large cells with glandular eosinophilic cytoplasm (oncocytes).

OTHER TYPES OF MONOMORPHIC ADENOMAS There are some uncommon forms of monomorphic adenomas:
i) Myoepithelioma
ii) Basal cell adenoma
iii) Clear cell adenoma

MISCELLANEOUS BENIGN TUMOURS

A number of mesenchymal tumours can rarely occur in salivary glands. These include: fibroma, lipoma, neurilemmomas, neurofibroma, haemangioma and lymphangioma.

B. MALIGNANT SALIVARY GLAND TUMOURS

MUCOEPIDERMOID CARCINOMA

Mucoepidermoid carcinoma has following peculiar features:
1. It is the most *common malignant* salivary gland tumour (both in the major and minor glands).
2. The *parotid gland* amongst the major salivary glands and the minor salivary glands in the *palate* are the most common sites.
3. Common age group affected is 30-60 years but it is also the most common malignant salivary gland tumour affecting *children and adolescents*.
4. It is the most common example of *radiation-induced* malignant tumour.

G/A The tumour is usually circumscribed but not encapsulated. It varies in size from 1 to 4 cm.

M/E The tumour is classified into low, intermediate and high grade depending upon the degree of differentiation and tumour invasiveness. The tumour is composed of combination of 4 types of cells: mucin-producing, squamous, intermediate and clear cells.

Malignant mixed tumour comprises three distinct clinicopathologic entities:
1.   Carcinoma arising in benign mixed salivary gland tumour (carcinoma *ex* pleomorphic adenoma)
2.   Carcinosarcoma
3.   Metastasising mixed salivary tumour.
Carcinoma *ex* pleomorphic adenoma is more common (3-5%) while the other two are rare tumours.

G/A   The tumour is poorly-circumscribed with irregular infiltrating margin. Cut section may show haemorrhages, necrosis and cystic degeneration.

M/E   Besides the typical appearance of pleomorphic adenoma, malignant areas show cytologic features of carcinoma such as anaplasia, nuclear hyperchromatism, large nucleolisation, mitoses and evidence of invasive growth.

ADENOID CYSTIC CARCINOMA (CYLINDROMA)

This is a highly malignant tumour due to its typical infiltrative nature, especially along the nerve sheaths.

M/E   Adenoid cystic carcinoma is characterised by cribriform appearance i.e. the epithelial tumour cells of duct-lining and myoepithelial cells are arranged in duct-like structures or masses of cells, having typical fenestrations.

ACINIC CELL CARCINOMA

This is a rare tumour composed of acinic cells resembling serous cells of normal salivary gland. These cells are arranged in sheets or acini and have characteristic basophilic granular cytoplasm.

ADENOCARCINOMA

Adenocarcinoma of the salivary gland does not differ from adenocarcinoma elsewhere in the body.

EPIDERMOID CARCINOMA

This rare tumour has features of squamous cell carcinoma with keratin formation and has intercellular bridges similar to its appearance elsewhere in the body.

UNDIFFERENTIATED CARCINOMA

This highly malignant tumour consists of anaplastic epithelial cells which are too poorly differentiated to be placed in any other known category.

MISCELLANEOUS MALIGNANT TUMOURS

Some rare malignant tumour of epithelial and mesenchymal origin are melanoma, sebaceous carcinoma, undifferentiated carcinoma, lymphoma, fibrosarcoma and leiomyosarcoma. All these tumours are similar in morphology to such tumours elsewhere in the body.

SELF ASSESSMENT

1.   **The following tissues are lined by keratinised stratified squamous epithelium <u>except</u>:**
     A. Hard palate   B. Soft palate
     C. Lips   D. Gingiva
2.   **Fordyce's granules are composed of the following:**
     A. Sebaceous glands   B. Sweat glands
     C. Fibrous tissue   D. Epithelial hyperplasia
3.   **Patients of AIDS have the following type of oral leukoplakia:**
     A. Speckled   B. Nodular
     C. Hairy   D. Wrinkled

4. The most common gross pattern of carcinoma of oral cavity is:
   - A. Papillary
   - B. Nodular
   - C. Ulcerative
   - D. Scirrhous

5. The following type of dental cyst is more often associated with development of ameloblastoma:
   - A. Radicular cyst
   - B. Dentigerous cyst
   - C. Primordial cyst
   - D. Gingival cysts

6. Which of the following conditions is not associated with oral pigmentation?
   - A. Addison's disease
   - B. Lichen planus
   - C. Albright syndrome
   - D. Haemochromatosis

7. The pseudocartilage or matrix in mixed salivary tumour is a product of:
   - A. Connective tissue mucin
   - B. Ductal epithelial cell origin
   - C. Myoepithelial cell origin
   - D. Combination of all mucins

8. Most common malignant salivary gland tumour is:
   - A. Malignant mixed tumour
   - B. Mucoepidermoid carcinoma
   - C. Adenoid cyst carcinoma
   - D. Adenocarcinoma

9. The most common malignant salivary gland tumour in children is:
   - A. Acinic cell tumour
   - B. Adenoid cystic carcinoma
   - C. Mucoepidermoid carcinoma
   - D. Adenocarcinoma

10. Malignant salivary gland tumour that commonly spreads along the nerves is:
    - A. Malignant mixed salivary tumour
    - B. Mucoepidermoid carcinoma
    - C. Acinic cell carcinoma
    - D. Adenoid cystic carcinoma

11. All of the following have strong association with oral squamous cell carcinoma except:
    - A. Tobacco smoking
    - B. Chronic alcoholism
    - C. Submucosal fibrosis
    - D. HPV 16 and 18

12. Secondary dentin is:
    - A. Reaction of the tooth to carious process
    - B. Mature form of dentin
    - C. Dentin formed with ageing
    - D. Mineralised primary dentin

13. Most common cyst arising from dental tissues is:
    - A. Radicular cyst
    - B. Dentigerous cyst
    - C. Eruption cyst
    - D. Gingival cyst

14. All the following are patterns of ameloblastoma except:
    - A. Follicular
    - B. Plexiform
    - C. Granular
    - D. Spindle

15. Which one of the following autosomal dominant disorders is characterised by the formation of multiple gastrointestinal polyps along with pigmented lesions around the oval cavity?
    - A. Cowden disease
    - B. Gardner syndrome
    - C. Peutz-Jeghers syndrome
    - D. Rotor syndrome

KEY

1 = B	2 = A	3 = C	4 = C	5 = B
6 = B	7 = C	8 = B	9 = C	10 = D
11 = C	12 = A	13 = A	14 = D	15 = C

18   The Gastrointestinal Tract

OESOPHAGUS *(p. 521)*

NORMAL STRUCTURE

The oesophagus is a muscular tube extending from the pharynx to the stomach. In an adult, this distance measures 25 cm. However, from the clinical point of view, the distance from the incisor teeth to the gastro-oesophageal (GE) junction is about 40 cm.

Histologically, the wall of the oesophagus consists of mucosa, submucosa, muscularis propria and adventitia/serosa.

◈   The **mucosa** is composed of non-keratinising stratified squamous epithelium overlying lamina propria except at the lower end for a distance of 0.5 to 1.5 cm. At the lower end of the oesophagus, there is sudden change from stratified squamous epithelium to mucin-secreting columnar epithelium; this is called the *junctional mucosa.*

◈   The **submucosa** consists of loose connective tissue with sprinkling of lymphocytes, plasma cells, and occasional eosinophil and mast cell.

◈   The **muscularis propria** is composed of 2 layers of smooth muscle—an inner circular coat and an outer longitudinal coat.

◈   The **adventitia/serosa** is the outer covering of oesophagus. Serosa is present in intra-abdominal part of oesophagus only.

CONGENITAL ANOMALIES *(p. 521)*

OESOPHAGEAL ATRESIA AND TRACHEO-OESOPHAGEAL FISTULA
In about 85% of cases, congenital atresia of the oesophagus is associated with tracheo-oesophageal fistula, usually at the level of tracheal bifurcation.

Morphologically, the condition is recognised by cord-like non-canalised segment of oesophagus having blind pouch at both ends.

MUSCULAR DYSFUNCTIONS *(p. 521)*

ACHALASIA (CARDIOSPASM)

Achalasia of the oesophagus is a neuromuscular dysfunction due to which the cardiac sphincter fails to relax during swallowing and results in progressive dysphagia and dilatation of the oesophagus *(mega-oesophagus).*

ETIOLOGY There is loss of intramural neurons in the wall of the oesophagus. Most cases are of primary idiopathic achalasia i.e. congenital. Secondary achalasia may occur from some other causes which includes: Chagas' disease (an epidemic parasitosis with *Trypanosoma cruzi*).

MORPHOLOGIC FEATURES There is dilatation above the short contracted terminal segment of the oesophagus. Muscularis propria of the wall may be of normal thickness, hypertrophied as a result of obstruction, or thinned out due to dilatation.

HIATUS HERNIA

Hiatus hernia is the herniation or protrusion of part of the stomach through the oesophageal hiatus of the diaphragm. Oesophageal hiatal hernia is the cause of diaphragmatic hernia in 98% of cases. In symptomatic cases, especially the elderly women, the clinical features are heartburn (retrosternal burning sensation) and regurgitation of gastric juice into the mouth, both of which are worsened due to heavy work, lifting weights and excessive bending.

ETIOLOGY   It may be congenital or acquired.

◈   **Congenitally short oesophagus** may be the cause of hiatus hernia in a small proportion of cases.

◈   More commonly, it is **acquired** due to secondary factors e.g.

a)   Degeneration of muscle due to ageing.

b)   Increased intra-abdominal pressure such as in pregnancy, abdominal tumours etc.

c)   Recurrent oesophageal regurgitation and spasm causing inflammation and fibrosis.

d)   Increase in fatty tissue in obese people causing decreased muscular elasticity of diaphragm.

MORPHOLOGIC FEATURES   There are 3 patterns in hiatus hernia:

i)   **Sliding or oesophago-gastric hernia** is the most common, occurring in 85% of cases.

ii)   **Rolling or para-oesophageal hernia** is seen in 10% of cases. This is a true hernia in which cardiac end of the stomach rolls up para-oesophageally.

iii)   **Mixed or transitional hernia** constitutes the remaining 5% cases in which there is combination of sliding and rolling hiatus hernia.

OESOPHAGEAL DIVERTICULA

Diverticula are the outpouchings of oesophageal wall at the point of weakness. They may be congenital or acquired.

◈   **Congenital diverticula** occur either at the upper end of the oesophagus or at the bifurcation of trachea.

◈   **Acquired diverticula** may be of 2 types:

a)   *Pulsion (Zenker's) type*—It is seen in the region of hypopharynx and occurs due to oesophageal obstruction such as due to chronic oesophagitis, carcinoma etc.

b)   *Traction type*—It occurs in the lower third of oesophagus from contraction of fibrous tissue.

OESOPHAGEAL WEBS AND RINGS

Radiological shadows in the oesophagus resembling 'webs' and 'rings' are observed in some patients complaining of dysphagia.

WEBS   These are located in the upper oesophagus, seen more commonly in adult women, and associated with dysphagia, iron deficiency anaemia and chronic atrophic glossitis (Plummer-Vinson syndrome).

RINGS   Those located in the lower oesophagus, not associated with iron-deficiency anaemia, nor occurring in women alone, are referred to as 'Schatzki's rings'.

MORPHOLOGIC FEATURES   The rings and webs are transverse folds of mucosa and submucosa encircling the entire circumference, or are localised annular thickenings of the muscle.

HAEMATEMESIS OF OESOPHAGEAL ORIGIN *(p. 522)*

Massive haematemesis (vomiting of blood) may occur due to vascular lesions in the oesophagus e.g.

1.   Oesophageal varices
2.   Mallory-weiss syndrome
3.   Rupture of the oesophagus
4.   Other causes
i)   Bursting of aortic aneurysm into the lumen of oesophagus
ii)   Vascular erosion by malignant growth in the vicinity
iii)   Hiatus hernia
iv)   Oesophageal cancer
v)   Purpuras
vi)   Haemophilia.

REFLUX (PEPTIC) OESOPHAGITIS

Reflux of the gastric juice is the commonest cause of oesophagitis.

PATHOGENESIS Gastro-oesophageal reflux, to an extent, may occur in normal healthy individuals after meals and in early pregnancy. In some clinical conditions, the gastro-oesophageal reflux is excessive e.g.

i) Sliding hiatus hernia
ii) Chronic gastric and duodenal ulcers
iii) Nasogastric intubation
iv) Persistent vomiting
v) Surgical vagotomy
vi) Neuropathy in alcoholics, diabetics
vii) Oesophagogastrostomy.

Endoscopically, the demarcation between normal squamous and columnar epithelium at the junctional mucosa is lost.

M/E The reflux changes in the distal oesophagus include basal cell hyperplasia and deep elongation of the papillae touching close to the surface epithelium. Inflammatory changes vary according to the stage of the disease. *In early stage,* mucosa and submucosa are infiltrated by some polymorphs and eosinophils; *in chronic stage,* there is lymphocytic infiltration and fibrosis of all the layers of the oesophageal wall.

BARRETT'S OESOPHAGUS

This is a condition in which, following reflux oesophagitis, stratified squamous epithelium of the lower oesophagus is replaced by columnar epithelium (columnar metaplasia). Barrett's oesophagus is a premalignant condition evolving sequentially-from Barrett's epithelium (columnar metaplasia with goblet cells) to dysplasia to carcinoma *in situ* and finally to oesophageal adenocarcinoma.

Endoscopically, the affected area is red and velvety. Hiatus hernia and peptic ulcer at squamocolumnar junction (Barrett's ulcer) are frequently associated.

M/E The changes are as under:

1. The most common finding is the replacement of squamous epithelium by metaplastic columnar cells, along with goblet cells and Paneth cells (intestinal metaplasia).
2. Intestinal metaplasia may be accompanied by dysplastic changes of the columnar epithelium or glands ranging from low to high grade.
3. There may be changes of peptic ulcer due to presence of fundic gastric glands, or cardiac mucous glands.

High-grade dysplasia may progress to invasive adenocarcinoma of the oesophagus in up to 20% cases: the reported risk of development of adenocarcinoma in Barrett's oesophagus is at the rate of 0.5% per year after diagnosis.

OTHER CAUSES OF OESOPHAGITIS

INFECTIVE CAUSES

i) Candida (Monilial) oesophagitis
ii) Herpes simplex (Herpetic) oesophagitis
iii) Cytomegalovirus
iv) Tuberculosis.

NON-INFECTIVE CAUSES

i) Eosinophilic oesophagitis caused by radiation, corrosives
ii) Intake of certain drugs (anticholinergic drugs, doxycycline, tetracycline)
iii) Ingestion of hot, irritating fluids
iv) Crohn's disease
v) Various vesiculobullous skin diseases.

CARCINOMA OF OESOPHAGUS

Carcinoma of the oesophagus is diagnosed late, after symptomatic oesophageal obstruction (dysphagia) has developed and the tumour has transgressed the anatomical limits of the organ. The tumour occurs more commonly in men over 50 years of age.

ETIOLOGY   Following conditions and factors are implicated.

1.   Diet and personal habits:

i)   Heavy smoking
ii)   Alcohol consumption
iii)   Intake of foods contaminated with fungus
iv)   Nutritional deficiency of vitamins and trace elements.

2.   Oesophageal disorders:

i)   Oesophagitis (especially Barrett's oesophagus in adenocarcinoma)
ii)   Achalasia
iii)   Hiatus hernia
iv)   Diverticula
v)   Plummer-Vinson syndrome.

3.   Other factors:

i)   *Race*—more common in the Chinese and Japanese than in Western races; more frequent in blacks than whites.
ii)   *Family history*—association with tylosis (keratosis palmaris et plantaris).
iii)   *Genetic factors*—predisposition with coeliac disease, epidermolysis bullosa, tylosis.
iv)   *HPV infection*—is a recent addition in etiologic factors.

MORPHOLOGIC FEATURES   Carcinoma of the oesophagus is mainly of 2 types—squamous cell (epidermoid) and adenocarcinoma.

SQUAMOUS CELL (EPIDERMOID) CARCINOMA   Squamous cell or epidermoid carcinoma comprises 90% of primary oesophageal cancers. The disease occurs in 6th to 7th decades of life. Half of the squamous cell carcinomas of oesophagus occur in the middle third, followed by lower third, and the upper third of oesophagus in that order of frequency.

G/A   3 types of patterns are recognised:
i)   *Polypoid fungating type*—is the most common form. It appears as a cauliflower-like friable mass protruding into the lumen.
ii)   *Ulcerating type*—is the next common form. It looks grossly like a necrotic ulcer with everted edges.
iii)   *Diffuse infiltrating type*—appears as an annular, stenosing narrowing of the lumen due to infiltration into the wall of oesophagus.

M/E   Majority of the squamous cell carcinomas of the oesophagus are well-differentiated or moderately-differentiated. An exophytic, slow-growing, extremely well-differentiated variant, *verrucous squamous cell carcinoma,* has also been reported in the oesophagus.

ADENOCARCINOMA   Adenocarcinoma of the oesophagus constitutes less than 10% of primary oesophageal cancer. It occurs predominantly in men in their 4th to 5th decades. The common locations are lower and middle third of the oesophagus. These tumours have a strong and definite association with Barrett's oesophagus in which there are foci of gastric or intestinal type of epithelium.

G/A   Oesophageal adenocarcinoma appears as nodular, elevated mass in the lower oesophagus.

M/E   Adenocarcinoma of the oesophagus can have 3 patterns:
i)   *Intestinal type*—is the adenocarcinoma with a pattern similar to that seen in adenocarcinoma of intestine or stomach.
ii)   *Adenosquamous type*—is the pattern in which there is an irregular admixture of adenocarcinoma and squamous cell carcinoma.

iii) *Adenoid cystic type*—is an uncommon variety and is akin to similar growth in salivary gland.

OTHER CARCINOMAS Besides the two main histological types of oesophageal cancer, a few other varieties are occasionally encountered e.g.
i) Mucoepidermoid carcinoma
ii) Malignant melanoma
iii) Small cell carcinoma
iv) Undifferentiated carcinoma
v) Carcinosarcoma
vi) Secondary tumours

SPREAD The oesophageal cancer spreads by following routes:
i) Local spread
ii) Lymphatic spread
iii) Haematogenous spread

STOMACH (p. 526)

NORMAL STRUCTURE

The stomach is 'gland with cavity', extending from its junction with lower end of the oesophagus (cardia) to its junction with the duodenum (pylorus). The *lesser curvature* is inner concavity on the right, while the *greater curvature* is the outer convexity on the left side of the stomach.

The stomach has 5 anatomical regions:

1. **Cardia** is the oesophagogastric junction and lacks the sphincter.

2. **Fundus** is the portion above the horizontal line drawn across the oesophagogastric junction.

3. **Body** is the middle portion of the stomach between the fundus and the pyloric antrum.

4. **Pyloric antrum** is the distal third of the stomach.

5. **Pylorus** is the junction of distal end of the stomach with the duodenum. It has powerful sphincter muscle.

Gastric canal is the relatively fixed portion of the pyloric antrum and the adjoining lesser curvature; it is the site for numerous pathological changes such as gastritis, peptic ulcer and gastric carcinoma.

M/E The wall of the stomach consists of 4 layers:

1. **Serosa** is derived from the peritoneum which is deficient in the region of lesser and greater curvatures.

2. **Muscularis** consists of 3 layers of smooth muscle fibres—the outer longitudinal, the middle circular and the inner oblique.

3. **Submucosa** is a layer of loose fibroconnective tissue binding the mucosa to the muscularis loosely and contains branches of blood vessels, lymphatics and nerve plexuses and ganglion cells.

4. **Mucosa** consists of 2 layers—superficial and deep. Between the two layers is the lamina propria.

i) Superficial layer: It consists of a single layer of surface epithelium composed of regular, mucin-secreting, tall columnar cells with basal nuclei.
a) *Cardiac mucosa* is the transition zone between the oesophageal squamous mucosa and the oxyntic mucosa of the fundus and body with which it gradually merges.
b) *Oxyntic mucosa* lines both gastric fundus and body.
c) *Antral mucosa* lines the pyloric antrum.

ii) Deep layer: It consists of glands that open into the bottom of the crypts. Depending upon the structure, these glands are of 3 types:
a) *Glands of the cardia* are simple tubular or compound tubulo-racemose
b) *Glands of the body-fundus* are long, tubular and tightly packed. There are 4 types of cells present in the glands of body-fundic mucosa:
◈ Parietal (Oxyntic) cells
◈ Chief (Peptic) cells

◈ Mucin-secreting neck cells
◈ Endocrine (Kulchitsky or Enterochromaffin) cells
c) *Glands of the pylorus* are much longer than the body-fundic glands.

The secretory products of the gastric mucosa are the *gastric juice* and the *intrinsic factor*, required for absorption of vitamin B_{12}.

The *control of gastric secretions* chiefly occurs in one of the following 3 ways:
1. Cephalic phase
2. Gastric phase
i) *Mechanical stimulation*
ii) *Chemical stimulation*
3. Intestinal phase

GASTRIC ANALYSIS *(p. 527)*

A. TESTS FOR GASTRIC SECRETIONS

1. TESTS FOR GASTRIC ACID SECRETIONS

These tests are based on the principle of measuring basal acid output (BAO) and maximal acid output (MAO) produced by the stomach under the influence of a variety of stimulants, and then comparing the readings of BAO and MAO with the normal values.

The tests for gastric acid secretion are named after the stimulants used for MAO. Some of the commonly used substances are as under:
i) Histamine
ii) Histalog (Betazole)
iii) Pentagastrin (Peptavlon)
iv) Insulin Meal (Hollander Test)
v) Tubeless Analysis

SIGNIFICANCE

Higher values are found in:
   i) duodenal ulcer;
   ii) Zollinger-Ellison syndrome (gastrinoma); and
   iii) anastomotic ulcer.

Low value or achlorhydria are observed in:
   i) pernicious anaemia (atrophic gastritis); and
   ii) achlorhydria in the presence of gastric ulcer is highly suggestive of gastric malignancy.

2. TESTS FOR PEPSIN

Pepsin inhibitors are used for analysis of pepsin derived from pepsinogen for research purposes. The levels of pepsin are low in atrophic gastritis.

3. TESTS FOR MUCUS

Protein content of gastric mucus is measured, normal value being 1.8 mg/ml. The level is increased in chronic hypertrophic gastritis (Ménétrier's disease).

4. TEST FOR INTRINSIC FACTOR

Intrinsic factor (IF) is essential for vitamin B_{12} absorption from the small intestine. In its absence, the absorption of vitamin B_{12} is impaired as occurs in chronic atrophic gastritis and gastric atrophy. *Schilling test* is used for evaluation of patients with suspected pernicious anaemia but can also be used as a diagnostic test for pancreatic insufficiency.

B. TESTS FOR GASTRIN

Circulating gastrin secreted by G-cells present in the antropyloric and proximal duodenal mucosa is normally 0-200 pg/ml. It can be tested by the following methods:

Section III

Systemic Pathology

1. **SERUM GASTRIN LEVELS**

Radioimmunoassay (RIA) is the commonly used method of measurement of serum gastrin levels. The levels are high in:
   i) atrophic gastritis (with low gastric acid secretion);
   ii) Zollinger-Ellison syndrome or gastrinoma (with high gastric acid secretion); and
   iii) following surgery on the stomach.

2. **GASTRIN PROVOCATION TESTS**

These tests are used to differentiate between hypergastrinaemia and gastric acid hypersecretion as follows:
i) Secretin test
ii) Calcium infusion test

CONGENITAL AND MISCELLANEOUS ACQUIRED CONDITIONS (p. 529)

PANCREATIC HETEROTOPIA

Heterotopic pancreatic tissue may present clinically as a gastric mass or may be an incidental finding. Symptomatic cases may present in newborn or later in life.

PYLORIC STENOSIS

Hypertrophy and narrowing of the pyloric lumen occurs predominantly in male children as a congenital defect (infantile pyloric stenosis). The adult form is rarely seen, either as a result of late manifestation of mild congenital anomaly or may be acquired type due to inflammatory fibrosis or invasion by tumours.

G/A & M/E There is hypertrophy as well as hyperplasia of the circular layer of muscularis in the pyloric sphincter accompanied by mild degree of fibrosis.

CLINICAL FEATURES Following clinical features may be present.
1. Vomiting, which may be projectile and occasionally contains bile or blood.
2. Visible peristalsis, usually noticed from left to right side of the upper abdomen.
3. Palpable lump, better felt after an episode of vomiting.
4. Constipation.
5. Loss of weight.

OTHER ACQUIRED CONDITIONS

BEZOARS Bezoars are foreign bodies in the stomach, usually in patients with mental illness who chew these substances.
i) Trichobezoars composed of a ball of hair.
ii) Phytobezoars composed of vegetable fibres, seeds or fruit skin.
iii) Trichophytobezoars combining both hair and vegetable matter.

ACUTE DILATATION Sudden and enormous dilatation of the stomach by gas or fluids due to paralysis of the gastric musculature may occur after abdominal operations, generalised peritonitis, and, in pyloric stenosis.

GASTRIC RUPTURE The stomach may rupture rarely and prove fatal e.g. due to blunt trauma, external cardiac massage, ingestion of heavy meal or large quantity of liquid intake like beer.

INFLAMMATORY CONDITIONS (p. 529)

The two important inflammatory conditions of the stomach are gastritis and peptic ulcer.

GASTRITIS

The term 'gastritis' is commonly employed for any clinical condition with upper abdominal discomfort like indigestion or dyspepsia in which the specific clinical signs and radiological abnormalities are absent.

ACUTE GASTRITIS

Acute gastritis is a transient acute inflammatory involvement of the stomach, mainly mucosa.

ETIOPATHOGENESIS

1. **Diet and personal habits:**
    i)   Highly spiced food
    ii) Excessive alcohol consumption
    iii) Malnutrition
    iv) Heavy smoking.

2. **Infections:**
    i)   *Bacterial infections* e.g. *Helicobacter pylori*, diphtheria, salmonellosis, pneumonia, staphylococcal food poisoning.
    ii) *Viral infections* e.g. viral hepatitis, influenza, infectious mononucleosis.

3. **Drugs:** Intake of drugs like non-steroidal anti-inflammatory drugs (NSAIDs), aspirin, cortisone, phenylbutazone, indomethacin, preparations of iron, chemotherapeutic agents.

4. **Chemical and physical agents:**
    i)   Intake of corrosive chemicals such as caustic soda, phenol, lysol
    ii) Gastric irradiation
    iii) Freezing.

5. **Severe stress:**
    i)   Emotional factors like shock, anger, resentment etc.
    ii) Extensive burns
    iii) Trauma
    iv) Surgery.

In acute gastritis, the mucosal injury by any of the above agents causes acute inflammation by one of the following mechanisms:
1. Reduced blood flow
2. Increased acid secretion
3. Decreased production of bicarbonate buffer.

G/A The gastric mucosa is oedematous with abundant mucus and haemorrhagic spots.

M/E Depending upon the stage, there is variable amount of oedema and infiltration by neutrophils in the lamina propria. In acute haemorrhagic and erosive gastritis, the mucosa is sloughed off and there are haemorrhages on the surface.

CHRONIC GASTRITIS

Chronic gastritis is the commonest histological change observed in biopsies from the stomach. The condition occurs more frequently with advancing age; average age for symptomatic chronic gastritis being 45 years which corresponds well with the age incidence of gastric ulcer.

ETIOPATHOGENESIS In the absence of clear etiology of chronic gastritis, a number of etiologic factors have been implicated. All the causative factors of acute gastritis described above may result in chronic gastritis too. Recurrent attacks of acute gastritis may result in chronic gastritis. Some additional causes are as under:
1. *Reflux of duodenal contents into the stomach*
2. *Infection with H. pylori*
3. *Associated disease of the stomach and duodenum*
4. *Chronic hypochromic anaemia*
5. *Immunological factors* such as autoantibodies to gastric parietal cells in atrophic gastritis and autoantibodies against intrinsic factor.

The *mechanism* of chronic gastric injury by any of the etiologic agents is by cytotoxic effect of the injurious agent on the gastric mucosal epithelium, thus breaking the barrier and then inciting the inflammatory response.

CLASSIFICATION Based on the type of mucosa affected (i.e. cardiac, body, pyloric, antral or transitional), a clinicopathologic classification has been proposed.

1. Type A gastritis (Autoimmune gastritis) Type A gastritis involves mainly the body-fundic mucosa. It is also called autoimmune gastritis due to the presence of circulating antibodies and is sometimes associated with other autoimmune diseases such as Hashimoto's thyroiditis and Addison's disease.

2. Type B gastritis (*H. pylori*-related) Type B gastritis mainly involves the region of antral mucosa and is more common. It is also called hypersecretory gastritis due to excessive secretion of acid, commonly due to infection with *H. pylori*.

3. Type AB gastritis (Mixed gastritis, Environmental gastritis, Chronic atrophic gastritis) Type AB gastritis affects the mucosal region of A as well as B types (body-fundic and antral mucosa). This is the most common type of gastritis in all age groups. It is also called environmental gastritis.

G/A The features of all forms of gastritis are inconclusive. The gastric mucosa may be normal, atrophied, or oedematous.

M/E The changes are:
i) Extent of inflammatory changes in the mucosa (i.e. superficial or deep).
ii) Activity of inflammation (i.e. quiescent or active; acute or chronic).
iii) Presence of and type of metaplasia (i.e. intestinal or pseudopyloric).
   Based on above, following simple morphologic classification has been proposed:
1. Chronic superficial gastritis
2. Chronic atrophic gastritis
3. Gastric atrophy
4. Chronic hypertrophic gastritis (Ménétrier's disease)
5. Uncommon forms of chronic gastritis.
   However, *Sydney system* of recording of histologic changes in gastritis is more acceptable since it takes into account following multiple parameters as well:
i) *Etiology* (*H. pylori*, autoimmune, NSAIDs, infections).
ii) *Location* (pangastritis, predominant antral, predominant body-fundic).
iii) *Morphology* (depth of inflammation—superficial or deep, severity of inflammation, type of inflammation, atrophy, metaplasia).
iv) *Some special features* (e.g. granulomas, eosinophilic gastritis, erosions, necrosis, haemorrhages).

1. CHRONIC SUPERFICIAL GASTRITIS As the name suggests there is an inflammatory infiltrate consisting of plasma cells and lymphocytes in the superficial layer of the gastric mucosa, *but there are no histological changes in the deep layer of mucosa containing gastric glands.*

Its most common etiologic agent is *H. pylori*, a spiral-shaped bacteria. It is now known that *H. pylori* is causative for almost all active cases of chronic superficial gastritis and about 65% of quiescent cases. The organism is identified on the epithelial layer on the luminal surface and does not invade the mucosa. It is not seen on areas with intestinal metaplasia.

H. pylori infection is now considered an independent risk factor for gastric cancer: 3-6 fold increased risk for gastric adenocarcinoma and 6-50 times risk of MALT lymphoma.

2. CHRONIC ATROPHIC GASTRITIS In this stage, *there is inflammatory cell infiltrate in the deeper layer of the mucosa and atrophy of the epithelial elements including destruction of the glands.* Two types of metaplasia are commonly associated with atrophic gastritis:

i) Intestinal metaplasia Intestinal metaplasia is more common and involves antral mucosa more frequently. However, areas of intestinal metaplasia are not colonised by *H. pylori*.

ii) Pseudopyloric metaplasia It involves the body glands which are replaced by proliferated mucus neck cells, conforming in appearance to normal pyloric glands.

3. GASTRIC ATROPHY In this, there is thinning of the gastric mucosa with loss of glands but no inflammation.

4. CHRONIC HYPERTROPHIC GASTRITIS (MÉNÉTRIER'S DISEASE) This is an uncommon condition characterised pathologically by enormous thickening of gastric rugal folds resembling cerebral convolutions, affecting mainly the region of fundic-body mucosa.

5. MISCELLANEOUS FORMS OF CHRONIC GASTRITIS A few other types are as under:

i) Eosinophilic gastritis This condition is characterised by diffuse thickening of the pyloric antrum due to oedema and extensive infiltration by eosinophils in all the layers of the wall of antrum.

ii) Chronic follicular gastritis This is a variant of chronic atrophic gastritis in which numerous lymphoid follicles are present in the mucosa and submucosa of the stomach.

iii) Haemorrhagic (Erosive) gastritis In this condition, there are superficial erosions and mucosal haemorrhages, usually following severe haematemesis.

iv) Granulomatous gastritis Rarely, granulomas may be present in the gastric mucosa such as in tuberculosis, sarcoidosis, Crohn's disease, syphilis, various mycoses, and as a reaction to endogenous substance or foreign material.

PEPTIC ULCERS

Peptic ulcers are the areas of degeneration and necrosis of gastrointestinal mucosa exposed to acid-peptic secretions. Though they can occur at any level of the alimentary tract that is exposed to hydrochloric acid and pepsin, they occur most commonly (98-99%) in either the duodenum or the stomach in the ratio of 4:1. Each of the two main types may be acute or chronic.

ACUTE PEPTIC (STRESS) ULCERS

Acute peptic ulcers or stress ulcers are multiple, small mucosal erosions, seen most commonly in the stomach but occasionally involving the duodenum.

ETIOLOGY Following factors are implicated:
1. *Psychological stress*
2. *Physiological stress* as in the following:
   i) Shock
   ii) Severe trauma
   iii) Septicaemia
   iv) Extensive burns (Curling's ulcers in the posterior aspect of the first part of the duodenum).
   v) Intracranial lesions (Cushing's ulcers developing from hyperacidity following excessive vagal stimulation).
   vi) Drug intake (e.g. aspirin, steroids, butazolidine, indomethacin).
   vii) Local irritants (e.g. alcohol, smoking, coffee etc).

PATHOGENESIS It is not clear how the mucosal erosions occur in stress ulcers because actual hypersecretion of gastric acid is demonstrable in only Cushing's ulcers occurring from intracranial conditions such as due to brain trauma, intracranial surgery and brain tumours.

G/A Acute stress ulcers are multiple (more than three ulcers in 75% of cases). They are more common anywhere in the stomach, followed in decreasing frequency by occurrence in the first part of duodenum. They may be oval or circular in shape, usually less than 1 cm in diameter.

M/E The stress ulcers are shallow and do not invade the muscular layer. The margins and base may show some inflammatory reaction depending upon the duration of the ulcers.

CHRONIC PEPTIC ULCERS (GASTRIC AND DUODENAL ULCERS)

If not specified, chronic peptic ulcers would mean gastric and duodenal ulcers, the two major forms of 'peptic ulcer disease' of the upper GI tract in which the acid-pepsin secretions are implicated in their pathogenesis.

INCIDENCE Peptic ulcers are more frequent in middle-aged adults. The peak incidence for duodenal ulcer is 5th decade, while for gastric ulcer it is a decade later (6th decade). Duodenal as well as gastric ulcers are more common in males than in females. Duodenal ulcer is almost four times more common than gastric ulcer.

ETIOLOGY The immediate cause of peptic ulcer disease is disturbance in normal protective mucosal 'barrier' by acid-pepsin, resulting in digestion of the mucosa. However, in contrast to duodenal ulcers, *the patients of gastric ulcer have low-to-normal gastric acid secretions, though true achlorhydria in response to stimulants never occurs in benign gastric ulcer.*

1. *Helicobacter pylori* **gastritis** About 15-20% cases infected with *H. pylori* in the antrum develop duodenal ulcer in their life time while gastric colonisation by *H. pylori* never develops ulceration and remain asymptomatic.

2. **NSAIDs-induced mucosal injury** Non-steroidal anti-inflammatory drugs are most commonly used medications in the developed countries and are responsible for direct toxicity, endothelial damage and epithelial injury to both gastric as well as duodenal mucosa.

3. **Acid-pepsin secretions** There is conclusive evidence that some level of acid-pepsin secretion is essential for the development of duodenal as well as gastric ulcer.

4. **Gastritis** Some degree of gastritis is always present in the region of gastric ulcer, though it is not clear whether it is the cause or the effect of ulcer.

5. **Other local irritants** Pyloric antrum and lesser curva-ture of the stomach are the sites most exposed for longer periods to local irritants and thus are the common sites for occurrence of gastric ulcers.

6. **Dietary factors** Nutritional deficiencies have been regarded as etiologic factors in peptic ulcers.

7. **Psychological factors** Psychological stress, anxiety, fatigue and ulcer-type personality may exacerbate as well as predispose to peptic ulcer disease.

8. **Genetic factors** People with blood group O appear to be more prone to develop peptic ulcers than those with other blood groups.

9. **Hormonal factors** Secretion of certain hormones by tumours is associated with peptic ulceration e.g. elaboration of gastrin by islet-cell tumour in Zollinger-Ellison syndrome, endocrine secretions in hyperplasia.

10. **Miscellaneous** Duodenal ulcers have been observed to occur in association with various other conditions such as alcoholic cirrhosis, chronic renal failure, hyperparathyroidism, chronic obstructive pulmonary disease, and chronic pancreatitis.

PATHOGENESIS There are distinct differences in the pathogenetic mechanisms involved in duodenal and gastric ulcers as under:

Duodenal ulcer There is conclusive evidence to support the role of high acid-pepsin secretions in the causation of duodenal ulcers:

1. There is generally *hypersecretion of gastric acid* into the fasting stomach at night which takes place under the influence of vagal stimulation.

2. Patients of duodenal ulcer have *rapid emptying* of the stomach so that the food which normally buffers and neutralises the gastric acid, passes down into the small intestine.

3. *Helicobacter* gastritis caused by *H. pylori* is seen in 95-100% cases of duodenal ulcers. The underlying mechanisms are as under:

Gastric ulcer The pathogenesis of gastric ulcer is mainly explained on the basis of impaired gastric mucosal defenses against acid-pepsin secretions.

1. Hyperacidity may occur in gastric ulcer due to *increased serum gastrin* levels in response to ingested food in an atonic stomach.

2. However, many patients of gastric ulcer have low-to-normal gastric acid levels. Ulcerogenesis in such patients is explained on the basis of damaging influence of *other factors* such as gastritis, bile reflux, cigarette smoke etc.

3. The normally protective *gastric mucus 'barrier'* against acid-pepsin is deranged in gastric ulcer. There is depletion in the quantity as well as quality of gastric mucus. One of the mechanisms for its depletion is colonisation of the gastric mucosa by *H. pylori* seen in 75-80% patients of gastric ulcer.

MORPHOLOGIC FEATURES *Gastric ulcers* are found predominantly along the lesser curvature in the region of pyloric antrum, more commonly on the posterior than the anterior wall. Most *duodenal ulcers* are found in the first part of the duodenum, usually immediate post-pyloric, more commonly on the anterior than the posterior wall.

G/A Typical peptic ulcers are commonly solitary (80%), small (1-2.5 cm in diameter), round to oval and characteristically 'punched out'. Benign ulcers usually have flat margins in level with the surrounding mucosa. *Chronic duodenal ulcer never turns malignant*, while chronic gastric ulcer may develop carcinoma in less than 1% of cases. Malignant gastric ulcers are larger, bowl-shaped with elevated and indurated mucosa at the margin.

M/E Chronic peptic ulcers have 4 histological zones.

1. *Necrotic zone*—lies in the floor of the ulcer and is composed of fibrinous exudate containing necrotic debris and a few leucocytes.
2. *Superficial exudative zone*—lies underneath the necrotic zone. The tissue elements here show coagulative necrosis giving eosinophilic, smudgy appearance with nuclear debris.
3. *Granulation tissue zone*—is seen merging into the necrotic zone. It is composed of nonspecific inflammatory infiltrate and proliferating capillaries.
4. *Zone of cicatrisation*—is seen merging into thick layer of granulation tissue.

COMPLICATIONS Acute and subacute peptic ulcers usually heal without leaving any visible scar. However, healing of chronic, larger and deeper ulcers may result in complications.

1. Obstruction
2. Haemorrhage
3. Perforation
4. Malignant transformation

CLINICAL FEATURES Peptic ulcers are remitting and relapsing lesions. Their chronic and recurrent behaviour is summed up the saying: *'once a peptic ulcer patient, always a peptic ulcer patient.'*

1. Age The peak incidence of duodenal ulcer is in 5th decade while that for gastric ulcer is a decade later.

2. People at risk Duodenal ulcer occurs more commonly in people faced with more stress and strain of life (e.g. executives, leaders), while gastric ulcer is seen more often in labouring groups.

3. Periodicity The attacks in gastric ulcers last from 2-6 weeks, with interval of freedom from 1-6 months. The attacks of duodenal ulcer, are classically worsened by *'work, worry and weather.'*

4. Pain In gastric ulcer, epigastric pain occurs immediately or within 2 hours after food and never occurs at night. In duodenal ulcer, pain is severe, occurs late at night ('hunger pain') and is usually relieved by food.

5. Vomiting Vomiting which relieves the pain is a conspicuous feature in patients of gastric ulcer. Duodenal ulcer patients rarely have vomiting but instead get heart-burn (retrosternal pain).

6. Haematemesis and melaena Haematemesis and melaena occur in gastric ulcers in the ratio of 60:40, while in duodenal ulcers in the ratio of 40:60.

7. Appetite The gastric ulcer patients, though have good appetite but are afraid to eat, while duodenal ulcer patients have very good appetite.

8. Diet Patients of gastric ulcer commonly get used to a bland diet consisting of milk, eggs etc and avoid taking fried foods, curries and heavily spiced foods. In contrast, duodenal ulcer patients usually take all kinds of diets.

9. Weight Loss of weight is a common finding in gastric ulcer patients while patients of duodenal ulcer tend to gain weight due to frequent ingestion of milk to avoid pain.

10. Deep tenderness Deep tenderness is demonstrable in both types of peptic ulcers. In the case of gastric ulcer it is in the midline of the epigastrium, while in the duodenal ulcer it is in the right hypochondrium.

HAEMATEMESIS AND MELAENA OF GASTRIC ORIGIN *(p. 537)*

- i) Chronic peptic ulcers (gastric as well as duodenal)
- ii) Acute peptic ulcers (stress ulcers)
- iii) Multiple gastric and duodenal erosions
- iv) Carcinoma of the stomach
- v) Peptic ulcer in Meckel's diverticulum
- vi) Mallory-Weiss syndrome
- vii) Anaemias
- viii) Purpuras
- ix) Haemophilia.

TUMOURS AND TUMOUR-LIKE LESIONS *(p. 537)*

A.   TUMOUR-LIKE LESIONS (POLYPS)

HYPERPLASTIC (INFLAMMATORY) POLYPS

Hyperplastic or inflammatory polyps are regenerative, non-neoplastic lesions which are the most common type (90%). They may be single or multiple and are more often located in the pyloric antrum.

G/A The lesions may be sessile or pedunculated, 1 cm or larger in size, smooth and soft.

M/E They are composed of irregular hyperplastic glands, which may show cystic change. The lining epithelium is mostly superficial gastric type but antral glands, chief cells and parietal cells may be present.

HAMARTOMATOUS POLYPS

Hamartomatous polyps are not true neoplasms but are malformations. They are of various types such as gastric polyps of the Peutz-Jeghers syndrome, juvenile polyp, pancreatic heterotopia, heterotopia of Brunner's glands and inflammatory fibroid polyps (eosinophilic granulomatous polyps).

B.   BENIGN TUMOURS

ADENOMAS (ADENOMATOUS OR NEOPLASTIC POLYPS)

Adenomas, also, referred to as adenomatous or neoplastic polyps, are true benign epithelial neoplasms and are much rare in the stomach than in the large intestine. They are also found more often in the region of pyloric antrum. They are commonly associated with atrophic gastritis and pernicious anaemia.

STROMAL TUMOURS

Stomach may be the site for occurrence of various uncommon benign tumours of stromal cell origin e.g. leiomyomas (being the most common); others are neurofibromas, schwannomas and lipomas.

The term *gastrointestinal stromal tumours (GISTs)* is used for a group of uncommon benign tumours composed of spindle cells or stromal cells but lacking the true phenotypic features of smooth muscle cells, neural cells or Schwann cells. They are uncommon but as compared to other sites in the GIT, are most common in the stomach. Their behaviour is generally benign but may be recurrent, aggressive or even metastasis may occur.

GASTRIC CARCINOMA

INCIDENCE Carcinoma of the stomach comprises more than 90% of all gastric malignancies and is the leading cause of cancer-related deaths in countries where its incidence is high. The highest incidence is between 4th to 6th decades of life.

ETIOLOGY Following factors are implicated:

1. *H. pylori* infection *H. pylori* infection of the stomach is an important risk factor for the development of gastric cancer. Epidemiologic studies throughout world have shown that a seropositivity with *H. pylori* is associated with 3 to 6 times higher risk of development of gastric cancer. It may be mentioned here that similar association of *H. pylori* infection exists with gastric lymphomas (MALT type) as well.

2. Dietary factors Epidemiological studies suggest that dietary factors are most significant in the etiology of gastric cancer. The evidences in support of this are multifold:

i) Occurrence of gastric cancer in the region of gastric canal (i.e. along the lesser curvature and the pyloric antrum) where irritating foods exert their maximum effect.

ii) Populations consuming certain foodstuffs have high risk of developing gastric cancer e.g. ingestion of smoked foods, high intake of salt, pickled raw vegetables, high intake of carcinogens as nitrates in foods and drinking water, nitrites as preservatives for certain meats etc.

iii) Tobacco smoke, tobacco juice and consumption of alcohol have all been shown to have carcinogenic effect on gastric mucosa.

3. Geographical factors The higher incidence in certain geographic regions is the result of environmental influences.

4. Racial factors Within the country, different ethnic groups may have variations in incidence of gastric cancer e.g. incidence is higher in Blacks, American Indians, Chinese in Indonesia, North Wales than other parts of Wales.

5. Genetic factors Genetic influences have some role in the etiology of gastric cancer. Not more than 4% of patients of gastric cancer have a family history of this disease. Individuals with blood group A have higher tendency to develop gastric cancer.

6. Pre-malignant changes in the gastric mucosa These are:

i) Hypo- or achlorhydria in atrophic gastritis of gastric mucosa with intestinal metaplasia.

ii) Adenomatous (neoplastic) polyps of the stomach.

iii) Chronic gastric ulcer (ulcer-cancer), and its association with achlorhydria.

iv) Stump carcinoma in patients who have undergone partial gastrectomy.

MORPHOLOGIC FEATURES Gastric carcinoma is most commonly located in the region of gastric canal (prepyloric region) formed by lesser curvature, pylorus and antrum. Other less common locations are the body, cardia and fundus.

Pathogenetically, a sequential evolution of all gastric carcinomas from an initial stage of *in situ* carcinoma confined to mucosal layers called early gastric carcinoma (EGC) has been found. Accordingly, gastric carcinomas are broadly classified into 2 main groups:

I. *Early gastric carcinoma (EGC)*.

II. *Advanced gastric carcinoma*, which has 5 further major gross subtypes:

i) Ulcerative carcinoma

ii) Fungating (Polypoid) carcinoma

iii) Scirrhous carcinoma (Linitis plastica)

iv) Colloid (Mucoid) carcinoma

v) Ulcer-cancer

In addition to the above classification, gastric carcinomas have been classified, *on the basis of extent of invasion*, into 2 groups:

I. *Expanding (formerly intestinal type) carcinomas* that grow laterally by an invasive margin.

II. *Infiltrating (formerly diffuse type) carcinomas* have poorly-defined invasive border.

I. EARLY GASTRIC CARCINOMA (EGC)

EGC is the term used to describe cancer limited to the mucosa and submucosa. The diagnosis of this condition has been made possible by extensive work on histogenesis of gastric cancer by Japanese pathologists by the use of fibreoptic endoscope and gastrocamera. In Japan, EGC comprises 35% of newly-diagnosed cases of gastric cancer.

G/A The lesion of EGC may have 3 patterns—polypoid (protruded), superficial and ulcerated.

M/E EGC is a typical glandular adenocarcinoma, usually well-differentiated type.

II. ADVANCED GASTRIC CARCINOMA

When the carcinoma crosses the basement membrane into the muscularis propria or beyond, it is referred to as advanced gastric carcinoma. Advanced gastric carcinoma has following 5 patterns:

i) Ulcerative carcinoma This is the most common pattern. The tumour appears as a flat, infiltrating and ulcerative growth with irregular necrotic base and raised margin. It is seen more commonly in the region of gastric canal.

M/E Ulcerative carcinoma are poorly-differentiated adenocarcinomas, which invade deeply into the stomach wall.

ii) Fungating (polypoid) carcinoma The second common pattern is a cauliflower growth projecting into the lumen. It is seen more often in the fundus.

M/E Fungating or polypoid carcinomas are well-differentiated adeno-carcinomas, commonly papillary type.

iii) Scirrhous carcinoma (Linitis plastica) In this pattern, the stomach wall is thickened due to extensive desmoplasia giving the appearance as 'leather-bottle stomach' or 'linitis plastica'. The lumen of the stomach is reduced.

M/E It may be an adenocarcinoma or signet-ring cell carcinoma, extensively infiltrating the stomach wall, but due to marked desmoplasia cancer cells may be difficult to find.

iv) Colloid (Mucoid) carcinoma This pattern is usually seen in the fundus.

M/E Mucoid carcinoma contains abundant pools of mucin in which are seen a small number of tumour cells, sometimes having signet-ring appearance.

v) Ulcer-cancer Development of cancer in chronic gastric ulcer is a rare occurrence (less than 1%). Majority of ulcer-cancers are malignant lesions from the beginning.

M/E Ulcer-cancers are adenocarcinomas without any specific features.

SPREAD Carcinoma of the stomach may spread by the following routes:

1. **Direct spread** Direct spread by local extension is the most common feature of gastric carcinoma. The spread occurs mainly from the loose submucosal layer but eventually muscularis and serosa are also invaded. After the peritoneal covering of the stomach has been invaded, transcoelomic dissemination may occur in any other part of the peritoneal cavity but ovarian masses (one sided or both-sided) occur more commonly, referred to as *Krukenberg tumours*.

2. **Lymphatic spread** Metastases to regional lymph nodes occur early, especially in the scirrhous carcinoma. The groups of lymph nodes

involved are along the lesser and greater curvature around the cardia and suprapancreatic lymph nodes. Involvement of left supraclavicular lymph node, *Virchow* or *Troisier's sign,* is sometimes the presenting feature of gastric carcinoma.

3. Haematogenous spread Blood spread of gastric carcinoma may occur to the liver, lungs, brain, bones, kidneys and adrenals.

CLINICAL FEATURES The usual clinical features are:

i)   Persistent abdominal pain
ii)   Gastric distension and vomiting
iii) Loss of weight (cachexia)
iv)   Loss of appetite (anorexia)
v)   Anaemia, weakness, malaise.

LEIOMYOSARCOMA

Leiomyosarcoma, though rare, is the commonest soft tissue sarcoma, the stomach being the more common site in the gastrointestinal tract.

G/A The tumour may be of variable size but is usually quite large, pedunculated and lobulated mass into the lumen.

M/E Leiomyosarcoma is characterised by high cellularity and presence of mitotic figures.

CARCINOID TUMOUR

Carcinoid tumours are rare in the stomach and are usually non-argentaffin type but argentaffinomas also occur. Their behaviour is usually malignant.

LYMPHOMAS OF GUT

Primary gastrointestinal lymphomas are defined as lymphomas arising in the gut without any evidence of systemic involvement at the time of presentation.

Secondary gastrointestinal lymphomas, on the other hand, appear in the gut after dissemination from other primary site.

Gastric lymphomas constitute over 50% of all bowel lymphomas; other sites being small and large bowel in decreasing order of frequency. Prognosis of primary gastric lymphoma is better than for intestinal lymphomas. Primary lymphoma of stomach is the most common malignant gastric tumour (4%) next to carcinoma.

Clinical manifestations of gastric lymphomas may be similar to gastric carcinoma. Relationship with long-standing chronic *H. pylori* gastritis with lymphoid hyperplasia has been strongly suggested.

G/A Gastric lymphomas have 2 types of appearances:
1. *Diffusely infiltrating type,* producing thickening of the affected gut wall, obliteration of mucosal folds and ulcerations.
2. *Polypoid type,* which produces large protruding mass into the lumen with ulcerated surface.

M/E Gastric lymphomas are most often non-Hodgkin's lymphomas of the following types:
❖ *High-grade* large cell immunoblastic lymphoma being the most common.
❖ *Low-grade* small lymphocytic well-differentiated B-cell lymphoma referred to as *MALToma* is the next in frequency (arising from *M*ucosa *A*ssociated *L*ymphoid *T*issue).

SMALL INTESTINE *(p. 544)*

NORMAL STRUCTURE

Anatomically, the small bowel having a length of 550-650 cm, includes the duodenum, jejunum and ileum and tends to become narrower throughout its course.

M/E The small bowel is identified by recognition of villi. The wall of the small intestine consists of 4 layers:

1. The **serosa** is the outer covering of the small bowel which is complete except over a part of the duodenum.

2. The **muscularis propria** is composed of 2 layers of smooth muscle tissue—outer thinner longitudinal and inner thicker circular layer.

3. The **submucosa** is composed of loose fibrous tissue with blood vessels and lacteals in it.

4. The **mucosa** consists of glandular epithelium overlying the lamina propria composed of loose connective tissue and contains phagocytic cells and abundance of lymphoid cells (Peyer's patches in the ileum) and plasma cells. It is supported externally by thin layer of smooth muscle fibres, *muscularis mucosae*. The absorptive surface is further increased by the intestinal villi. *Villi* are finger-like or leaf-like projections which contain 3 types of cells:

i) *Simple columnar cells*

ii) *Goblet cells*

iii) *Endocrine cells*, or *Kulchitsky cells*, or *enterochromaffin cells*, or *argentaffin cells*. These specialised cells are considered to be part of APUD cell system.

The duodenum contains distinctively branched *Brunner's glands* present in the submucosa and going up to muscularis mucosae.

CONGENITAL ANOMALIES AND INTESTINAL OBSTRUCTION (p. 544)

MECKEL'S DIVERTICULUM

Meckel's diverticulum is the most common congenital anomaly of the gastrointestinal tract, occurring in 2% of population. It is more common in males. The anomaly is commonly situated on the antimesenteric border of the ileum, about 1 meter above the ileocaecal valve. Like other true diverticula, Meckel's diverticulum is an outpouching containing all the layers of the intestinal wall in their normal orientation. It is almost always lined by small intestinal type of epithelium; rarely it may contain islands of gastric mucosa and ectopic pancreatic tissue. Embryologic origin of Meckel's diverticulum is from incomplete obliteration of vitellointestinal duct (Other anomalies resulting from the remnants of vitellointestinal duct are vitelline sinus and vitelline cyst).

The common *complications* of Meckel's diverticulum are perforation, haemorrhage and diverticulitis.

OTHER ANOMALIES

There are a few uncommon anomalies of small intestine e.g.

◈ Intestinal atresia

◈ Intestinal stenosis

◈ Intestinal malrotation

INTESTINAL OBSTRUCTION

The causes of intestinal obstruction can be classified under the following 3 broad groups:

1. Mechanical obstruction

i) *Internal obstruction (intramural and intraluminal):*

    a) Inflammatory strictures (e.g. Crohn's disease)

    b) Congenital stenosis, atresia, imperforate anus

    c) Tumours

    d) Meconium in mucoviscidosis

    e) Roundworms

    f) Gallstones, faecoliths, foreign bodies

    g) Ulceration induced by potassium chloride tablets prescribed to counter hypokalaemia.

ii) *External compression*:
   a) Peritoneal adhesions and bands
   b) Strangulated hernias
   c) Intussusception
   d) Volvulus
   e) Intra-abdominal tumour.

2. Neurogenic obstruction It occurs due to paralytic ileus i.e. paralysis of muscularis of the intestine as a result of shock after abdominal operation or by acute peritonitis.

3. Vascular obstruction Obstruction of the superior mesenteric artery or its branches may result in infarction causing paralysis e.g.
   i) Thrombosis
   ii) Embolism
   iii) Accidental ligation.

Out of the various causes listed above, conditions producing external compression on the bowel wall are the most common causes of intestinal obstruction (80%).

PERITONEAL ADHESIONS AND BANDS Adhesions and bands in the peritoneum composed of fibrous tissue result following healing in peritonitis.

HERNIA Hernia is protrusion of portion of a viscus through an abnormal opening in the wall of its natural cavity.
◈ **External hernia** is the protrusion of the bowel through a defect or weakness in the peritoneum.
◈ **Internal hernia** is the term applied for herniation that does not present on the external surface.

Two major factors involved in the formation of a hernia are as under:
i) *Local weakness*
ii) *Increased intra-abdominal pressure*

Inguinal hernias are more common, followed in decreasing frequency, by femoral and umbilical hernias. Inguinal hernias may be of 2 types:
◈ **Direct** when hernia passes medial to the inferior epigastric artery and it appears through the external abdominal ring.
◈ **Indirect** when it follows the inguinal canal lateral to the inferior epigastric artery.

When the contents of hernia such as loop of intestine can be returned to the abdominal cavity, it is called *reducible*. When it is not possible to reduce hernia due to large contents or due to adhesions in the hernial sac, it is referred to as *irreducible*.

When the blood flow in the hernial sac is obstructed, it results in *strangulated hernia*. Obstruction to the venous drainage and arterial supply may result in infarction or gangrene of the affected loop of intestine.

INTUSSUSCEPTION Intussusception is the telescoping of a segment of intestine into the segment below due to peristalsis. The telescoped segment is called the *intussusceptum* and lower receiving segment is called the *intussuscipiens*. The condition occurs more commonly in infants and young children, more often in the ileocaecal region when the portion of ileum invaginates into the ascending colon without affecting the position of the ileocaecal valve.

The main *complications* of intussusception are intestinal obstruction, infarction, gangrene, perforation and peritonitis.

VOLVULUS Volvulus is the twisting of loop of intestine upon itself through 180° or more. This leads to obstruction of the intestine as well as cutting off of the blood supply to the affected loop. The usual causes are bands and adhesions (congenital or acquired) and long mesenteric attachment.

ISCHAEMIC BOWEL DISEASE (ISCHAEMIC ENTEROCOLITIS) *(p. 546)*

Ischaemic lesions of the gastrointestinal tract may occur in the small intestine and/or colon; the latter is called *ischaemic colitis or ischaemic enterocolitis* and is commonly referred to as ischaemic bowel disease. In either case, the cause of ischaemia is compromised mesenteric circulation.

Depending upon the extent and severity of ischaemia, 3 patterns of pathologic lesions can occur:

1. *Transmural infarction,* characterised by full thickness involvement i.e. transmural ischaemic necrosis and gangrene of the bowel.

2. *Mural infarction,* characterised by haemorrhagic gastroenteropathy (haemorrhage and necrosis).

3. *Ischaemic colitis,* due to chronic colonic ischaemia causing fibrotic narrowing of the affected bowel.

TRANSMURAL INFARCTION

Ischaemic necrosis of the full-thickness of the bowel wall is more common in the small intestine than the large intestine.

ETIOPATHOGENESIS

1. *Mesenteric arterial thrombosis* e.g.
   i) Atherosclerosis (most common)
   ii) Aortic aneurysm
   iii) Vasospasm
   iv) Fibromuscular hyperplasia
   v) Invasion by the tumour
   vi) Use of oral contraceptives
   vii) Arteritis of various types

2. *Mesenteric arterial embolism* arising from
   i) Mural thrombi in the heart
   ii) Endocarditis (infective and nonbacterial thrombotic)
   iii) Atherosclerotic plaques
   iv) Atrial myxoma

3. *Mesenteric venous occlusion*
   i) Intestinal sepsis e.g. appendicitis
   ii) Portal venous thrombosis in cirrhosis of the liver
   iii) Tumour invasion
   iv) Use of oral contraceptives

4. *Miscellaneous causes*:
   i) Strangulated hernia
   ii) Torsion
   iii) Fibrous bands and adhesions.

G/A Irrespective of the underlying etiology, infarction of the bowel is haemorrhagic (red) type. A varying length of the small bowel may be affected. The wall is thickened, oedematous and haemorrhagic. The lumen is dilated and contains blood and mucus.

M/E There is coagulative necrosis and ulceration of the mucosa and there are extensive submucosal haemorrhages. Subsequently, inflammatory cell infiltration and secondary infection occur, leading to gangrene of the bowel.

MURAL AND MUCOSAL INFARCTION (HAEMORRHAGIC GASTROENTEROPATHY)

Mural and mucosal infarctions are limited to superficial layers of the bowel wall, sparing the deeper layer of the muscularis and the serosa. The condition is also referred to as *haemorrhagic gastroenteropathy,* and in the case of colon as *membranous colitis.*

ETIOPATHOGENESIS Haemorrhagic gastroenteropathy results from conditions causing non-occlusive hypoperfusion e.g.

1. Shock
2. Cardiac failure
3. Infections
4. Intake of drugs causing vasoconstriction e.g. digitalis, norepinephrine.

G/A The lesions affect variable length of the bowel. The affected segment of the bowel is red or purple but without haemorrhage and exudation on the serosal surface. The mucosa is oedematous at places, sloughed and ulcerated at other places. The lumen contains haemorrhagic fluid.

M/E There is patchy ischaemic necrosis of mucosa, vascular congestion, haemorrhages and inflammatory cell infiltrate. Secondary bacterial infection may supervene resulting in pseudomembranous enterocolitis.

ISCHAEMIC COLITIS

Ischaemic colitis is characterised by chronic segmental colonic ischaemia followed by chronic inflammation and healing by fibrosis and scarring causing obstruction (ischaemic stricture).

G/A Most frequently affected site is the splenic flexure; other site is rectum. Ischaemic colitis passes through 3 stages: infarct, transient ischaemia and ischaemic stricture.

M/E The ulcerated areas of the mucosa show granulation tissue. The submucosa is characteristically thickened due to inflammation and fibrosis. The muscularis may also show inflammatory changes and patchy replacement by fibrosis.

NECROTISING ENTEROCOLITIS

Necrotising enterocolitis is an acute inflammation of the terminal ileum and ascending colon, occurring primarily in premature and low-birth-weight infants within the first week of life and less commonly in full-term infants.
1. Ischaemia
2. Hypoxia/anoxia of the bowel
3. Bacterial infection and endotoxins
4. Establishment of feeding
5. Infants fed on commercial formulae than breast-fed.

G/A The affected segment of the bowel is dilated, necrotic, haemorrhagic and friable. Bowel wall may contain bubbles of air (pneumatosis intestinalis).

M/E The changes are variable depending upon the stage. Initial changes are confined to mucosa and show oedema, haemorrhage and coagulative necrosis. A *pseudomembrane* composed of necrotic epithelium, fibrin and inflammatory cells may develop.

INFLAMMATORY BOWEL DISEASE (CROHN'S DISEASE AND ULCERATIVE COLITIS) *(p. 548)*

DEFINITION The term 'inflammatory bowel disease (IBD)' is commonly used to include 2 idiopathic bowel diseases having many similarities but the conditions usually have distinctive morphological appearance:

1. **Crohn's disease or Regional enteritis** is an idiopathic chronic ulcerative IBD, characterised by transmural, non-caseating granulomatous inflammation, affecting most commonly the segment of terminal ileum and/or colon, though any part of the gastrointestinal tract may be involved.

2. **Ulcerative colitis** is an idiopathic form of acute and chronic ulcero-inflammatory colitis affecting chiefly the mucosa and submucosa of the rectum and descending colon, though sometimes it may involve the entire length of the large bowel.

Both these disorders primarily affect the bowel but may have systemic involvement in the form of polyarthritis, uveitis, ankylosing spondylitis, skin lesions and hepatic involvement.

ETIOPATHOGENESIS

The exact etiology of IBD remains unknown. However, multiple factors are implicated which can be considered under the following 3 groups:

1. **Genetic factors**
i) There is about 3 to 20 times higher incidence of occurrence of IBD in first-degree relatives.
ii) Overall, there is approximately 50% chance of development of IBD (Crohn's disease about 60% concordance, ulcerative colitis about 6% concordance) in monozygotic twins.

iii) Although no specific and consistent gene association with IBD has been seen, genome-wide search has revealed that disease-predisposing loci are present in chromosomes 16q, 12p, 6p, 14q and 5q.

iv) HLA studies show that ulcerative colitis is more common in HLA-DRB1-alleles while Crohn's disease is more common in HLA-DR7 and DQ4 alleles.

2.   Immunologic factors Defective immunologic regulation in IBD has been shown to play significant role in the pathogenesis of IBD:

i)   *Defective regulation of immune suppression* In IBD, immune mechanism of suppression of inflammation is defective and thus results in uncontrolled inflammation.

ii)   *Transgenic mouse experimental model studies.* Gene 'knock out' studies on colitis in mice have revealed that multiple immune abnormalities may be responsible for IBD as under:

a)   Deletion of inflammation inhibitory cytokines.

b)   Deletion of molecules responsible for T cell recognition.

c)   Interference with normal epithelial barrier function in the intestine.

iii) *Type of inflammatory cells* In both types of IBD, activated CD4+ T cells are present in the lamina propria and in the peripheral blood.

◈   *TH1 cells* secrete proinflammatory cytokines IFN-γ and TNF which induce transmural granulomatous inflammation seen in Crohn's disease.

◈   *TH2 cells* secrete IL-4, IL-5 and IL-13 which induce superficial mucosal inflammation characteristically seen in ulcerative colitis.

3. Exogenous factors In addition to role of genetic factors and deranged T-cell mediated immunity, a role for several exogenous and environmental factors has been assigned e.g.

i)   Microbial factors

ii)   Psychosocial factors

iii)   Smoking

iv)   Oral contraceptives

Consensus hypothesis in *pathogenesis* of IBD combines the role of above three major groups of etiologic factors i.e. in a *genetically predisposed individual*, the effects of exogenous and endogenous host factors result in dysregulation of mucosal immune function, which gets further modified by *certain environmental factors*.

MORPHOLOGIC FEATURES

CROHN'S DISEASE Crohn's disease may involve any portion of the gastrointestinal tract but affects most commonly 15-25 cm of the terminal ileum which may extend into the caecum and sometimes into the ascending colon:

G/A Characteristic feature is the multiple, well-demarcated segmental bowel involvement with intervening uninvolved 'skip areas'. The lumen of the affected segment is markedly narrowed. The mucosa shows 'serpiginous ulcers', while intervening surviving mucosa is swollen giving 'cobblestone appearance'. There may be deep fissuring into the bowel wall.

M/E Main features are as under:

1. .*Transmural inflammatory cell infiltrate* consisting of chronic inflammatory cells (lymphocytes, plasma cells and macrophages).

2. *Non-caseating, sarcoid-like granulomas* are present in all the layers of the affected bowel wall in 60% of cases.

3. There is *patchy ulceration* of the mucosa which may take the form of deep fissures.

4. *Widening of the submucosa* due to oedema and foci of lymphoid aggregates.

5. In more *chronic cases*, fibrosis becomes increasingly prominent.

ULCERATIVE COLITIS Classically, ulcerative colitis begins in the rectum, and in continuity extends upwards into the sigmoid colon, descending colon, transverse colon, and sometimes may involve the entire colon.

G/A The characteristic feature is the continuous involvement of the rectum and colon without any uninvolved skip areas compared to Crohn's disease. The appearance of colon may vary depending upon the stage and intensity of the disease because of remissions and exacerbations. Mucosa shows linear and superficial ulcers, usually not penetrating the muscular layer. The intervening intact mucosa may form inflammatory 'pseudopolyps.'

M/E Ulcerative colitis because of remission and exacerbations, is characterised by alternating 'active disease process' and 'resolving colitis.' The changes in the 'active disease process' are as under:

1. *Crypt distortion, cryptitis* and focal accumulations of neutrophils forming *crypt abscesses.*
2. Marked *congestion, dilatation and haemorrhages* from mucosal capillaries.
3. *Superficial mucosal ulcerations,* usually not penetrating into the muscle coat, and is accompanied by nonspecific inflammatory cell infiltrate of lymphocytes, plasma cells, neutrophils, some eosinophils and mast cells in the lamina propria.
4. *Goblet cells* are markedly *diminished* in cases of active disease.
5. Areas of *mucosal regeneration and mucodepletion* of lining cells.
6. In long-standing cases, epithelial *cytologic atypia* ranging from mild to marked dysplasia and sometimes developing into carcinoma *in situ* and frank adenocarcinoma.

COMPLICATIONS

Crohn's disease:
1. *Malabsorption*
2. *Fistula formation*
3. *Stricture formation*
4. *Development of malignancy* lymphoma may develop more often in Crohn's disease than adenocarcinoma.

Ulcerative colitis:
1. *Toxic megacolon (Fulminant colitis)* is the acute fulminating colitis in which the affected colon is thin-walled and dilated and is prone to perforation and faecal peritonitis. There is deep penetration of the inflammatory cell infiltrate into muscle layer which is disrupted.
2. *Perianal fistula* formation may occur rarely.
3. *Carcinoma* may develop in long-standing cases of ulcerative colitis of more than 10 years duration.
4. *Stricture formation* almost never occurs in ulcerative colitis.

INFECTIVE AND OTHER ENTEROCOLITIS *(p. 552)*

Besides IBD, a variety of other acute and chronic inflammatory conditions affect small bowel (enteritis), large bowel (colitis), or both (enterocolitis).

INFECTIVE ENTEROCOLITIS

These are a group of acute and chronic inflammatory lesions of small intestine and/or colon caused by microorganisms (bacteria, viruses, fungi, protozoa and helminths). All these are characterised by diarrhoeal syndromes. Pathogenetically speaking, these microorganisms can cause enterocolitis by 2 mechanisms—by *enteroinvasive bacteria* producing ulcerative lesions, and by *enterotoxin-producing bacteria* resulting in non-ulcerative lesions.

INTESTINAL TUBERCULOSIS

Intestinal tuberculosis can occur in 3 forms—primary, secondary and hyperplastic caecal tuberculosis.

1. PRIMARY INTESTINAL TUBERCULOSIS Though an uncommon disease in the developed countries of the world, primary tuberculosis of the ileocaecal region is quite common in developing countries including India. Virtually all cases of intestinal tuberculosis are caused by *M. tuberculosis.* The predominant changes are in the mesenteric lymph nodes without any significant intestinal lesion.

G/A The affected lymph nodes are enlarged, matted and caseous (tabes mesenterica). Eventually, there is healing by fibrosis and calcification.

M/E In the initial stage, there is primary complex or Ghon's focus in the intestinal mucosa as occurs elsewhere in primary tuberculous infection. Subsequently, the mesenteric lymph nodes are affected which show typical tuberculous granulomatous inflammatory reaction with caseation necrosis.

2. SECONDARY INTESTINAL TUBERCULOSIS Self-swallowing of sputum in patients with active pulmonary tuberculosis may cause secondary intestinal tuberculosis, most commonly in the terminal ileum.

G/A The intestinal lesions are prominent than the lesions in regional lymph nodes as in secondary pulmonary tuberculosis. The lesions begin in the Peyer's patches or the lymphoid follicles with formation of small ulcers that spread through the lymphatics to form large ulcers which are *transverse to the long axis of the bowel*, (*c.f.* typhoid ulcers of small intestine, described below).

M/E The tuberculous lesions in the intestine are similar to those observed elsewhere i.e. presence of tubercles. Mucosa and submucosa show ulceration and the muscularis may be replaced by variable degree of fibrosis.

3. HYPERPLASTIC ILEOCAECAL TUBERCULOSIS This is a variant of occurring secondary to pulmonary tuberculosis.

G/A The terminal ileum, caecum and/or ascending colon are thick-walled with mucosal ulceration. Clinically, the lesion is palpable and may be mistaken for carcinoma.

M/E The presence of caseating tubercles distinguishes the condition from Crohn's disease in which granulomas are non-caseating.

ENTERIC FEVER

The term enteric fever is used to describe acute infection caused by *Salmonella typhi* (typhoid fever) or *Salmonella paratyphi* (paratyphoid fever). Besides these 2 salmonellae, *Salmonella typhimurium* causes food poisoning.

PATHOGENESIS The typhoid bacilli are ingested through contaminated food or water. During the initial asymptomatic incubation period of about 2 weeks, the bacilli invade the lymphoid follicles and Peyer's patches of the small intestine and proliferate. Following this, the bacilli invade the blood-stream causing bacteraemia, and the characteristic clinical features of the disease like continuous rise in temperature and 'rose spots' on the skin are observed. Immunological reactions (Widal's test) begin after about 10 days and peak titres are seen by the end of the third week.

MORPHOLOGIC FEATURES The lesions are observed in the intestines as well as in other organs.

1. INTESTINAL LESIONS *G/A* Terminal ileum is affected most often, but lesions may be seen in the jejunum and colon. Peyer's patches show oval typhoid ulcers with their *long axis along the length of the bowel* (c.f. tuberculous ulcers of small intestine, described above). The base of the ulcers is black due to sloughed mucosa. The margins of the ulcers are slightly raised due to inflammatory oedema and cellular proliferation.

M/E There is hyperaemia, oedema and cellular proliferation consisting of phagocytic histiocytes (showing characteristic erythrophagocytosis), lymphocytes and plasma cells.

The main **complications** of the intestinal lesions of typhoid are perforation of the ulcers and haemorrhage.

2. OTHER LESIONS Various other organ involvements produce following changes:

    i) *Mesenteric lymph nodes*—haemorrhagic lymphadenitis.
    ii) *Liver*—foci of parenchymal necrosis.
    iii) *Gallbladder*—typhoid cholecystitis.
    iv) *Spleen*—splenomegaly with reactive hyperplasia.
    v) *Kidneys*—nephritis.
    vi) *Abdominal muscles*—Zenker's degeneration.
    vii) *Joints*—arthritis.

viii) *Bones*—osteitis.
ix) *Meninges*—Meningitis.
x) *Testis*—Orchitis.

BACTERIAL FOOD POISONING

This is a form of acute bacterial illness that occurs following ingestion of food or water contaminated with bacteria other than those that cause specific acute intestinal infections like typhoid, paratyphoid, cholera or dysentery bacilli.

The commonest causes of bacterial food poisoning resulting in enteritis or enterocolitis are as under:
1. Staphylococcal food poisoning
2. Clostridial food poisoning
3. Botulism
4. *Salmonella* food poisoning (Salmonellosis)

DYSENTERIES

The term 'dysentery' is used to mean diarrhoea with abdominal cramps, tenesmus and passage of mucus in the stools. Based on etiology, there are 2 main forms of dysenteries.

1. BACILLARY DYSENTERY Bacillary dysentery is the term used for infection by *Shigella* species: *S. dysenteriae, S. flexneri, S. boydii and S. sonnei.* Infection occurs by faeco-oral route and is seen with poor personal hygiene, in densely populated areas, and with contaminated food and water. The common housefly plays a role in spread of infection.

G/A The lesions are mainly found in the colon and occasionally in the ileum. Superficial transverse ulcerations of mucosa of the bowel wall occur in the region of lymphoid follicles but perforation is seldom seen.

M/E The mucosa overlying the lymphoid follicles is necrosed. The surrounding mucosa shows congestion, oedema and infiltration by neutrophils and lymphocytes. The mucosa may be covered by greyish-yellow *'pseudomembrane'* composed of fibrinosuppurative exudate.

2. AMOEBIC DYSENTERY This is due to infection by *Entamoeba histolytica.* It is more prevalent in the tropical countries and primarily affects the large intestine. Infection occurs from ingestion of cyst form of the parasite.

G/A Early intestinal lesions appear as small areas of elevation on the mucosal surface. In advanced cases, typical flask-shaped ulcers having narrow neck and broad base are seen. They are more conspicuous in the caecum, rectum and in the flexures.

M/E The ulcerated area shows chronic inflammatory reaction consisting of lymphocytes, plasma cells, macrophages and eosinophils. The trophozoites of *Entamoeba* are seen in the inflammatory exudate and are concentrated at the advancing margin of the lesion.

Complications of intestinal amoebic ulcers are: amoebic liver abscess or amoebic hepatitis, perforation, haemorrhage and formation of amoeboma which is a tumour-like mass.

PSEUDOMEMBRANOUS ENTEROCOLITIS (ANTIBIOTIC-ASSOCIATED DIARRHOEA)

Pseudomembranous enterocolitis is a form of acute inflammation of colon and/or small intestine characterised by formation of *'pseudomembrane'* over the site of mucosal injury.

ETIOLOGY Numerous studies have established the overgrowth of *Clostridium difficile* with production of its toxin in the etiology of antibiotic-associated diarrhoea culminating in pseudomembranous colitis. Oral anti-biotics such as clindamycin, ampicillin and the cephalosporins are more often (20%) associated with antibiotic-associated diarrhoea.

G/A   The lesions may be confined, to the large intestine or small intestine, or both may be involved. The mucosa of the bowel is covered by patchy, raised yellow-white plaques.

M/E   The '*pseudomembrane*' is composed of network of fibrin and mucus, in which are entangled inflammatory cells and mucosal epithelial cells. There is focal necrosis of surface epithelial cells.

MALABSORPTION SYNDROME *(p. 556)*

DEFINITION AND CLASSIFICATION

The malabsorption syndrome (MAS) is characterised by impaired intestinal absorption of nutrients especially of fat; some other substances are proteins, carbohydrates, vitamins and minerals. MAS is subdivided into 2 broad groups.

CLINICAL FEATURES

1. Steatorrhoea (pale, bulky, foul-smelling stools)
2. Chronic diarrhoea
3. Abdominal distension
4. Barborygmi and flatulence
5. Anorexia
6. Weight loss
7. Muscle wasting
8. Dehydration
9. Hypotension
10. Specific malnutrition and vitamin deficiencies depending upon the cause.

INVESTIGATIONS

I.   LABORATORY TESTS

1.   Tests for fat malabsorption:
i)   Faecal analysis for fat content
ii)   Microscopic analysis for faecal fat
iii) Blood lipid levels after a fatty meal
iv)   Tests based on absorption of radioactive-labelled fat.

2.   Tests for protein malabsorption:
i)   Bile acid malabsorption
ii)   Radioactive-labelled glycine breath test.
iii) Prothrombin time (vitamin K deficiency)
iv)   Secretin and other pancreatic tests.

3.   Tests for carbohydrate malabsorption:
i)   D-xylose tolerance test
ii)   Lactose tolerance test
iii) Hydrogen breath test
iv)   Bile acid breath test

4.   Vitamin B_{12}, malabsorption:
i)   Schilling test.

II.   INTESTINAL MUCOSAL BIOPSY

Mucosal biopsy of small intestine is essential for making the diagnosis of MAS and also evaluation of a patient on follow-up. The availability of endoscopes has enabled easy viewing of affected mucosa directly and taking mucosal biopsy under vision.

Villous atrophy   Variable degree of flattening of intestinal mucosa in MAS is the commonest pathological change in mucosal pattern and is referred to as villous atrophy. It may be of 2 types—partial and subtotal/total type.
◈   *Partial villous atrophy* is the mild form of the lesion in which villi fuse with each other and thus become short and broad, commonly called as convolutions and irregular ridges. The epithelial cells show compensatory hyperplasia suggesting a turnover of these cells.

❖ *Subtotal/Total villous atrophy* is the severe form of the lesion in which there is flattening of mucosa due to more advanced villous fusion. The surface epithelium is cuboidal and there is increased plasma cell infiltrate in the lamina propria.

Subtotal and total villous atrophy is exhibited by a number of conditions such as nontropical sprue, tropical sprue, intestinal lymphomas, carcinoma, protein-calorie malnutrition etc.

IMPORTANT TYPES OF MAS

COELIAC SPRUE (NON-TROPICAL SPRUE, GLUTEN-SENSITIVE ENTEROPATHY, IDIOPATHIC STEATORRHOEA)

This is the most important cause of primary malabsorption occurring in temperate climates. The condition is characterised by significant loss of villi in the small intestine and therefore diminished absorptive surface area. The condition occurs in 2 forms:

Childhood form, seen in infants and children and is commonly referred to as *coeliac disease.*

Adult form, seen in adolescents and early adult life and used to be called *idiopathic steatorrhoea.*

In either case, there is genetic abnormality resulting in sensitivity to gluten (a protein) and its derivative, gliadin, present in diets such as grains of wheat, barley and rye. Serum antibodies—IgA antigliadin and IgA antiendomysial, have been found.

The symptoms are usually relieved on elimination of gluten from the diet. The role of heredity is further supported by the observation of familial incidence and HLA association of the disease. Following hypotheses have been proposed in causing mucosal cell damage:

1. *Hypersensitivity reaction* as seen by gluten-stimulated antibodies.
2. Toxic effect of gluten due to *inherited enzyme deficiency* in the mucosal cells.

M/E There are no differences in the pathological findings in children and adults. There is variable degree of flattening of the mucosa, particularly of the upper jejunum, and to some extent of the duodenum and ileum. The surface epithelial cells are cuboidal or low columnar type. There may be *partial villous atrophy* which is replacement of normal villous pattern by convolutions, or *subtotal villous atrophy* characterised by flat mucosal surface.

COLLAGENOUS SPRUE

This entity is regarded as the end-result of coeliac sprue in which the villi are totally absent *(total villous atrophy)* and there are unique and diagnostic broad bands of collagen under the basal lamina of surface epithelium.

TROPICAL SPRUE

This disease, as the name suggests, occurs in individuals living in or visiting tropical areas such as Caribbean countries, South India, Sri Lanka and Hong Kong. Pathogenesis of the condition is not clear but there is evidence to support enterotoxin production by some strains of *E. coli* which causes the intestinal injury.

M/E There is usually *partial villous atrophy* and sometimes *subtotal atrophy.*

WHIPPLE'S DISEASE (INTESTINAL LIPODYSTROPHY)

This is an uncommon bacterial disease involving not only the intestines but also various other systems such as central nervous system, heart, blood vessels, skin, joints, lungs, liver, spleen and kidneys. Patients may present with features of malabsorption or may have atypical presentation in the form of migratory polyarthritis, neurological disturbances and focal hyperpigmentation of the skin.

M/E The affected tissues show presence of characteristic macrophages containing PAS-positive granules and rod-shaped micro-organisms (Whipple's bacilli). These macrophages are predominantly present in the lamina propria of the small intestine and mesenteric lymph nodes.

PROTEIN-LOSING ENTEROPATHIES

i) Whipple's disease
ii) Crohn's disease
iii) Ulcerative colitis
iv) Sprue
v) Intestinal lymphangiectasia
vi) Ménétrier's disease (Hypertrophic gastritis).

SMALL INTESTINAL TUMOURS *(p. 559)*

Although small intestine is about 6 meter long, but for obscure reasons, benign as well as malignant tumours in it are surprisingly rare.

◆ Most common *benign tumours,* in descending order of frequency, are: gastrointestinal stromal tumours (GIST), leiomyomas, adenomas and vascular tumours (haemangioma, lymphangioma).

◆ Amongst the *malignant tumours,* the most frequently encountered, in descending frequency, are: carcinoid tumours, lymphomas and adenocarcinoma.

CARCINOID TUMOUR (ARGENTAFFINOMA)

Carcinoid tumour or argentaffinoma is a generic term applied to tumours originating from endocrine cells belonging to APUD cell system and are therefore also called as apudomas. The endocrine cells are distributed throughout the mucosa of GI tract. These cells have secretory granules which stain positively with silver salts (argentaffin granules) or many stain after addition of exogenous reducing agent (non-argentaffin or argyrophil granules). Accordingly, carcinoid tumour may be argentaffin or argyrophil type. Depending upon the embryologic derivation of the tissues where the tumour is located, these are classified as follows:

◆ **Midgut carcinoids,** seen in terminal ileum and appendix are the most common (60-80%) and are more often argentaffin positive.

◆ **Hindgut carcinoids,** occurring in rectum and colon are more commonly argyrophil type, and comprise about 10-20% of carcinoids.

◆ **Foregut carcinoids,** located in the stomach, duodenum and oesophagus are also argyrophil type and are encountered as frequently as in the hindgut (10-20%).

Appendix and terminal ileum, the two most common sites for carcinoids, depict variation in their age and sex incidence and biologic behaviour.

G/A All carcinoids are small, button-like submucosal elevations with intact or ulcerated overlying mucosa. They are usually small; those larger than 2 cm are more often metastasising. Ileal and gastric carcinoids are commonly multiple, whereas appendiceal carcinoids commonly involve the tip of the organ and are solitary. Cut section of all the carcinoids is bright yellow.

M/E The tumour cells may be arranged in a variety of patterns—solid nests, sheets, cords, trabeculae and clusters, all of which show characteristic palisading of the peripheral cells. Acinar arrangement and rosettes are rarely seen. The tumour cells are classically small, monotonous, having uniform nuclei and poorly-defined cell boundaries.

CARCINOID SYNDROME Carcinoid tumours that metastasise, especially to the liver, are sometimes associated with the carcinoid syndrome. The syndrome consists of the following features:

1. Intermittent attacks of flushing of the skin of face
2. Episodes of watery diarrhoea
3. Abdominal pain
4. Attacks of dyspnoea due to bronchospasm
5. Right-sided heart failure due to involvement of tricuspid and pulmonary valves and endocardium.

5-HT and its degradation product, 5-HIAA, are particularly significant in **367** the production of *carcinoid syndrome*.

Chapter 18

The Gastrointestinal Tract

LYMPHOMA

Malignant lymphoma of the small intestine has a few peculiarities:

1. Presence and type of an underlying disorder: e.g. long-term malabsorption syndrome, AIDS, Crohn's disease.

2. Primary versus secondary lymphoma: Extranodal lymphoma is more common in gastrointestinal tract than elsewhere, it is important to rule out spread of primary nodal lymphoma to the intestine.

3. Type of lymphoma and its cell lineage: NHL of various types, particularly B-cell type include: immunoproliferative small intestinal diease (IPSID), low-grade B-cell NHL of MALT type, follicular lymphoma, diffuse large B-cell lymphoma (DBCL), Burkitt's lymphoma, mantle zone lymphoma.

APPENDIX (p. 561)

NORMAL STRUCTURE

Appendix is a vestigial organ which serves no useful purpose in human beings but instead becomes the site of trouble at times. It is like a diverticulum of the caecum, usually lying behind the caecum and varies in length from 4 to 20 cm (average 7 cm).

M/E Appendix has four layers in its wall—*mucosa, submucosa, muscularis* and *serosa*. The muscularis of the appendix has two layers (inner circular and outer longitudinal) as elsewhere in the alimentary tract.

Two important diseases involving the appendix are appendicitis and appendiceal carcinoids.

APPENDICITIS (p. 561)

Acute inflammation of the appendix, acute appendicitis, is the most common acute abdominal condition confronting the surgeon. The condition is seen more commonly in older children and young adults, and is uncommon at the extremes of age.

ETIOPATHOGENESIS Common causes are as under:

A. Obstructive:
1. Faecolith
2. Calculi
3. Foreign body
4. Tumour
5. Worms (especially *Enterobius vermicularis*)
6. Diffuse lymphoid hyperplasia, especially in children.

B. Non-obstructive:
1. Haematogenous spread of generalised infection
2. Vascular occlusion
3. Inappropriate diet lacking roughage.

G/A The appearance depends upon the stage at which the acutely-inflamed appendix is examined. In *early acute appendicitis*, the organ is swollen and serosa shows hyperaemia. In well-developed acute inflammation called *acute suppurative appendicitis*, the serosa is coated with fibrinopurulent exudate and engorged vessels on the surface. In further advanced cases called *acute gangrenous appendicitis*, there is necrosis and ulcerations of mucosa which extend through the wall.

M/E The most important diagnostic histological criterion is the *neutrophilic infiltration of the muscularis*. In early stage, other changes besides acute inflammatory changes, are congestion and oedema of the appendiceal wall. In later stages, the mucosa is sloughed off, the wall becomes necrotic, the blood vessels may get thrombosed and there may be neutrophilic abscesses in the wall.

CLINICAL COURSE The patient presents with features of acute abdomen as under:
1. Colicky pain, initially around umbilicus, later localised to right iliac fossa
2. Nausea and vomiting
3. Pyrexia of mild grade
4. Abdominal tenderness
5. Increased pulse rate
6. Neutrophilic leucocytosis with toxic granules in neutrophils.

COMPLICATIONS If the condition is not adequately managed, the following complications may occur:
1. Peritonitis
2. Appendix abscess
3. Adhesions
4. Portal pylephlebitis
5. Mucocele

TUMOURS OF APPENDIX *(p. 562)*

Tumours of the appendix are quite rare.

CARCINOID TUMOUR Both argentaffin and argyrophil types are encountered, the former being more common.

G/A Carcinoid tumour of the appendix is mostly situated near the tip of the organ and appears as a circumscribed nodule, usually less than 1 cm in diameter.

M/E Carcinoid tumour of the appendix resembles other carcinoids of the midgut.

ADENOCARCINOMA It is an uncommon tumour in the appendix and is morphologically similar to adenocarcinoma elsewhere in the alimentary tract.

PSEUDOMYXOMA PERITONEI Pseudomyxoma peritonei is accumulation of gelatinous mucinous ascites. Mucinous collection is generally secondary to an appendiceal neoplasm and may be acellular or may contain tumour cells (either benign or signet ring cells). The associated appendiceal tumour is frequently benign mucinous cystadenoma of the appendix but occasionally invasive carcinoma of the appendix are also encountered. In assessing an ovarian mucinous tumour associated with pseudomyxoma peritonei, the state of appendix is important.

LARGE BOWEL *(p. 563)*

NORMAL STRUCTURE

The large bowel consists of 6 parts—the caecum, ascending colon, transverse colon, descending colon, sigmoid colon and rectum, and in all measures about 1.5 meters in length. The serosal surface of the large intestine except the rectum is studded with *appendices epiploicae* which are small, rounded collections of fatty tissue covered by peritoneum.

M/E The wall of large bowel consists of 4 layers as elsewhere in the alimentary tract—serosa, muscularis, submucosa and mucosa.

The *blood supply* to the right colon is from the superior mesenteric artery which also supplies blood to the small bowel. The remaining portion of large bowel except the lower part of rectum receives blood supply from inferior mesenteric artery. The lower rectum is supplied by haemorrhoidal branches.

The *innervation* of the large bowel consists of 3 plexuses of ganglion cells—*Auerbach's* or *myenteric plexus* lying between the two layers of muscularis, *Henle's plexus* lying in the deep submucosa inner to circular muscle layer, and *Meissner plexus* that lies in the superficial mucosa just beneath the muscularis mucosae.

Anal canal, 3-4 cm long tubular structure, begins at the lower end of the rectum, though is not a part of large bowel, but is included here to cover simultaneously lesions pertaining to this region. It is lined by keratinised or nonkeratinised stratified squamous epithelium.

Chapter 18

The Gastrointestinal Tract

CONGENITAL AND OTHER MISCELLANEOUS CONDITIONS *(p. 563)*

HIRSCHSPRUNG'S DISEASE (CONGENITAL MEGACOLON)

The term 'megacolon' is used for any form of marked dilatation of the entire colon or its segment and may occur as a congenital or acquired disorder. *Congenital form* characterised by congenital absence of ganglion cells in the bowel wall (enteric neurons) is called Hirschsprung's disease. Genetically, Hirschsprung's disease is a heterogeneous disorder as under:
1. Autosomal dominant inheritance with mutation in *RET* proto-oncogene in some cases.
2. Autosomal recessive form with mutation in endothelin-B receptor gene in many other cases.

Clinically, the condition manifests shortly after birth with constipation, gaseous distension and sometimes with acute intestinal obstruction. Its frequency is 1 in 5,000 live-births, has familial tendency in about 4% of cases and has predilection for development in Down's syndrome.

MORPHOLOGIC FEATURES Two types of biopsies may be done on infants suspected of having Hirschsprung's disease—full-thickness rectal biopsy, and suction biopsy that includes mucosa and submucosa.

G/A Typical case of Hirschsprung's disease shows 2 segments—a *distal narrow segment* that is aganglionic and a *dilated proximal segment* that contains normal number of ganglion cells.

M/E The distal narrow segment shows total absence of ganglion cells of all the three plexuses (Auerbach's or myenteric plexus present between the two layers of muscularis, deep submucosal or Henle's plexus, and superficial mucosal or Meissner's plexus) and prominence of non-myelinated nerve fibres.

In addition to congenital megacolon discussed above, megacolon may occur from certain *acquired causes* as under:
i. *Obstructive* e.g. due to tumour, post-inflammatory strictures.
ii. *Endocrine* e.g. in myxoedema, cretinism.
iii. *CNS disorders* e.g. spina bifida, paraplegia, parkinsonism.
iv. *Psychogenic* e.g. emotional disturbances, psychiatric disorders.
v. *Chagas' disease* due to infection with *Trypanosoma cruzi* is the only example resulting in acquired loss of ganglion cells.

COLITIS

Colitis may occur in isolation but more commonly involvement of small intestine is also present (enterocolitis). In view of the considerable overlapping of enteritis and colitis, these lesions have already been described under small intestine.

DIVERTICULOSIS COLI

Diverticula are the outpouchings or herniations of the mucosa and submucosa of the colon through the muscle wall. *Diverticular disease*, as it is commonly known, is rare under 30 years of age and is seen more commonly as the age advances. Multiple diverticula of the colon are very common in the Western societies, probably due to ingestion of low-fibre diet but is seen much less frequently in tropical countries and in Japan.

Based on the etiologic role of low fibre diet, pathogenesis of diverticular disease of the colon can be explained as under:
1. *Increased intraluminal pressure* such as due to low fibre content of the diet causing hyperactive peristalsis and thereby sequestration, of mucosa and submucosa.
2. *Muscular weakness* of the colonic wall at the junction of the muscularis with submucosa.

G/A Diverticulosis is seen most commonly in the sigmoid colon (95%) but any other part of the entire colon may be involved. They may vary in number from a few to several hundred. They appear as small, spherical or flask-shaped outpouchings, usually less than 1 cm in diameter, commonly extend into appendices epiploicae and may contain inspissated faeces.

M/E The flask-shaped structures extend from the intestinal lumen through the muscle layer. The colonic wall in the affected area is thin and is composed of atrophic mucosa, compressed submucosa and thin or deficient muscularis.

The *complications* of diverticulosis and diverticulitis are perforation, haemorrhage, intestinal obstruction and fistula formation.

HAEMORRHOIDS (PILES)

Haemorrhoids or piles are varicosities of the haemorrhoidal veins. They are called *internal piles* if dilatation is of superior haemorrhoidal plexus covered over by mucous membrane, and *external piles* if they involve inferior haemorrhoidal plexus covered over by the skin. Their possible causes include the following:
1. Portal hypertension
2. Chronic constipation and straining at stool
3. Cardiac failure
4. Venous stasis of pregnancy
5. Hereditary predisposition
6. Tumours of the rectum.

MELANOSIS COLI

Melanosis coli is a peculiar condition in which mucosa of the large intestine acquires brown-black colouration. The condition is said to occur in individuals who are habitual users of cathartics of anthracene type.

ANGIODYSPLASIA

Angiodysplasia is a submucosal telangiectasia affecting caecum and right colon that causes recurrent acute and chronic haemorrhage. The condition is more common in the elderly past 6th decade. The pathogenesis is obscure but is possibly due to mechanical obstruction of the veins.

MISCELLANEOUS INFLAMMATORY CONDITIONS

◈ **Fistula-in-ano** It is a well known and common condition in which one or more fistulous tracts pass from the internal opening at the pectinate line through the internal sphincter on to the skin surface.

◈ **Anal fissure** It is an ulcer in the anal canal below the level of the pectinate line, mostly in midline and posteriorly.

◈ **Solitary rectal ulcer syndrome** It is a condition characterised usually by solitary, at times multiple, rectal ulcers with prolapse of rectal mucosa and development of proctitis. Besides ulceration and inflammation of the rectal mucosa, lamina propria is occupied by spindle-shaped fibroblasts and smooth muscle cells.

POLYPS AND TUMOURS OF LARGE BOWEL (p. 566)

Large bowel is the most common site for a variety of benign and malignant tumours, majority of which are of epithelial origin. Most of the benign tumours present clinically as polyps. A classification of polyps, along with benign tumours and malignant tumours, is presented below.
I.   COLORECTAL POLYPS
A.   *Non-neoplastic polyps*
     1. Hyperplastic (metaplastic) polyps
     2. Hamartomatous polyps
          (i) Peutz-Jeghers polyps and polyposis
          (ii) Juvenile (Retention) polyps and polyposis

3. Inflammatory polyps (Pseudopolyps)
4. Lymphoid polyps
B. *Neoplastic polyps (Adenomas)*
 1. Tubular adenoma (Adenomatous polyp)
 2. Villous adenoma (Villous papilloma)
 3. Tubulovillous adenoma (Papillary adenoma, villoglandular adenoma)
C. *Familial polyposis syndromes*
 1. Familial polyposis coli (Adenomatosis)
 2. Gardner's syndrome
 3. Turcot's syndrome
 4. Juvenile polyposis syndrome
II. OTHER BENIGN COLORECTAL TUMOURS
 (Leiomyomas, leiomyoblastoma, neurilemmoma, lipoma and vascular tumours)
III. MALIGNANT COLORECTAL TUMOURS
A. *Carcinoma*
 1. Adenocarcinoma
 2. Other carcinomas
  (Mucinous adenocarcinoma, signet-ring cell carcinoma, adenosquamous carcinoma, undifferentiated carcinoma)
B. *Other malignant tumours*
 (Leiomyosarcoma, malignant lymphoma, carcinoid tumours)
IV. TUMOURS OF THE ANAL CANAL
A. *Benign* (viral warts or condyloma acuminata)
B. *Malignant* (squamous cell carcinoma, basaloid carcinoma, muco-epidermoid carcinoma, adenocarcinoma, undifferentiated carcinoma, malignant melanoma)

COLORECTAL POLYPS

A polyp is defined as any growth or mass protruding from the mucous membrane into the lumen. Polyps are much more common in the large intestine than in the small intestine and are more common in the recto-sigmoid colon than the proximal colon. Polyps are broadly classified into 2 groups—non-neoplastic and neoplastic.

A. NON-NEOPLASTIC POLYPS

HYPERPLASTIC (METAPLASTIC) POLYPS

The hyperplastic or metaplastic polyps are the most common amongst all epithelial polyps, particularly in the rectosigmoid. They are called 'hyperplastic' because there is epithelial hyperplasia at the base of the crypts, and 'metaplastic' as there are areas of cystic metaplasia. They may be seen at any age but are more common in the elderly (6th-7th decade).

G/A Hyperplastic polyps are generally multiple, sessile, smooth-surfaced and small (less than 0.5 cm).

M/E They are composed of long and cystically dilated glands and crypts lined by normal epithelial cells. Their lining is partly flat and partly papillary. The luminal border of the lining epithelium is often serrated or saw-toothed.

Hyperplastic polyps are usually symptomless and have no malignant potential unless there is a coexistent adenoma.

HAMARTOMATOUS POLYPS

These are tumour-like lesions composed of abnormal mixture of tissues indigenous to the part. They are further of 2 types:

PEUTZ-JEGHERS POLYPS AND POLYPOSIS Peutz-Jeghers syndrome is autosomal dominant defect, characterised by hamartomatous intestinal polyposis and melanotic pigmentation of lips, mouth and genitalia. The polyps may be located in the stomach, small intestine or colon but are most common in the jejunum and ileum. The most common age is adolescence and early childhood.

G/A These polyps are of variable size but are often large, multiple and pedunculated and more commonly situated in the small intestine.

M/E The most characteristic feature is the tree-like branching of muscularis mucosae. The lining epithelium is by normal-appearing epithelial cells. The glands may show hyperplasia and cystic change.

Peutz-Jeghers polyps do not undergo malignant transformation unless a coexistent adenoma is present.

JUVENILE (RETENTION) POLYPS Juvenile or retention polyps, another form of hamartomatous polyps, occur more commonly in children below 5 years of age. Solitary juvenile polyps occur more often in the rectum, while juvenile polyposis may be present anywhere in the large bowel.

G/A Juvenile polyps are spherical, smooth-surfaced, about 2 cm in diameter and are often pedunculated.

M/E The classical appearance is of cystically dilated glands containing mucus and lined by normal mucus-secreting epithelium.

Most cases, on becoming symptomatic in the form of rectal bleeding, are removed. In common with other non-neoplastic polyps, they are also not precancerous.

INFLAMMATORY POLYPS (PSEUDOPOLYPS)

Inflammatory polyps or pseudopolyps appear due to re-epithelialisation of the undermined ulcers and overhanging margins in inflammatory bowel disease, most frequently in ulcerative colitis (colitis polyposa) and sometimes in Crohn's disease.

G/A They are usually multiple, cylindrical to rounded overgrowths of mucosa and may vary from minute nodules to several centimeters in size.

M/E The centre of inflammatory polyp consists of connective tissue core that shows some inflammatory cell infiltrate and is covered superficially by regenerating epithelial cells and some cystically-dilated glands.

These lesions have no malignant potential; carcinomas seen in long-standing cases of ulcerative colitis arise in the region of epithelial dysplasia and not from the polyps.

LYMPHOID POLYPS

Reactive hyperplasia of lymphoid tissue that is normally also more prominent in the rectum and terminal ileum, gives rise to localised or diffuse lymphoid polyps, also called *rectal tonsils*.

G/A They are solitary or multiple, tiny elevated lesions.

M/E They are composed of prominent lymphoid follicles with germinal centres located in the submucosa and mucosa.

They are benign lesions and have to be distinguished from malignant lymphoma.

B. NEOPLASTIC POLYPS (ADENOMAS)

Neoplastic polyps are colorectal adenomas which have potential for malignant change while polypoid carcinoma is the term used for invasive epithelial tumours. Adenomas have 3 main varieties (tubular, villous and tubulovillous).

TUBULAR ADENOMA (ADENOMATOUS POLYP)

Tubular adenomas or adenomatous polyps are the most common neoplastic polyps (75%). They are common beyond 3rd decade of life and have slight male preponderance. They occur most often in the distal colon and rectum. They may be found singly as sporadic cases, or multiple tubular adenomas as part of familial polyposis syndrome with autosomal dominant inheritance pattern.

G/A Adenomatous polyps may be single or multiple, sessile or pedun- culated, vary in size from less than 1 cm to large, spherical masses with an irregular surface.

M/E The usual appearance is of benign tumour overlying muscularis mucosa and is composed of branching tubules which are embedded in the lamina propria. The lining epithelial cells are of large intestinal type with diminished mucus secreting capacity, large nuclei and increased mitotic activity. However, tubular adenomas may show variable degree of cytologic atypia ranging from atypical epithelium restricted within the glandular basement membrane called as 'carcinoma *in situ*' to invasion into the fibrovascular stromal core.

Malignant transformation is present in about 5% of tubular adenomas; the incidence being higher in larger adenomas.

VILLOUS ADENOMA (VILLOUS PAPILLOMA)

Villous adenomas or villous papillomas of the colon are much less common than tubular adenomas. The mean age at which they appear is 6th decade of life with approximatey equal sex incidence.

G/A Villous adenomas are round to oval exophytic masses, usually sessile, varying in size from 1 to 10 cm or more in diameter.

M/E The characteristic histologic feature is the presence of many slender, finger-like villi, which appear to arise directly from the area of muscularis mucosae. Each of the papillae has fibrovascular stromal core that is covered by epithelial cells varying from apparently benign to anaplastic cells.

Villous adenomas are invariably symptomatic; rectal bleeding, diarrhoea and mucus being the common features. The presence of severe atypia, carcinoma *in situ* and invasive carcinoma are seen more frequently. Invasive carcinoma has been reported in 30% of villous adenomas.

TUBULOVILLOUS ADENOMA
(PAPILLARY ADENOMA, VILLOGLANDULAR ADENOMA)

Tubulovillous adenoma is an intermediate form of pattern between tubular adenoma and villous adenoma.

G/A Tubulovillous adenomas may be sessile or pedunculated and range in size from 0.5-5 cm.

M/E They show intermediate or mixed pattern, characteristic vertical villi and deeper part showing tubular pattern.

The behaviour of tubulovillous adenoma is intermediate between tubular and villous adenomas.

C. FAMILIAL POLYPOSIS SYNDROMES

Familial polyposis syndromes are a group of disorders with multiple polyposis of the colon with autosomal dominant inheritance pattern. Important conditions included in familial polyposis are discussed below:

FAMILIAL POLYPOSIS COLI (ADENOMATOSIS)

This hereditary disease is defined as the presence of more than 100 neoplastic polyps (adenomas) on the mucosal surface of the colon; the average number is about 1000. Adenomatosis can be distinguished from multiple adenomas in which the number of adenomas is fewer, not exceeding 100. The condition has autosomal dominant transmission and is due to germline mutations in *APC* gene which results in occurrence of hundreds of adenomas which progress to invasive cancer. The average age at diagnosis is 2nd and 3rd decades of life with equal incidence in both the sexes.

G/A & M/E The commonest pattern is that of adenomatous polyps (tubular adenomas) discussed above.

The malignant potential of familial polyposis coli is very high. Colorectal cancer develops virtually in 100% of cases by age of 50 years if not treated with colectomy.

GARDNER'S SYNDROME

Gardner's syndrome is combination of familial polyposis coli and certain extra-colonic lesions such as multiple osteomas (particularly of the mandible and maxilla), sebaceous cysts and connective tissue tumours.

TURCOT'S SYNDROME

Turcot's syndrome is combination of familial polyposis coli and malignant neoplasms of the central nervous system.

JUVENILE POLYPOSIS SYNDROME

Juvenile polyposis is appearance of multiple juvenile polyps in the colon, stomach and small intestine but their number is not as high as in familial polyposis coli. Family history in some cases may show autosomal dominant inheritance pattern, while it may be negative in others. They resemble the typical juvenile polyps as regards their age (under 5 years), sex distribution and morphology.

MALIGNANT COLORECTAL TUMOURS

COLORECTAL CARCINOMA

Colorectal cancer comprises 98% of all malignant tumours of the large intestine. It is the commonest form of visceral cancer accounting for deaths from cancer in the United States, next only to lung cancer. The incidence of carcinoma of the large intestine rises with age; average age of patients is about 60 years. Cancer in the rectum is more common in males than females in the ratio of 2:1.

ETIOLOGY A few etiological factors have been implicated:

1. Geographic variations It is much more common in North America and Northern Europe than in South America, Africa and Asia. Colorectal cancer is generally thought to be a disease of affluent societies because its incidence is directly correlated with the socioeconomic status of the countries.

2. Dietary factors Diet plays a significant part in the causation of colorectal cancer:
i) A low intake of vegetable fibre-diet
ii) Consumption of large amounts of fatty foods
iii) Excessive consumption of refined carbohydrates

3. Adenoma-carcinoma sequence There is strong evidence to suggest that colonic adenocarcinoma evolves from pre-existing adenomas, referred to as adenoma-carcinoma sequence. The following evidences are cited to support this hypothesis:
i) In a case with early invasive cancer, the surrounding tissue often shows *preceding changes* of evolution from adenoma→ hyperplasia → dysplasia → carcinoma *in situ* → invasive carcinoma.
ii) *Incidence* of adenomas in a population is directly proportionate to the prevalence of colorectal cancer.
iii) The risk of adenocarcinoma colon declines with *endoscopic removal* of all identified adenomas.
iv) Peak incidence of adenomas generally *precedes* by some years to a few decades the peak incidence for colorectal cancer.
v) The risk of malignancy increases with the following *adenoma-related factors*:
a) *Number of adenomas*: familial polyposis coli syndrome almost certainly evolves into malignancy.
b) *Size of adenomas*: large size increases the risk.
c) *Type of adenomas*: greater villous component associated with higher prevalence.

4. **Hereditary non-polyposis colonic cancer (HNPCC or Lynch syndrome)** HNPCC is an autosomal dominant condition associated with multiple primary cancers at different sites (endometrium, ovary) including colorectal cancer without evidence of familial polyposis coli. In HNPCC, colorectal cancer is seen in at least two generations of first-degree relatives, occurs at a relatively early age (≤ 50 years), located more often in proximal colon, and has better prognosis than sporadic colon cancer cases.

5. **Other factors** Presence of certain pre-existing diseases and some other factors, e.g.:
i)   Inflammatory bowel disease (especially ulcerative colitis).
ii)   Diverticular disease for long duration.
iii) Role of tobacco smoking.

GENETIC BASIS OF COLORECTAL CARCINOGENESIS Studies by molecular genetics have revealed that there are sequential multistep mutations in evolution of colorectal cancer from adenomas by one of the following two mechanisms:

1. **APC mutation/β-catenin mechanism** This pathway of multiple mutations is generally associated with morphologically identifiable changes as described earlier in adenoma-carcinoma sequence. These changes are as under:

i)   *Loss of tumour suppressor APC* (adenomatous polyposis coli) gene located on the long arm of chromosome 5 (5q) is observed in 80% cases of sporadic colon cancer.
ii)   *Point mutation in K-RAS gene*
iii) *Deletion of DCC gene* located on long arm of chromosome 18.
iv)   *Loss of p53 tumour suppressor gene.*

2. **Microsatellite instability mechanism** In this pathway also, there are multiple mutations but of different genes, and unlike APC mutation/β-catenin mechanism, there are no morphologically identifiable changes. This pathway accounts for 10-15% cases of colon cancer. Basic mutation is loss of DNA repair gene. This results in a situation in which repetitive DNA sequences (i.e. microsatellites) become unstable during replication cycle, termed microsatellite instability, which is the hallmark of this pathway. The significant DNA repair genes which are mutated in colon cancer are as under:
i)   *TGF-β receptor gene*
ii)   *BAX gene*

MORPHOLOGIC FEATURES *Distribution* of the primary colorectal cancer reveals that about 60% of the cases occur in the rectum, followed in descending order, by sigmoid and descending colon (25%), caecum and ileocaecal valve (10%); ascending colon, hepatic and splenic flexures (5%); and quite uncommonly in the transverse colon.

G/A There are distinct differences between the growth on the right and left half of the colon.
◈   **Right-sided colonic growths** tend to be large, cauliflower-like, soft and friable masses projecting into the lumen *(fungating polypoid carcinoma).*
◈   **Left-sided colonic growths,** on the other hand, have napkin-ring configuration i.e. they encircle the bowel wall circumferentially with increased fibrous tissue forming annular ring, and have central ulceration on the surface with slightly elevated margins *(carcinomatous ulcers).*

M/E The appearance of right and left-sided growths is similar. About 95% of colorectal carcinomas are adenocarcinomas of varying grades of differentiation, out of which approximately 10% are mucin-secreting colloid carcinomas.

SPREAD Carcinoma of the large intestine may spread by the following routes:

1. **Direct spread** The tumour spreads most commonly by direct extension in both ways—*circumferentially* into the bowel wall as well as *directly* into the depth of the bowel wall.

2. **Lymphatic spread** Spread via lymphatics occurs rather commonly and involves, firstly the regional lymph nodes in the vicinity of the tumour, and then into other groups of lymph nodes.

3. Haematogenous spread Blood spread of large bowel cancer occurs relatively late and involves the liver, lungs, brain, bones and ovary.

CLINICAL FEATURES These appear after considerable time.
i)   Occult bleeding (melaena)
ii)   Change in bowel habits, more often in left-sided growth
iii) Loss of weight (cachexia)
iv) Loss of appetite (anorexia)
v)   Anaemia, weakness, malaise.

The most common *complications* are obstruction and haemorrhage; less often perforation and secondary infection may occur. Aside from the diagnostic methods like stool test for occult blood, PR examination, proctoscopy, radiographic contrast studies and CT scan, recently the role of tumour-markers has been emphasised. Of particular importance is the estimation of carcinoembryonic antigen (CEA) level which is elevated in 100% cases of metastatic colorectal cancers. CEA levels are elevated in some non-neoplastic conditions also like in ulcerative colitis, pancreatitis and alcoholic cirrhosis.

STAGING AND PROGNOSIS The *prognosis* of colorectal cancer depends upon a few variables:
i)   Extent of the bowel involvement
ii)   Presence or absence of metastases
iii) Histologic grade of the tumour
iv) Location of the tumour

The most important prognostic factor in colorectal cancer is, however, the *stage* of the disease at the time of diagnosis. Three staging systems are in use:
1.   *Dukes' ABC staging* (modified Duke's includes stage D as well).
2.   *Astler-Coller staging* which is a further modification of Duke's staging and is most widely used.
3.   *TNM staging* described by American Joint Committee is also used.

TUMOURS OF THE ANAL CANAL

Epithelial tumours of the anal canal are uncommon and may be combination of several histological types. Amongst the *benign tumours* of the anal canal, multiple viral warts called as condyloma acuminata are the only tumours of note. *Malignant tumours* of the anal canal include the following:
1.   Squamous cell carcinoma
2.   Basaloid carcinoma
3.   Mucoepidermoid carcinoma
4.   Adenocarcinoma (rectal, of anal glands, within anorectal fistulas)
5.   Undifferentiated carcinoma
6.   Malignant melanoma.

PERITONEUM (p. 574)

NORMAL STRUCTURE

The peritoneal cavity is lined by a layer of surface mesothelium derived from mesoderm. The lining rests on vascularised subserosal fibrous tissue. Other structures topographically related to peritoneum are retroperitoneum, omentum, mesentery and umbilicus. These structures are involved in a variety of pathologic states but a few important conditions as follows.

PERITONITIS (p. 574)

1.   Chemical peritonitis can be caused by the following:
◈   *Bile* extravasated due to trauma or diseases of the gallbladder.
◈   *Pancreatic secretions* released from pancreas in acute haemorrhagic pancreatitis.
◈   *Gastric juice* leaked from perforation of stomach.
◈   *Barium sulfate* from perforation of bowel during radiographic studies.

❖ Chemical peritonitis is localised or generalised sterile inflammation of the peritoneum.

2. Bacterial peritonitis may be primary or secondary; the latter being more common.

Primary form is caused by streptococcal infection, especially in children. *Secondary* bacterial peritonitis may occur from the following disorders:

- i) Appendicitis
- ii) Cholecystitis
- iii) Salpingitis
- iv) Rupture of peptic ulcer
- v) Gangrene of bowel
- vi) Tuberculosis (specific inflammation).

TUMOUR-LIKE LESIONS AND TUMOURS *(p. 575)*

Idiopathic Retroperitoneal Fibrosis

This rare entity of unknown etiology is characterised by diffuse fibrous overgrowth and chronic inflammation. The condition is, therefore, more like inflammatory rather than neoplastic in origin. It may be associated with similar process in the mediastinum, sclerosing cholangitis and Riedel's thyroiditis and termed *multifocal fibrosclerosis*. Though idiopathic, the etiologic role of ergot derivative drugs and autoimmune reaction has been suggested.

Mesenteric Cysts

Mesenteric cysts of unknown etiology and varying sizes may be found in the peritoneal cavity. On the basis of their possible origin, they are of various types:

1. Chylous cyst
2. Pseudocysts
3. Neoplastic cysts

Tumours

Peritoneum may be involved in malignant tumours—primary and metastatic.

❖ **Mesothelioma** is an example of primary peritoneal tumour (benign and malignant) and is similar in morphology as in pleural cavity.

❖ **Intra-abdominal desmoplastic small cell tumour** is a recently described highly malignant tumour belonging to the group of other round cell or blue cell tumours such as small cell carcinoma lung, Ewing's sarcoma, rhabdomyosarcoma, neuroblastoma and others.

❖ **Metastatic peritoneal tumours** are quite common and may occur from dissemination from any intra-abdominal malignancy.

SELF ASSESSMENT

1. **The distance from the incisor teeth to the gastro-oesophageal junction is:**
   A. 25 cm   B. 30 cm
   C. 35 cm   D. 40 cm
2. **Oesophageal webs have the following features <u>except</u>:**
   A. They are located at lower oesophagus
   B. They are associated with dysphagia
   C. They are associated with chronic atrophic glossitis
   D. They are associated with iron deficiency anaemia
3. **Some of the common causes of haematemesis of oesophageal origin are as follows <u>except</u>:**
   A. Oesophageal varices
   B. Mallory-Weiss syndrome
   C. Reflux oesophagitis
   D. Oesophageal rupture

4. Some common conditions predisposing to reflux oesophagitis are as follows except:
   A. Hiatus hernia
   B. Mallory-Weiss syndrome
   C. Peptic ulcers
   D. Persistent vomiting

5. The nature of lesion in Barrett's oesophagus is:
   A. Congenital anomaly
   B. Inflammatory disease
   C. Metaplastic process
   D. Neoplastic lesion

6. Barrett's oesophagus predisposes to development of:
   A. Reflux oesophagitis
   B. Oesophageal varices
   C. Squamous cell carcinoma
   D. Adenocarcinoma

7. The most frequent anatomic site for squamous cell carcinoma of the oesophagus is:
   A. Upper third
   B. Middle third
   C. Lower third
   D. Gastro-oesophageal junction

8. H. pylori gastritis has the following features except:
   A. H. pylori is seen on the epithelial layer of the luminal surface
   B. H. pylori is seen on areas with intestinal metaplasia
   C. H. pylori does not invade the mucosa
   D. H. pylori gastritis may lead to malignant transformation

9. Patients of benign gastric ulcer generally have:
   A. High gastric acid
   B. Normal-to-high gastric acid
   C. Normal-to-low gastric acid
   D. Absence of gastric acid

10. Duodenal ulcers are found most commonly at:
    A. First part, anterior surface
    B. First part, posterior surface
    C. Second part, anterior surface
    D. Second part, posterior surface

11. The most common location for gastric colloid carcinoma is:
    A. Cardia
    B. Fundus
    C. Body
    D. Pylorus

12. The most common gross growth pattern of gastric carcinoma is:
    A. Scirrhous
    B. Fungating
    C. Ulcerative
    D. Colloid

13. Meckel's diverticulum is commonly located at:
    A. Mesenteric border of small intestine one meter above ileocaecal valve
    B. Mesenteric border of small intestine two meter above ileocaecal valve
    C. Antimesenteric border of small intestine one meter above ileocaecal valve
    D. Antimesenteric border of small intestine two meter above ileocaecal valve

14. The remnants of vitellointestinal duct are in the form of following lesions except:
    A. Vitelline sinus
    B. Vitelline cyst
    C. Omphalocele
    D. Meckel's diverticulum

15. Following humoral factors are implicated in the etiology of inflammatory bowel disease except:
    A. Anti-colon antibodies to E. coli
    B. Decreased synthesis of IgG
    C. IgE-mediated hypersensitivity
    D. Circulating immune complexes

16. Crohn's disease is characterised by the following histopathologic features **except**:
    A. Non-caseating sarcoid like granulomas
    B. Superficial mucosal ulceration
    C. Stricture formation in chronic cases
    D. Widening of submucosa due to oedema

17. The following features characterise ulcerative colitis **except**:
    A. Formation of crypt abscess and cryptitis
    B. Superficial mucosal ulceration
    C. Depletion of goblet cells and mucus
    D. Stricture formation in chronic cases

18. Long-standing cases of Crohn's disease may develop the following complications **except**:
    A. Malabsorption
    B. Toxic megacolon
    C. Fistula formation
    D. Stricture formation

19. Tuberculous ulcers in bowel have the following features **except**:
    A. They begin in the Peyer's patches
    B. They are transverse to the long axis
    C. Advanced cases may cause intestinal obstruction
    D. Tuberculous ulcers often cause intestinal perforation

20. The major complication of typhoid ulcer is:
    A. Intestinal obstruction
    B. Intestinal perforation
    C. Malabsorption
    D. Fistula formation

21. Pseudomembranous enterocolitis occurs most often in association with the following:
    A. Shigella dysentery
    B. Candida enterocolitis
    C. Cephalosporin antibiotics
    D. Clostridial food poisoning

22. Common causes of total/subtotal villous atrophy are as follows **except**:
    A. Crohn's disease
    B. Tropical sprue
    C. Nontropical sprue
    D. Intestinal lymphoma

23. The nature of Whipple's disease is:
    A. Genetic defect
    B. Familial occurrence
    C. Bacterial infection
    D. Hypersensitivity reaction

24. The most common location for carcinoid tumour is:
    A. Foregut
    B. Midgut
    C. Hindgut
    D. Equal at all these three sites

25. The histologic hallmark of diagnosis of acute appendicitis is:
    A. Mucosal ulceration
    B. Impacted foreign body
    C. Neutrophilic infiltrate in muscularis
    D. Thrombosed blood vessels

26. Out of various patterns of Hirschsprung's disease, the most common is:
    A. Total colonic aganglionosis
    B. Long segment disease
    C. Short segment disease
    D. Ultra short segment disease

27. The following type of colorectal polyps has the maximum incidence of malignant transformation:
    A. Hyperplastic polyp
    B. Adenomatous
    C. Villous adenoma
    D. Tubulovillous adenoma

28. The most common location for primary colorectal carcinoma is:
    A. Rectum
    B. Sigmoid and descending colon
    C. Caecum and ileocaecal valve
    D. Ascending colon

29. Elevation of carcinoembryonic antigen (CEA) level is particularly significant in:
   A. Early lesion of colorectal carcinoma
   B. Advanced primary colorectal carcinoma
   C. Metastatic colorectal carcinoma
   D. Ulcerative colitis

30. Intra-abdominal desmoplastic small cell tumour is a:
   A. Benign tumour
   B. Fibromatosis
   C. Tumour-like lesion
   D. Highly malignant tumour

31. The significant genetic mutations in adenoma-carcinoma sequence are all the following except:
   A. Loss of APC gene
   B. Deletion of DCC gene
   C. Mutated RB gene
   D. Mutation in K-RAS gene

32. H. pylori colonisation of gastric mucosa is implicated in the following diseases except:
   A. Gastritis
   B. Gastric carcinoma
   C. MALT lymphoma
   D. Intestinal metaplasia

33. Which of the following is not implicated in oesophageal carcinoma?
   A. HPV infection
   B. Mallory-Weiss Syndrome
   C. Plummer-Vinson Syndrome
   D. Heavy smoking

34. In gastric ulcer, BAO and MAO are:
   A. Normal
   B. Elevated
   C. Absent
   D. Markedly decreased but not absent

35. Which classification system is used for gastritis?
   A. Bethesda system
   B. Geneva system
   C. Sydney system
   D. WHO system

36. Partial villous atrophy is seen in all except:
   A. Crohn's disease
   B. Parasitic infestation
   C. Drugs
   D. Tropical sprue

37. Most common malignant tumour of the small intestine is:
   A. Carcinoid tumour
   B. Lymphoma
   C. Adenocarcinoma
   D. Malignant GIST

38. All are hamartomatous polyps except:
   A. Juvenile polyps
   B. Peutz-Jeghers polyps
   C. Retention polyps
   D. Metaplastic polyps

39. Which of the following is not familial polyposis syndrome?
   A. Cronkhite Canada syndrome
   B. Gardner's syndrome
   C. Turcot's syndrome
   D. Juvenile polyposis syndrome

40. Disease predisposing locus implicated in Crohn's disease:
   A. CARD 15
   B. CARD 14
   C. CARD 24
   D. CARD 25

KEY

1 = D	2 = A	3 = C	4 = B	5 = C
6 = D	7 = B	8 = B	9 = C	10 = A
11 = B	12 = C	13 = C	14 = C	15 = B
16 = B	17 = D	18 = B	19 = D	20 = B
21 = C	22 = A	23 = C	24 = B	25 = C
26 = C	27 = C	28 = A	29 = C	30 = D
31 = C	32 = D	33 = B	34 = A	35 = C
36 = D	37 = A	38 = D	39 = A	40 = A

19 The Liver, Biliary Tract and Exocrine Pancreas

LIVER (p. 577)

NORMAL STRUCTURE

ANATOMY The liver is the largest organ in the body weighing 1400-1600 gm in the males and 1200-1400 gm in the females. There are 2 main anatomical lobes—right and left, the right being about six times the size of the left lobe. The right and left lobes are separated anteriorly by a fold of peritoneum called the *falciform ligament,* inferiorly by the fissure for the *ligamentum teres,* and posteriorly by the fissure for the *ligamentum venosum.*

The *porta hepatis* is the region on the inferior surface of the right lobe where blood vessels, lymphatics and common hepatic duct form the hilum of the liver. A firm smooth layer of connective tissue called *Glisson's capsule* encloses the liver and is continuous with the connective tissue of the porta hepatis forming a sheath around the structures in the porta hepatis. The liver has a double blood supply—the portal vein brings the venous blood from the intestines and spleen, and the hepatic artery coming from the coeliac axis supplies arterial blood to the liver. This dual blood supply provides sufficient protection against infarction in the liver.

HISTOLOGY The hepatic parenchyma is composed of numerous hexagonal or pyramidal *classical lobules,* each with a diameter of 0.5 to 2 mm. Each classical lobule has a central tributary from the hepatic vein and at the periphery are 4 to 5 portal tracts or triads containing branches of bile duct, portal vein and hepatic artery. Cords of hepatocytes and blood-containing sinusoids radiate from the central vein to the peripheral portal triads.

The blood supply to the liver parenchyma flows from the portal triads to the central veins. Accordingly, the hepatic parenchyma of liver lobule is divided into 3 zones:

◆ **Zone 1** or the *periportal (peripheral) area* is closest to the arterial and portal blood supply and hence bears the brunt of all forms of toxic injury.

◆ **Zone 3** or the *centrilobular area* surrounds the central vein and is most remote from the blood supply and thus suffers from the effects of hypoxic injury.

◆ **Zone 2** is the intermediate *midzonal area.*

The **hepatocytes** are polygonal cells with a round single nucleus and a prominent nucleolus. The liver cells have a remarkable capability to undergo mitosis and regeneration. A hepatocyte has 3 surfaces: *one* facing the sinusoid and the space of Disse, the *second* facing the canaliculus, and the *third* facing neighbouring hepatocytes.

The blood-containing *sinusoids* between cords of hepatocytes are lined by discontinuous endothelial cells and scattered flat Kupffer cells belonging to the reticuloendothelial system.

The *space of Disse* is the space between hepatocytes and sinusoidal lining endothelial cells. A few scattered fat storing *Ito cells* lie within the space of Disse.

The *portal triad or tract* besides containing portal vein radicle, the hepatic arteriole and bile duct, has a few mononuclear cells and scanty connective tissue considered to be extension of Glisson's capsule. The portal triads are surrounded by a limiting plate of hepatocytes.

The *intrahepatic biliary system* begins with the bile canaliculi interposed between the adjacent hepatocytes.

FUNCTIONS The liver performs multifold functions:

1. Manufacture and excretion of bile.
2. Manufacture of several major plasma proteins such as albumin, fibrinogen and prothrombin.
3. Metabolism of proteins, carbohydrates and lipids.
4. Storage of vitamins (A, D and B_{12}) and iron.
5. Detoxification of toxic substances such as alcohol and drugs.

LIVER FUNCTION TESTS (p. 578)

In view of multiplicity and complexity of the liver functions, it is obvious that no single test can establish the disturbance in liver function. Thus a battery of liver function tests is employed for accurate diagnosis, to assess the severity of damage, to judge prognosis and to evaluate therapy. A summary of various liver function tests is given below:

	TESTS	SIGNIFICANCE
I.	TESTS FOR MANUFACTURE AND EXCRETION OF BILE	
1.	*Bilirubin:*	
	i) Serum bilirubin (0.3-1.3 mg/dl)	Increased in hepatocellular, obstructive and haemolytic disease, Gilbert's disease
	ii) In faeces	Absent in biliary obstruction
	iii) In urine	Conjugated bilirubinuria in patients of hepatitis
2.	*Urobilinogen:*	Increased in hepatocellular and haemolytic diseases, absent in biliary obstruction
3.	*Bile acid (Bile salts):*	Increased in serum and detectable in urine in cholestasis
II.	SERUM ENZYME ASSAYS	
1.	*Alkaline phosphatase* (33-96 U/L)	Increased in hepatobiliary disease (highest in biliary obstruction), bone diseases, pregnancy
2.	*γ-Glutamyl transpeptidase (γ-GT)* (9-58 IU/L)	Rise parallels alkaline phosphatase but is specific for hepatobiliary diseases
3.	*Transaminases:*	
	i) SGOT (AST) (12-38 U/L)	Increased in tissue injury to liver as well as to other tissues like in MI
	ii) SGPT (ALT) (7-41 U/L)	Increase is fairly specific for liver cell injury
4.	*Other enzymes:*	
	i) 5'-Nucleotidase	Rise parallels alkaline phosphatase but more specific for diseases of hepatic origin
	ii) Lactate dehydrogenase (115-221 U/L)	Increased in tumours involving the liver
	iii) Cholinesterase	Decreased in hepatocellular disease, malnutrition
III.	TESTS FOR METABOLIC FUNCTIONS	
1.	*Amino acid and protein metabolism:*	
	i) Serum proteins (total = 6.7-8.6 g/dl; A/G ratio = 1.5-3:1)	Hypoalbuminaemia in hepatocellular diseases; hyperglobulinaemia in cirrhosis and chronic active hepatitis
	ii) Immuno-globulins	Nonspecific alterations in IgA, IgG and IgM

	iii)	Clotting factors	PT and APTT prolonged in hepatocellular disease
	iv)	Plasma ammonia (19-60 µg/dl)	Increased in acute fulminant hepatitis, cirrhosis, hepatic encephalopathy
	v)	Aminoaciduria	In fulminant hepatitis

2. *Lipid and lipoprotein metabolism:*

Blood lipids (total serum cholesterol <200 mg/dl; triglycerides < 150 mg/dl; and lipoprotein fractions)	Increased in cholestasis, decreased in acute and chronic diffuse liver disease

3. *Carbohydrate metabolism:*

Blood glucose and GTT	Decreased in hepatic necrosis

IV. IMMUNOLOGIC TESTS

1. *Nonspecific immunologic reactions:*

	i)	Smooth muscle antibody	In hepatic necrosis
	ii)	Mitochondrial antibody	In primary biliary cirrhosis
	iii)	Antinuclear antibody and LE cell test	In chronic active hepatitis

2. *Antibodies to specific etiologic agents:*

	i)	Antibodies to hepatitis B (HBsAg, HBc, HBeAg)	In hepatitis B
	ii)	Amoeba antibodies	Amoebic liver abscess

V. ANCILLARY DIAGNOSTIC TESTS

1.	*Ultrasound examination*	Cholestasis of various etiologies; SOLs, US-guided-FNAC/liver biopsy
2.	*FNAC and/ or percutaneous liver biopsy*	Unknown cause of hepatocellular disease, hepatomegaly and splenomegaly; long-standing hepatitis; PUO and SOLs of the liver

JAUNDICE—GENERAL *(p. 581)*

Jaundice or icterus refers to the yellow pigmentation of the skin or sclerae by bilirubin. Bilirubin pigment has high affinity for elastic tissue and hence jaundice is particularly noticeable in tissues rich in elastin content. Jaundice is the result of elevated levels of bilirubin in the blood termed hyperbilirubinaemia. Normal serum bilirubin concentration ranges from 0.3-1.3 mg/dl, about 80% of which is unconjugated. Jaundice becomes clinically evident when the total serum bilirubin exceeds 2 mg/dl. A rise of serum bilirubin between the normal and 2 mg/dl is generally not accompanied by visible jaundice and is called *latent jaundice*.

Normal metabolism of bilirubin can be conveniently described under 4 main headings:

1. SOURCE OF BILIRUBIN About 80-85% of the bilirubin is derived from the catabolism of haemoglobin present in senescent red blood cells. The remaining 15-20% of the bilirubin comes partly from non-haemoglobin haem-containing pigments such as myoglobin, catalase and cytochromes, and partly from ineffective erythropoiesis.

2. TRANSPORT OF BILIRUBIN Bilirubin on release from macrophages circulates as unconjugated bilirubin in plasma tightly bound to albumin.

3. HEPATIC PHASE On coming in contact with the hepatocyte surface, unconjugated bilirubin is preferentially metabolised which involves 3 steps:

i) Hepatic uptake Albumin-bound unconjugated bilirubin upon entry into the hepatocyte, is dissociated into bilirubin and albumin. The bilirubin gets bound to cytoplasmic protein *glutathione-S-transferase (GST)* (earlier called ligandin).

ii) Conjugation Unconjugated bilirubin is not water-soluble but is alcohol-soluble and is converted into water-soluble compound by conjugation. Conjugation occurs in endoplasmic reticulum and involves conversion to bilirubin mono- and diglucuronide by the action of microsomal enzyme, *bilirubin- UDP-glucuronosyl transferase*.

iii) Secretion into bile Conjugated (water-soluble) bilirubin is rapidly transported directly into bile canaliculi by energy-dependent process and then excreted into the bile.

4. INTESTINAL PHASE Appearance of conjugated bilirubin in the intestinal lumen is followed by either direct excretion in the stool as stercobilinogen which imparts the normal yellow colour to stool, or may be metabolised to urobilinogen by the action of intestinal bacteria. Some of the absorbed urobilinogen in resecreted by the liver into the bile while the rest is excreted in the urine as urobilinogen.

The major differences between unconjugated and conjugated bilirubin are as under:

	FEATURE	UNCONJUGATED BILIRUBIN	CONJUGATED BILIRUBIN
1.	Normal serum level	More	Less (less than 0.25 mg/dl)
2.	Water solubility	Absent	Present
3.	Affinity to lipids (alcohol solubility)	Present	Absent
4.	Serum albumin binding	High	Low
5.	van den Bergh reaction	Indirect (Total minus direct)	Direct
6.	Renal excretion	Absent	Present
7.	Bilirubin albumin covalent complex formation	Absent	Present
8.	Affinity to brain tissue	Present (Kernicterus)	Absent

TYPES OF LIVER CELL NECROSIS

All forms of injury to the liver such as microbiologic, toxic, circulatory or traumatic, result in necrosis of liver cells. The extent of involvement of hepatic lobule in necrosis varies. Accordingly, liver cell necrosis is divided into 3 types:

1. **DIFFUSE (SUBMASSIVE TO MASSIVE) NECROSIS** When there is extensive and diffuse necrosis of the liver involving all the cells in groups of lobules, it is termed diffuse, or submassive to massive necrosis. It is most commonly caused by viral hepatitis or drug toxicity.

2. **ZONAL NECROSIS** Zonal necrosis is necrosis of hepatocytes in 3 different zones of the hepatic lobule. Accordingly, it is of 3 types; each type affecting respective zone is caused by different etiologic factors:

i) **Centrilobular necrosis** is the commonest type involving hepatocytes in zone 3 (i.e. located around the central vein). Centrilobular necrosis is characteristic feature of ischaemic injury such as in shock and CHF since zone 3 is farthest from the blood supply.

ii) **Midzonal necrosis** is uncommon and involves zone 2 of the hepatic lobule. This pattern of necrosis is seen in yellow fever and viral hepatitis.

iii) **Periportal (peripheral) necrosis** is seen in zone 1 involving the parenchyma closest to the arterial and portal blood supply. Since zone 1 is most well perfused, it is most vulnerable to the effects of circulating hepato-toxins.

3. **FOCAL NECROSIS** This form of necrosis involves small groups of hepatocytes irregularly distributed in the hepatic lobule. Focal necrosis is most often caused by microbiologic infections.

CLASSIFICATION AND FEATURES OF JAUNDICE

Based on pathophysiology, jaundice may result from one or more of the following mechanisms:
1. Increased bilirubin production
2. Decreased hepatic uptake
3. Decreased hepatic conjugation
4. Decreased excretion of bilirubin into bile

Accordingly, a simple age-old classification of jaundice was to divide it into 3 predominant types: *pre-hepatic (haemolytic), hepatic,* and *post-hepatic cholestatic.* However, hyperbilirubinaemia due to first three mechanisms is *mainly unconjugated* while the last variety yields *mainly conjugated* hyper-bilirubinaemia. Hence, currently pathophysiologic classification of jaundice is based on predominance of the type of hyperbilirubinaemia. The presence of bilirubin in the urine is evidence of conjugated hyperbilirubinaemia.

I. *PREDOMINANTLY UNCONJUGATED HYPERBILIRUBINAEMIA*

This form of jaundice can result from the following three sets of conditions:

1. **INCREASED BILIRUBIN PRODUCTION (HAEMOLYTIC, ACHOL-URIC OR PREHEPATIC JAUNDICE)** This results from excessive red cell destruction as occurs in intra- and extravascular haemolysis or due to ineffective erythropoiesis. There is increased release of haemoglobin from excessive breakdown of red cells that leads to overproduction of bilirubin.

Laboratory data in haemolytic jaundice, in addition to predominant unconjugated hyperbilirubinaemia, reveal normal serum levels of transaminases, alkaline phosphatase and proteins. Bile pigment being unconjugated type is absent from urine (acholuric jaundice). However, there is dark brown colour of stools due to excessive faecal excretion of bile pigment and there is increased urinary excretion of urobilinogen.

2. **DECREASED HEPATIC UPTAKE** The uptake of bilirubin by the hepatocyte that involves dissociation of the pigment from albumin and its binding to cytoplasmic protein, GST or ligandin, may be deranged in certain conditions e.g. due to drugs, prolonged starvation and sepsis.

3. **DECREASED BILIRUBIN CONJUGATION** This mechanism involves deranged hepatic conjugation due to defect or deficiency of the enzyme,

glucuronosyl transferase. This can occur in certain inherited disorders of the enzyme, or acquired defects in its activity. However, hepatocellular damage causes deranged excretory capacity of the liver more than its conjugating capacity.

II. PREDOMINANTLY CONJUGATED HYPERBILIRUBINAEMIA (CHOLESTASIS)

This form of hyperbilirubinaemia is defined as failure of normal amounts of bile to reach the duodenum. Morphologically, cholestasis means accumulation of bile in liver cells and biliary passages. The defect in excretion may be within the biliary canaliculi of the hepatocyte and in the microscopic bile ducts *(intrahepatic cholestasis or medical jaundice)*, or there may be mechanical obstruction to the extrahepatic biliary excretory apparatus *(extrahepatic cholestasis or obstructive jaundice)*.

1. INTRAHEPATIC CHOLESTASIS Intrahepatic cholestasis is due to impaired hepatic excretion of bile and may occur from hereditary or acquired disorders.

i) **Hereditary disorders** producing intrahepatic obstruction to biliary excretion are characterised by *'pure cholestasis'* e.g. in Dubin-Johnson syndrome, Rotor syndrome, fibrocystic disease of pancreas, benign familial recurrent cholestasis, intrahepatic atresia and cholestatic jaundice of pregnancy.

ii) **Acquired disorders** with intrahepatic excretory defect of bilirubin are largely due to hepatocellular diseases and hence are termed *'hepatocellular cholestasis'* e.g. in viral hepatitis, alcoholic hepatitis, and drug-induced cholestasis such as from administration of chlorpromazine and oral contraceptives.

The **features** of intrahepatic cholestasis include: predominant conjugated hyperbilirubinaemia due to regurgitation of conjugated bilirubin into blood, bilirubinuria, elevated levels of serum bile acids and consequent pruritus, elevated serum alkaline phosphatase, hyperlipidaemia and hypoprothrombinaemia. 'Pure cholestasis' can be distinguished from 'hepatocellular cholestasis' by elevated serum levels of transaminases in the latter due to liver cell injury.

◈ **Liver biopsy** in cases with intrahepatic cholestasis reveals milder degree of cholestasis than the extrahepatic disorders. The biliary canaliculi of the hepatocytes are dilated and contain characteristic elongated green-brown *bile plugs*.

2. EXTRAHEPATIC CHOLESTASIS Extrahepatic cholestasis results from mechanical obstruction to large bile ducts outside the liver or within the porta hepatis. The common causes are gallstones, inflammatory strictures, carcinoma head of pancreas, tumours of bile duct, sclerosing cholangitis and congenital atresia of extrahepatic ducts.

The **features** of extrahepatic cholestasis (obstructive jaundice), like in intrahepatic cholestasis, are: predominant conjugated hyperbilirubinaemia, bilirubinuria, elevated serum bile acids causing intense pruritus, high serum alkaline phosphatase and hyperlipidaemia. However, there are certain features which help to distinguish extrahepatic from intrahepatic cholestasis. In obstructive jaundice, there is malabsorption of fat-soluble vitamins (A, D, E and K) and steatorrhoea resulting in vitamin K deficiency. Prolonged prothrombin time in such cases shows improvement following parenteral administration of vitamin K.

◈ **Liver biopsy** in cases with extrahepatic cholestasis shows more marked changes of cholestasis. Since the obstruction is in the extrahepatic bile ducts, there is progressive retrograde extension of bile stasis into intrahepatic duct system. This results in dilatation of bile ducts and rupture of canaliculi with extravasation of bile producing *bile lakes*.

NEONATAL JAUNDICE (p. 585)

Jaundice appears in neonates when the total serum bilirubin is more than 3 mg/dl. It may be the result of unconjugated or conjugated

A. UNCONJUGATED HYPERBILIRUBINAEMIA
1. Physiologic and prematurity jaundice
2. Haemolytic disease of the newborn and kernicterus
3. Congenital haemolytic disorders
4. Perinatal complications (e.g. haemorrhage, sepsis)
5. Gilbert's syndrome
6. Crigler-Najjar syndrome (type I and II)

B. CONJUGATED HYPERBILIRUBINAEMIA
1. Hereditary (Dubin-Johnson syndrome, Rotor's syndrome)
2. Infections (e.g. hepatitis B, hepatitis C or non-A non-B hepatitis, rubella, coxsackievirus, cytomegalovirus, echovirus, herpes simplex, syphilis, toxoplasma, gram-negative sepsis)
3. Metabolic (e.g. galactosaemia, alpha-1-antitrypsin deficiency, cystic fibrosis, Niemann-Pick disease)
4. Idiopathic (neonatal hepatitis, congenital hepatic fibrosis)
5. Biliary atresia (intrahepatic and extrahepatic)
6. Reye's syndrome

HEREDITARY NON-HAEMOLYTIC HYPERBILIRUBINAEMIAS

Hereditary non-haemolytic hyperbilirubinaemias are a small group of uncommon familial disorders of bilirubin metabolism when haemolytic causes have been excluded. The commonest is Gilbert's syndrome; others are Crigler-Najjar syndrome, Dubin-Johnson syndrome, Rotor's syndrome, benign recurrent intrahepatic cholestasis and progressive familial intrahepatic cholestasis. The features common to all these conditions are presence of icterus but almost normal liver function tests and no well-defined morphologic changes except in Dubin-Johnson syndrome. Gilbert's syndrome and Crigler-Najjar syndrome are examples of *hereditary non-haemolytic unconjugated hyperbilirubinaemia*, whereas Dubin-Johnson syndrome, Rotor's syndrome and benign familial recurrent cholestasis are conditions with *hereditary conjugated hyperbilirubinaemia*.

NEONATAL HEPATITIS

Neonatal hepatitis, also termed giant cell hepatitis or neonatal hepatocellular cholestasis, is a general term used for the constant morphologic change seen in conjugated hyperbilirubinaemia as a result of known infectious and metabolic causes, or may have an idiopathic etiology. 'Idiopathic' neonatal hepatitis is more common and accounts for 75% of cases. The condition usually presents in the first week of birth with jaundice, bilirubinuria, pale stools and high serum alkaline phosphatase.

MORPHOLOGIC FEATURES These are as under:
1. Loss of normal lobular architecture of the liver.
2. Presence of prominent multinucleate giant cells derived from hepatocytes.
3. Mononuclear inflammatory cell infiltrate in the portal tracts with some periportal fibrosis.
4. Haemosiderosis.
5. Cholestasis in small proliferated ductules in the portal tract and between necrotic liver cells.

BILIARY ATRESIAS

Biliary atresias, also called as *infantile cholangiopathies*, are a group of intrauterine developmental abnormalities of the biliary system. Depending upon the portion of biliary system involved, biliary atresias may be extrahepatic or intrahepatic.

EXTRAHEPATIC BILIARY ATRESIA

The extrahepatic bile ducts fail to develop normally so that in some cases the bile ducts are *absent* at birth, while in others the ducts may have been formed but start undergoing sclerosis in the perinatal period. Cholestatic jaundice appears by the first week after birth. The baby has severe pruritus, pale stools, dark urine and elevated serum transaminases. Death is usually due to intercurrent infection, liver failure, and bleeding due to vitamin K deficiency or oesophageal varices. Cirrhosis and ascites are late complications appearing within 2 years of age.

INTRAHEPATIC BILIARY ATRESIA

Intrahepatic biliary atresia is characterised by biliary hypoplasia so that there is *paucity of bile ducts* rather than their complete absence. The condition probably has its origin in viral infection acquired during intrauterine period or in the neonatal period. Cholestatic jaundice usually appears within the first few days of birth and is characterised by high serum bile acids with associated pruritus, and hypercholesterolaemia with appearance of xanthomas by first year of life.

REYE'S SYNDROME

Reye's syndrome is defined as an acute postviral syndrome of encephalo-pathy and fatty change in the viscera. The syndrome may follow almost any known viral disease but is most common after influenza A or B and varicella. Viral infection may act singly, but more often its effect is modified by certain exogenous factors such as by administration of salicylates, aflatoxins and insecticides.

The patients are generally children between 6 months and 15 years of age. Within a week after a viral illness, the child develops intractable vomiting and progressive neurological deterioration due to encephalopathy, eventually leading to stupor, coma and death.

G/A The liver is enlarged and yellowish-orange.

M/E Hepatocytes show small droplets of neutral fat in their cytoplasm (microvesicular fat). Similar fatty change is seen in the renal tubular epithelium and in the cells of skeletal muscles and heart.

HEPATIC FAILURE (p. 587)

Though the liver has a marked regenerative capacity and a large functional reserve, hepatic failure may develop from severe acute and fulminant liver injury with massive necrosis of liver cells *(acute hepatic failure)*, or from advanced chronic liver disease *(chronic hepatic failure)*.

ETIOLOGY Acute and chronic hepatic failure result from different causes:

◈ **Acute (fulminant) hepatic failure** occurs most frequently in *acute viral hepatitis*. Other causes are hepatotoxic drug reactions (e.g. anaesthetic agents, nonsteroidal anti-inflammatory drugs, anti-depressants), carbon tetrachloride poisoning, acute alcoholic hepatitis, mushroom poisoning and pregnancy complicated with eclampsia.

◈ **Chronic hepatic failure** is most often due to *cirrhosis*. Other causes include chronic active hepatitis, chronic cholestasis (cholestatic jaundice) and Wilson's disease.

MANIFESTATIONS In view of the diverse functions performed by the liver, the syndrome of acute or chronic hepatic failure produces complex manifestations.

1. Jaundice
2. Hepatic encephalopathy (Hepatic coma)
3. Hyperkinetic circulation
4. Hepatorenal syndrome
5. Hepatopulmonary syndrome
6. Coagulation defects
7. Ascites and oedema
8. Endocrine changes
9. Skin changes
10. Foetor hepaticus

I. HEPATIC VENOUS OBSTRUCTION

The central veins of lobules of the liver are tributaries of the hepatic veins. In the normal liver, there are no anastomoses between hepatic vein and portal vein but in cirrhotic liver there are such anastomoses.

Three uncommon diseases produced by obstruction of the hepatic veins: are Budd-Chiari syndrome (hepatic vein thrombosis), hepatic veno-occlusive disease and bacillary angiomatosis-peliosis hepatis.

BUDD-CHIARI SYNDROME (HEPATIC VEIN THROMBOSIS)

Budd-Chiari syndrome in its pure form consists of slowly developing thrombosis of the hepatic veins and the adjacent inferior vena cava, while some workers include hepatic veno-occlusive disease in this syndrome.

ETIOLOGY The etiology of hepatic venous thrombosis in about a third of cases is unknown (idiopathic), while in the remaining cases various causes associated with increased thrombotic tendencies are attributed:
i) Polycythaemia vera
ii) Paroxysmal nocturnal haemoglobinuria
iii) Use of oral contraceptives
iv) Pregnancy and postpartum state
v) Intra-abdominal cancers (e.g. hepatocellular carcinoma)
vi) Chemotherapy and radiation
vii) Myeloproliferative diseases
viii) Formation of membranous webs in the suprahepatic portion of inferior vena cava (either congenital or as a consequence of organised thrombosis).

CLINICAL FEATURES Budd-Chiari syndrome is clinically characterised by either an acute form or chronic form depending upon the speed of occlusion.
❖ In the *acute form,* the features are abdominal pain, vomiting, enlarged liver, ascites and mild icterus.
❖ In the more usual *chronic form,* the patients present with pain over enlarged tender liver, ascites and other features of portal hypertension.

HEPATIC VENO-OCCLUSIVE DISEASE

Hepatic veno-occlusive disease consists of intimal thickening, stenosis and obliteration of the terminal central veins and medium-sized hepatic veins. The venous occlusion results in pathologic changes similar to those of Budd-Chiari syndrome and can be distinguished from the latter by demonstration of absence of thrombosis in the major hepatic veins.

The etiology of hepatic veno-occlusive disease can be explained by following associations:
i) Hepatotoxic alkaloids.
ii) High doze chemotherapy administered before bone marrow transplantation.
iii) As part of a rare hereditary veno-occlusive disease with immuno-deficiency.

BACILLARY ANGIOMATOSIS AND PELIOSIS HEPATIS

Although sinusoidal dilatation can occur secondary to many liver diseases, peliosis hepatis is an uncommon condition of primary sinusoidal dilatation that results in blockage of blood outflow and may result in massive intraperitoneal haemorrhage. Although exact etiology is not known, peliosis hepatis and another related condition, bacillary angiomatosis, have been found to occur in HIV-infected patients whose CD4+ T cell counts fall below 100/μl. Opportunistic infection with *Bartonella henselae* in poor hygienic conditions in these cases results in blood-filled cysts in liver partly lined by endothelial cells and having mixed inflammatory cells in a fibromyxoid background.

Obstruction of the portal vein may occur within the intrahepatic course or in extrahepatic site.

❖   **Intrahepatic cause** of portal venous occlusion is hepatic cirrhosis as the commonest and most important, followed in decreasing frequency by tumour invasion, congenital hepatic fibrosis and schistosomiasis.

❖   **Extrahepatic causes** of portal vein obstruction are intra-abdominal cancers, intra-abdominal sepsis, direct invasion by tumour, myeloproliferative disorders and upper abdominal surgical procedure followed by thrombosis.

The **effects** of portal venous obstruction depend upon the site of obstruction. The most important effect, irrespective of the site of occlusion or cause, is portal hypertension and its manifestations.

III.   HEPATIC ARTERIAL OBSTRUCTION

Diseases from obstruction of the hepatic artery are uncommon. Rarely, accidental ligation of the main hepatic artery or its branch to right lobe may be followed by fatal infarction.

VIRAL HEPATITIS (p. 590)

The term viral hepatitis is used to describe infection of the liver caused by hepatotropic viruses. Currently there are 5 main varieties of these viruses causing distinct types of viral hepatitis:

❖   *Hepatitis A virus (HAV),* causing a faecally-spread self-limiting disease.

❖   *Hepatitis B virus (HBV),* causing a parenterally transmitted disease that may become chronic.

❖   *Hepatitis C virus (HCV),* previously termed non-A, non-B (NANB) hepatitis virus involved chiefly in transfusion-related hepatitis.

❖   *Hepatitis delta virus (HDV)* which is sometimes associated as superinfection with hepatitis B infection.

❖   *Hepatitis E virus (HEV),* causing water-borne infection.

While HBV is a DNA virus, all other human hepatitis viruses are RNA viruses.

ETIOLOGIC CLASSIFICATION

Based on the etiologic agent, viral hepatitis is currently classified into 6 etiologic types—hepatitis A, hepatitis B, hepatitis C, hepatitis D, hepatitis E and hepatitis G.

HEPATITIS A

Infection with HAV causes hepatitis A (infectious hepatitis). Hepatitis A is responsible for 20-25% of clinical hepatitis in the developing countries of the world. Hepatitis A is usually a benign, self-limiting disease and has an incubation period of 15-45 days. The disease occurs in epidemic form as well as sporadically. It is almost exclusively spread by faeco-oral route. The spread is related to close personal contact such as in overcrowding, poor hygienic and sanitary conditions.

HEPATITIS A VIRUS (HAV)   The etiologic agent for hepatitis A, HAV, is a small, 27 nm diameter, icosahedral non-enveloped, single-stranded RNA virus. Viral genome has been characterised but only a single serotype has been identified. Chronic carriers have not been identified for HAV infection.

PATHOGENESIS   Hepatitis A virus is present in the liver and replicates there. Evidence that hepatitis caused by HAV has an immunologic basis comes from demonstration of following antibodies acting as serum markers for hepatitis A infection:

1.   *IgM anti-HAV antibody* appears in the serum at the onset of symptoms of acute hepatitis A.

2.   *IgG anti-HAV antibody* is detected in the serum after acute illness and remains detectable indefinitely. It gives life-long protective immunity against reinfection with HAV.

Hepatitis B (serum hepatitis) caused by HBV infection has a longer incubation period (30-180 days) and is transmitted parenterally such as in recipients of blood and blood products, intravenous drug addicts, patients treated by renal dialysis and hospital workers exposed to blood, and by intimate physical contact such as from mother to child and by sexual contact. HBV infection causes more severe form of illness that includes: acute hepatitis B, chronic hepatitis, progression to cirrhosis, fulminant hepatitis and an asymptomatic carrier stage. HBV plays some role in the development of hepatocellular carcinoma as discussed later.

HEPATITIS B VIRUS (HBV)   The etiologic agent for hepatitis B, HBV, is a DNA virus which has been extensively studied. Electron microscopic studies on serum of patients infected with HBV show 3 forms of viral particles of 2 sizes: small (spheres and tubules/filaments) and large (spheres) as under:

i)   *Small particles* are most numerous and exist in two forms— as 22 nm spheres, and as tubules 22 nm in diameter and 100 nm long. These are antigenically identical to envelope protein of HBV and represent excess of viral envelope protein referred to as hepatitis B surface antigen (HBsAg).

ii)   *Large particles,* 42 nm in diameter, are double-shelled spherical particles, also called as *Dane particles.* These are about 100 to 1000 times less in number in serum compared to small 22 nm particles and represent intact virion of HBV.

The genomic structure of HBV is quite compact and complex. The HBV DNA consists of 4 overlapping genes which encode for multiple proteins:

1.   *S gene* codes for the surface envelope protein, hepatitis B surface antigen (HBsAg); this product is major protein.

2.   *P gene* is the largest and codes for DNA polymerase.

3.   *C gene* codes for two nucleocapsid proteins, HBeAg and a core protein termed HBcAg.

4.   *X gene* codes for HBxAg which is a small non-particulate protein. Expression of HBxAg and its antibodies associated with enhanced HBV DNA replication has been implicated in hepatocellular carcinoma in patients of chronic hepatitis.

PATHOGENESIS   There is strong evidence linking immune pathogenesis with hepatocellular damage:

i)   Since a carrier state of hepatitis B without hepatocellular damage exists, it means that HBV is not directly cytopathic.

ii)   Individuals with defect or deficiency of cellular immunity have more persistent hepatitis B disease.

iii)   Viral antigens (in particular nucleocapsid proteins HbcAg and HbeAg) are attacked by host cytotoxic CD8+T lymphocytes.

iv)   The host response of CD8+T lymphocytes by elaboration of antiviral cytokines is variable in different individuals.

Serologic and viral markers. In support of immune pathogenesis is the demonstration of several immunological markers in the serum and in hepatocytes indicative of presence of HBV infection.

1.   **HBsAg**   In 1965, Blumberg and colleagues in Philadelphia found a lipoprotein complex in the serum of a multiple-transfused haemophiliac of Australian aborigine which was subsequently shown by them to be associated with serum hepatitis. This antigen was termed *Australia antigen* by them. The term Australia antigen is now used synonymous with hepatitis B surface antigen (HBsAg). HBsAg appears early in the blood after about 6 weeks of infection and its detection is an indicator of active HBV infection. It usually disappears in 3-6 months. Its persistence for more than 6 months implies a carrier state.

2.   **Anti-HBs**   Specific antibody to HBsAg in serum called anti-HBs appears late, about 3 months after the onset. Anti-HBs response may be both IgM and IgG type.

3.   **HBeAg**   HBeAg derived from core protein is present transiently (3-6 weeks) during an acute attack. Its persistence beyond 10 weeks is indicative of development of chronic liver disease and carrier state.

4. Anti-HBe Antibody to HBeAg called anti-HBe appears after disappearance of HBeAg. Seroconversion from HBeAg to anti-HBe during acute stage of illness is a prognostic sign for resolution of infection.

5. HBcAg HBcAg derived from core protein cannot be detected in the blood. But HBcAg can be demonstrated in the nuclei of hepatocytes in carrier state and in chronic hepatitis patients.

6. Anti-HBc Antibody to HBcAg called anti-HBc can, however, be detected in the serum of acute hepatitis B patients during pre-icteric stage. In the initial period, it is IgM class antibody which persists for 4-6 months and is followed later by IgG anti-HBc.

7. HBV-DNA Detection of HBV-DNA by molecular hybridisation using the Southern blot technique is the most sensitive index of hepatitis B infection.

HEPATITIS D

Infection with delta virus (HDV) in the hepatocyte nuclei of HBsAg-positive patients is termed hepatitis D. HDV is a defective virus for which HBV is the helper. Thus, hepatitis D develops when there is concomitant hepatitis B infection. HDV infection and hepatitis B may be simultaneous *(co-infection)*, or HDV may infect a chronic HBsAg carrier *(superinfection)*.

The high-risk individuals for HDV infection are the same as for HBV infection i.e. intravenous drug abusers, homosexuals, transfusion recipients, and health care workers.

HEPATITIS DELTA VIRUS (HDV) The etiologic agent, HDV, is a small single-stranded RNA particle with a diameter of 36 nm. It is double-shelled—the outer shell consists of HBsAg and the inner shell consists of delta antigen provided by a circular RNA strand. It is highly infectious and can induce hepatitis in any HBsAg-positive host. HDV replication and proliferation takes place within the nuclei of liver cells. Markers for HDV infection include the following:

1. *HDV identification* in the blood and in the liver cell nuclei.
2. *HDAg* detectable in the blood and on fixed liver tissue specimens.
3. *Anti-HD antibody* in acute hepatitis which is initially IgM type and later replaced by IgG type anti-HD antibody.

PATHOGENESIS HDV, unlike HBV, is thought to cause direct cytopathic effect on hepatocytes.

HEPATITIS C

Hepatitis C infection is acquired by blood transfusions, blood products, haemodialysis, parenteral drug abuse and accidental cuts and needle-pricks in health workers. About 90% of post-transfusion hepatitis is of hepatitis C type. About 1-2% of volunteer blood donors and up to 5% of professional blood donors are carriers of HCV. Hepatitis C has an incubation period of 20-90 days (mean 50 days). Clinically, acute HCV hepatitis is milder than HBV hepatitis but HCV has a higher rate of progression to chronic hepatitis than HBV. Occurrence of cirrhosis after 5 to 10 years and progression to hepatocellular carcinoma are other late consequences of HCV infection. Currently, HCV is considered more important cause of chronic liver disease worldwide than HBV.

HEPATITIS C VIRUS (HCV) HCV is a single-stranded, enveloped RNA virus, having a diameter of 30-60 nm. The genomic organisation of HCV shows a 5' terminal end, C (capsid) region and the envelope regions E1 and E2 in the exons.

The viral proteins result in corresponding serologic and virologic markers for HCV infection as under:

1. *Anti-HCV antibodies.* Three generations of anti-HCV IgG assays are available:

i) First generation antibodies are against C100-3 region proteins and appear 1 to 3 months after infection.

ii) Second generation antibodies are against C200 and C33c proteins and appear about one month earlier than the first generation.

iii) Third generation antibodies are against C22-3 and NS-5 region proteins and are detected even earlier.

2. *HCV-RNA*. HCV infection is, however, confirmed by HCV-RNA employing PCR technique.

PATHOGENESIS HCV induces hepatocellular injury by cell-mediated immune mechanism is supported by the following:

i) It is possible that the host lymphoid cells are infected by HCV.

ii) HCV-activated CD4+ helper T lymphocytes stimulate CD8+ T lymphocytes via cytokines elaborated by CD4+ helper T cells.

iii) The stimulated CD8+T lymphocytes, in turn, elaborate antiviral cytokines against various HCV antigens.

iv) Further support to this T- cell mediated mechanism comes from the observation that immune response is stronger in those HCV-infected persons who recover.

v) There is some role of certain HLA alleles and innate immunity.

vi) Natural killer (NK) cells also seem to contribute to containment of HCV infection.

vii) In a subset of patients, there is crossreactivity between viral antigens of HCV and host autoantibodies to liver-kidney microsomal antigen (anti-LKM).

HEPATITIS E

Hepatitis E is an enterically-transmitted virus, previously labelled as epidemic or enterically transmitted variant of non-A non-B hepatitis. The infection occurs in young or middle-aged individuals, primarily seen in India, other Asian countries, Africa and central America.

The infection is generally acquired by contamination of water supplies such as after monsoon flooding. HEV infection has a particularly high mortality in pregnant women but is otherwise a self-limited disease and has not been associated with chronic liver disease.

HEPATITIS E VIRUS (HEV) HEV is a single-stranded 32-34 nm, icosahedral non-enveloped virus. The virus has been isolated from stools, bile and liver of infected persons. Serologic markers for HEV include the following:

1. Anti-HEV antibodies of both IgM and IgG class.
2. HEV-RNA.

CLINICOPATHOLOGIC SPECTRUM

Among the various etiologic types of hepatitis, evidence linking HBV and HCV infection with the spectrum of clinicopathologic changes is stronger than with other hepatotropic viruses. The typical pathologic changes of hepatitis by major hepatotropic viruses are virtually similar. HAV and HEV, however, do not have a carrier stage nor cause chronic hepatitis. The various clinical patterns and pathologic consequences of different hepatotropic viruses can be considered under the following headings:

i) Carrier state
ii) Asymptomatic infection
iii) Acute hepatitis
iv) Chronic hepatitis
v) Fulminant hepatitis (Submassive to massive necrosis)

In addition, progression to cirrhosis and association with hepatocellular carcinoma are known to occur in certain types of hepatitis.

I. CARRIER STATE

An asymptomatic individual without manifest disease, harbouring infection with hepatotropic virus and capable of transmitting it is called carrier state. There can be 2 types of carriers:

1. An *'asymptomatic healthy carrier'* who does not suffer from ill-effects of the virus infection but is capable of transmitting.

2. An *'asymptomatic carrier with chronic disease'* capable of transmitting the organisms.

Hepatitis B is responsible for the largest number of carriers in the world, while concomitant infection with HDV more often causes progressive disease rather than an asymptomatic carrier state. An estimated 2-3% of the general population are asymptomatic carriers of HCV. Data on HBV carrier state reveal role of 2 important factors rendering the individual more vulnerable to harbour the organisms—*early age at infection* and *impaired immunity*.

Clinical recognition of HBV carrier state is done by persistence of HBsAg in the serum of an infected person who fails to clear HBsAg from blood for more than 6 months.

II. ASYMPTOMATIC INFECTION

These are cases who are detected incidentally to have infection with one of the hepatitis viruses as revealed by their raised serum transaminases or by detection of the presence of antibodies but are otherwise asymptomatic.

III. ACUTE HEPATITIS

The most common consequence of all hepatotropic viruses is acute inflammatory involvement of the entire liver. In general, type A, B, C, D and E run similar clinical course and show identical pathologic findings.

Clinically, acute hepatitis is categorised into 4 phases: incubation period, pre-icteric phase, icteric phase and post-icteric phase.

1. Incubation period It varies among different hepatotropic viruses: for hepatitis A it is about 4 weeks (15-45 days); for hepatitis B the average is 10 weeks (30-180 days); for hepatitis D about 6 weeks (30-50 days); for hepatitis C the mean incubation period is about 7 weeks (20-90 days), and for hepatitis E it is 2-8 weeks (15-60 days).

2. Pre-icteric phase This phase is marked by prodromal constitutional symptoms that include anorexia, nausea, vomiting, fatigue, malaise, distaste for smoking, arthralgia and headache. There may be low-grade fever preceding the onset of jaundice, especially in hepatitis A.

3. Icteric phase The prodromal period is heralded by the onset of clinical jaundice and the constitutional symptoms diminish. Other features include dark-coloured urine due to bilirubinuria, clay-coloured stools due to cholestasis, pruritus as a result of elevated serum bile acids, loss of weight and abdominal discomfort due to enlarged, tender liver.

4. Post-icteric phase The icteric phase lasting for about 1 to 4 weeks is usually followed by clinical and biochemical recovery in 2 to 12 weeks. Up to 1% cases of acute hepatitis may develop severe form of the disease (fulminant hepatitis); and 5-10% of cases progress on to chronic hepatitis.

G/A The liver is slightly enlarged, soft and greenish.

M/E The changes are as follows:

1. Hepatocellular injury There may be variation in the degree of liver cell injury but it is most marked in zone 3 (centrilobular zone):
i) Mildly injured hepatocytes appear swollen with granular cytoplasm which tends to condense around the nucleus *(ballooning degeneration)*.
ii) Others show acidophilic degeneration in which the cytoplasm becomes intensely eosinophilic, the nucleus becomes small and pyknotic and is eventually extruded from the cell, leaving behind necrotic, acidophilic mass called *Councilman body* or *acidophil body* by the process of apoptosis.
iii) Another type of hepatocellular necrosis is *dropout necrosis*.
iv) *Bridging necrosis* is a more severe form of hepatocellular injury in acute viral hepatitis and is characterised by bands of necrosis linking portal tracts to central hepatic veins, one central hepatic vein to another, or a portal tract to another tract.

2. Inflammatory infiltrate There is infiltration by mononuclear inflammatory cells, usually in the portal tracts, but may permeate into the lobules.

3. Kupffer cell hyperplasia There is reactive hyperplasia of Kupffer cells many of which contain phagocytosed cellular debris, bile pigment and lipofuscin granules.

4. Cholestasis Biliary stasis is usually not severe in viral hepatitis and may be present as intracytoplasmic bile pigment granules.

5. Regeneration As a result of necrosis of hepatocytes, there is lobular disarray. Surviving adjacent hepatocytes undergo regeneration and hyperplasia.

IV. CHRONIC HEPATITIS

Chronic hepatitis is defined as continuing or relapsing hepatic disease for more than 6 months with symptoms along with biochemical, serologic and histopathologic evidence of inflammation and necrosis. Majority of cases of chronic hepatitis are the result of infection with hepatotropic viruses—hepatitis B, hepatitis C and combined hepatitis B and hepatitis D infection. However, some non-viral causes of chronic hepatitis include: Wilson's disease, α-1-antitrypsin deficiency, chronic alcoholism, drug-induced injury and autoimmune diseases. The last named gives rise to *autoimmune or lupoid hepatitis* which is characterised by positive serum autoantibodies (e.g. antinuclear, anti-smooth muscle and anti-mitochondrial) and a positive LE cell test but negative for serologic markers of viral hepatitis.

Currently, chronic hepatitis is classified on the basis of etiology and hepatitis activity score (described below).

M/E Common features are as under:

1. Piecemeal necrosis Piecemeal necrosis is defined as periportal destruction of hepatocytes at the limiting plate (*piecemeal* = piece by piece). Its features in chronic hepatitis are as under:
i)   Necrosed hepatocytes at the limiting plate in periportal zone.
ii) Interface hepatitis due to expanded portal tract by infiltration of lymphocytes, plasma cells and macrophages.
iii) Expanded portal tracts are often associated with proliferating bile ductules as a response to liver cell injury.

2. Portal tract lesions All forms of chronic hepatitis are characterised by variable degree of changes in the portal tract.
i)   Inflammatory cell infiltration by lymphocytes, plasma cells and macrophages (triaditis).
ii) Proliferated bile ductules in the expanded portal tracts.
iii) Additionally, chronic hepatitis C may show lymphoid aggregates or follicles with reactive germinal centre and infiltration of inflammatory cells in the damaged bile duct epithelial cells.

3. Intralobular lesions Generally, the architecture of lobule is retained in mild to moderate chronic hepatitis.
i)   There are focal areas of necrosis and inflammation within the hepatic parenchyma.
ii) Scattered acidophilic bodies in the lobule.
iii) Kupffer cell hyperplasia.
iv) More severe form of injury shows bridging necrosis.
v)   Regenerative changes in hepatocytes in cases of persistent hepatocellular necrosis.
vi) Cases of chronic hepatitis C show moderate fatty change.

4. Bridging fibrosis The onset of fibrosis in chronic hepatitis from the area of interface hepatitis and bridging necrosis is a feature of irreversible damage.
i)   At first, there is periportal fibrosis at the sites of interface hepatitis giving the portal tract stellate-shaped appearance.
ii) Progressive cases show bridging fibrosis connecting portal tract-to-portal tract or portal tract-to-central vein traversing the lobule.
iii) End-stage of chronic hepatitis is characterised by dense collagenous septa destroying lobular architecture and forming nodules resulting in postnecrotic cirrhosis.

As prognostic indicator of chronic hepatitis, a histologic grading of chronic hepatitis (ranging from none to minimal/mild to moderate and severe) was originally described by Knodell and Ishak. A combined histologic grade leads to hepatitis activity index (HAI) and takes the following features into consideration:

A. *Necroinflammatory activity:*
◈ Periportal necrosis i.e. piecemeal necrosis and/or bridging necrosis.
◈ Intralobular necrosis, focal or confluent.
◈ Extent and depth of portal inflammation.

B. *Stage of fibrosis:*
◈ Extent and density of fibrosis.

CLINICAL FEATURES The clinical features of chronic hepatitis are quite variable ranging from mild disease to full-blown picture of cirrhosis.
i) Mild chronic hepatitis shows only slight but persistent elevation of transaminases ('transaminitis') with fatigue, malaise and loss of appetite.
ii) Other cases may show mild hepatomegaly, hepatic tenderness and mild splenomegaly.
iii) Laboratory findings may reveal prolonged prothrombin time, hyperbilirubinaemia, hyperglobulinaemia and markedly elevated alkaline phosphatase.

V. *FULMINANT HEPATITIS (SUBMASSIVE TO MASSIVE NECROSIS)*

Fulminant hepatitis is the most severe form of acute hepatitis in which there is rapidly progressive hepatocellular failure. Two patterns are recognised—*submassive necrosis* having a less rapid course extending up to 3 months; and *massive necrosis* in which the liver failure is rapid and fulminant occurring in 2-3 weeks.

Fulminant hepatitis of either of the two varieties can occur from viral and non-viral etiologies:

◈ *Acute viral hepatitis* accounts for about half the cases, most often from HBV and HCV; less frequently from combined HBV-HDV and rarely from HAV. However, HEV infection is a serious complication in pregnant women. In addition, herpesvirus can also cause serious viral hepatitis.

◈ *Non-viral causes* include acute hepatitis due to drug toxicity (e.g. acetaminophen, non-steroidal anti-inflammatory drugs, isoniazid, halothane and anti-depressants), poisonings, hypoxic injury and massive infiltration of malignant tumours into the liver.

G/A The liver is small and shrunken, often weighing 500-700 gm. The capsule is loose and wrinkled. The sectioned surface shows diffuse or random involvement of hepatic lobes.

M/E Two forms of fulminant necrosis are distinguished:
i) In **submassive necrosis,** large groups of hepatocytes in zone 3 (centrilobular area) and zone 2 (mid zone) are wiped out leading to a collapsed reticulin framework. Regeneration in submassive necrosis is more orderly and may result in restoration of normal architecture.
ii) In **massive necrosis,** the entire liver lobules are necrotic. As a result of loss of hepatic parenchyma, all that is left is the collapsed and condensed reticulin framework and portal tracts with proliferated bile ductules plugged with bile. Inflammatory infiltrate is scanty. Regeneration, if it takes place, is disorderly forming irregular masses of hepatocytes.

IMMUNOPROPHYLAXIS AND HEPATITIS VACCINES

Best prophylaxis against the viral hepatitis remains prevention of its spread to the contacts after detection and identification of route by which infection is acquired such as from food or water contamination, sexual spread or parenteral spread. Of late, however, immunoprophylaxis and a few hepatitis vaccines have been developed and some more are under development.

1. **Hepatitis A** Passive immunisation with immune globulin as well as active immunisation with a killed vaccine are available.

2. **Hepatitis B** Current recommendations include pre-exposure and post-exposure prophylaxis with recombinant hepatitis B vaccine:
◈ *Pre-exposure prophylaxis* is done for individuals at high-risk e.g. health care workers, haemodialysis patients and staff, haemophiliacs, intravenous drug users etc. Three intramuscular injections of hepatitis vaccine at 0, 1 and 6 months are recommended.

◈ *Post-exposure prophylaxis* is carried out for unvaccinated persons exposed to HBV infection and includes prophylaxis with combination of hepatitis B immune globulin and hepatitis B vaccine.

3. Hepatitis D Hepatitis D infection can also be prevented by hepatitis B vaccine.

4. Hepatitis C Currently, hepatitis C vaccine has yet not been feasible though antibodies to HCV envelope have been developed.

5. Hepatitis E It is not certain whether immune globulin (like for HAV) prevents hepatitis E infection or not but a vaccine against HEV is yet to be developed.

OTHER INFECTIONS AND INFESTATIONS (p. 599)

CHOLANGITIS

Cholangitis is the term used to describe inflammation of the extrahepatic or intrahepatic bile ducts, or both. There are two main types of cholangitis—pyogenic and primary sclerosing; the latter is discussed on page 403.

PYOGENIC CHOLANGITIS

Cholangitis occurring secondary to obstruction of a major extrahepatic duct causes pyogenic cholangitis. Most commonly, the obstruction is from impacted gallstone; other causes are carcinoma arising in the extrahepatic ducts, carcinoma head of pancreas, acute pancreatitis and inflammatory strictures in the bile duct.

PYOGENIC LIVER ABSCESS

Most liver abscesses are of bacterial (pyogenic) origin; less often they are amoebic, hydatid and rarely actinomycotic. Pyogenic liver abscesses have become uncommon due to improved diagnostic facilities and the early use of antibiotics. However, their incidence is higher in old age and in immunosuppressed patients such as in AIDS, transplant recipients and those on intensive chemotherapy.

Pyogenic liver abscesses can occur by following modes of entry:
1. Ascending cholangitis.
2. Portal pyaemia
3. Septicaemia
4. Direct infection
5. Iatrogenic causes
6. Cryptogenic.

Liver abscesses are clinically characterised by pain in the right upper quadrant, fever, tender hepatomegaly and sometimes jaundice. Laboratory examination reveals leucocytosis, elevated serum alkaline phosphatase, hypoalbuminaemia and a positive blood culture.

G/A Depending upon the cause for pyogenic liver abscess, they occur as single or multiple yellow abscesses, 1 cm or more in diameter, in an enlarged liver. A single abscess generally has a thick fibrous capsule. The abscesses are particularly common in right lobe of the liver.

M/E Typical features of abscess are seen. There are multiple small neutrophilic abscesses with areas of extensive necrosis of the affected liver parenchyma. The adjacent viable area shows pus and blood clots in the portal vein, inflammation, congestion and proliferating fibroblasts.

AMOEBIC LIVER ABSCESS

Amoebic liver abscesses are less common than pyogenic liver abscesses and have many similar features. They are caused by the spread of *Entamoeba histolytica* from intestinal lesions. The trophozoite form of amoebae in the colon invade the colonic mucosa forming flask-shaped ulcers from where they are carried to the liver in the portal venous system.

G/A Amoebic liver abscesses are usually solitary and more often located in the right lobe in the posterosuperior portion. Amoebic liver abscess may vary greatly in size but is generally of the size of an orange. The centre of the abscess contains large necrotic area having reddish-brown, thick pus resembling anchovy or chocolate sauce.

M/E The necrotic area consists of degenerated liver cells, leucocytes, red blood cells, strands of connective tissue and debris. Amoebae are most easily found in the liver tissue at the margin of abscess. PAS-staining is employed to confirm the trophozoites of *E. histolytica*.

HEPATIC TUBERCULOSIS

Tuberculosis of the liver occurs as a result of miliary dissemination from primary complex or from chronic adult pulmonary tuberculosis. The diagnosis is possible by liver biopsy.

M/E The basic lesion is the epithelioid cell granuloma characterised by central caseation necrosis with destruction of the reticulin framework and peripheral cuff of lymphocytes. Ziehl-Neelsen staining for AFB or culture of the organism from the biopsy tissue is confirmatory.

HYDATID DISEASE (ECHINOCOCCOSIS)

Hydatid disease occurs as a result of infection by the larval cyst stage of the tapeworm, *Echinococcus granulosus*. The dog is the common definite host, while man, sheep and cattle are the intermediate hosts. Man can acquire infection by handling dogs as well as by eating contaminated vegetables. The ova ingested by man are liberated from the chitinous wall by gastric juice and pass through the intestinal mucosa from where they are carried to the liver by portal venous system. These are trapped in the hepatic sinusoids where they eventually develop into hydatid cyst. About 70% of hydatid cysts develop in the liver which acts as the first filter for ova. However, ova which pass through the liver enter the right side of the heart and are caught in the pulmonary capillary bed and form pulmonary hydatid cysts. Some ova which enter the systemic circulation give rise to hydatid cysts in the brain, spleen, bone and muscles.

Complications of hydatid cyst include its rupture (e.g. into the peritoneal cavity, bile ducts and lungs), secondary infection and hydatid allergy due to sensitisation of the host with cyst fluid.

MORPHOLOGIC FEATURES Hydatid cyst grows slowly and may eventually attain a size over 10 cm in diameter in about 5 years. *E. granulosus* generally causes unilocular hydatid cyst while *E. multilocularis* results in multilocular or alveolar hydatid disease in the liver.

M/E The cyst wall is composed of 3 distinguishable zones:

1. Pericyst is the outer host inflammatory reaction consisting of fibroblastic proliferation, mononuclear cells, eosinophils and giant cells, eventually developing into dense fibrous capsule which may even calcify.

2. Ectocyst is the intermediate layer composed of characteristic acellular, chitinous, laminated hyaline material.

3. Endocyst is the inner germinal layer bearing daughter cysts (brood-capsules) and scolices projecting into the lumen.

Hydatid sand is the grain-like material composed of numerous scolices present in the hydatid fluid.

CHEMICAL AND DRUG INJURY *(p. 601)*

HEPATIC DRUG METABOLISM The liver plays a central role in the metabolism of a large number of organic and inorganic chemicals and drugs which gain access to the body by inhalation, injection, or most commonly, via the intestinal tract. The main drug metabolising system resides in the microsomal fraction of the smooth endoplasmic reticulum of the liver cells via P-450 cytochrome and cytochrome reductase enzyme systems.

HEPATOTOXICITY Toxic liver injury produced by drugs and chemicals may virtually mimic any form of naturally-occurring liver disease. In fact, any patient presenting with liver disease or unexplained jaundice is

Hepatotoxicity from drugs and chemicals is the commonest form of iatrogenic disease.

Among the various *inorganic compounds* producing hepatotoxicity are arsenic, phosphorus, copper and iron. *Organic agents* include certain naturally-occurring plant toxins such as pyrrolizidine alkaloids, mycotoxins and bacterial toxins.

In general, drug reactions affecting the liver are divided into two main classes:

1. Direct or predictable, when the drug or one of its metabolites is either directly toxic to the liver or it lowers the host immune defense mechanism.

2. Indirect or unpredictable or idiosyncratic, when the drug or one of its metabolites acts as a hapten and induces hypersensitivity in the host. In many instances, drug hepatotoxicity is associated with appearance of autoantibodies to liver-kidney microsomes (i.e. anti-LKM2) directed against cytochrome P450 enzyme. The hepatotoxicity by this group does not occur regularly in all individuals and the effects are usually not dose-related e.g. acetaminophen.

The pathologic changes by hepatotoxins include 2 large categories:
1. *Acute liver disease* characterised by cholestasis, hepatocellular necrosis, fatty change, granulomatous reaction or vascular disease.
2. *Chronic liver disease* characterised by variable degree of fibrosis, cirrhosis or neoplasia.

CIRRHOSIS *(p. 603)*

Cirrhosis of the liver is one of the ten leading causes of death in the Western world. It represents the irreversible end-stage of several diffuse diseases causing hepatocellular injury and is characterised by the following 4 features:
1. It involves the entire liver.
2. The normal lobular architecture of hepatic parenchyma is disorganised.
3. There is formation of nodules separated from one another by irregular bands of fibrosis.
4. It occurs following hepatocellular necrosis of varying etiology so that there are alternate areas of necrosis and regenerative nodules.

PATHOGENESIS

Irrespective of the etiology, cirrhosis involves a combination of a few processes:

FIBROGENESIS Continued destruction of hepatocytes causes collapse of normal lobular hepatic parenchyma followed by fibrosis around necrotic liver cells. Fibrosis in the liver lobules may be portal-central, portal-portal, or both. The mechanism of fibrosis is by increased synthesis of type I and III collagen in the space of Disse. Besides collagen, two glycoproteins, fibronectin and laminin, are deposited in excessive amounts in area of liver cell damage. Stimulants for fibrosis are several growth factors, vasoactive factors, cytokines, lymphokines and chemokines.

REGENERATIVE NODULES The surviving hepatocytes act as stimulants for growth and proliferation of more hepatocytes under influence of growth factors. This compensatory proliferation of hepatocytes is restricted within fibrous nodules forming regenerative nodules.

VASCULAR REORGANISATION Due to damaged hepatic parenchyma and formation of fibrous nodules, the new vessels formed in the fibrous septa are connected to the vessels in the portal triad (i.e. branches of hepatic artery and portal vein) and then the blood is drained into hepatic vein. This way, the blood bypasses the hepatic parenchyma.

CLASSIFICATION

Cirrhosis can be classified on the basis of morphology and etiology.

A. MORPHOLOGIC CLASSIFICATION There are 3 morphologic types of cirrhosis—micronodular, macronodular and mixed. Each of these forms may have an active and inactive form.

❖ An *active form* is characterised by continuing hepatocellular necrosis and inflammatory reaction.

❖ An *inactive form,* on the other hand, has no evidence of continuing hepatocellular necrosis and has sharply-defined nodules of surviving hepatic parenchyma.

1. Micronodular cirrhosis In micronodular cirrhosis, the nodules are usually regular and small, *less than 3 mm* in diameter. There is diffuse involvement of all the hepatic lobules forming nodules by thick fibrous septa which may be portal-portal, portal-central, or both. The micronodular cirrhosis includes etiologic type of alcoholic cirrhosis.

2. Macronodular cirrhosis In this type, the nodules are of variable size and are generally *larger than 3 mm* in diameter. The pattern of involvement is more irregular than in micronodular cirrhosis, sparing some portal tracts and central veins, and more marked evidence of regeneration. Macronodular cirrhosis corresponds to post-necrotic (or post-hepatitis) cirrhosis of the etiologic classification.

3. Mixed cirrhosis In mixed type, some parts of the liver show micronodular appearance while other parts show macronodular pattern.

B. ETIOLOGIC CLASSIFICATION Based on the etiologic agent for cirrhosis, various categories of cirrhosis are described below.

SPECIFIC TYPES OF CIRRHOSIS

ALCOHOLIC LIVER DISEASE AND CIRRHOSIS

Alcoholic liver disease is the term used to describe the spectrum of liver injury associated with acute and chronic alcoholism. There are three sequential stages in alcoholic liver disease: *alcoholic steatosis (fatty liver), alcoholic hepatitis* and *alcoholic cirrhosis.*

ETHANOL METABOLISM One gram of alcohol gives 7 calories. But alcohol cannot be stored in the body and must undergo obligatory oxidation, chiefly in the liver.

Ethanol after ingestion and absorption from the small bowel circulates through the liver where about 90% of it is oxidised to acetate by a *two-step enzymatic process* involving two enzymes: *alcohol dehydrogenase (ADH)* present in the cytosol, and *acetaldehyde dehydrogenase (ALDH)* in the mitochondria of hepatocytes. The remaining 10% of ethanol is oxidised elsewhere in the body.

First step: Ethanol is catabolised to acetaldehyde in the liver by the following three pathways, one major and two minor:

i) *In the cytosol,* by the major rate-limiting pathway of alcohol dehydrogenase (ADH).

ii) *In the smooth endoplasmic reticulum,* via microsomal P-450 oxidases, where only part of ethanol is metabolised.

iii) *In the peroxisomes,* minor pathway via catalase such as H_2O_2.

Acetaldehyde is toxic and may cause membrane damage and cell necrosis.

Second step: The second step occurs in the mitochondria where acetaldehyde is converted to acetate with ALDH acting as a co-enzyme. Most of the acetate on leaving the liver is finally oxidised to carbon dioxide and water. A close estimate of NADH:NAD ratio is measured by the ratio of its oxidised and reduced metabolites in the form of *lactate-pyruvate ratio* and β-*hydroxy butyrate-acetoacetate ratio.*

RISK FACTORS FOR ALCOHOLIC LIVER DISEASE All those who indulge in alcohol abuse do not develop liver damage. The incidence of cirrhosis among alcoholics at autopsy is about 10-15%. Why some individuals are predisposed to alcoholic cirrhosis is not clearly known, but a few risk factors have been implicated.

1. **Drinking patterns** Most epidemiologic studies have attributed alcoholic cirrhosis to chronic alcoholism. Available evidence suggests that chronic and excessive consumption of alcohol invariably leads to fatty liver in >90% of chronic alcoholics, progression to alcoholic hepatitis in 10-20% cases, and eventually to alcoholic cirrhosis in more than 10 years.

2. **Gender** Women have increased susceptibility to develop advanced alcoholic liver disease with much lesser alcohol intake (20-40 g/day).

3. **Malnutrition** Absolute or relative malnutrition of proteins and vitamins is regarded as a contributory factor in the evolution of cirrhosis. The combination of chronic alcohol ingestion and impaired nutrition leads to alcoholic liver disease and not malnutrition *per se*.

4. **Infections** Intercurrent bacterial infections are common in cirrhotic patients and may accelerate the course of the disease.

5. **Genetic factors** The rate of ethanol metabolism is under genetic control. It is chiefly related to altered rates of elimination of ethanol due to genetic polymorphism for the two main enzyme systems, MEOS and ADH.

6. **Hepatitis B and C infection** Concurrent infection with either HBV or HCV is an important risk factor for progression of alcoholic liver disease. HBV or HCV infection in chronic alcoholic leads to development of alcoholic liver disease with much less alcohol consumption, disease progression at a younger age, having greater severity, and increased risk to develop cirrhosis and hepatocellular carcinoma, and overall poorer survival.

PATHOGENESIS Exact pathogenesis of alcoholic liver injury is yet unclear as to why only some chronic alcoholics develop the complete sequence of changes in the liver while others don't. However, knowledge and understanding of the ethanol metabolism has resulted in discarding the old concept of liver injury due to malnutrition. Instead, it is now known that ethanol and its metabolites are responsible for ill-effects on the liver in a susceptible chronic alcoholic having above-mentioned risk factors. Briefly, the biomedical and cellular pathogenesis due to chronic alcohol consumption culminating in morphologic lesions of alcoholic steatosis (fatty liver), alcoholic hepatitis and alcoholic cirrhosis is as under:

1. Direct hepatotoxicity by ethanol
2. Hepatotoxicity by ethanol metabolites i.e. *production of protein-aldehyde adducts* and *formation of malon-di-aldehyde-acetaldehyde (MAA) adducts*.
3. Oxidative stress
4. Immunological mechanism
5. Inflammation
6. Fibrogenesis Main event facilitating hepatic fibrogenesis is activation of stellate cells by various stimuli:
i) by damaged hepatocytes,
ii) by malon-di-aldehyde-acetaldehyde adducts,
iii) by activated Kupffer cells, and
iv) direct stimulation by acetaldehyde.
7. Increased redox ratio
8. Retention of liver cell water and proteins
9. Hypoxia
10. Increased liver fat.

MORPHOLOGIC FEATURES Three types of lesions are described.

1. ALCOHOLIC STEATOSIS (FATTY LIVER) This is the initial stage.

G/A The liver is enlarged, yellow, greasy and firm with a smooth and glistening capsule.

M/E The features consist of initial *microvesicular* droplets of fat in the hepatocyte cytoplasm followed by more common and pronounced feature of *macrovesicular* large droplets of fat displacing the nucleus to the periphery. *Fat cysts* may develop due to coalescence and rupture of fat-containing hepatocytes. Less often, *lipogranulomas* consisting of collection of lymphocytes, macrophages and some multinucleate giant cells may be found.

2. ALCOHOLIC HEPATITIS Alcoholic hepatitis develops acutely, usually following a bout of heavy drinking. Repeated episodes of alcoholic hepatitis superimposed on pre-existing fatty liver are almost certainly a forerunner of alcoholic cirrhosis.

M/E The features are as under:

i) **Hepatocellular necrosis:** Single or small clusters of hepatocytes, especially in the centrilobular area (zone 3), undergo ballooning degeneration and necrosis.

ii) **Mallory bodies or alcoholic hyalin:** These are eosinophilic, intracytoplasmic inclusions seen in perinuclear location within swollen and ballooned hepatocytes. They represent aggregates of cytoskeletal intermediate filaments (prekeratin). Mallory bodies are also found in certain other conditions such as: primary biliary cirrhosis, Indian childhood cirrhosis, cholestatic syndromes, Wilson's disease, intestinal bypass surgery, focal nodular hyperplasia and hepatocellular carcinoma.

iii) **Inflammatory response:** The areas of hepatocellular necrosis and regions of Mallory bodies are associated with an inflammatory infiltrate, chiefly consisting of polymorphs and some scattered mononuclear cells.

iv) **Fibrosis:** Most cases of alcoholic hepatitis are accompanied by pericellular and perivenular fibrosis, producing a web-like or chickenwire-like appearance. This is also termed as *creeping collagenosis.*

3. ALCOHOLIC CIRRHOSIS Alcoholic cirrhosis is the most common form of lesion, constituting 60-70% of all cases of cirrhosis. Several terms have been used for this type of cirrhosis such as *Laennec's cirrhosis, portal cirrhosis, hobnail cirrhosis, nutritional cirrhosis, diffuse cirrhosis* and *micronodular cirrhosis.*

G/A Alcoholic cirrhosis classically begins as micronodular cirrhosis (nodules less than 3 mm diameter), the liver being large, fatty and weighing usually above 2 kg. The nodules of the liver due to their fat content are tawny-yellow. The surface of liver in alcoholic cirrhosis is studded with diffuse nodules which vary little in size, producing hobnail liver. On cut section, spheroidal or angular nodules of fibrous septa are seen.

M/E This is a progressive alcoholic liver disease.

i) **Nodular pattern:** Normal lobular architecture is effaced in which central veins are hard to find and is replaced with nodule formation.

ii) **Fibrous septa:** The fibrous septa that divide the hepatic parenchyma into nodules are initially delicate and extend from central vein to portal regions, or portal tract to portal tract, or both.

iii) **Hepatic parenchyma:** The hepatocytes in the islands of surviving parenchyma undergo slow proliferation forming regenerative nodules having disorganised masses of hepatocytes.

iv) **Necrosis, inflammation and bile duct proliferation:** The etiologic clue to diagnosis in the form of Mallory bodies is hard to find in a fully-developed alcoholic cirrhosis.

LABORATORY DIAGNOSIS Progressive form of the disease generally presents the following biochemical and haematological alterations:

1. Elevated transaminases; increase in SGOT (AST) is more than that of SGPT (ALT).
2. Rise in serum γ-glutamyl transpeptidase (γ-GT).
3. Elevation in serum alkaline phosphatase.
4. Hyperbilirubinaemia.
5. Hypoproteinaemia with reversal of albumin-globulin ratio.
6. Prolonged prothrombin time and partial thromboplastin time.
7. Anaemia.
8. Neutrophilic leucocytosis in alcoholic hepatitis and in secondary infections.

POST-NECROTIC CIRRHOSIS

Post-necrotic cirrhosis, also termed *post-hepatitic cirrhosis, macronodular cirrhosis* and *coarsely nodular cirrhosis,* is characterised by large and irregular nodules with broad bands of connective tissue and occurring most commonly after previous viral hepatitis.

ETIOLOGY Based on epidemiologic and serologic studies, the following factors have been implicated in the etiology of post-necrotic cirrhosis.

1. Viral hepatitis About 25% of patients give history of recent or remote attacks of acute viral hepatitis followed by chronic viral hepatitis. Most common association is with hepatitis B and C; hepatitis A is not known to evolve into cirrhosis.

2. Drugs and chemical hepatotoxins A small percentage of cases may have origin from toxicity due to chemicals and drugs such as phosphorus, carbon tetrachloride, mushroom poisoning, acetaminophen and α-methyl dopa.

3. Others Certain infections (e.g. brucellosis), parasitic infestations (e.g. clonorchiasis), metabolic diseases (e.g. Wilson's disease or hepatolenticular degeneration) and advanced alcoholic liver disease may produce a picture of post-necrotic cirrhosis.

4. Idiopathic After all these causes have been excluded, a group of cases remain in which the etiology is unknown.

MORPHOLOGIC FEATURES Typically, post-necrotic cirrhosis is macronodular type.

G/A The liver is usually small, weighing less than 1 kg, having distorted shape with irregular and coarse scars and nodules of varying size. Sectioned surface shows scars and nodules varying in diameter from 3 mm to a few centimeters.

M/E The features are as follows:

1. Nodular pattern: The normal lobular architecture of hepatic parenchyma is mostly lost and is replaced by nodules larger than those in alcoholic cirrhosis.

2. Fibrous septa: The fibrous septa dividing the variable-sized nodules are generally thick.

3. Necrosis, inflammation and bile duct proliferation: Active liver cell necrosis is usually inconspicuous. Fibrous septa contain prominent mono-nuclear inflammatory cell infiltrate which may even form follicles, especially in cases following HCV chronic hepatitis.

4. Hepatic parenchyma: Liver cells vary considerably in size and multiple large nuclei are common in regenerative nodules. Fatty change may or may not be present in the hepatocytes.

CLINICAL FEATURES Besides the general clinical features, post-necrotic cirrhosis is seen as frequent in women as in men, especially in the younger age group. Splenomegaly and hypersplenism are other prominent features. The results of haematologic and liver function test are similar to those of alcoholic cirrhosis.

BILIARY CIRRHOSIS

Biliary cirrhosis is defined as a chronic disorder characterised by clinical, biochemical and morphological features of long-continued cholestasis of intrahepatic or extrahepatic origin. Biliary cirrhosis is of following types:

A. *Primary biliary cirrhosis* in which the destructive process of unknown etiology affects intrahepatic bile ducts.

B. *Secondary biliary cirrhosis* resulting from prolonged mechanical obstruction of the extrahepatic biliary passages.

C. *Primary sclerosing cholangitis and autoimmune cholangiopathy* causing biliary cirrhosis.

ETIOLOGY The etiology of these forms of biliary cirrhosis is distinctive:

A. Primary biliary cirrhosis The etiology of this type remains unknown. However, a few factors have been implicated:

1. The possible *endocrine origin*.

2. *Familial incidence* has been observed.

3. There is *elevated cholesterol* level.

4. *Autoimmune origin* of the disease e.g.
i) increased incidence of associated autoimmune diseases;
ii) circulating anti-mitochondrial antibody of IgG class detected in more than 90% cases;
iii) elevated levels of immunoglobulins, particularly of IgM;
iv) increased levels of circulating immune complexes;
v) decreased number of circulating T-cells; and
vi) accumulation of T cells around bile ducts.

B. Secondary biliary cirrhosis   Most cases of secondary biliary cirrhosis result from prolonged obstruction of extrahepatic biliary passages:
1. Extrahepatic gallsone formation, most common
2. Biliary atresia
3. Cancer of biliary tree and of head of pancreas
4. Postoperative strictures with superimposed ascending cholangitis.

C. Cirrhosis due to primary sclerosing cholangitis   Primary or idio-pathic sclerosing cholangitis is a chronic cholestatic syndrome of unknown etiology. It is characterised by progressive, inflammatory, sclerosing and obliterative process affecting the entire biliary passages, both extra-hepatic and intrahepatic ducts.

G/A   In biliary cirrhosis of all types, the liver is initially enlarged and characteristically *greenish* in appearance, but later becomes smaller, firmer and coarsely micronodular.

M/E   The salient features of various forms are as under:

A. Primary biliary cirrhosis: The diagnostic histologic feature is a chronic, non-suppurative, destructive cholangitis involving intrahepatic bile ducts. The disease evolves through the following 4 histologic states:
Stage I: There are *florid bile duct lesions* confined to portal tracts.
Stage II: There is *ductular proliferation.*
Stage III: This stage is characterised by *fibrous scarring* interconnecting the portal areas.
Stage IV: Well-formed *micronodular pattern* of cirrhosis develops in a period of a few years.

B. Secondary biliary cirrhosis: Prolonged obstruction of extrahepatic bile ducts may produce the following histologic changes:
1. *Bile stasis*
2. Formation of *bile lakes*
3. *Cholangitis,* sterile or pyogenic
4. *Progressive expansion* of the portal tract by fibrosis.

C. Cirrhosis due to primary sclerosing cholangitis:
1. *Fibrosing cholangitis*
2. *Periductal fibrosis*
3. *Intervening bile ducts* are dilated, tortuous and inflamed.
4. Late cases show *cholestasis.*

CLINICAL FEATURES   Clinical features of the three types of biliary cirrhosis are variable:
❖   **Primary biliary cirrhosis** may remain asymptomatic for months to years. Symptoms develop insidiously. Basically, it is a cholestatic disorder. The patients present with persistent pruritus, dark urine, pale stools, steator-rhoea, jaundice and skin pigmentation.
❖   The diagnosis of **secondary biliary cirrhosis** is considered in patients with previous history of gallstones, biliary tract surgery or clinical features of ascending cholangitis.
❖   The patients of **primary sclerosing cholangitis** may remain asymptomatic or may show features of cholestatic jaundice (raised alkaline phosphatase, pruritus, fatigue).

PIGMENT CIRRHOSIS IN HAEMOCHROMATOSIS

Haemochromatosis is an iron-storage disorder in which there is excessive accumulation of iron in parenchymal cells with eventual tissue damage and functional insufficiency of organs such as the liver, pancreas, heart and pituitary gland. The condition is characterised by a triad of features—*micronodular pigment cirrhosis, diabetes mellitus* and *skin pigmentation*. On the basis of the last two features, the disease has also come to be termed as *'bronze diabetes'*. Haemochromatosis exists in 2 main forms:

1. *Idiopathic (primary, genetic) haemochromatosis* is an autosomal recessive disorder of excessive accumulation of iron. It is associated with overexpression of HFE gene located on chromosome 6 close to the HLA gene locus, and normally regulates intestinal absorption of iron. Mutated (overexpressed) HFE gene complexes with transferrin receptor on intestinal crypt epithelial cells and results in excessive absoption of dietary iron throughout life.

2. *Secondary (acquired) haemochromatosis* is gross iron overload with tissue injury arising secondary to other diseases such as thalassaemia, sideroblastic anaemias, alcoholic cirrhosis or multiple transfusions.

ETIOPATHOGENESIS It is distinct in the two forms:

◆ In **idiopathic or hereditary haemochromatosis,** the primary mechanism of disease appears to be the genetic basis in which the defect may either lie at the intestinal mucosal level causing excessive iron absorption, or at the post-absorption excretion level leading to excessive accumulation of iron. The excess iron in primary haemochromatosis is deposited mainly in the cytoplasm of parenchymal cells of organs such as the liver, pancreas, spleen, heart and endocrine glands.

◆ In **secondary or acquired haemochromatosis,** there is excessive accumulation of iron due to acquired causes like ineffective erythropoiesis, defective haemoglobin synthesis, multiple blood transfusions and enhanced absorption of iron due to alcohol consumption. Cases of secondary haemochromatosis have increased iron storage within the reticuloendothelial system and liver.

MORPHOLOGIC FEATURES Excessive deposition of iron in organs and tissues is ferritin and haemosiderin, both of which appear as golden-yellow pigment granules in the cytoplasm of affected parenchymal cells and haemosiderin stains positively with Prussian blue reaction. The organs most frequently affected are the liver and pancreas, and to a lesser extent, the heart, endocrine glands, skin, synovium and testis.

CLINICAL FEATURES The major clinical manifestations of haemochromatosis include skin pigmentation, diabetes mellitus, hepatic and cardiac dysfunction, arthropathy and hypogonadism. Characteristic bronze pigmentation is the presenting feature in about 90% of cases. Demonstration of excessive parenchymal iron stores is possible by measurement of serum iron, determination of percent saturation of transferrin, measurement of serum ferritin concentration, estimation of chelatable iron stores using chelating agent (e.g. desferrioxamine), and finally, by liver biopsy.

CIRRHOSIS IN WILSON'S DISEASE

Wilson's disease, also termed by a more descriptive designation of *hepatolenticular degeneration,* is an autosomal recessive inherited disease of copper metabolism, characterised by toxic accumulation of copper in many tissues, chiefly the liver, brain and eye. These accumulations lead to the *triad* of features:

1. Cirrhosis of the liver.
2. Bilateral degeneration of the basal ganglia of the brain.
3. Greenish-brown pigmented rings in the periphery of the cornea (Kayser-Fleischer rings).

The disease manifests predominantly in children and young adults (5-30 years). Initially, the clinical manifestations are referable to liver involvement such as jaundice and hepatomegaly *(hepatic form)* but later progressive *neuropsychiatric changes* and *Kayser-Fleischer rings* in the cornea appear.

PATHOGENESIS In Wilson's disease, the initial steps of dietary absorption and transport of copper to the liver are normal but copper accumulates in the liver rather than being excreted by the liver. Eventually, capacity of hepatocytes to store copper is exceeded and copper is released into circulation which then gets deposited in extrahepatic tissues such as the brain, eyes and others. However, increased copper in the kidney does not produce any serious renal dysfunction.

Biochemical abnormalities in Wilson's disease include the following:
1. Decreased serum ceruloplasmin
2. Increased hepatic copper in liver biopsy
3. Increased urinary excretion of copper.
4. However, serum copper level estimation is of no diagnostic help and may vary from low-to-normal-to-high depending upon the stage of disease.

MORPHOLOGIC FEATURES The **liver** shows varying grades of changes that include fatty change, acute and chronic active hepatitis, submassive liver necrosis and macronodular cirrhosis. Mallory bodies are present in some cases. Copper is usually deposited in the periportal hepatocytes in the form of reddish granules in the cytoplasm or as reddish cytoplasmic coloration, stainable by rubeanic acid or rhodamine stains for copper.

Involvement of basal ganglia in the **brain** is seen in the form of toxic injury to neurons, in the **cornea** as greenish-brown deposits of copper in Descemet's membrane, and in the **kidney** as fatty and hydropic change.

CIRRHOSIS IN α-1-ANTITRYPSIN DEFICIENCY

Alpha-1-antitrypsin deficiency is an autosomal codominant condition in which the homozygous state produces liver disease (cirrhosis), pulmonary disease (emphysema), or both. The most frequent abnormal phenotype in α-1-antitrypsin deficiency leading to liver and/or lung disease is PiZZ in homozygote form.

The patients may present with respiratory disease due to the development of emphysema, or may develop liver dysfunction, or both.

MORPHOLOGIC FEATURES The hepatic changes vary according to the age at which the deficiency becomes apparent. At birth or in neonates, the histologic features consist of neonatal hepatitis that may be acute or 'pure' cholestasis. Micronodular or macronodular cirrhosis may appear in childhood or in adolescence in which the diagnostic feature is the presence of intracellular, acidophilic, PAS-positive globules in the periportal hepatocytes.

CARDIAC CIRRHOSIS

Cardiac cirrhosis is an uncommon complication of severe right-sided congestive heart failure of long-standing duration. The common causes culminating in cardiac cirrhosis are cor pulmonale, tricuspid insufficiency or constrictive pericarditis. The pressure in the right ventricle is elevated which is transmitted to the liver via the inferior vena cava and hepatic veins. The patients generally have enlarged and tender liver with mild liver dysfunction. Splenomegaly occurs due to simple passive congestion.

G/A The liver is enlarged and firm with stretched Glisson's capsule.

M/E In acute stage, the hepatic sinusoids are dilated and congested with haemorrhagic necrosis of centrilobular hepatocytes *(central haemorrhagic necrosis)*. Severe and more prolonged heart failure results in delicate fibrous strands radiating from the central veins.

INDIAN CHILDHOOD CIRRHOSIS

Indian childhood cirrhosis (ICC) is an unusual form of cirrhosis seen in children between the age of 6 months and 3 years in rural, middle class, Hindus in India and in parts of South-East Asia and in the Middle-East. There is no role of viral infection in its etiology. Instead, a combination of some common toxic effects and inherited abnormality of copper metabolism has been suggested. Death occurs due to hepatic failure within a year of diagnosis.

M/E Following features are generally seen:

i) Liver cell injury ranging from ballooning degeneration to significant damage to hepatocytes.

ii) Prominent Mallory bodies in some hepatocytes without fatty change.

iii) Neutrophilic and sometimes alongwith lymphocytic infiltrate.

iv) Creeping pericellular fibrosis which may eventually lead to fine micro-macro-nodular cirrhosis.

v) There is significant deposition of copper and copper-associated proteins in hepatocytes, often more than what is seen in Wilson's disease.

CIRRHOSIS IN AUTOIMMUNE HEPATITIS

Autoimmune hepatitis (also called lupoid hepatitis) is a form of chronic hepatitis characterised by continued hepatocellular injury, inflammation and fibrosis which may progress to cirrhosis. The condition may run a variable natural history ranging from indolent to severe rapid course. This form of hepatitis has prominent autoimmune etiology is supported by immunologic abnormalities and a few other characteristic diagnostic criteria as under:

1. Female gender predisposition.
2. Predominant elevation of aminotransferases (AST and ALT).
3. Hyperglobulinaemia (elevated IgG and γ-globulin).
4. High serum titres of nuclear (ANA), smooth muscle (SMA), and liver-kidney microsomal (LKM1) autoantibodies, and absence of antimitochondrial antibodies.
5. Concurrent presence of other autoimmune diseases.
6. Presence of HLA DR3 or HLA DR4 markers.
7. Lack of prominent elevation of alkaline phosphatase.
8. Exclusion of chronic hepatitis of other known etiologies (viral, toxic, genetic etc).

M/E Autoimmune hepatitis is morphologically indistinguishable from chronic hepatitis of viral etiology. Patients who survive active disease develop cirrhosis. There are features of burnt out chronic autoimmune hepatitis accompanied with cirrhosis.

CIRRHOSIS IN NON-ALCOHOLIC STEATOHEPATITIS

Non-alcoholic steatohepatitis (NASH) or non-alcoholic fatty liver disease (NAFLD) is a form of hepatitis resembling alcoholic liver disease but seen in nondrinkers of alcohol. The condition is seen more commonly in affluent western societies, has a strong association with obesity, dyslipidaemia and type 2 diabetes mellitus.

NON-CIRRHOTIC PORTAL FIBROSIS

Non-cirrhotic portal fibrosis (NCPF) is a group of congenital and acquired diseases in which there is localised or generalised hepatic fibrosis without nodular regenerative activity and there is absence of clinical and functional evidence of cirrhosis. Besides, the patients of NCPF are relatively young as compared to those of cirrhosis and develop repeated bouts of haematemesis in the course of disease. Similar condition described from Japan has been named as *idiopathic (primary) portal hypertension with splenomegaly*.

The type common in India, particularly in young males, is related to following etiologic factors:

1. Exposure to trace elements, particularly chronic arsenic ingestion in drinking water.
2. Intake of orthodox medicines.
3. Infections, particularly of umbilical cord, infective diarrhoea and sepsis, causing infection in portal circulation and leading to thrombophelebitis.
4. Familial aggegation of disease and its relationship to HLA-DR3.

G/A The liver is small, fibrous and shows prominent fibrous septa on both external as well as on cut surface.

M/E The salient features are as under:

i) Standing out of portal tracts due to their increased amount of fibrous tissue in triad without significant inflammation.

ii) Obliterative sclerosis of portal vein branches in the portal tracts (obliterative portovenopathy).

CLINICAL MANIFESTATIONS AND COMPLICATIONS OF CIRRHOSIS

The range of clinical features in cirrhosis varies widely, from an asymptomatic state to progressive liver failure and death. The onset of disease is insidious. Advanced cases develop a number of complications which are as follows:
1. Portal hypertension
2. Progressive hepatic failure
3. Development of hepatocellular carcinoma
4. Chronic relapsing pancreatitis
5. Steatorrhoea
6. Gallstones
7. Infections
8. Haematologic derangements
9. Cardiovascular complications
10. Musculoskeletal abnormalities
11. Endocrine disorders
12. Hepatorenal syndrome.

The ultimate *causes of death* are hepatic coma, massive gastro-intestinal haemorrhage from oesophageal varices (complication of portal hypertension), intercurrent infections, hepatorenal syndrome and development of hepatocellular carcinoma.

PORTAL HYPERTENSION (p. 615)

Increase in pressure in the portal system usually follows obstruction to the portal blood flow anywhere along its course. Portal veins have no valves and thus obstruction anywhere in the portal system raises pressure in all the veins proximal to the obstruction. However, unless proved otherwise, portal hypertension means obstruction to the portal blood flow by cirrhosis of the liver. The normal portal venous pressure is quite low (10-15 mm saline). Portal hypertension occurs when the portal pressure is above 30 mm saline.

CLASSIFICATION Based on the site of obstruction to portal venous blood flow, portal hypertension is categorised into 3 main types—*intrahepatic, posthepatic* and *prehepatic*. Rare cases of idiopathic portal hypertension showing non-cirrhotic portal fibrosis are encountered.

1. Intrahepatic portal hypertension Cirrhosis is by far the commonest cause of portal hypertension. Other less frequent intrahepatic causes are metastatic tumours, non-cirrhotic nodular regenerative conditions, hepatic venous obstruction (Budd-Chiari syndrome), veno-occlusive disease, schistosomiasis, diffuse granulomatous diseases and extensive fatty change.

2. Posthepatic portal hypertension This is uncommon and results from obstruction to the blood flow through hepatic vein into inferior vena cava. The causes are neoplastic occlusion and thrombosis of the hepatic vein or of the inferior vena cava (including Budd-Chiari syndrome).

3. Prehepatic portal hypertension Blockage of portal flow before portal blood reaches the hepatic sinusoids results in prehepatic portal hypertension. Such conditions are thrombosis and neoplastic obstruction of the portal vein before it ramifies in the liver, myelofibrosis, and congenital absence of portal vein.

MAJOR SEQUELAE OF PORTAL HYPERTENSION Irrespective of the mechanisms involved in the pathogenesis of portal hypertension, there are 4 major clinical consequences—*ascites, varices, splenomegaly* and *hepatic encephalopathy.*

1. Ascites Ascites is the accumulation of excessive volume of fluid within the peritoneal cavity. It frequently accompanies cirrhosis and other diffuse liver diseases. The development of ascites is associated with haemodilution, oedema and decreased urinary output. Ascitic fluid is generally transudate with specific gravity of 1.010, protein content below

3 gm/dl and electrolyte concentrations like those of other extracellular fluids.

Pathogenesis The ascites becomes clinically detectable when more than 500 ml of fluid has accumulated in the peritoneal cavity. Briefly, the systemic and local factors favouring ascites formation are as under:

A. Systemic Factors:
i)   Decreased plasma colloid oncotic pressure
ii) Hyperaldosteronism
iii) Impaired renal excretion

B. Local Factors:
i)   Increased portal pressure
ii) Increased hepatic lymph formation

2. Varices (Collateral channels or Porto-systemic shunts) As a result of rise in portal venous pressure and obstruction in the portal circulation within or outside the liver, the blood tends to bypass the liver and return to the heart by development of porto-systemic collateral channels (or shunts or varices). These varices develop at sites where the systemic and portal circulations have common capillary beds. The principal sites are as under:
i)   Oesophageal varices
ii) Haemorrhoids
iii) Caput medusae
iv) Retroperitoneal anastomoses

3. Splenomegaly The enlargement of the spleen in prolonged portal hypertension is called congestive splenomegaly. The spleen may weigh 500-1000 gm and is easily palpable. The spleen is larger in young people and in macronodular cirrhosis than in micronodular cirrhosis.

4. Hepatic encephalopathy Porto-systemic venous shunting may result in a complex metabolic and organic syndrome of the brain characterised by disturbed consciousness, neurologic signs and flapping tremors.

HEPATIC TUMOURS AND TUMOUR-LIKE LESIONS (p. 617)

TUMOUR-LIKE LESIONS

These include cysts in the liver and focal nodular hyperplasia.

HEPATIC CYSTS

1. CONGENITAL CYSTS These are uncommon. They are usually small (less than 1 cm in diameter) and are lined by biliary epithelium. They may be single, or occur as polycystic liver disease, often associated with polycystic kidney. On occasions, these cysts have abundant connective tissue and numerous ducts, warranting the designation of *congenital hepatic fibrosis*.

2. SIMPLE (NON-PARASITIC) CYSTS Simple cysts are solitary non-parasitic cysts seen more frequently in middle-aged women. The cyst is usually large (up to 20 cm in diameter), lying underneath the Glisson's capsule and filled with serous fluid.

3. HYDATID (ECHINOCOCCUS) CYSTS Hydatid cyst has already been discussed.

FOCAL NODULAR HYPERPLASIA

The *etiology* of focal nodular hyperplasia is not known but these lesions are more common in women taking oral contraceptives.

G/A Focal nodular hyperplasia is a well-demarcated tumour-like nodule occurring underneath the Glisson's capsule. The nodules may be single or multiple, measuring about 5 cm in diameter. The sectioned surface shows a central fibrous scar.

M/E It is composed of collagenous septa radiating from the central fibrous scar which separate nodules of normal hepatocytes without portal triads or central hepatic veins.

HEPATOCELLULAR (LIVER CELL) ADENOMA

Adenomas arising from hepatocytes are rare and are reported in women in reproductive age group in association with use of oral contraceptives, sex hormone therapy and with pregnancy.

G/A The tumour usually occurs singly but about 10% are multiple. It is partly or completely encapsulated and slightly lighter in colour than adjacent liver or may be bile-stained. The tumours vary from a few centimetres up to 30 cm in diameter. On cut section, many of the tumours have varying degree of infarction and haemorrhage.

M/E Liver cell adenomas are composed of sheets and cords of hepatocytes which may be normal-looking or may show slight variation in size and shape but no mitoses. Numerous blood vessels are generally present in the tumour which may be thrombosed.

BILE DUCT ADENOMA (CHOLANGIOMA)

Intrahepatic or extrahepatic bile duct adenoma is a rare benign tumour. The tumour may be small, composed of acini lined by biliary epithelium and separated by variable amount of connective tissue, or are larger cystadenomas having loculi lined by biliary epithelium.

HAEMANGIOMA

Haemangioma is the commonest benign tumour of the liver. Majority of them are asymptomatic and discovered incidentally. Rarely, a haemangioma may rupture into the peritoneal cavity.

G/A Haemangiomas appear as solitary or multiple, circumscribed, red-purple lesions, commonly subcapsular and varying from a few millimetres to a few centimetres in diameter. They are commonly cavernous type giving the sectioned surface a spongy appearance.

M/E Haemangioma of the liver shows characteristic large, cavernous, blood-filled spaces, lined by a single layer of endothelium and separated by connective tissue.

MALIGNANT HEPATIC TUMOURS

Among the primary malignant tumours of the liver, hepatocellular (liver cell) carcinoma accounts for approximately 85% of all primary malignant tumours, cholangiocarcinoma for about 5-10%, and infrequently mixed pattern is seen. The remainder are rare tumours that include hepatoblastoma, haemangiosarcoma (angiosarcoma) and embryonal sarcoma.

HEPATOCELLULAR CARCINOMA

Hepatocellular carcinoma (HCC) or liver cell carcinoma, also termed as hepatoma, is the most common primary malignant tumour of the liver. The tumour shows marked geographic variations in incidence which is closely related to HBV and HCV infection in the region. Liver cell cancer is more common in males than in females in the ratio of 4:1. The peak incidence occurs in 5th to 6th decades of life. The tumour supervenes on cirrhosis in 70-80% of cases.

ETIOPATHOGENESIS A number of etiologic factors are implicated in the etiology of HCC, most important being *HBV and HCV infection, and association with cirrhosis.*

1. Relation to HBV infection Genesis of HCC is linked to prolonged infection with HBV.

i) The incidence of HBsAg positivity is higher in HCC patients.

ii) In African and Asian patients, 95% cases of HCC have anti-HBc.

iii) There is more direct evidence of integration of HBV-DNA genome in the genome of tumour cells of HCC.

2. Relation to HCV infection Long-standing HCV infection has emereged as a major factor in the etiology of HCC, generally after more than 30 years of infection. The evidences in support are as under:

i) In developed countries where higher incidence of HCC was earlier attributed to endemic HBV infection (e.g. in Japan) has shown a remarkable shift to HCV infection.

ii) The patients having anti-HCV and anti-HBc antibodies together have three times higher risk of developing HCC than in those with either antibody alone.

iii) HCV infection after a long interval produces cirrhosis more often prior to development of HCC, while in HCC following HBV infection half the cases have cirrhosis and remainder have chronic hepatitis.

iv) It is also possible that HBV and HCV infection may act synergistically to predispose to HCC.

3. Relation to cirrhosis Cirrhosis of all etiologic types is more commonly associated with HCC but the most frequent association is with macronodular post-necrotic cirrhosis. *Liver cell dysplasia* identified by cellular enlargement, nuclear hyperchromatism and multinucleate cells, is found in 60% of cirrhotic livers with HCC.

4. Relation to alcohol It has been observed that alcoholics have about four-fold increased risk of developing HCC. It is possible that alcohol may act as co-carcinogen with HBV or HCV infection, but alcohol does not appear to be a hepatic carcinogen *per se*.

5. Mycotoxins An important mycotoxin, aflatoxin B1, produced by a mould *Aspergillus flavus*, can contaminate poorly stored wheat grains or groundnuts, in hot and humid palces. Aflatoxin B1 is carcinogenic; it may act as a co-carcinogen with hepatitis B or may suppress the cellular immune response.

6. Chemical carcinogens These include:

i) Butter-yellow, saffrole and nitrosamines used as common food additives.

ii) Bush trees containing pyrrolizidine, tannin acid.

iii) Pollutants such as pesticides and insecticides.

7. Miscellaneous factors Various other factors are:

i) Haemochromatosis

ii) α-1-antitrypsin deficiency

iii) Prolonged immunosuppressive therapy in renal transplant patients

iv) Other types of viral hepatitis

v) Non-alcoholic steatohepatitis (NASH)

vi) Tobacco smoking

vii) Parasitic infestations such as clonorchiasis and schistosomiasis

viii) Glycogen storage diseases.

Molecular pathogenesis of HCC can be explained on the basis of genetic mutations induced by one or more of the above major etiologic factors which damage the DNA of hepatocye and results in neoplastic tranformation. These mutated genes are as under:

i) Inactivation of tumour suppressor oncogene *p53* by HBV.

ii) Binding of X-protein (HBxAg) generated from X-gene of HBV to *p53*.

iii) Mutations of oncogenes such as *KRAS*

iv) Mutations in receptors for hepatocyte growth factors e.g. *c-MYC*, *c-MET*.

v) Activation of *WNT* and *AKT* pathways.

G/A HCC may form one of the following 3 patterns of growth, in decreasing order of frequency:

i) *Expanding type:* Most frequently, it forms a *single*, yellow-brown, *large mass*, most often in the right lobe of the liver with central necrosis, haemorrhage and occasional bile-staining.

ii) *Multifocal type:* Less often, *multifocal, multiple masses,* 3-5 cm in diameter, scattered throughout the liver are seen.

iii) *Infiltrating (Spreading) type:* Rarely, the HCC forms diffusely infiltrating tumour mass.

M/E The tumour cells in the typical HCC resemble hepatocytes but vary with the degree of differentiation, ranging from well-differentiated to highly anaplastic lesions.

1. Histologic patterns: These include the following:

i) *Trabecular or sinusoidal pattern* is the most common. The trabeculae are made up of 2-8 cell wide layers of tumour.

ii) *Pseudoglandular or acinar pattern* is seen sometimes. The tumour cells are disposed around central cystic space.

iii) *Compact pattern* resembles trabecular pattern but the tumour cells form large solid masses.

iv) *Scirrhous pattern* is characterised by more abundant fibrous stroma.

2. Cytologic features: The typical cytologic features in the HCC consist of cells resembling hepatocytes having vesicular nuclei with prominent nucleoli. The cytoplasm is granular and eosinophilic but becomes increasingly basophilic with increasing malignancy. Aside from these features, a few other cellular features are: pleomorphism, bizarre giant cell formation, spindle-shaped cells, tumour cells with clear cytoplasm, presence of bile within dilated canaliculi, and intracytoplasmic Mallory's hyalin.

FIBROLAMELLAR CARCINOMA A clinicopathologic variant of the HCC is fibrolamellar carcinoma of the liver found in young people of both sexes. The tumour forms a single large mass which may be encapsulated and occurs in the absence of cirrhosis.

M/E The tumour is composed of eosinophilic polygonal cells (oncocytes) forming cords and nests which are separated by bands of fibrous stroma.

The prognosis of fibrolamellar carcinoma is better than other forms of HCC.

CLINICAL FEATURES The usual features consist of hepatomegaly with palpable mass in the liver, right upper quadrant pain or tenderness, and less often, jaundice, fever and haemorrhage from oesophageal varices. Ascites with RBCs and malignant cells is found in about half the patients. Rarely, systemic endocrine manifestations due to paraneoplastic syndrome are obsereved such as hypercalcaemia, hypoglycaemia, gynaecomastia and acquired porphyria.

Laboratory findings yield nonspecific results like anaemia, markedly elevated serum alkaline phosphatase as found in cirrhosis, and high serum alpha-foetoprotein (AFP). Elevated AFP level is quite specific; very high levels of AFP (above 500 ng/ml) are observed in 70-80% cases of HCC but lacks sensitivity since AFP is also found elevated in yolk sac tumour, cirrhosis, chronic hepatitis, massive liver necrosis and normal pregnancy.

SPREAD The HCC can have both intrahepatic and extrahepatic spread which faithfully reproduces the structure of the primary tumour:

The causes of death from the HCC are cachexia, massive bleeding from oesophageal varices, and liver failure with hepatic coma. Usually, survial after dignosis of HCC is less than 2 years.

CHOLANGIOCARCINOMA

Cholangiocarcinoma is the designation used for carcinoma arising from bile duct epithelium within the liver *(peripheral cholangiocarcinoma)*. Carcinomas arising from the large hilar ducts *(hilar cholangiocarcinoma)* and from extrahepatic ducts are termed *bile duct carcinomas*. None of the etiologic factors related to HCC have any role in the genesis of cholangiocarcinoma. However, the etiological factors involved in it are exposure to radio-opaque dye thorotrast, anabolic steroids, clonorchiasis and fibrocystic disease.

G/A The tumour is firm to hard and whitish.

M/E The tumour has glandular structure. The tumour cells resemble biliary epithelium but without bile secretion. They form various patterns such as tubular, ductular or papillary. The stroma consists of fibrous tissue with little or no capillary formation.

Hepatoblastoma is a rare malignant tumour arising from primitive hepatic parenchymal cells. It presents before the age of 2 years as progressive abdominal distension with anorexia, failure to thrive, fever and jaundice. It is more common in boys. The concentration of serum AFP is high.

G/A The tumour is circumscribed and lobulated mass measuring 5-25 cm in size, having areas of cystic degeneration, haemorrhage and necrosis.

M/E Hepatoblastoma consists of 2 components:

i) **Epithelial component** contains 2 types of cells—*'embryonal' hepatocytes* are small with dark-staining, hyperchromatic nuclei and scanty cytoplasm, while *'foetal' hepatocytes* are larger with more cytoplasm that may be granular or clear.

ii) **Mesenchymal component** includes fibrous connective tissue, cartilage and osteoid of variable degree of maturation.

SECONDARY HEPATIC TUMOURS

Metastatic tumours in the liver are more common than the primary hepatic tumours. Most frequently, they are blood-borne metastases, irrespective of whether the primary tumour is drained by portal vein or systemic veins. Most frequent primary tumours metastasising to the liver, in descending order of frequency, are those of stomach, breast, lungs, colon, oesophagus, pancreas, malignant melanoma and haematopoietic malignancies. Sarcomas rarely metastasise to the liver.

G/A Most metastatic carcinomas form multiple, spherical, nodular masses which are of variable size. The tumour deposits are white, well-demarcated, soft or haemorrhagic.

M/E The metastatic tumours generally reproduce the structure of the primary lesions.

BILIARY TRACT (p. 623)

NORMAL STRUCTURE

ANATOMY The gallbladder is a pear-shaped organ, 9 cm in length and has a capacity of approximately 50 ml. It consists of the *fundus, body* and *neck* that tapers into the cystic duct. The two hepatic ducts from right and left lobes of the liver unite at the porta hepatis to form the common hepatic duct which is joined by the cystic duct from the gallbladder to form the common bile duct. The common bile duct enters the second part of the duodenum posteriorly.

M/E The gallbladder, unlike the rest of gastrointestinal tract, lacks the muscularis mucosae and submucosa. The wall of the gallbladder is composed of the following 4 layers:
1. Mucosal layer
2. Smooth muscle layer
3. Perimuscular layer
4. Serosal layer

FUNCTIONS The main function of the gallbladder is to store and concentrate the bile secreted by the liver and then deliver it into the intestine for digestion and absorption of fat.

CHOLELITHIASIS (GALLSTONES) (p. 623)

Gallstones are formed from constituents of the bile (viz. cholesterol, bile pigments and calcium salts) along with other organic components. Accordingly, the gallstones commonly contain cholesterol, bile pigment and calcium salts in varying proportions. They are usually formed in the gallbladder, but sometimes may develop within extrahepatic biliary passages, and rarely in the larger intrahepatic bile duct.

These factors which largely pertain to cholesterol stones can be summed up in the old saying that gallstones are common in 4F's acronym for—'fat, female, fertile (multipara) and forty'. Some of the risk factors in lithogenesis are as under:

1. **Geography** Gallstones are quite prevalent in almost the entire Western world.

2. **Genetic factors** There is increased frequency of gallstones in first-degree relatives of patients with cholelithiasis.

3. **Age** There is steady increase in the prevalence of gallstones with advancing age which may be related to increased cholesterol content in the bile.

4. **Sex** Gallstones are twice more frequent in women than in men.

5. **Drugs** Women on oestrogen therapy or on birth control pills have higher incidence of gallstones.

6. **Obesity** Obesity is associated with increased cholesterol synthesis and its excretion resulting in higher incidence of gallstones in obese patients.

7. **Diet** Deficiency of dietary fibre content is linked to higher prevalence of gallstones.

8. **Gastrointestinal diseases** Certain gastrointestinal disorders such as Crohn's disease, ileal resection, ileal bypass surgery etc are associated with interruption in enterohepatic circulation followed by gallstone formation.

9. **Factors in pigment gallstones** All the above factors apply largely to cholesterol stones. Pigment stones, whether pure or mixed type, are more frequently associated with haemolytic anaemias which lead to increased content of unconjugated bilirubin in the bile.

PATHOGENESIS

The mechanism is explained separately below for mixed and pigment gallstones.

PATHOGENESIS OF CHOLESTEROL, MIXED GALLSTONES AND BILIARY SLUDGE

Formation of lithogenic (stone-forming) bile is explained by the following mechanisms:

1. **Supersaturation of bile** Two other disturbances which may contribute to supersaturation of the bile with cholesterol are:
i) Reduced bile acid pool
ii) Increased conversion of cholic acid to deoxycholic acid

2. **Cholesterol nucleation** Initiation of cholesterol stones occurs by nucleation of cholesterol monohydrate crystals. Accelerated nucleation of cholesterol monohydrate may occur either from pro-nucleating factors or from deficiency of anti-nucleating factors:

3. **Gallbladder hypomotility** Normally, the gallbladder is capable of emptying and clearing any sludge or debris which might initiate stone formation. This takes place under the influence of *cholecystokinin* secreted from small intestine. However, the motility of gallbladder may be impaired due to decrease in cholecystokinin receptors in the gallbladder resulting in stasis of biliary sludge and lithogenesis.

PATHOGENESIS OF PIGMENT GALLSTONES

i) Chronic haemolysis resulting in increased level of unconjugated bilirubin in the bile.
ii) Alcoholic cirrhosis.
iii) Chronic biliary tract infection e.g. by parasitic infestations of the biliary tract such as by *Clonorchis sinensis* and *Ascaris lumbricoides*.
iv) Demographic and genetic factors e.g. in rural setting and prevalence in Asian countries.

As stated before, gallstones contain cholesterol, bile pigment and calcium carbonate, either in pure form or in various combinations. Accordingly, gallstones are of 3 major types—*pure gallstones, mixed gallstones* and *combined gallstones*. Mixed gallstones are the most common (80%) while pure and combined gallstones comprise 10% each. In general, gallstones are formed most frequently in the gallbladder but may occur in extrahepatic as well as intrahepatic biliary passages. Presence of calcium salts renders gallstones radio-opaque, while cholesterol stones appear as radiolucent filling defects in the gallbladder.

1. PURE GALLSTONES They constitute about 10% of all gallstones. They are further divided into 3 types according to the component of bile forming them.

i) Pure cholesterol gallstones: They are usually solitary, oval and fairly large (3 cm or more) filling the gallbladder. Their surface is hard, smooth, whitish-yellow and glistening. On cut section, the pure cholesterol stone shows radiating glistening crystals.

ii) Pure pigment gallstones: These stones composed primarily of bile pigment, calcium bilirubinate, and contain less than 20% cholesterol. They are generally multiple, jet-black and small (less than 1 cm in diameter). They have mulberry like external surface.

iii) Pure calcium carbonate gallstones: They are rare. Calcium carbonate gallstones are usually multiple, grey-white, small (less than 1 cm in diameter), faceted and fairly hard due to calcium content.

2. MIXED GALLSTONES Mixed gallstones are the most common (80%) and contain more than 50% cholesterol monohydrate plus an admixture of calcium salts, bile pigments and fatty acids. They are always multiple, multifaceted so that they fit together and vary in size from as tiny as sand-grain to 1 cm or more in diameter.

3. COMBINED GALLSTONES They comprise about 10% of all gallstones. Combined gallstones are usually solitary, large and smooth-surfaced. It has a *pure gallstone nucleus* (cholesterol, bile pigment or calcium carbonate) and outer shell of mixed gallstone; or a *mixed gallstone nucleus* with pure gallstone shell.

CLINICAL MANIFESTATIONS AND COMPLICATIONS

In about 50% cases, gallstones cause no symptoms and may be diagnosed by chance during investigations for some other condition *(silent gallstones)*. Symptomatic gallstone disease appears only when complications develop:
1. Cholecystitis
2. Choledocholithiasis
3. Mucocele and empyema
4. Biliary fistula
5. Gallstone ileus
6. Pancreatitis
7. Gallbladder cancer

CHOLECYSTITIS *(p. 626)*

Cholecystitis or inflammation of the gallbladder may be acute, chronic, or acute superimposed on chronic.

ACUTE CHOLECYSTITIS

In many ways, acute cholecystitis is similar to acute appendicitis.

ETIOPATHOGENESIS Based on the initiating mechanisms, acute cholecystitis occurs in two types of situations.

◈ **Acute calculous cholecystitis** In 90% of cases, acute cholecystitis is caused by obstruction in the neck of the gallbladder or in the cystic duct by a gallstone. The commonest location of impaction of a gallstone is in Hartmann's pouch.

◈ **Acute acalculous cholecystitis** The remaining 10% cases of acute cholecystitis do not contain gallstones. In such cases, a variety of causes have been assigned such as previous nonbiliary surgery, multiple injuries, burns, recent childbirth, severe sepsis, dehydration, torsion of the gallbladder and diabetes mellitus.

G/A The gallbladder is distended and tense. The serosal surface is coated with fibrinous exudate with congestion and haemorrhages. The mucosa is bright red. The lumen is filled with pus mixed with green bile. When obstruction of the cystic duct is complete, the lumen is filled with purulent exudate and the condition is known as *empyema of the gallbladder.*

M/E Wall of the gallbladder shows marked inflammatory oedema, congestion and neutrophilic exudate. There may be frank abscesses in the wall and gangrenous necrosis.

CLINICAL FEATURES The patients of acute cholecystitis of either type have similar clinical features. They present with severe pain in the upper abdomen with features of peritoneal irritation such as guarding and hyperaesthesia. The gallbladder is tender and may be palpable. Fever, leucocytosis with neutrophilia and slight jaundice are generally present.

CHRONIC CHOLECYSTITIS

Chronic cholecystitis is the commonest type of clinical gallbladder disease.

ETIOPATHOGENESIS The association of chronic cholecystitis with mixed and combined gallstones is virtually always present. However, it is not known what initiates the inflammatory response in the gallbladder wall. In some patients, repeated attacks of mild acute cholecystitis result in chronic cholecystitis.

G/A The gallbladder is generally contracted but may be normal or enlarged. The wall of the gallbladder is thickened which on cut section is grey-white due to dense fibrosis or may be even calcified.

M/E The features are as under:
1. Thickened and congested mucosa but occasionally mucosa may be totally destroyed.
2. Penetration of the mucosa deep into the wall of the gallbladder up to muscularis layer to form *Rokitansky-Aschoff'sinuses.*
3. Variable degree of chronic inflammatory reaction, consisting of lymphocytes, plasma cells and macrophages, present in the lamina propria and subserosal layer.
4. Variable degree of fibrosis in the subserosal and subepithelial layers.
   A few morphologic variants of chronic cholecystitis are:
◈ Cholecystitis glandularis
◈ Porcelain gallbladder
◈ Acute on chronic cholecystitis.

CLINICAL FEATURES Chronic cholecystitis has ill-defined and vague symptoms. Generally, the patient—*a fat, fertile, female of forty or fifty,* presents with abdominal distension or epigastric discomfort, especially after a fatty meal. There is a constant dull ache in the right hypochondrium and epigastrium and tenderness over the right upper abdomen. Nausea and flatulence are common.

TUMOURS OF BILIARY TRACT *(p. 628)*

BENIGN TUMOURS

Benign tumours such as papilloma, adenoma, adenomyoma, fibroma, lipoma, myxoma, and haemangioma have been described in the biliary tract but all of them are exceedingly rare. *Adenomyoma* is more common benign tumour than the rest.

MALIGNANT TUMOURS

CARCINOMA OF THE GALLBLADDER

Primary carcinoma of the gallbladder is more prevalent than other cancers of the extrahepatic biliary tract. Like cholelithiasis and cholecystitis, it is

more frequent in women than in men (ratio 4:1) with a peak incidence in 7th
decade of life.

ETIOLOGY   Following factors have been implicated:

1.   Cholelithiasis and cholecystitis   The most significant association of cancer of the gallbladder is with cholelithiasis and cholecystitis, though there is no definite evidence of causal relationship.

2.   Chemical carcinogens   These include methyl cholanthrene, various nitrosamines and pesticides. Workers engaged in rubber industry have higher incidence of gallbladder cancer.

3.   Genetic factors   There is higher incidence of cancer of the gallbladder in certain populations living in the same geographic region suggesting a strong genetic component in the disease.

4.   Miscellaneous   Patients who have undergone previous surgery on the biliary tract have higher incidence of subsequent gallbladder cancer. Patients with inflammatory bowel disease (ulcerative colitis and Crohn's disease) have high incidence of gallbladder cancer.

MORPHOLOGIC FEATURES   The commonest site is the fundus, followed next in frequency by the neck of the gallbladder.

G/A   Cancer of the gallbladder is of 2 types—
1. Infiltrating type appears as an irregular area of diffuse thickening and induration of the gallbladder wall.
2. Fungating type grows like an irregular, friable, papillary or cauliflower-like growth into the lumen as well as into the wall of the gallbladder and beyond.

M/E   Following patterns are observed:
1. Most gallbladder cancers are *adenocarcinomas* (90%). They may be papillary or infiltrative, well-differentiated or poorly-differentiated.
2. About 5% of gallbladder cancers are *squamous cell carcinomas* arising from squamous metaplastic epithelium.
3. A few cases show both squamous and adenocarcinoma pattern of growth called *adenosquamous carcinoma*.

CLINICAL FEATURES   Carcinoma of the gallbadder is slow-growing and causes symptoms late in the course of disease. Quite often, the diagnosis is made when gallbladder is removed for cholelithiasis. The symptomatic cases have pain, jaundice, noticeable mass, anorexia and weight loss.

CARCINOMA OF AMPULLA OF VATER AND EXTRAHEPATIC BILE DUCTS

In its pure form, the term *ampullary carcinoma* is used for adenocarcinoma located in the ampulla of Vater, and often its origin from pre-existing villous or tubulovillous adenoma of the ampulla may be demonstrable. However, when the tumour is advanced, it is indistinguishable from 3 other cancers in the vicinity:
i)   cancer of adjacent duodenal mucosa with secondary involvement of ampulla;
ii)   cancer of terminal third of bile duct infiltrating in the ampulla; and
iii) carcinoma of the head of pancreas merging into the ampulla.
   Therefore, in adavanced cancer involving the ampulla, the term *periampullary carcinoma* is used that encompasses cancer from all 4 anatomic sites: i) ampulla of Vater, ii) duodenum, iii) terminal part of common bile duct, and iv) the head of pancreas.

ETIOLOGY   There is no association between carcinoma of common bile duct and gallstones. Bile duct cancers are associated with a number of other conditions such as ulcerative colitis, sclerosing cholangitis, parasitic infestations of the bile ducts with *Fasciola hepatica* (liver fluke), *Ascaris lumbricoides* and *Clonorchis sinensis*.

MORPHOLOGIC FEATURES   Ampullary carcinoma may be centered on the ampulla bulging into the duodenum *(intraampullary carcinoma)* or may form circumferential growth around the ampulla *(periampullary carcinoma)*.

G/A Ampullary carcinoma projects into the duodenal lumen and has a papillary surface. Bile duct carcinoma is usually small, extending for 1-2 cm along the duct.

M/E The tumour is usually adenocarcinoma varying from well-differentiated to poorly differentiated and may or may not be mucin-secreting.

CLINICAL FEATURES   Obstructive jaundice is the usual presenting feature which is characterised by intense pruritus. Pain, steatorrhoea, weight loss and weakness may be present. The tumour usually metastasises to the regional lymph nodes. Prognosis of ampullary carcinoma is better than than pancreatic cancer and bile duct carcinoma.

EXOCRINE PANCREAS *(p. 630)*

NORMAL STRUCTURE

The human pancreas, though anatomically a single organ, histologically and physiologically has 2 distinct parts—the *exocrine* and *endocrine parts.*

ANATOMY   The pancreas lies obliquely in the concavity of the duodenum as an elongated structure about 15 cm in length and 100 gm in weight. It is subdivided into 3 topographic zones: *head, body, tail.*

HISTOLOGY   The exocrine pancreas constitutes 80 to 85% of the total gland, while the endocrine pancreas comprises the remaining part. The exocrine part is divided into rhomboid lobules separated by thin fibrous tissue septa containing blood vessels, lymphatics, nerves and ducts. Each lobule is composed of numerous acini.

FUNCTIONS   The main functions of the exocrine pancreas is the alkaline secretion of digestive enzymes prominent among which are trypsin, chymotrypsin, elastase, amylase, lipase and phospholipase.

DEVELOPMENTAL ANOMALIES *(p. 631)*

CYSTIC FIBROSIS

Cystic fibrosis of the pancreas or fibrocystic disease is a hereditary disorder characterised by viscid mucous secretions in all the exocrine glands of the body *(mucoviscidosis)* and is associated with increased concentrations of electrolytes in the eccrine glands.

The disease has an *autosomal recessive inheritance* but clinical features are apparent in homozygotes only with apparent clinical features in homozygotes only. It is quite common in the whites (1 per 2000 livebirths). The clinical manifestations may appear at birth or later in adolescence and pertain to multiple organs and systems such as pancreatic insufficiency, intestinal obstruction, steatorrhoea, malnutrition, hepatic cirrhosis and respiratory complications.

MORPHOLOGIC FEATURES   Depending upon the severity of involvement and organs affected, the changes are variable.

1. Pancreas   The pancreas is almost invariably involved in cystic fibrosis.

G/A Pancreatic lobules are ovoid rather than rhomboid. Fatty replacement of the pancreas and grossly visible cysts may be seen.

M/E The lobular architecture of pancreatic parenchyma is maintained. There is increased interlobular fibrosis. The acini are atrophic and many of the acinar ducts contain laminated, eosinophilic concretions.

2. Liver   The bile canaliculi are plugged by viscid mucous which may cause diffuse fatty change, portal fibrosis and ductular proliferation.

3. Respiratory tract   Changes in the respiratory passages are seen in almost all typical cases of cystic fibrosis. The viscid mucous secretions of the submucosal glands of the respiratory tract cause obstruction, dilatation and infection of the airways.

4. Salivary glands   Pathologic changes in the salivary glands are similar to those in pancreas and include obstruction of the ducts, dilatation, fibrosis and glandular atrophy.

5. Sweat glands Hypersecretion of sodium and chloride in the sweat observed in these patients may be reflected pathologically by diminished vacuolation of the cells of eccrine glands.

PANCREATITIS *(p. 631)*

Pancreatitis is inflammation of the pancreas with acinic cell injury. It is classified into acute and chronic forms.

ACUTE PANCREATITIS

Acute pancreatitis is an acute inflammation of the pancreas presenting clinically with 'acute abdomen'. The severe form of the disease associated with macroscopic haemorrhages and fat necrosis in and around the pancreas is termed *acute haemorrhagic pancreatitis* or *acute pancreatic necrosis*. The condition occurs in adults between the age of 40 and 70 years and is commoner in females than in males.

The onset of acute pancreatitis is sudden, occurring after a bout of alcohol or a heavy meal. The patient presents with abdominal pain, vomiting and collapse and the condition must be differentiated from other diseases producing acute abdomen. Characteristically, there is elevation of *serum amylase* level within the first 24 hours and elevated *serum lipase* level after 3 to 4 days, the latter being more specific for pancreatic disease.

ETIOLOGY The two leading causes associated with acute pancreatitis are *alcoholism* and *cholelithiasis,* both of which are implicated in more than 80% of cases. Less common causes of acute pancreatitis include trauma, ischaemia, shock, extension of inflammation from the adjacent tissues, blood-borne bacterial infection, viral infections, certain drugs (e.g. thiazides, sulfonamides, oral contraceptives), hypothermia, hyperlipoproteinaemia and hypercalcaemia from hyperparathyroidism.

PATHOGENESIS The destructive changes in the pancreas are attributed to the liberation and activation of pancreatic enzymes. Though more than 20 enzymes are secreted by exocrine pancreas, 3 main groups of enzymes which bring about destructive effects on the pancreas are:
1. Proteases
2. Lipases and phospholipases
3. Elastases.

The activation and release of these enzymes is brought about by one of the following mechanisms:
i) Acinic cell damage
ii) Duct obstruction
iii) Block in exocytosis.

G/A In the early stage, the pancreas is swollen and oedematous. Subsequently, in a day or two, characteristic variegated appearance of grey-white pancreatic necrosis, chalky-white fat necrosis and blue-black haemorrhages are seen.

M/E Following features in varying grades are seen:
1. Necrosis of pancreatic lobules and ducts.
2. Necrosis of the arteries and arterioles with areas of haemorrhages.
3. Fat necrosis.
4. Inflammatory reaction, chiefly by polymorphs, around the areas of necrosis and haemorrhages.

COMPLICATIONS A patient of acute pancreatitis who survives may develop a variety of systemic and local complications.

Systemic complications:
1. Chemical and bacterial peritonitis.
2. Endotoxic shock.
3. Acute renal failure.

Local sequelae:
1. Pancreatic abscess.
2. Pancreatic pseudocyst.
3. Duodenal obstruction.

Mortality in acute pancreatitis is high (20-30%). Patients succumb to hypotensive shock, infection, acute renal failure, and DIC.

CHRONIC PANCREATITIS

Chronic pancreatitis or *chronic relapsing pancreatitis* is the progressive destruction of the pancreas due to repeated mild and subclinical attacks of acute pancreatitis. Most patients present with recurrent attacks of severe abdominal pain at intervals of months to years. Weight loss and jaundice are often associated.

ETIOLOGY Most cases of chronic pancreatitis are caused by the same factors as for acute pancreatitis. Thus, most commonly, chronic pancreatitis is related to *chronic alcoholism* with protein-rich diet, and less often to *biliary tract disease.*

PATHOGENESIS Acute haemorrhagic pancreatitis seldom develops into chronic pancreatitis, but instead develops pancreatic pseudocysts following recovery. Pathogenesis of alcoholic and non-alcoholic chronic pancreatitis is explained by different mechanisms:
1. Chronic pancreatitis due to *chronic alcoholism* accompanied by a high-protein diet results in increase in protein concentration in the pancreatic juice which obstructs the ducts and causes damage.
2. *Non-alcoholic cases* of chronic pancreatitis seen in tropical countries (tropical chronic pancreatitis) result from protein-calorie malnutrition.

G/A The pancreas is enlarged, firm and nodular. The cut surface shows a smooth grey appearance with loss of normal lobulation. Foci of calcification and tiny pancreatic concretions to larger visible stones are frequently found.

M/E Depending upon the stage, following changes are seen:
1. Obstruction of the ducts
2. Squamous metaplasia and dilatation of some inter- and intralobular ducts.
3. Chronic inflammatory infiltrate around the lobules as well as the ducts.
4. Atrophy of the acinar tissue.
5. Islet tissue is involved in late stage only.

COMPLICATIONS Late stage of chronic pancreatitis may be complicated by diabetes mellitus, pancreatic insufficiency with steatorrhoea and malabsorption and formation of pancreatic pseudocysts.

TUMOURS AND TUMOUR-LIKE LESIONS (p. 633)

PANCREATIC PSEUDOCYST

Pancreatic pseudocyst is a localised collection of pancreatic juice, necrotic debris and haemorrhages. It develops following either acute pancreatitis or trauma. The patients generally present with abdominal mass producing pain, intraperitoneal haemorrhage and generalised peritonitis.

G/A The pseudocyst may be present within or adjacent to the pancreas. Usually it is solitary, unilocular, measuring up to 10 cm in diameter with thin or thick wall.

M/E The cyst wall is composed of dense fibrous tissue with marked inflammatory reaction. There is evidence of preceding haemorrhage and necrosis in the form of deposits of haemosiderin pigment, calcium and cholesterol crystals.

CARCINOMA OF PANCREAS

Pancreatic cancer is the term used for cancer of the exocrine pancreas. It is one of the common cancers, particularly in the Western countries and Japan. It is commoner in males than in females and the incidence increases progressively after the age of 50 years.

ETIOLOGY Following factors have been implicated in its etiology:
1. *Smoking:* Heavy cigarette smokers have higher incidence than the non-smokers.

2. *Diet and obesity:* Diet with high total caloric value and high consumption of animal proteins and fats is related to higher incidence of pancreatic cancer.

3. *Chemical carcinogens:* Individuals exposed to β-naphthylamine, benzidine and nitrosamines have higher incidence of cancer of the pancreas.

4. *Diabetes mellitus:* Patients of long-standing diabetes mellitus have a higher incidence.

5. *Chronic pancreatitis* patients are at increased risk.

6. *H. pylori infection* has been reported to have association with pancreatic cancer.

7. *Genetic factors* have been found to have association with pancreatic cancer e.g. its occurrence in first-degree relatives.

MORPHOLOGIC FEATURES The most common location of pancreatic cancer is the head of pancreas (70%), followed in decreasing frequency, by the body and the tail of pancreas.

G/A Carcinoma of the head of pancreas is generally small, homogeneous, poorly-defined, grey-white mass without any sharp demarcation between the tumour and the surrounding pancreatic parenchyma. The tumour of the head extends into the ampulla of Vater, common bile duct and duodenum, producing obstructive biliary symptoms and jaundice early in the course of illness.

M/E Following patterns are seen:

1. *Well-differentiated adenocarcinoma,* both mucinous and non-mucin secreting type, is the most common pattern. Perineural invasion is commonly present and is diagnostic of malignancy.

2. *Adenoacanthoma* consisting of glandular carcinoma and benign squamous elements is seen in a proportion of cases.

3. Rarely, peculiar *tumour giant cell formation* is seen with marked anaplasia, pleomorphism and numerous mitoses.

4. *Acinar cell carcinoma* occurs rarely and reproduces the pattern of acini in normal pancreas.

CLINICAL FEATURES Clinical symptoms depend upon the site of origin of the tumour. Generally, the following features are present:

1. *Obstructive jaundice* More often and early in the course of disease in cases with carcinoma head of the pancreas (80%).

2. *Other features* These include: abdominal pain, anorexia, weight loss, cachexia, weakness and malaise, nausea and vomiting, and migratory thrombophlebitis (Trousseau's syndrome).

The prognosis of pancreatic cancer is dismal.

SELF ASSESSMENT

1. **All are features of extrahepatic biliary atresia (EHBA) <u>except</u>:**
   A. Ductular proliferation
   B. Giant cells
   C. Cholestasis
   D. Increased hepatic copper

2. **Centrilobular necrosis is seen in all <u>except</u>:**
   A. Yellow fever
   B. Ischaemia
   C. Chloroform
   D. Carbon tetrachloride

3. **The form of bilirubin which remains detectable in serum for sufficient time after recovery from the disease is:**
   A. Biliverdin
   B. Unconjugated bilirubin
   C. Unbound conjugated bilirubin
   D. Delta bilirubin

4. **Acute viral hepatitis by the following hepatotropic virus is characterised by fatty change in liver:**
   A. HAV
   B. HBV
   C. HCV
   D. HDV

5. **Extrahepatic cholestasis can be distinguished from intrahepatic cholestasis by the following tests in the former:**
   A. Bilirubinuria
   B. Hypoprothrombinaemia showing improvement following parenteral administration of vitamin K

C. Elevated serum alkaline phosphatase

D. Elevated serum bile acids

6. The following conditions have unconjugated hyperbilirubinaemia **except**:
   A. Dubin-Johnson syndrome
   B. Crigler-Najjar syndrome
   C. Jaundice of prematurity
   D. Gilbert syndrome

7. Kernicterus often develops in the following type of hereditary hyperbilirubinaemia:
   A. Gilbert syndrome
   B. Crigler-Najjar syndrome, type I
   C. Dubin-Johnson syndrome
   D. Rotor syndrome

8. Reye's syndrome is characterised by the following features **except**:
   A. It is a form of hereditary hyperbilirubinaemia
   B. There is microvesicular fatty change in hepatocytes
   C. Patients have a rapidly downhill course
   D. There is decreased activity of mitochondrial enzymes in the liver

9. Hepatic encephalopathy is due to:
   A. Hypoxic damage from ischaemia
   B. Toxic damage from ammonia
   C. Thromboembolic phenomena
   D. Hepatopulmonary syndrome

10. Following etiologic factors are implicated in Budd-Chiari syndrome **except**:
    A. Pulmonary embolism
    B. Hepatocellular carcinoma
    C. Polycythaemia vera
    D. Pregnancy

11. Councilman bodies in viral hepatitis are a form of apoptosis seen commonly at the following site:
    A. Submassive
    B. Centrilobular
    C. Midzonal
    D. Periportal

12. The following hepatotropic virus is a DNA virus:
    A. HAV
    B. HBV
    C. HCV
    D. HEV

13. Chronic carrier state of the following hepatotropic virus infection is observed in the following **except**:
    A. HAV
    B. HBV
    C. HCV
    D. HDV

14. In hepatitis A, life-long protective immunity against reinfection is given by the following class of antibody:
    A. IgA
    B. IgE
    C. IgG
    D. IgM

15. Hepatitis B surface antigen (HBsAg) is present as the following structures **except**:
    A. Viral spheres
    B. Viral tubules
    C. Surface envelope of Dane particle
    D. Inner core of Dane particle

16. HBsAg can be demonstrated at the following sites **except**:
    A. Serum of HBV-infected patient
    B. Carrier state of HBV
    C. Hepatocyte cell membrane in acute stage of illness
    D. Hepatocyte cell membrane in chronic hepatitis B

17. In chronic hepatitis B and carrier state of HBV infection, the following antigen is detected on the nuclei of infected hepatocytes:
    A. HBsAg
    B. HBeAg
    C. HBcAg
    D. HBV-DNA

18. In an HDV-infected individual, HDV antigen is detected at the following sites **except**:
    A. Serum in acute illness
    B. Serum in carrier state
    C. Hepatocyte cell membrane
    D. Hepatocyte nuclei

19. Vast majority (more than 90%) of cases of post-transfusion hepatitis are caused by:
   A. HBV
   B. HCV
   C. HDV
   D. HGV

20. The most progressive form of chronic hepatitis is caused by:
   A. Hepatitis A
   B. Hepatitis B
   C. Hepatitis C
   D. Hepatitis D

21. The following genetic component of HBV is considered responsible for its carcinogenic influence:
   A. HBsAg
   B. HBeAg
   C. HBcAg
   D. HBxAg

22. In amoebic liver abscess, trophozoites of E. histolytica are best demonstrated at:
   A. Necrotic centre of abscess
   B. Margin of abscess with viable liver tissue
   C. Granulation tissue in the abscess wall
   D. Fibrous wall of the abscess

23. The most common site for hydatid cyst is:
   A. Liver
   B. Lungs
   C. Spleen
   D. Brain

24. Micronodular cirrhosis includes the following etiologic types except:
   A. Laennec's cirrhosis
   B. Nutritional cirrhosis
   C. Post-necrotic cirrhosis
   D. Portal cirrhosis

25. The major hepatotoxic effect of ethanol is exerted by:
   A. Direct hepatotoxicity of ethanol
   B. Free radical injury
   C. Hepatotoxicity of acetaldehyde
   D. Immunologic mechanisms

26. Mallory's hyalin is seen in the following conditions except:
   A. Alcoholic hepatitis
   B. Hepatocellular carcinoma
   C. Post-necrotic cirrhosis
   D. Primary biliary cirrhosis

27. Primary biliary cirrhosis has the following features except:
   A. There is elevated cholesterol level in blood
   B. It has familial occurrence
   C. The condition is more common in men
   D. The disease has autoimmune origin

28. Patients of following type of cirrhosis more often may develop hepatocellular carcinoma as a late complication:
   A. Biliary cirrhosis
   B. Haemochromatosis-induced cirrhosis
   C. Cirrhosis in $\alpha 1$ antitrypsin deficiency
   D. Cardiac cirrhosis

29. Biochemical abnormalities in Wilson's disease include the following except:
   A. Increased serum ceruloplasmin
   B. Increased urinary copper excretion
   C. Increased hepatic copper
   D. Serum copper low-to-normal-to-high

30. Intrahepatic causes of portal hypertension include the following except:
   A. Cirrhosis
   B. Budd-Chiari syndrome
   C. Portal vein thrombosis
   D. Metastatic tumours

31. In developed countries the major risk factor in the pathogenesis of hepatocellular carcinoma is:
   A. Long-standing HBV infection
   B. Long-standing HCV infection
   C. Alcoholic cirrhosis
   D. Aflatoxin B1

32. Risk factors implicated in the etiology of cholesterol gallstones include the following <u>except</u>:
    - A. Family history
    - B. Obesity
    - C. Haemolytic anaemia
    - D. Oral contraceptives

33. The following type of gallstones are generally unassociated with changes in the gallbladder wall:
    - A. Cholesterol
    - B. Mixed
    - C. Combined
    - D. Pigment

34. The most common site for cancer of the gallbladder is:
    - A. Fundus
    - B. Body
    - C. Neck
    - D. Cystic duct

35. Pancreatic carcinoma of the following site more often produces obstructive jaundice:
    - A. Head
    - B. Body
    - C. Tail
    - D. Uncinate process

36. Which of the following hepatotropic viruses is not transmitted by transfusion?
    - A. HAV
    - B. HBV
    - C. HCV
    - D. HGV

37. Which of the following hepatotropic viruses does not cause chronic hepatitis?
    - A. HBV
    - B. HCV
    - C. HDV
    - D. HEV

38. All are true for fibrolamellar HCC <u>except</u>:
    - A. Found in young
    - B. Not preceded by cirrhosis
    - C. Encapsulated
    - D. Worse prognosis than classic HCC

39. A 40 years old woman presents with fever, malaise, signs of jaundice, clay-coloured stools, and high-coloured urine for 10 days. A liver biopsy reveals hepatocyte drop out necrosis, focal inflammation and ballooning degeneration and a few intensely eosinophilic oval bodies are found. What are these microscopic bodies called?
    - A. Councilman bodies
    - B. Mallory bodies
    - C. Psammoma bodies
    - D. Russell bodies

40. Which of the following abnormalities is most likely to be observed in a known case of hereditary haemochromatosis?
    - A. Ochronosis
    - B. Blue sclera
    - C. Bronze skin
    - D. Cherry-red pupils

KEY

1 = D	2 = B	3 = D	4 = C	5 = B
6 = A	7 = B	8 = A	9 = B	10 = A
11 = C	12 = B	13 = A	14 = C	15 = D
16 = C	17 = C	18 = C	19 = B	20 = C
21 = D	22 = B	23 = A	24 = C	25 = C
26 = C	27 = C	28 = B	29 = A	30 = C
31 = C	32 = C	33 = D	34 = A	35 = A
36 = C	37 = D	38 = D	39 = A	40 = C

KIDNEY (p. 636)

NORMAL STRUCTURE

ANATOMY The kidneys are bean-shaped paired organs, each weighing about 150 gm in the adult male and about 135 gm in the adult female. The hilum of the kidney is situated at the midpoint on the medial aspect where the artery, vein, lymphatics and ureter are located. The kidney is surrounded by a thin fibrous capsule which is adherent at the hilum.

Cut surface of the kidney shows 3 main structures: well-demarcated *peripheral cortex, inner medulla* and the innermost *renal pelvis*:

◈ The **renal cortex** forms the outer rim of the kidney and is about 1 cm in thickness. It contains all the glomeruli and about 85% of the nephron tubules.

◈ The **renal medulla** is composed of 8-18 cone-shaped renal pyramids. The base of a renal pyramid lies adjacent to the outer cortex and forms the cortico-medullary junction, while the apex of each called the *renal papilla* contains the opening of each renal pyramid for passage of urine.

◈ The **renal pelvis** is the funnel-shaped collection area of the urine for drainage into the ureter. The minor calyces (8-18 in number in a normal kidney) collect urine from renal papillae and drain into major calyces (2-3 in a normal kidney).

HISTOLOGY The parenchyma of each kidney is composed of approximately one million microstructures called nephrons. A nephron, in turn, consists of 5 major parts, each having a functional role in the formation of urine: the glomerular capsule (glomerulus and Bowman's capsule), the proximal convoluted tubule (PCT), the loop of Henle, the distal convoluted tubule (DCT), and the collecting ducts. From point of view of diseases of the kidneys, 4 components of renal parenchyma require further elaboration: renal vasculature, glomeruli, tubules and interstitium.

1. Renal vasculature Each kidney is supplied with blood by a main *renal artery* which arises from the aorta at the level of the 2nd lumbar vertebra. It is from the interlobular arteries that the *afferent arterioles* take their origin, each one supplying a single glomerulus. From the glomerulus emerge the *efferent arterioles*. The following important inferences can be drawn from the peculiarities of the renal vasculature:

i) The renal cortex receives about 90% of the total renal blood supply and that the pressure in the glomerular capillaries is high. Therefore, renal cortex is more prone to the effects of hypertension.

ii) The renal medulla, on the other hand, is poorly perfused and any interference in blood supply to it results in medullary necrosis.

iii) The divisions and subdivisions of the renal artery up to arterioles are end-arteries and have no anastomoses. Thus, occlusion of any of the branches results in infarction of the renal parenchyma supplied by it.

iv) Since the tubular capillary beds are derived from the efferent arterioles leaving the glomeruli, diseases affecting the blood flow through glomerular tuft have significant effects on the tubules as well.

2. Glomerulus The glomerulus consists of invagination of the blind end of the proximal tubule and contains a *capillary tuft* fed by the afferent arteriole and drained by efferent arteriole. The capillary tuft is covered by visceral epithelial cells (podocytes) which are continuous with those of the parietal epithelium at the *vascular pole*. The transition to proximal tubular cells occurs at the *urinary pole* of the glomerulus. The visceral and parietal epithelial cells are separated by the urinary space or *Bowman's space.*

Subdivisions of capillaries derived from the afferent arterioles result in the formation of *lobules* (up to 8 in number) within a glomerulus. Each lobule of a glomerular tuft consists of a centrilobular supporting stalk composed of mesangium containing *mesangial cells* (≤ 3 per lobule) and *mesangial matrix.*

The major *function* of glomerulus is complex filtration from the capillaries to the urinary space. Normally, glomerular filtration rate (GFR) is about 125 ml/minute. The barrier to glomerular filtration consists of the following 3 components:

i) Fenestrated endothelial cells lining the capillary loops.
ii) Glomerular basement membrane (GBM) on which the endothelial cells rest. It further consists of 3 layers—the central lamina densa, bounded by lamina rara interna on endothelial side of the capillary and lamina rara externa on visceral epithelial side of the capillary.
iii) Filtration slit pores between the foot processes of the visceral epithelial cells (podocytes) external to GBM.

The barrier to filtration of macromolecules of the size and molecular weight of albumin and larger depends upon the following:

a) A normal lamina densa.
b) Maintenance of negative charge on both lamina rarae.
c) A healthy covering of glomerular epithelial cells.

Juxtaglomerular apparatus The juxtaglomerular apparatus (JGA) is situated at the vascular pole of the glomerulus and is made up of 3 parts:

i) The juxtaglomerular cells
ii) The macula densa
iii) The lacis cells or non-granular cells

The JGA is intimately concerned with sodium metabolism and is the principal source of renin production.

3. Tubules The tubules of the kidney account for the greatest amount of the renal parenchyma. The structure of renal tubular epithelium varies in different parts of the nephron and is correlated with the functional capacity of that part of the tubule.

i) Proximal convoluted tubule (PCT) This is the first part arising from the glomerulus and is highly specialised part functionally.
ii) Loop of Henle The PCT drains into the straight part of loop of Henle that consists of thin descending, and thin and thick ascending limbs, both of which have different structure and function.
iii) Distal convoluted tubule (DCT) The DCT represents a transition from thick ascending limb from the point where the ascending limb meets the vascular pole of the glomerulus of its origin, to the early collecting ducts.
iv) Collecting ducts The system of collecting ducts is the final pathway by which urine reaches the tip of renal papilla.

4. Interstitium In health, the renal cortical interstitium is scanty and consists of a small number of fibroblast-like cells.

RENAL FUNCTION TESTS *(p. 639)*

In order to assess renal function, a number of tests have been devised which give information regarding the following parameters:

a) Renal blood flow
b) Glomerular filtration
c) Renal tubular function
d) Urinary outflow unhindered by any obstruction.

Renal function tests are broadly divided into 4 groups:

1. Urine analysis.
2. Concentration and dilution tests.
3. Blood chemistry.
4. Renal clearance tests.

In addition, renal biopsy is performed to confirm the diagnosis of renal disease. Renal biopsy is ideally fixed in alcoholic Bouin's solution and examined by routine morphology combined with special stains and for further studies as under:

1. *Periodic acid-Schiff* stain for highlighting glomerular basement membrane.
2. *Silver impregnation* to outline the glomerular and tubular basement membrane.
3. *Immunofluorescence* to localise the antigens, complements and immunoglobulins.
4. *Electron microscopy* to see the ultrastructure of glomerular changes.

1. URINE ANALYSIS The simplest diagnostic tests for renal function is the physical, chemical, bacteriologic and microscopic examination of the urine.

i) The *physical examination* includes 24-hour urinary output, colour, specific gravity and osmolality.

ii) The *chemical tests* are carried out to detect the presence of protein, glucose, red cells and haemoglobin to assess the permeability of glomerular membrane.

iii) The *bacteriologic examination* of the urine is done by proper and aseptic collection of midstream specimen of urine.

iv) *Urine microscopy* is undertaken on a fresh unstained sample. Various components observed on microscopic examination of the urine in renal disease are red cells, pus cells, epithelial cells, crystals and urinary casts.

2. CONCENTRATION AND DILUTION TESTS Concentration and dilution tests are designed to evaluate functional capacity of the renal tubules.

Traditionally, urinary concentration is determined by specific gravity of the urine (normal range 1.003 to 1.030, average 1.018). The tubular disease can be diagnosed in its early stage by *water deprivation* (concentration) or *water excess* (dilution) tests.

i) In **concentration test,** an artificial fluid deprivation is induced in the patient for more than 20 hours. If the nephron is normal, water is selectively reabsorbed resulting in excretion of urine of high solute concentration (specific gravity of 1.025 or more). However, if the tubular cells are nonfunctional, the solute concentration of the urine will remain constant regardless of stress of water deprivation.

ii) In **dilution test,** an excess of fluid is given to the patient. Normally, renal compensation should result in excretion of urine with high water content and lower solute concentration (specific gravity of 1.003 or less). If the renal tubules are diseased, the concentration of solutes in the urine will remain constant irrespective of the excess water intake.

3. BLOOD CHEMISTRY Impairment of renal function results in elevation of end-products of protein metabolism. This includes increased accumulation of certain substances in the blood, chiefly urea (normal range 20-40 mg/dl), blood urea nitrogen (BUN) (normal range 10-20 mg/dl) and creatinine (normal range 0.6-1.2 mg/dl). An increase of these end-products in the blood is called *azotaemia*.

4. RENAL CLEARANCE TESTS A clearance test is employed to assess the rate of glomerular filtration and the renal blood flow. The rate of this filtration can be measured by determining the excretion rate of a substance which is filtered through the glomerulus but subsequently is neither reabsorbed nor secreted by the tubules.

The substances which are used for clearance tests include inulin, mannitol, creatinine and urea.

PATHOPHYSIOLOGY OF RENAL DISEASE: RENAL FAILURE (p. 640)

Major groups of renal diseases are as under:

1. *Glomerular diseases:* These are most often immunologically-mediated and may be acute or chronic.

2. *Tubular diseases:* These are more likely to be caused by toxic or infectious agents and are often acute.

3. *Interstitial diseases:* These are likewise commonly due to toxic or infectious agents and quite often involve interstitium as well as tubules (tubulo-interstitial diseases).

4. *Vascular diseases:* These include changes in the nephron as a consequence of increased intra-glomerular pressure such as in hypertension or impaired blood flow.

Regardless of cause, renal disease usually results in the evolution of one of the two major pathological syndromes: *acute renal failure* and *chronic renal failure (or chronic kidney disease, CKD).*

ACUTE RENAL FAILURE (ARF)

Acute renal failure (ARF) is a syndrome characterised by rapid onset of renal dysfunction, chiefly oliguria or anuria, and sudden increase in metabolic waste-products (urea and creatinine) in the blood with consequent development of uraemia.

ETIOPATHOGENESIS The causes of ARF may be classified as pre-renal, intra-renal and post-renal in nature.

1. Pre-renal causes These causes include inadequate cardiac output and hypovolaemia or vascular disease causing reduced perfusion of the kidneys.

2. Intra-renal causes These include vascular disease of the arteries and arterioles within the kidney, diseases of glomeruli, acute tubular necrosis due to ischaemia, or the effect of a nephrotoxin, acute tubulointerstitial nephritis and pyelonephritis.

3. Post-renal causes Post-renal disease is characteristically caused by obstruction to the flow of urine anywhere along the renal tract distal to the opening of the collecting ducts.

CLINICAL FEATURES The clinical features will depend to a large extent on the underlying cause of ARF and on the stage of the disease at which the patient presents. However, one of the following three major patterns usually emerge:

1. Syndrome of acute nephritis The characteristic features are: mild proteinuria, haematuria, oedema and mild hypertension.

2. Syndrome accompanying tubular pathology When the ARF is caused by destruction of the tubular cells of the nephron as occurs in acute tubular necrosis, the disease typically progresses through 3 characteristic stages from oliguria to diuresis to recovery.

3. Pre-renal syndrome Typically, this pattern is seen in marginal ischaemia caused by renal arterial obstruction, hypovolaemia, hypotension or cardiac insufficiency. Due to depressed renal blood flow, there is decrease in GFR causing oliguria, azotaemia (elevation of BUN and creatinine) and possible fluid retention and oedema.

CHRONIC RENAL FAILURE (CRF)

Chronic renal failure is a syndrome characterised by progressive and irreversible deterioration of renal function due to slow destruction of renal parenchyma, eventually terminating in death when sufficient number of nephrons have been damaged.

ETIOPATHOGENESIS All chronic nephropathies can lead to CRF. The diseases leading to CRF can generally be classified into two major groups:

1. Diseases causing glomerular pathology A number of glomerular diseases associated with CRF have their pathogenesis in immune mechanisms. Glomerular destruction results in changes in filtration process and leads to development of the nephrotic syndrome characterised by proteinuria, hypoalbuminaemia and oedema. The important examples of chronic glomerular diseases causing CRF are covered under two headings:

i) *Primary glomerular pathology:* The major cause of CRF is chronic glomerulonephritis, usually initiated by various types of *glomerulonephritis* such as membranous glomerulonephritis, membranoproliferative glomerulonephritis, lipoid nephrosis (minimal change disease) and anti-glomerular basement membrane nephritis.

ii) *Systemic glomerular pathology:* Certain conditions originate outside the renal system but induce changes in the nephrons secondarily. Major examples of this type are systemic lupus erythematosus, serum sickness nephritis and diabetic nephropathy.

2. Diseases causing tubulointerstitial pathology Tubulointerstitial diseases can be categorised according to initiating etiology into 4 groups:

i) *Vascular causes:* Long-standing primary or essential hypertension produces characteristic changes in renal arteries and arterioles referred to as nephrosclerosis.

ii) *Infectious causes:* A good example of chronic renal infection causing CRF is chronic pyelonephritis.

iii) *Toxic causes:* Some toxic substances induce slow tubular injury, eventually culminating in CRF. The most common example is intake of high doses of analgesics such as phenacetin, aspirin and acetaminophen (chronic analgesic nephritis).

iv) *Obstructive causes:* The examples of this type of chronic injury are stones, blood clots, tumours, strictures and enlarged prostate.

Regardless of the initiating cause, CRF evolves progressively through 4 stages:

◆ **Decreased renal reserve** At this stage, damage to renal parenchyma is marginal and the kidneys remain functional. The GFR is about 50% of normal, BUN and creatinine values are normal.

◆ **Renal insufficiency** At this stage, about 75% of functional renal parenchyma has been destroyed. The GFR is about 25% of normal accompanied by elevation in BUN and serum creatinine.

◆ **Renal failure** At this stage, about 90% of functional renal tissue has been destroyed. The GFR is approximately 10% of normal. Tubular cells are essentially nonfunctional.

◆ **End-stage kidney (chronic kidney disease)** The GFR at this stage is less than 5% of normal and results in complex clinical picture of uraemic syndrome with progressive primary (renal) and secondary systemic (extra-renal) symptoms.

CLINICAL FEATURES Clinical manifestations of full-blown CRF culminating in uraemic syndrome are described under 2 main headings:

A. Primary uraemic (renal) manifestations Primary symptoms of uraemia develop when there is slow and progressive deterioration of renal function. The resulting imbalances cause the following manifestations:

1. Metabolic acidosis
2. Hyperkalaemia
3. Sodium and water imbalance
4. Hyperuricaemia
5. Azotaemia

B. Secondary uraemic (extra-renal) manifestations A number of extra-renal systemic manifestations develop secondarily following fluid-electrolyte and acid-base imbalances.

1. Anaemia
2. Integumentary system
3. Cardiovascular system
4. Respiratory system
5. Digestive system
6. Skeletal system
i) *Osteomalacia*
ii) *Osteitis fibrosa*

Approximately 10% of all persons are born with potentially significant malformations of the urinary system. About half of all patients with malformations of the kidneys have coexistent anomalies either elsewhere in the urinary tract or in other organs.

Malformations of the kidneys are classified into 3 broad groups:

I.   Abnormalities in amount of renal tissue Anomalies with deficient renal parenchyma (e.g. unilateral or bilateral renal hypoplasia) or with excess renal tissue (e.g. renomegaly, supernumerary kidneys).

II.   Anomalies of position, form and orientation Renal ectopia (pelvic kidney), renal fusion (horseshoe kidney) and persistent foetal lobation.

III.   Anomalies of differentiation Cystic diseases of the kidney.

CYSTIC DISEASES OF KIDNEY

Cystic lesions of the kidney may be *congenital or acquired, non-neoplastic or neoplastic*. Majority of these lesions are congenital non-neoplastic. Cystic lesions in the kidney may occur at any age, extending from foetal life (detected on ultrasonography) to old age.

Potter divided developmental renal cystic lesions into three types—I, II and III. As per current nomenclatures, common types are discussed below:

I. MULTICYSTIC RENAL DYSPLASIA

The term 'multicystic renal dysplasia' or Potter type II is used for disorganised metanephrogenic differentiation with persistence of structures in the kidney which are not represented in normal nephrogenesis. Renal dysplasia is the most common form of cystic renal disease in the newborn and infants.

MORPHOLOGIC FEATURES Renal dysplasia may be unilateral or bilateral. The dysplastic process may involve the entire renal mass or a part of it.

G/A The dysplastic kidney is almost always cystic. The kidney or its affected part is replaced by disorderly mass of multiple cysts resembling a bunch of grapes.

M/E The characteristic feature is the presence of undifferentiated mesenchyme that contains smooth muscle, cartilage and immature collecting ducts. The cysts in the mass represent dilated tubules lined by flattened epithelium which are surrounded by concentric layers of connective tissue.

CLINICAL FEATURES Unilateral renal dysplasia is frequently discovered in newborn or infants as a flank mass.

The prognosis of unilateral renal dysplasia following removal of the abnormal kidney is excellent.

II. POLYCYSTIC KIDNEY DISEASE

Polycystic disease of the kidney (PKD) is a disorder in which major portion of the renal parenchyma is converted into cysts of varying size. The disease occurs in two forms:

A. ADULT POLYCYSTIC KIDNEY DISEASE

Adult (autosomal dominant) polycystic kidney disease (ADPKD) is relatively common (incidence 1:400 to 1: 1:1000) and is the cause of end-stage renal failure in approximately 4% of haemodialysis patients. The pattern of inheritance is *autosomal dominant* with mutation in *PKD* gene. Family history of similar renal disease may be present. The true adult polycystic renal disease is always bilateral and diffuse. Though the kidneys are abnormal at birth, renal function is retained, and symptoms appear in adult life, mostly between the age of 30 and 50 years.

G/A Kidneys in ADPKD are always bilaterally enlarged, usually symmetrically, heavy (weighing up to 4 kg) and give it a lobulated appearance on external surface due to underlying cysts. The cut surface shows cysts throughout the renal parenchyma varying in size from tiny cysts to 4-5 cm in diameter. The contents of the cysts vary from clear straw-yellow fluid to reddish-brown material. The renal pelvis and calyces are present but are greatly distorted by the cysts and may contain concretions. The cysts, however, do not communicate with the pelvis of the kidney.

M/E The cysts arise from all parts of nephron. It is possible to find some cysts containing recognisable glomerular tufts reflecting their origin from Bowman's capsule, while others have epithelial lining like that of distal or proximal tubules or collecting ducts.

CLINICAL FEATURES The condition may become clinically apparent at any age. The most frequent and earliest presenting feature is a dull-ache in the lumbar regions. In others, the presenting complaints are haematuria or passage of blood clots in urine, renal colic, hypertension, urinary tract infection and progressive CRF with polyuria and proteinuria.

B. INFANTILE POLYCYSTIC KIDNEY DISEASE

The infantile (autosomal recessive) form of polycystic kidney disease (ARPKD) is distinct from the adult form and is less common (incidence 1:20,000 births). It is transmitted as an *autosomal recessive* trait and the family history of similar disease is usually not present. The condition occurs due to a mutation in chromosome 6. It is invariably bilateral. The age at presentation may be perinatal, neonatal, infantile or juvenile, but frequently serious manifestations are present at birth and result in death from renal failure in early childhood.

G/A The kidneys are bilaterally enlarged with smooth external surface and retained normal reniform shape. Cut surface reveals small, fusiform or cylindrical cysts radiating from the medulla and extend radially to the outer cortex. This gives the sectioned surface of the kidney *sponge-like appearance.*

M/E The total number of nephrons is normal. Since the cysts are formed from dilatation of collecting tubules, all the collecting tubules show cylindrical or saccular dilatations and are lined by cuboidal to low columnar epithelium.

CLINICAL FEATURES The clinical manifestations depend on age of the child. In severe form, the gross bilateral cystic renal enlargement may interfere with delivery. In infancy, renal failure may manifest early. Almost all cases of infantile polycystic kidney disease have associated multiple epithelium-lined cysts in the liver or proliferation of portal bile ductules.

III. MEDULLARY CYSTIC DISEASE

Cystic disease of the renal medulla has two main types:

A. MEDULLARY SPONGE KIDNEY

Medullary sponge kidney consists of multiple cystic dilatations of the papillary ducts in the medulla. It has an autosomal dominant transmission. The condition occurs in adults and may be recognised as an incidental radiographic finding in asymptomatic cases, or the patients may complain of colicky flank pain, dysuria, haematuria and passage of sandy material in the urine.

G/A The kidneys may be enlarged, normal or shrunken in size depending upon the extent of secondary pyelonephritis. On cut surface, the characteristic feature is the presence of several, small (less than 0.5 cm diameter), cystically dilated papillary ducts, which may contain spherical calculi.

M/E The cysts are lined by tall columnar, cuboidal, transitional or squamous epithelium.

B. NEPHRONOPHTHIASIS-MEDULLARY CYSTIC DISEASE COMPLEX

This form of medullary cystic disease, also called *juvenile nephronophthiasis or uraemic sponge kidney,* is a progressive renal disease. It is classified into infantile, juvenile and adolescent type depending upon the age at presentation.

G/A The kidneys are moderately reduced in size and granular and have narrow cortices. Cut surface reveals minute cysts, majority of which are present at the cortico-medullary junction.

M/E The cysts are lined by flattened or cuboidal epithelium. There is widespread nonspecific chronic inflammatory infiltrate and interstitial fibrosis.

IV. SIMPLE RENAL CYSTS

Simple renal cysts or cortical cysts are a very common postmortem finding. They are seen in about half of all persons above the age of 50 years.

G/A Simple renal cysts are usually solitary but may be multiple. They are commonly located in the cortex. Their size varies from a few millimeters to 10 cm in diameter.

M/E The lining of the cyst is by flattened epithelium.

GLOMERULAR DISEASES *(p. 647)*

DEFINITION AND CLASSIFICATION

Glomerular diseases encompass a large and clinically significant group of renal diseases. Glomerulonephritis (GN) or Bright's disease is the term used for diseases that primarily involve the renal glomeruli. It is convenient to classify glomerular diseases into 2 broad groups:

I. PRIMARY GLOMERULONEPHRITIS
1. Acute GN
    i) Post-streptococcal
    ii) Non-streptococcal
2. Rapidly progressive GN
3. Minimal change disease
4. Membranous GN
5. Membrano-proliferative GN
6. Focal and diffuse proliferative GN
7. Focal segmental glomerulosclerosis (FSGS)
8. IgA nephropathy
9. Chronic glomerulonephritis

II. SECONDARY SYSTEMIC GLOMERULAR DISEASES
1. Lupus nephritis (SLE)
2. Diabetic nephropathy
3. Amyloidosis
4. Polyarteritis nodosa
5. Wegener's granulomatosis
6. Goodpasture's syndrome
7. Henoch-Schönlein purpura
8. Systemic infectious diseases (*bacterial* e.g. bacterial endocarditis, syphilis, leprosy; *viral* e.g. HBV, HCV, HIV; *parasitic* e.g. falciparum malaria, filariasis)
9. Idiopathic mixed cryoglobulinaemia

III. HEREDITARY NEPHRITIS
1. Alport's syndrome
2. Fabry's disease
3. Nail-patella syndrome

CLINICAL MANIFESTATIONS

The clinical presentation of glomerular disease is quite variable but in general four features—proteinuria, haematuria, hypertension and disturbed excretory function, are present in varying combinations depending upon the underlying condition. A firm diagnosis, however, can be established by examination of renal biopsy under light, electron and immunofluorescence **433** microscopy.

Chapter 20

The Kidney and Lower Urinary Tract

Following six major glomerular syndromes are commonly found in different glomerular diseases:

I. ACUTE NEPHRITIC SYNDROME This is the acute onset of microscopic haematuria, mild proteinuria, hypertension, oedema and oliguria following an infective illness about 10 to 20 days earlier.

The underlying causes of acute nephritic syndrome may be primary glomerulonephritic diseases (classically acute glomerulonephritis and rapidly progressive glomerulonephritis) or certain systemic diseases.

II. NEPHROTIC SYNDROME Nephrotic syndrome is a constellation of features in different diseases having varying pathogenesis; it is characterised by findings of massive proteinuria, hypoalbuminaemia, oedema, hyper-lipidaemia, lipiduria, and hypercoagulability.

◈   In *children,* primary glomerulonephritis is the cause in majority of cases of the nephrotic syndrome; most frequent being *lipoid nephrosis (65%).*

◈   In *adults,* on the other hand, systemic diseases (diabetes, amyloidosis and SLE) are more frequent causes of nephrotic syndrome. The most common primary glomerular disease in adults is *membranous glomerulo-nephritis (40%).*

III. ACUTE RENAL FAILURE Acute renal failure (ARF) is characterised by rapid decline in renal function. ARF has many causes including glomerular disease, principally rapidly progressive GN and acute diffuse proliferative GN.

IV. CHRONIC RENAL FAILURE These cases have advanced renal impairment progressing over years and is detected by significant proteinuria, haematuria, hypertension and azotaemia. Such patients generally have small contracted kidneys due to chronic glomerulonephritis.

V. ASYMPTOMATIC PROTEINURIA Presence of proteinuria unexpec-tedly in a patient may be unrelated to renal disease (e.g. exercise-induced, extreme lordosis and orthostatic proteinuria), or may indicate an underlying mild glomerulonephritis.

VI. ASYMPTOMATIC HAEMATURIA Asymptomatic microscopic haematuria is common in children and young adolescents and has many diverse causes such as diseases of the glomerulus, renal interstitium, calyceal system, ureter, bladder, prostate, urethra, and underlying bleeding disorder, congenital abnormalities of the kidneys or neoplasia.

PATHOGENESIS OF GLOMERULAR INJURY *(p. 649)*

Most forms of primary GN and many of the secondary glomerular diseases in human beings have immunologic pathogenesis. This view is largely based on immunofluorescence studies of GN in humans which have revealed glomer-ular deposits of immunoglobulins and complement in patterns that closely resemble those of experimental models.

I. IMMUNOLOGIC MECHANISMS

A. ANTIBODY-MEDIATED GLOMERULAR INJURY

1. IMMUNE COMPLEX DISEASE Majority of cases of glomerular disease result from deposits of immune complexes (antigen-antibody complexes). The immune complexes are represented by *irregular or granular glomerular deposits* of immunoglobulins (IgG, IgM and IgA) and complement (mainly C3). Based on the experimental models and studies in human beings, the following 3 patterns of glomerular deposits of immune complexes in various glomerular diseases have been observed:

i)   *Exclusive mesangial deposits* are characterised by very mild form of glomerular disease.

ii)   *Extensive subendothelial deposits* along the GBM are accompanied by severe hypercellular sclerosing glomerular lesions.

iii) *Subepithelial deposits* are seen between the outer surface of the GBM and the podocytes.

Now, it has been shown that glomerular deposits are formed by one of the following two mechanisms:

i) Local immune complex deposits Classic experimental model to understand human *in situ* immune complex GN is Heymann nephritis.

Similar phenomenon is seen in human *membranous glomerulonephritis*. In non-basement membrane antigen is identified as gp330 (*glyco protein* with a mass of 330 kD) or nonglomerular antigens planted on glomeruli (e.g. certain drugs, endotoxins, parasitic products etc). It is located on the podocytes and coated on pits of proximal tubular epithelial cells. Antibodies are formed against such planted antigens. Main antigen-antibody reaction takes place at soles of the foot processes of podocytes and the immune complexes get deposited at the lamina rara externa of the basement membrane. Correspondingly, in membranous glomerulonephritis, granular IgG deposits are found along the subepithelial side of basement membrane. Similarly, electron dense deposits are found on the epithelial side of basement membrane.

Currently, this mechanism is considered responsible for most cases of immune complex GN.

ii) Circulating immune complex deposits It is believed that circulating immune complexes cause glomerular damage under certain circumstances only. These situations are: their presence in high concentrations for prolonged periods, or when they possess special properties that cause their binding to glomeruli, or when host mechanisms are defective and fail to eliminate immune complexes. The antigens evoking antibody response may be endogenous (e.g. in SLE) or may be exogenous (e.g. Hepatitis B virus, *Treponema pallidum*, *Plasmodium falciparum* and various tumour antigens). The antigen-antibody complexes are formed in the circulation and then trapped in the glomeruli where they produce glomerular injury after combining with complement.

Immune complex GN by either of the above mechanisms is observed in the following human diseases:

i) *Primary GN* e.g. acute diffuse proliferative GN, membranous GN, membranoproliferative GN, IgA nephropathy and some cases of rapidly progressive GN and focal GN.

ii) *Systemic diseases* e.g. glomerular disease in SLE, malaria, syphilis, hepatitis, Henoch-Schonlein purpura and idiopathic mixed cryoglobulinaemia.

2. ANTI-GBM DISEASE Less than 5% cases of human GN are associated with anti-GBM antibodies. The constituent of GBM acting as antigen appears to be a component of collagen IV of the basement membrane. The experimental model of anti-GBM disease is *Masugi nephritis* (nephrotoxic serum nephritis).

Anti-GBM disease is classically characterised by *interrupted linear deposits* of anti-GBM antibodies (mostly IgG; rarely IgA and IgM) and complement (mainly C3) along the glomerular basement membrane. These deposits are detected by immunofluorescence microscopy or by electron microscopy.

Anti-GBM disease is characteristically exemplified by glomerular injury in Goodpasture's syndrome in some cases of rapidly progressive GN. About half to two-third of the patients with renal lesions in Goodpasture's syndrome have pulmonary haemorrhage mediated by cross-reacting autoantibodies against alveolar basement membrane.

3. ALTERNATE PATHWAY DISEASE The complement system, in particular C3, contributes to glomerular injury in most forms of GN. Deposits of C3 are associated with the early components C1, C2 and C4 which are evidence of classic pathway activation of complement. But in alternate pathway activation, there is decreased serum C3 level, decreased serum levels of factor B and properdin, normal serum levels of C1, C2 and C4 but C3 and properdin are found deposited in the glomeruli without immunoglobulin deposits, reflecting activation of alternate pathway of complement. Such

The deposits in alternate pathway disease are characteristically electron-dense under electron microscopy; glomerular lesions in such cases are referred to as *dense-deposit disease.*

Alternate pathway disease occurs in most cases of type II membranoproliferative GN, some patients of rapidly progressive GN, acute diffuse proliferative GN, IgA nephropathy and in SLE.

4. OTHER MECHANISMS OF ANTIBODY-MEDIATED INJURY A few autoantibodies have been implicated in some patients of focal segmental glomerulosclerosis and few other types of GN. These antibodies include the following:

i) **Anti-neutrophil cytoplasmic antibodies (ANCA)** About 40% cases of rapidly progressive GN are deficient in immunoglobulins in glomeruli (pauci-immune GN) and are positive for ANCA against neutrophil cytoplasmic antigens in their circulation.

ii) **Anti-endothelial cell antibodies (AECA)** Autoantibodies against endothelial antigens have been detected in circulation in several inflammatory vasculitis and glomerulonephritis.

B. CELL-MEDIATED GLOMERULAR INJURY (DELAYED-TYPE HYPERSENSITIVITY)

There is evidence to suggest that cell-mediated immune reactions may be involved in causing glomerular injury, particularly in cases with deficient immunoglobulins (e.g. in pauci-immune type glomerulonephritis in RPGN). Cytokines and other mediators released by activated T cells stimulate cytotoxicity, recruitment of more leucocytes and fibrogenesis. CD4+ T lymphocytes recruit more macrophages while CD8+ cytotoxic T lymphocytes and natural killer cells cause further glomerular cell injury by antibody-dependent cell toxicity.

C. SECONDARY PATHOGENETIC MECHANISMS (MEDIATORS OF IMMUNOLOGIC INJURY)

Secondary pathogenetic mechanisms are a number of mediators of immunologic glomerular injury operating in man and in experimental models.

1. Neutrophils Neutrophils are conspicuous in certain forms of glomerular disease such as in acute diffuse proliferative GN, and may also be present in membranoproliferative GN and lupus nephritis.

2. Mononuclear phagocytes Many forms of human and experimental proliferative GN are associated with glomerular infiltration by monocytes and macrophages.

3. Complement system Besides the components of complement which mediate glomerular injury via neutrophils already mentioned, C5bC6789 (MAC, acronym for membrane attack complex, also called terminal complex) is capable of inducing damage to GBM directly.

4. Platelets Platelet aggregation and release of mediators play a role in the evolution of some forms of GN.

5. Mesangial cells There is evidence to suggest that mesangial cells present in the glomeruli may be stimulated to produce mediators of inflammation and take part in glomerular injury.

6. Coagulation system The presence of fibrin in early crescents in certain forms of human and experimental GN suggests the role of coagulation system in glomerular damage.

II. NON-IMMUNOLOGIC MECHANISMS

Though most forms of GN are mediated by immunologic mechanisms, a few examples of glomerular injury by non-immunologic mechanisms are found:

1. *Metabolic glomerular injury* e.g. in diabetic nephropathy (due to hyperglycaemia), Fabry's disease (due to sulfatidosis).
2. *Haemodynamic glomerular injury* e.g. systemic hypertension, intraglomerular hypertension in FSGS.
3. *Deposition diseases* e.g. amyloidosis.
4. *Infectious diseases* e.g. HBV, HCV, HIV, *E. coli*-derived nephrotoxin.
5. *Drugs* e.g. minimal change disease due to NSAIDs.
6. *Inherited glomerular diseases* e.g. Alport's syndrome, nail-patella syndrome.

SPECIFIC TYPES OF GLOMERULAR DISEASES *(p. 652)*

I. PRIMARY GLOMERULONEPHRITIS

ACUTE GLOMERULONEPHRITIS (SYNONYMS: ACUTE DIFFUSE PROLIFERATIVE GN, DIFFUSE ENDOCAPILLARY GN)

Acute GN is known to follow acute infection and characteristically presents as acute nephritic syndrome. Based on etiologic agent, acute GN is subdivided into 2 main groups:

ACUTE POST-STREPTOCOCCAL GN

Acute post-streptococcal GN, though uncommon and sporadic in the Western countries, is a common form of GN in developing countries, mostly affecting children between 2 to 14 years of age but 10% cases are seen in adults above 40 years of age. The onset of disease is generally sudden after 1-2 weeks of streptococcal infection, most frequently of the throat (e.g. streptococcal pharyngitis) and sometimes of the skin (e.g. streptococcal impetigo).

ETIOPATHOGENESIS Particularly nephritogenic are types 12,4,1 and Red Lake of group A β-haemolytic streptococci. The glomerular lesions appear to result from deposition of immune complexes in the glomeruli.
i) There is *epidemiological* evidence of preceding streptococcal sore throat or skin infection.
ii) The *latent period* between streptococcal infection and onset of clinical manifestations of the disease is compatible with the period required for building up of antibodies.
iii) Streptococcal infection may be identified by *culture* or may be inferred from elevated titres of *antibodies* against streptococcal antigens.
   a) anti-streptolysin O (ASO);
   b) anti-deoxyribonuclease B (anti-DNAse B);
   c) anti-streptokinase (ASKase);
   d) anti-nicotinyl adenine dinucleotidase (anti-NADase); and
   e) anti-hyaluronidase (AHase).
iv) There is usually *hypocomplementaemia*
v) It has also been possible to identify antigenic component of streptococci which is cytoplasmic antigen, *endostreptosin*.

G/A The kidneys are symmetrically enlarged, weighing one and a half to twice the normal weight. The cortical as well as sectioned surface show petechial haemorrhages giving the characteristic appearance of flea-bitten kidney.

M/E Light microscopic findings are as under:

i) Glomeruli They are enlarged and hypercellular. The diffuse hyper-cellularity of the tuft is due to proliferation of mesangial, endothelial and occasionally epithelial cells *(acute proliferative lesions)* as well as by infiltration of leucocytes, chiefly polymorphs and sometimes monocytes *(acute exudative lesion)*.

ii) Tubules There may be swelling and hyaline droplets in tubular cells, and tubular lumina may contain red cell casts.

iii) Interstitium There may be some degree of interstitial oedema and leucocytic infiltration.

EM demonstrates the characteristic electron-dense irregular deposits *('humps')* on the epithelial side of the GBM.

IF reveals that the irregular deposits along the GBM consist principally of IgG and complement C3.

CLINICAL FEATURES Typically, the patient is a young child, presenting with acute nephritic syndrome, having sudden and abrupt onset following an episode of sore throat or skin infection 1-2 weeks prior to the development of symptoms. The features include microscopic or intermittent haematuria, red cell casts, mild non-selective proteinuria (less than 3 gm per 24 hrs), hypertension, periorbital oedema and variably oliguria. Development of hypertension in either case is a poor prognostic sign.

Prognosis varies with the age of the patient. Children almost always (95%) recover completely with reversal of proliferative glomerular changes. Complications arise more often in adults and occasionally in children.

ACUTE NON-STREPTOCOCCAL GN

About one-third cases of acute GN are caused by organisms other than haemolytic streptococci. These include other bacteria (e.g. staphylococci, pneumococci, meningococci, *Salmonella* and *Pseudomonas),* viruses (e.g. hepatitis B virus, mumps, infectious mononucleosis and varicella), parasitic infections (e.g. malaria, toxoplasmosis and schistosomiasis) and syphilis.

RAPIDLY PROGRESSIVE GLOMERULONEPHRITIS (SYNONYMS: RPGN, CRESCENTIC GN, EXTRACAPILLARY GN)

RPGN presents with an acute reduction in renal function resulting in acute renal failure in a few weeks or months. It is characterised by formation of 'crescents' *(crescentic GN)* outside the glomerular capillaries *(extracapillary GN).* 'Crescents' are formed from the proliferation of parietal epithelial cells lining Bowman's capsule with contribution from visceral epithelial cells and the invading mononuclear cells. The stimulus for crescent formation appears to be the presence of fibrin in the capsular space.

ETIOPATHOGENESIS Patients with RPGN are divided into 3 groups as under:

Following three serologic markers are used for categorising RPGN:
i)   serum C3 level,
ii)   anti-GBM antibody; and
iii) anti-neutrophil cytoplasmic antibody (ANCA).

Type I RPGN: Anti-GBM disease A number of systemic diseases such as Goodpasture's syndrome, SLE, vasculitis, Wegener's granulomatosis, Henoch-Schonlein purpura and idiopathic mixed cryoglobulinaemia are associated with crescentic GN.

Goodpasture's syndrome Goodpasture's syndrome is characterised by acute renal failure due to RPGN and pulmonary haemorrhages. The condition is more common in males in 3rd decade of life. The disease results from damage to the glomeruli by anti-GBM antibodies which cross-react with alveolar basement membrane and hence, produce renal as well as pulmonary lesions. The evidences in support are the characteristic linear deposits of anti-GBM antibodies consisting of IgG and complement along the GBM, detection of circulating anti-GBM antibodies.

Type II RPGN: Immune complex disease A small proportion of cases of post-streptococcal GN, particularly in adults and sometimes of non-streptococcal origin, develop RPGN. The evidences in support of post-infectious RPGN having immune complex pathogenesis are granular deposits of immune complexes of IgG and C3 along the glomerular capillary walls, lowering of blood complement level and demonstration of circulating complexes.

Type III RPGN: Pauci-immune GN These include cases of Wegener's granulomatosis and microscopic polyarteritis nodosa. Majority of these patients are ANCA-positive, implying a defect in humoral immunity. Serum complement levels are normal and anti-GBM antibody is negative. There is little or no glomerular immune deposit (i.e. pauci-immune).

G/A The kidneys are usually enlarged and pale with smooth outer surface *(large white kidney)*. Cut surface shows pale cortex and congested medulla.

M/E General light microscopic findings are as under:

i) Glomeruli Irrespective of the underlying etiology, all forms of RPGN show pathognomonic *'crescents'* on the inside of Bowman's capsules. These are collections of pale-staining polygonal cells which commonly tend to be elongated. Eventually, crescents obliterate the Bowman's space and compress the glomerular tuft.

ii) Tubules Tubular epithelial cells may show hyaline droplets. Tubular lumina may contain casts, red blood cells and fibrin.

iii) Interstitium The interstitium is oedematous and may show early fibrosis. Inflammatory cells, usually lymphocytes and plasma cells, are commonly distributed in the interstitial tissue.

iv) Vessels Arteries and arterioles may show no change, but cases associated with hypertension usually show severe vascular changes.

EM findings vary according to the type of RPGN. Post-infectious RPGN cases show electron-dense subepithelial granular deposits similar to those seen in acute GN, while cases of RPGN in Goodpasture's syndrome show characteristic linear deposits along the GBM.

IF shows following patterns:

i) linear pattern of RPGN in Goodpasture's syndrome (type I RPGN), containing IgG accompanied by C3 along the capillaries.

ii) Granular pattern of post-infectious RPGN (type II RPGN) consisting of IgG and C3 along the capillary wall.

iii) Scanty or no deposits of immunoglobulin and C3 in pauci-immune GN (type III RPGN).

CLINICAL FEATURES Generally, the features of post-infectious RPGN are similar to those of acute GN, presenting as acute renal failure. The patients of Goodpasture's syndrome may present as acute renal failure and/or associated intrapulmonary haemorrhage producing recurrent haemoptysis. Prognosis of all forms of RPGN is poor. However, post-infectious cases have somewhat better outcome and may show recovery.

MINIMAL CHANGE DISEASE (SYNONYMS: MCD, LIPOID NEPHROSIS, FOOT PROCESS DISEASE, NIL DEPOSIT DISEASE)

Minimal change disease (MCD) is a condition in which the nephrotic syndrome is accompanied by no apparent change in glomeruli by light microscopy. Its other synonyms, lipoid nephrosis and foot process disease, are descriptive terms for fatty changes in the tubules and electron microscopic appearance of flattened podocytes respectively. Minimal change disease accounts for 80% cases of nephrotic syndrome in children under 16 years of age with preponderance in boys (ratio of boys to girls 2:1).

ETIOPATHOGENESIS The etiology of MCD remain elusive. However, following two groups have been identified:

i) Idiopathic (majority of cases).

ii) Cases associated with systemic diseases (Hodgkin's disease, HIV infection) and drug therapy (e.g. NSAIDs, rifampicin, interferon-α).

The following features point to possible immunologic pathogenesis for MCD:

i) Absence of deposits by immunofluorescence microscopy.

ii) Normal circulating levels of complement but presence of circulating immune complexes in many cases.

iii) Universal satisfactory response to steroid therapy.

iv) Evidence of increased suppressor T cell activity with elaboration of cytokines (interleukin-8, tumour necrosis factor).

v) Detection of a mutation in nephrin gene in cases of congenital MCD.

Nephrotic syndrome in MCD *in children* is characterised by *selective proteinuria* containing mainly albumin, and minimal amounts of high molecular weight proteins such as α2-macroglobulin. The basis for selective proteinuria appears to be as under:

i)   Reduction of normal negative charge on GBM due to loss of heparan sulfate proteoglycan from the GBM.

ii)   Change in the shape of epithelial cells producing foot process flattening due to reduction of sialoglycoprotein cell coat.

Adults having MCD, however, have *non-selective proteinuria*, suggesting more extensive membrane permeability defect.

G/A   The kidneys are of normal size and shape.

M/E   Light microscopic findings are as under:

i) Glomeruli   The most characteristic feature is no apparent abnormality in the glomeruli except for slight increase in the mesangial matrix at the most (minimal change disease or nil lesion).

ii) Tubules   There is presence of fine lipid vacuolation and hyaline droplets in the cells of proximal convoluted tubules and, hence, the older name of the condition as 'lipoid nephrosis'.

iii) Interstitium   There may be oedema of the interstitium.

iv) Vessels   Do not show any significant change.

EM   The most characteristic feature of the disease is identified which is diffuse flattening of foot processes of the visceral epithelial cells (podocytes) and, hence, the name foot process disease or podocytopathy.

IF does not show deposits of complement or immunoglobulins (nil deposit disease).

CLINICAL FEATURES   The classical presentation of MCD is of fully-developed nephrotic syndrome with massive and *highly selective proteinuria*; hypertension is unusual. Most frequently, the patients are children under 16 years (peak incidence at 6-8 years of age). The onset may be preceded by an upper respiratory infection, atopic allergy or immunisation.

The disease characteristically responds to steroid therapy. In spite of remissions and relapses, long-term prognosis is very good and most children become free of albuminuria after several years.

MEMBRANOUS GLOMERULONEPHRITIS
(SYNONYM: EPIMEMBRANOUS NEPHROPATHY)

Membranous GN is characterised by widespread thickening of the glomerular capillary wall and is the most common cause of nephrotic syndrome in adults. In majority of cases (85%), membranous GN is truly *idiopathic*, while in about 15% of cases it is *secondary* to an underlying condition (e.g. SLE, malignancies, infections such as chronic hepatitis B and C, syphilis, malaria and drugs).

ETIOPATHOGENESIS   *Idiopathic membranous GN* is an immune complex disease. The deposits of immune complex are formed locally because circulating immune complexes are detected in less than a quarter of cases. While nephritogenic antigen against which autoantibodies are formed in *idiopathic membranous* GN is not known yet, the antigen in cases of *secondary membranous GN* is either an endogenous (e.g. DNA in SLE) or exogenous one (e.g. hepatitis B virus, tumour antigen, treponema antigen, drug therapy with penicillamine). Currently, pathogenesis of membrane alteration in membranous GN is believed to be by MAC (membrane attack complex i.e. C35b-C9) terminal complex on podocytes.

G/A   The kidneys are enlarged, pale and smooth.

M/E   Light microscopy shows the following findings:
i) Glomeruli   The characteristic finding is diffuse thickening of the glomerular capillary walls with all the glomeruli being affected more or less uniformly. As the disease progresses, the deposits are incorporated into enormously thickened basement membrane, producing 'duplication' of GBM

which is actually formation of a new basement membrane. These basement membrane changes are best appreciated by silver impregnation stains (black colour) or by periodic acid-Schiff stain (pink colour).

ii) Tubules The renal tubules remain normal except in the early stage when lipid vacuolation of the proximal convoluted tubules may be seen.

iii) Interstitium The interstitium may show fine fibrosis and scanty chronic inflammatory cells.

iv) Vessels In the early stage, vascular changes are not prominent, while later hypertensive changes of arterioles may occur.

EM shows characteristic electron-dense deposits in subepithelial location. The basement membrane material protrudes between deposits as *'spikes'*.

IF reveals granular deposits of immune complexes consisting of IgG associated with complement C3.

CLINICAL FEATURES The presentation in majority of cases is insidious onset of nephrotic syndrome in an adult. The proteinuria is usually of *non-selective* type. In addition, microscopic haematuria and hypertension may be present at the onset or may develop during the course of the disease. Progression to impaired renal function and end-stage renal disease with progressive azotaemia occurs in approximately 50% cases within a span of 2 to 20 years.

MEMBRANOPROLIFERATIVE GLOMERULONEPHRITIS (SYNONYMS: MPGN, MESANGIOCAPILLARY GN)

Membranoproliferative GN is another important cause of nephrotic syndrome in children and young adults. As the name implies, it is characterised by two histologic features—increase in cellularity of the mesangium associated with increased lobulation of the tuft, and irregular thickening of the capillary wall.

ETIOPATHOGENESIS Etiology of MPGN is unknown though in some cases there is evidence of preceding streptococcal infection. Three types of MPGN are recognised:

◈ **Type I or classic form** is an example of immune complex disease and comprises more than 70% cases. It is characterised by immune deposits in the subendothelial position. Immune-complex MPGN is seen in association with systemic immune-complex diseases (e.g. SLE, mixed cryoglobulinaemia, Sjögren's syndrome), chronic infections (e.g. bacterial endocarditis, HIV, hepatitis B and C) and malignancies (e.g. lymphomas and leukaemias).

◈ **Type II or dense deposit disease** is the example of alternate pathway disease. The capillary wall thickening is due to the deposition of electron-dense material in the lamina densa of the GBM. Type II MPGN is an autoimmune disease in which patients have IgG autoantibody termed C3 nephritic factor.

◈ **Type III** is rare and shows features of type I MPGN and membranous nephropathy in association with systemic diseases or drugs.

G/A The kidneys are usually pale in appearance and firm in consistency.

M/E Light microscopic features are as under:

i) Glomeruli Glomeruli show highly characteristic changes. They are enlarged with accentuated lobular pattern. The enlargement is due to variable degree of mesangial cellular proliferation and increase in mesangial matrix. The GBM is considerably thickened; with silver stains it shows two basement membranes with a clear zone between them. This is commonly referred to as *'double contour', splitting, or 'tram track'* appearance.

ii) Tubules Tubular cells may show vacuolation and hyaline droplets.

iii) Interstitium There may be scattered chronic inflammatory cells and some finely granular foam cells in the interstitium.

iv) Vessels Hypertensive vascular changes are prominent in cases in which hypertension develops.

Type I: It shows *electron-dense deposits* in subendothelial location conforming to immune-complex character of the disease. These deposits reveal positive fluorescence for C3 and slightly fainter staining for IgG.

Type II: The hallmark of type II MPGN is the presence of *dense amorphous deposits* within the lamina densa of the GBM and in the mesangium. Immuno-fluorescence studies reveal the universal presence of C3 and properdin in the deposits but the immunoglobulins are usually absent.

Type III: This rare form has *electron-dense deposits* within the GBM as well as in subendothelial and subepithelial regions of the GBM. Immunofluores-cence studies show the presence of C3, IgG and IgM.

CLINICAL FEATURES Clinically, there are many similarities between the main forms of MPGN. The most common age at diagnosis is between 15 and 20 years. Approximately 50% of the patients present with nephrotic syndrome; about 30% have asymptomatic proteinuria; and 20% have nephritic syndrome at presentation. The proteinuria is non-selective. Haema-turia and hypertension are frequently present. Hypocomplementaemia is a common feature. With time, majority of patients progress to renal failure, while some continue to have proteinuria, haematuria and hypertension with stable renal function.

FOCAL PROLIFERATIVE GLOMERULONEPHRITIS (SYNONYM: MESANGIAL PROLIFERATIVE GN)

Focal proliferative GN is characterised by pathologic changes in fewer than 50% glomeruli *(focal)*, often confined to one or two lobules of the affected glomeruli while other glomeruli are normal.

ETIOPATHOGENESIS It may occur in following diverse conditions:
i)   As an early manifestation of a number of *systemic diseases* such as SLE (class III), Henoch-Schonlein purpura, subacute bacterial endocarditis, Wegener's granulomatosis, and polyarteritis nodosa, Goodpasture's syndrome.
ii)   As a component of a known *renal disease* such as in IgA nephropathy.
iii) As a primary *idiopathic* glomerular disease unrelated to systemic or other renal disease.

M/E The single most important feature in focal GN is the abnormality seen in certain number of glomeruli and generally confined to one or two lobules of the affected glomeruli i.e. *focal and segmental glomerular involvement*. The pathologic change most frequently consists of focal and segmental cellular proliferation of mesangial cells and endothelial cells but sometimes necrotising changes can be seen.

IF shows widespread mesangial deposits of immunoglobulins (mainly IgA with or without IgG), complement (C3) and fibrin are demonstrated in most cases of focal GN.

CLINICAL FEATURES The clinical features vary according to the condition causing it. Haematuria is one of the most common clinical manifestation. Proteinuria is frequently mild to moderate but hypertension is uncommon.

DIFFUSE PROLIFERATIVE GLOMERULONEPHRITIS (SYNONYM: DPGN)

DPGN is similar to focal proliferative GN in terms of etiology and pathogenesis.

M/E It is similar to focal proliferative GN but in its advanced form. It differs from focal GN in following ways:
1. The number of glomeruli involved is more than 50% i.e. diffuse proliferation.
2. The cells partaking in DPGN are more diffuse type and not mesangial cells alone; it also includes proliferation of epithelial, endothelial and inflammatory cells.

Focal segmental glomerulosclerosis (FSGS) is a condition in which there is sclerosis and hyalinosis of some glomeruli and portions of their tuft (less than 50% in a tissue section), while the other glomeruli are normal by light microscopy i.e. involvement is focal and segmental.

ETIOPATHOGENESIS The condition is divided into 3 groups:

i) Idiopathic type It is found in children and young adults with presentation of nephrotic syndrome. It differs from minimal change disease in having non-selective proteinuria, in being steroid-resistant, and may progress to chronic renal failure. Immunofluorescence microscopy reveals deposits of IgM and C3 in the sclerotic segment.

ii) With superimposed primary glomerular disease There may be cases of FSGS with superimposed MCD or IgA nephropathy.

iii) Secondary type This group consists of focal segmental sclerotic lesions as a secondary manifestation of certain diseases such as HIV, diabetes mellitus, reflux nephropathy, heroin abuse and analgesic nephropathy.

M/E Depending upon the severity of the disease, variable number of glomeruli are affected focally and segmentally, while others are normal. The affected glomeruli show solidification or *sclerosis* of one or more lobules of the tuft. *Hyalinosis* refers to collection of eosinophilic, homogeneous, PAS-positive, hyaline material present on the inner aspect of a sclerotic peripheral capillary loop. Mesangial hypercellularity is present in appreciable number of cases.

Besides the lesions of focal and segmental scarring, a variant of FSGS, *collapsing glomerulopathy*, has been described in HIV patients.

EM shows diffuse loss of foot processes as seen in minimal change disease.

IF reveals the deposits in the lesions as containing IgM and C3.

CLINICAL FEATURES The condition may affect all ages including children and has male preponderance. The most common presentation is in the form of nephrotic syndrome with heavy proteinuria. Haematuria and hypertension tend to occur more frequently than in minimal change disease.

IgA NEPHROPATHY (SYNONYMS: BERGER'S DISEASE, IgA GN)

IgA nephropathy is emerging as the most common form of glomerulopathy worldwide and its incidence has been rising. It is characterised by aggregates of IgA, deposited principally in the mesangium.

ETIOPATHOGENESIS Etiology remains unclear.
i) It is idiopathic in most cases.
ii) Seen as part of Henoch-Schonlein purpura.
iii) Association with chronic inflammation in various body systems (e.g. chronic liver disease, inflammatory bowel disease, interstitial pneumonitis, leprosy, dermatitis herpetiformis, uveitis, ankylosing spondylitis, Sjögren's syndrome, monoclonal IgA gammopathy).

Pathogenesis of IgA nephropathy is explained on the basis of following mechanisms:
i) In view of exclusive mesangial deposits of IgA and elevated serum levels of IgA and IgA-immune complexes, IgA nephropathy has been considered to arise from *entrapment* of these complexes in the mesangium.
ii) There is absence of early components of the complement but presence of C3 and properdin in the mesangial deposits, which point towards activation of *alternate complement pathway*.
iii) Since there is close association between mucosal infections (e.g. of the respiratory, gastrointestinal or urinary tract), it is suggested that IgA deposited in the mesangium could be due to increased *mucosal secretion of IgA*.
iv) HLA-B35 association has been reported in some cases. Another possibility is *genetically-determined* abnormality of the immune system.

M/E The pattern of involvement varies. These include: focal proliferative GN, focal segmental glomerulosclerosis, membranoproliferative GN, and rarely RPGN.

EM shows finely granular electron-dense deposits in the mesangium.

IF The diagnosis is firmly established by demonstration of mesangial deposits of IgA, with or without IgG, and usually with C3 and properdin.

CLINICAL FEATURES The disease is common in children and young adults. The clinical picture is usually characterised by recurrent bouts of haematuria that are often precipitated by mucosal infections. Mild proteinuria is usually present and occasionally nephrotic syndrome may develop.

CHRONIC GLOMERULONEPHRITIS
(SYNONYM: END-STAGE KIDNEY, CHRONIC KIDNEY DISEASE)

Chronic GN is the final stage of a variety of glomerular diseases which result in irreversible impairment of renal function. The conditions which may progress to chronic GN, in descending order of frequency, are as under:
i)   Rapidly progressive GN (90%)
ii)   Membranous GN (50%)
iii) Membranoproliferative GN (50%)
iv)   Focal segmental glomerulosclerosis (50%)
v)   IgA nephropathy (40%)
vi)   Acute post-streptococcal GN (1%).

G/A The kidneys are usually small and contracted weighing as low as 50 gm each. The capsule is adherent to the cortex. The cortical surface is generally diffusely granular. On cut section, the cortex is narrow and atrophic, while the medulla is unremarkable.

M/E Changes vary depending upon underlying renal disease.

i) Glomeruli Glomeruli are reduced in number and most of those present show completely hyalinised tufts, giving the appearance of acellular, eosinophilic masses which are PAS-positive. Evidence of underlying glomerular disease may be present.

ii) Tubules Many tubules completely disappear and there may be atrophy of tubules close to scarred glomeruli.

iii) Interstitium There is fine and delicate fibrosis of the interstitial tissue and varying number of chronic inflammatory cells are often seen.

iv) Vessels Advanced cases which are frequently associated with hypertension show conspicuous arterial and arteriolar sclerosis.

Patients of chronic kidney disease on dialysis show a variety of dialysis associated changes that include acquired cystic disease, occurrence of adenomas and adenocarcinomas of the kidney, calcification of tufts and deposition of calcium oxalate crystals in tubules.

CLINICAL FEATURES The patients are usually adults. The terminal stage of chronic GN is characterised by hypertension, uraemia and progressive deterioration of renal function. These patients eventually die if they do not receive a renal transplant.

II. SECONDARY GLOMERULAR DISEASES

Glomerular involvement may occur secondary to certain systemic diseases or a few hereditary diseases. In some of these, renal involvement may be the initial presentation, while in others clinical evidence of renal disease appears long after other manifestations have appeared.

LUPUS NEPHRITIS

Renal manifestations of systemic lupus erythematosus (SLE) are termed lupus nephritis. The incidence of renal involvement in SLE ranges from 40 to 75%. The two cardinal clinical manifestations of lupus nephritis are proteinuria and haematuria.

Pathogenesis of lesions in lupus nephritis is linked to genes related to major histocompatibility complex and B-cell signaling pathways such as TNF superfamily members.

M/E According to the WHO, six patterns of mutually-merging renal lesions are seen in lupus nephritis:

Class I: Minimal lesions On light microscopy, these cases do not show any abnormality. But examination by electron microscopy and immuno-fluorescence microscopy shows deposits within the mesangium which consist of IgG and C3.

Class II: Mesangial lupus nephritis By light microscopy, there is increase in the number of mesangial cells and amount of mesangial matrix. Ultra-structural and immunofluorescence studies reveal granular mesangial deposits of IgG and C3; sometimes IgA and IgM are also present in the deposits.

Class III: Focal segmental lupus nephritis This is characterised by focal and segmental proliferation of endothelial and mesangial cells, together with infiltration by macrophages and sometimes neutrophils. Haematoxylin bodies of Gross may be present. Subendothelial and subepithelial deposits of IgG, often with IgM or IgA and C3, are seen.

Class IV: Diffuse proliferative lupus nephritis There is diffuse proliferation of endothelial, mesangial, and sometimes epithelial cells, involving most or all glomeruli. Electron microscopy shows large electron-dense deposits in the mesangium and in the subendothelial region which on immunofluorescence are positive for IgG; sometimes also for IgA or IgM, and C3.

Class V: Membranous lupus nephritis These consist of diffuse thickening of glomerular capillary wall on light microscopy and show sub-endothelial deposits of immune complexes containing IgG, IgM and C3 on ultrastructural studies. Mesangial hypercellularity is present in some cases.

Class VI: Sclerosing lupus nephritis Most glomeruli are sclerosed and hyalinised and there may be remnants of preceding lesions.

DIABETIC NEPHROPATHY

Renal involvement is an important complication of diabetes mellitus. Chronic kidney disease with renal failure accounts for deaths in more than 10% of all diabetics. Renal complications are more severe, develop early and more frequently in type 1 diabetes mellitus (30-40% cases) than in type 2 diabetics (about 20% cases). Cardiovascular disease is 40 times more common in patients of chronic kidney disease in diabetes mellitus than in non-diabetics and more diabetics die from cardiovascular complications than from uraemia.

M/E Diabetic nephropathy encompasses 4 types of renal lesions in diabetes mellitus:

1. DIABETIC GLOMERULOSCLEROSIS Glomerular lesions in diabetes mellitus are particularly common and account for majority of abnormal findings referable to the kidney.

Glomerulosclerosis in diabetes may take one of the 2 forms:

i) Diffuse glomerulosclerosis Diffuse glomerular lesions are the most common. There is involvement of all parts of glomeruli. The pathologic changes consist of thickening of the GBM and diffuse increase in mesangial matrix with mild proliferation of mesangial cells. Various exudative lesions such as capsular hyaline drops and fibrin caps may also be present. *Capsular drop* is an eosinophilic hyaline thickening of the parietal layer of Bowman's capsule and bulges into the glomerular space. *Fibrin cap* is homogeneous, brightly eosinophilic material appearing on the wall of a peripheral capillary of a lobule.

ii) Nodular glomerulosclerosis Nodular lesions of diabetic glomerulo-sclerosis are also called as *Kimmelstiel-Wilson (KW) lesions* or *intercapillary glomerulosclerosis*. The pathologic changes consist of one or more nodules in a few or many glomeruli. *Nodule* is an ovoid or spherical, laminated, hyaline, acellular mass located within a lobule of the glomerulus. The nodules are surrounded peripherally by glomerular capillary loops which may have normal or thickened GBM. The nodules are PAS-positive and contain lipid and fibrin. As the nodular lesions enlarge, they compress the glomerular capillaries and obliterate the glomerular tuft. As a result of glomerular and arteriolar involvement, renal ischaemia occurs leading to tubular atrophy and interstitial fibrosis and results in grossly small, contracted kidney.

2. VASCULAR LESIONS   *Atheroma* of renal arteries is very common and severe in diabetes mellitus. *Hyaline arteriolosclerosis* affecting the afferent and efferent arterioles of the glomeruli is also often severe in diabetes.

3. DIABETIC PYELONEPHRITIS   Poorly-controlled diabetics are particularly susceptible to bacterial infections. Papillary necrosis (necrotising papillitis) is an important complication of diabetes that may result in acute pyelonephritis. Chronic pyelonephritis is 10 to 20 times more common in diabetics than in others.

4. TUBULAR LESIONS (ARMANNI-EBSTEIN LESIONS)   In untreated diabetics who have extremely high blood sugar level, the epithelial cells of the proximal convoluted tubules develop extensive glycogen deposits appearing as vacuoles. These are called Armanni-Ebstein lesions.

HEREDITARY NEPHRITIS

A group of hereditary diseases principally involving the glomeruli are termed hereditary nephritis.

1.   Alport's syndrome   Out of various hereditary nephritis, Alport's syndrome is relatively more common and has been extensively studied. This is an X-linked dominant disorder having mutation in α-5 chain of type IV collagen located on X-chromosome. It affects males more severely than females. The syndrome consists of sensori-neural deafness and ophthalmic complications (lens dislocation, posterior cataracts and corneal dystrophy) associated with hereditary nephritis. The condition is slowly progressive, terminating in chronic kidney disease in the 2nd to 3rd decades of life.

M/E   The glomeruli have predominant involvement and show segmental proliferation of mesangial cells with increased mesangial matrix and occasional segmental sclerosis. Another prominent feature is the presence of *lipid-laden foam cells* in the interstitium. As the disease progresses, there is increasing sclerosis of glomeruli, tubular atrophy and interstitial fibrosis.

2.   Fabry's disease,   another hereditary nephritis, is characterised by accumulation of neutral glycosphingolipids in lysosomes of glomerular, tubular, vascular and interstitial cells.

3.   Nail-patella syndrome   or osteonychodysplasia is a rare hereditary disease having abnormality in α-1 chain of collagen V on chromosome 9 associated with multiple osseous defects of elbows, knees and nail dysplasia.

TUBULAR AND TUBULOINTERSTITIAL DISEASES *(p. 666)*

This group parenchymal of diseases is discussed under 2 headings:

I.   Primary tubular diseases that include tubular injury by ischaemic or toxic agents i.e. acute tubular necrosis.

II.   Tubulointerstitial diseases that include inflammatory involvement of the tubules and the interstitium i.e. pyelonephritis (acute and chronic).

ACUTE TUBULAR NECROSIS

Acute tubular necrosis (ATN) is the term used for acute renal failure (ARF) resulting from destruction of tubular epithelial cells. ATN is the most common and most important cause of ARF characterised by sudden cessation of renal function. Based on etiology and morphology, two forms of ATN are distinguished—ischaemic and toxic; however both forms have a somewhat common pathogenesis.

PATHOGENESIS OF ATN The pathogenesis of both types of ATN resulting in ARF is explained on the basis of the following sequential mechanism:

i) Renal tubules are highly *susceptible* to injury by ischaemia and toxic agents.

ii) *Tubular damage* in ischaemic ATN is initiated by arteriolar vasoconstriction induced by renin-angiotensin system, while in toxic ATN by direct damage to tubules by the agent.

iii) Debris of the desquamated epithelium due to necrosis causes *tubular obstruction* and may block urinary outflow with consequent reduction of GFR.

iv) These events cause *increased intratubular pressure*.

v) Due to increased intratubular pressure, there is *tubular rupture*.

vi) Damage to tubules is accompanied with leakage of fluid into the interstitium causing *interstitial oedema*.

vii) Leakage of tubular fluid into the interstitium increases *interstitial pressure*.

viii) Leaked fluid incites host *inflammatory response*.

ix) Increased interstitial pressure causes *compression of tubules and blood vessels* and setting up a vicious cycle of accentuated ischaemia and necrosis.

x) Ultimately, it leads to reduced GFR and consequently *oliguria*.

ISCHAEMIC ATN

Ischaemic ATN, also called tubulorrhectic ATN, lower (distal) nephron nephrosis, anoxic nephrosis, or shock kidney, occurs due to hypoperfusion of the kidneys resulting in focal damage to the distal parts of the convoluted tubules.

ETIOLOGY Ischaemic ATN is more common than toxic ATN and accounts for more than 80% cases of tubular injury e.g.

1. Shock (post-traumatic, surgical, burns, dehydration, obstetrical and septic type).

2. Crush injuries.

3. Non-traumatic rhabdomyolysis induced by alcohol, coma, muscle disease or extreme muscular exertion (myoglobinuric nephrosis).

4. Mismatched blood transfusions, black-water fever (haemoglobinuric nephrosis).

G/A The kidneys are enlarged and swollen. On cut section, the cortex is often widened and pale, while the medulla is dark.

M/E Predominant changes are seen in the tubules, while glomeruli remain unaffected.

1. Dilatation of the proximal and distal convoluted tubules.

2. Focal tubular necrosis at different points along the nephron.

3. Flattened epithelium lining the tubules suggesting epithelial regeneration.

4. Eosinophilic hyaline casts or pigmented haemoglobin and myoglobin casts in the tubular lumina.

5. Disruption of tubular basement membrane adjacent to the cast may occur (tubulorrhexis).

In general, cases that follow severe trauma, surgical procedures, extensive burns and sepsis have much worse outlook than the others.

TOXIC ATN

Toxic ATN, also called nephrotoxic ATN or toxic nephrosis or upper (proximal) nephron nephrosis, occurs as a result of direct damage to tubules, more marked in proximal portions, by ingestion, injection or inhalation of a number of toxic agents.

ETIOLOGY Toxic agents causing ATN are as under:

1. General poisons such as mercuric chloride, carbon tetrachloride, ethylene glycol, mushroom poisoning and insecticides.

2. Heavy metals (mercury, lead, arsenic, phosphorus and gold).

3. Drugs such as sulfonamides, certain antibiotics (gentamycin, cephalosporin), anaesthetic agents (methoxyflurane, halothane), barbiturates, salicylates.

4. Radiographic contrast material.

M/E In general, it involves the segment of tubule diffusely (unlike ischaemic ATN where the involvement of nephron is focal). In mercuric chloride poisoning, the features are as follows:

1. Epithelial cells of mainly proximal convoluted tubules are necrotic and desquamated into the tubular lumina.

2. The desquamated cells may undergo dystrophic calcification.

3. Tubular basement membrane is generally intact.

4. The regenerating epithelium, which is flat and thin with few mitoses, may be seen lining the tubular basement membrane.

Prognosis of toxic ATN is good if there is no serious damage to other organs such as heart and liver.

TUBULOINTERSTITIAL DISEASES

The term tubulointerstitial nephritis is used for inflammatory process that predominantly involves the renal interstitial tissue and is usually accompanied by some degree of tubular damage.

ACUTE PYELONEPHRITIS

Acute pyelonephritis is an acute suppurative inflammation of the kidney caused by pyogenic bacteria.

ETIOPATHOGENESIS Most cases of acute pyelonephritis follow infection of the lower urinary tract. The most common pathogenic organism in urinary tract infection (UTI) is *Escherichia coli* (in 90% of cases), followed in decreasing frequency, by *Enterobacter, Klebsiella, Pseudomonas* and *Proteus*. The bacteria gain entry into the urinary tract, and then into the kidney by one of the two routes:

1. **Ascending infection** This is the most common route of infection. The common pathogenic organisms are inhabitants of the colon and may cause faecal contamination of the urethral orifice, especially in females in reproductive age group. Ascending infection may occur in a normal individual but the susceptibility is increased in patients with diabetes mellitus, pregnancy, urinary tract obstruction or instrumentation. Bacteria multiply in the urinary bladder. After having caused urethritis and cystitis, the bacteria in susceptible cases ascend further up into the ureters against the flow of urine, extend into the renal pelvis and then the renal cortex. The role of vesico-ureteral reflux is not a significant factor in the pathogenesis of acute pyelonephritis as it is in chronic pyelonephritis.

2. **Haematogenous infection** Less often, acute pyelonephritis may result from blood-borne spread of infection. This occurs more often in patients with obstructive lesions in the urinary tract, and in debilitated or immunosuppressed patients.

G/A Well-developed cases of acute pyelonephritis show enlarged and swollen kidney that bulges on section. The cut surface shows small, yellow-white abscesses with a haemorrhagic rim.

M/E Acute pyelonephritis is characterised by extensive acute inflammation involving the interstitium and causing destruction of the tubules. Generally, the glomeruli and renal blood vessels show considerable resistance to infection and are spared. The acute inflammation may be in the form of large number of neutrophils in the interstitial tissue and bursting into tubules, or may form focal neutrophilic abscesses in the renal parenchyma.

CLINICAL FEATURES Classically, acute pyelonephritis has an acute onset with chills, fever, loin pain, lumbar tenderness, dysuria and frequency of micturition.

COMPLICATIONS Complications of acute pyelonephritis are encountered more often in patients with diabetes mellitus or with urinary tract obstruction.

1. **Papillary necrosis** Papillary necrosis or necrotising papillitis develops more commonly in analgesic abuse nephropathy and in sickle cell disease but may occur as a complication of acute pyelonephritis as well.

2. Pyonephrosis Rarely, the abscesses in the kidney in acute pyelonephritis are extensive, particularly in cases with obstruction. This results in inability of the abscesses to drain and this transforms the kidney into a multilocular sac filled with pus.

3. Perinephric abscess The abscesses in the kidney may extend through the capsule of the kidney into the perinephric tissue and form perinephric abscess.

CHRONIC PYELONEPHRITIS

Chronic pyelonephritis is a chronic tubulointerstitial disease resulting from repeated attacks of inflammation and scarring.

ETIOPATHOGENESIS Depending upon the etiology and pathogenesis, two types of chronic pyelonephritis are described.

1. Reflux nephropathy Reflux of urine from the bladder into one or both the ureters during micturition is the major cause of chronic pyelonephritis. *Vesicoureteric reflux* is particularly common in children, especially in girls. Reflux results in increase in pressure in the renal pelvis so that the urine is forced into renal tubules which is eventually followed by damage to the kidney and scar formation. Vesicoureteric reflux is more common in patients with urinary tract infection.

2. Obstructive pyelonephritis Obstruction to the outflow of urine at different levels predisposes the kidney to infection. Recurrent episodes of such obstruction and infection result in renal damage and scarring.

G/A The kidneys are usually small and contracted (weighing less than 100 gm) showing unequal reduction, which distinguishes it from other forms of contracted kidney. The surface of the kidney is irregularly scarred; the capsule can be stripped off with difficulty due to adherence to scars. There is generally blunting and dilatation of calyces (*calyectasis*) and dilated pelvis of the kidney.

M/E Predominant changes are seen in the interstitium.

i) Interstitium There is chronic interstitial inflammatory reaction, chiefly composed of lymphocytes, plasma cells and macrophages with pronounced interstitial fibrosis. *Xanthogranulomatous pyelonephritis* is an uncommon variant characterised by collection of foamy macrophages admixed with other inflammatory cells and giant cells.

ii) Tubules The tubules show varying degree of atrophy and dilatation. Dilated tubules may contain eosinophilic colloid casts producing thyroidisation of tubules.

iii) Pelvicalyceal system The renal pelvis and calyces are dilated. The walls of pelvis and calyces show marked chronic inflammation and fibrosis.

iv) Blood vessels Blood vessels entrapped in the scarred areas show obliterative endarteritis.

v) Glomeruli Though glomerular tuft in the scarred area is usually intact, there is often periglomerular fibrosis. In advanced cases, there may be hyalinisation of glomeruli.

CLINICAL FEATURES Chronic pyelonephritis often has an insidious onset. The patients present with clinical picture of chronic renal failure or with symptoms of hypertension. Sometimes, the patients may present with features of acute recurrent pyelonephritis with fever, loin pain, lumbar tenderness, dysuria, pyuria, bacteriuria and frequency of micturition.

TUBERCULOUS PYELONEPHRITIS

Tuberculosis of the kidney occurs due to haematogenous spread of infection from another site, most often from the lungs. The renal lesions in tuberculosis may be in the form of tuberculous pyelonephritis or appear as multiple miliary tubercles.

G/A The lesions in tuberculous pyelonephritis are often bilateral, usually involving the medulla with replacement of the papillae by caseous tissue.

M/E Typical caseating epithelioid cell granulomatous reaction is seen. Acid-fast bacilli can often be demonstrated in the lesions.

CLINICAL FEATURES Most patients are young to middle-aged adults. The clinical presentation is extremely variable but it should always be considered as a possibility in a patient in whom there is persistent sterile pyuria, microscopic haematuria and mild proteinuria after effective antibiotic therapy for urinary tract infection.

MYELOMA NEPHROPATHY

Renal involvement in multiple myeloma is referred to as myeloma nephropathy or myeloma kidney. Functional renal impairment in multiple myeloma is a common manifestation, developing in about 50% of patients. The pathogenesis of myeloma kidney is related to excess filtration of Bence Jones proteins through the glomerulus, usually *kappa (k)* light chains. These light chain proteins are precipitated in the distal convoluted tubules in combination with Tamm-Horsfall proteins, the urinary glycoproteins.

G/A The kidneys may be normal or small and shrunken.

M/E There are some areas of tubular atrophy while many other tubular lumina are dilated and contain characteristic bright pink laminated cracked or fractured casts consisting of Bence-Jones proteins called fractured casts.

NEPHROCALCINOSIS

Nephrocalcinosis is a diffuse deposition of calcium salts in renal tissue in a number of renal diseases, in hypercalcaemia, hyperphosphataemia and renal tubular acidosis. Most commonly, it develops as a complication of severe hypercalcaemia such as due to hyperparathyroidism, hypervitaminosis D, excessive bone destruction in metastatic malignancy, hyperthyroidism, excessive calcium intake such as in milk-alkali syndrome and sarcoidosis.

M/E Nephrocalcinosis due to hypercalcaemia characteristically shows deposition of calcium in the tubular epithelial cells in the basement membrane, within the mitochondria and in the cytoplasm.

OBSTRUCTIVE UROPATHY *(p. 672)*

Obstruction in the urinary tract is common and important because it increases the susceptibility to infection and stone formation. Obstruction can occur at any age and in either sex. The cause of obstruction may lie at any level of the urinary tract—renal pelvis, ureters, urinary bladder and urethra. The obstruction at any of these anatomic locations may be intraluminal, intramural or extramural as under:

A. INTRALUMINAL
1. Calculi
2. Tumours (e.g. cancer of kidney and bladder)
3. Sloughed renal papilla
4. Blood clots
5. Foreign body

B. INTRAMURAL
1. Pelvi-ureteric junction (PUJ) obstruction
2. Vesicoureteric obstruction
3. Urethral stricture
4. Urethral valves
5. Inflammation (e.g. phimosis, cystitis etc)
6. Neuromuscular dysfunction

C. EXTRAMURAL
1. Pregnant uterus
2. Retroperitoneal fibrosis
3. Tumours (e.g. carcinoma of cervix, rectum, colon, caecum etc)
4. Prostatic enlargement, prostatic carcinoma and prostatitis
5. Trauma

The obstruction may be unilateral or bilateral, partial or complete, sudden or insidious. There are three important anatomic sequelae of obstruction, namely: *hydronephrosis, hydroureter and hypertrophy of the bladder.*

NEPHROLITHIASIS

Nephrolithiasis or urolithiasis is formation of urinary calculi at any level of the urinary tract. Urinary calculi are worldwide in distribution but are particularly common in some geographic locations such as in parts of the United States, South Africa, India and South-East Asia. Renal calculi are characterised clinically by colicky pain *(renal colic)* as they pass down along the ureter and manifest by haematuria.

TYPES OF URINARY CALCULI

There are 4 main types of urinary calculi:

1. CALCIUM STONES Calcium stones are the most common comprising about 75% of all urinary calculi. They may be pure stones of calcium oxalate (50%) or calcium phosphate (5%), or mixture of calcium oxalate and calcium phosphate (45%).

Etiology It is variable.
i) About 50% of patients with calcium stones have *idiopathic hypercalciuria without hypercalcaemia.*
ii) Approximately 10% cases are associated with *hypercalcaemia and hypercalciuria*, most commonly due to hyperparathyroidism, or a defect in the bowel (i.e. absorptive hypercalciuria), or in the kidney (i.e. renal hypercalciuria).
iii) About 15% of patients with calcium stones have *hyperuricosuria with a normal blood uric acid level* and without any abnormality of calcium metabolism.
iv) In about 25% of patients with calcium stones, the cause is unknown *'idiopathic calcium stone disease'.*

Pathogenesis The mechanism of calcium stone formation is explained on the basis of imbalance between the degree of supersaturation of the ions forming the stone and the concentration of inhibitors in the urine.

Morphology Calcium stones are usually small (less than a centimeter), ovoid, hard, with granular rough surface. They are dark brown due to old blood pigment deposited in them as a result of repeated trauma caused to the urinary tract by these sharp-edged stones.

2. MIXED (STRUVITE) STONES About 15% of urinary calculi are made of magnesium-ammonium-calcium phosphate, often called *struvite;* hence mixed stones are also called as *'struvite stones'* or *'triple phosphate stones'.*

Etiology Struvite stones are formed as a result of infection of the urinary tract with urea-splitting organisms that produce urease such as by species of *Proteus,* and occasionally *Klebsiella, Pseudomonas* and *Enterobacter.* These are, therefore, also known as infection-induced stones. However, *E. coli* does not form urease.

Morphology Struvite stones are yellow-white or grey. They tend to be soft and friable and irregular in shape. 'Staghorn stone' which is a large, solitary stone that takes the shape of the renal pelvis where it is often formed is an example of struvite stone.

3. URIC ACID STONES Approximately 6% of urinary calculi are made of uric acid. Uric acid calculi are *radiolucent* unlike radio-opaque calcium stones.

Etiology Uric acid stones are frequently formed in cases with hyperuricaemia and hyperuricosuria such as due to primary gout or secondary gout due to myeloproliferative disorders (e.g. in leukaemias), especially those on chemotherapy, and administration of uricosuric drugs (e.g. salicylates, probenecid).

Pathogenesis Hyperuricosuria is the most important factor in the production of uric acid stones, while hyperuricaemia is found in about half the cases.

Morphology Uric acid stones are smooth, yellowish-brown, hard and often multiple. On cut section, they show laminated structure.

4. CYSTINE STONES Cystine stones comprise less than 2% of urinary calculi.

Etiology Cystine stones are associated with cystinuria due to a genetically-determined defect in the transport of cystine and other amino acids across the cell membrane of the renal tubules and the small intestinal mucosa.

Morphology Cystine stones are small, rounded, smooth and often multiple. They are yellowish and waxy.

HYDRONEPHROSIS

Hydronephrosis is the term used for dilatation of renal pelvis and calyces due to partial or intermittent obstruction to the outflow of urine. Hydronephrosis develops if one or both the pelviureteric sphincters are incompetent, as otherwise there will be dilatation and hypertrophy of the urinary bladder but no hydronephrosis. Hydroureter nearly always accompanies hydronephrosis. Hydronephrosis may be *unilateral or bilateral.*

UNILATERAL HYDRONEPHROSIS

This occurs due to some form of ureteral obstruction at the level of pelviureteric junction (PUJ). The causes are:
1. *Intraluminal* e.g. a calculus in the ureter or renal pelvis.
2. *Intramural* e.g. congenital PUJ obstruction, atresia of ureter, inflammatory stricture, trauma, neoplasm of ureter or bladder.
3. *Extramural* e.g. obstruction of upper part of the ureter by inferior renal artery or vein, pressure on ureter from outside such as carcinoma cervix, prostate, rectum, colon or caecum and retroperitoneal fibrosis.

BILATERAL HYDRONEPHROSIS

This is generally the result of some form of urethral obstruction but can occur from the various causes listed above if the lesions involve both sides. Based on this, hydronephrosis may be of following types:
1. *Congenital* e.g. atresia of the urethral meatus, congenital posterior urethral valve.
2. *Acquired* e.g. bladder tumour involving both ureteric orifices, prostatic enlargement, prostatic carcinoma and prostatitis, bladder neck stenosis, inflammatory or traumatic urethral stricture and phimosis.

G/A The kidneys may have moderate to marked enlargement. Initially, there is *extrarenal hydronephrosis* characterised by dilatation of renal pelvis medially in the form of a sac. Eventually, the dilated pelvi-calyceal system extends deep into the renal cortex so that a thin rim of renal cortex is stretched over the dilated calyces and the external surface assumes lobulated appearance. This advanced stage is called as *intrarenal hydronephrosis.*

M/E The wall of hydronephrotic sac is thickened due to fibrous scarring and chronic inflammatory cell infiltrate. There is progressive atrophy of tubules and glomeruli alongwith interstitial fibrosis. Stasis of urine in hydronephrosis causes infection *(pyelitis)* resulting in filling of the sac with pus, a condition called *pyonephrosis.*

RENAL VASCULAR DISEASES *(p. 675)*

HYPERTENSIVE VASCULAR DISEASE

An elevated arterial blood pressure is a major health problem, particularly in developed countries. A persistent and sustained high blood pressure has damaging effects on the heart (e.g. hypertensive heart disease), brain (e.g. cerebrovascular accident or stroke) and kidneys (benign and malignant nephrosclerosis).

Hypertension is a common disease in industrialised countries and accounts for 6% of death worldwide. Epidemiologic studies have revealed that with elevation in systolic and diastolic blood pressure above normal in adults, there is a continuous increased risk of cardiovascular disease, stroke and renal disease. Criteria for normal blood pressure, prehypertension and hypertension (stage 1 and stage 2) have been laid by the National Institutes of Health (NIH), US as below:

CATEGORY	SYSTOLIC (mmHg)	DIASTOLIC (mmHg)
Normal	< 120	and < 80
Prehypertension	120-139	or 80-89
Hypertension		
Stage 1	140-159	or 90-99
Stage 2	>160	or >100
Isolated systolic hypertension	≥140	and < 90
Malignant hypertension	> 200 (sudden onset)	≥ 140 (sudden onset)

Hypertension is generally classified into 2 types:

1. Primary or essential hypertension in which the cause of increase in blood pressure is unknown. Essential hypertension constitutes about 80-95% patients of hypertension.

2. Secondary hypertension in which the increase in blood pressure is caused by diseases of the kidneys, endocrines or some other organs. Secondary hypertension comprises remaining 5-20% cases of hypertension.

According to the clinical course, both essential and secondary hypertension may be benign or malignant.

❖ *Benign hypertension* is moderate elevation of blood pressure and the rise is slow over the years. About 90-95% patients of hypertension have benign hypertension.

❖ *Malignant hypertension* is marked and sudden increase of blood pressure to 200/140 mmHg or more in a known case of hypertension or in a previously normotensive individual; the patients develop papilloedema, retinal haemorrhages and hypertensive encephalopathy.

ETIOLOGY AND PATHOGENESIS

The etiology and pathogenesis of secondary hypertension that comprises less than 10% cases has been better understood, whereas the mechanism of essential hypertension, that constitutes about 90% of cases, remains largely obscure. In general, normal blood pressure is regulated by 2 haemodynamic forces—*cardiac output* and *total peripheral vascular resistance.*

ESSENTIAL (PRIMARY) HYPERTENSION A number of factors are related to its development.

1. Genetic factors The role of heredity in the etiology of essential hypertension has long been suspected. The evidences in support are the familial aggregation, occurrence of hypertension in twins, epidemiologic data.

2. Racial and environmental factors A number of environmental factors have been implicated in the development of hypertension including salt intake, obesity, skilled occupation, higher living standards and individuals under high stress.

3. Risk factors modifying the course of essential hypertension There is sufficient evidence to show that the course of essential hypertension that begins in middle life is modified by a number of factors e.g.

i)   Age Younger the age at which hypertension is first noted but left untreated, lower the life expectancy.

ii) *Sex* Females with hypertension appear to do better than males.

iii) *Atherosclerosis* Accelerated atherosclerosis invariably accompanies essential hypertension. This could be due to contributory role of other independent factors like cigarette smoking, elevated serum cholesterol, glucose intolerance and obesity.

iv) *Other risk factors* e.g. smoking, excess of alcohol intake, diabetes mellitus.

SECONDARY HYPERTENSION The mechanisms of this less common type are better known.

1. Renal hypertension Hypertension produced by renal diseases is called renal hypertension. Renal hypertension is subdivided into 2 groups:

i) *Renal vascular hypertension* e.g. in occlusion of a major renal artery, pre-eclampsia, eclampsia, polyarteritis nodosa and fibromuscular dysplasia of renal artery.

ii) *Renal parenchymal hypertension* e.g. in various types of glomerulo-nephritis, pyelonephritis, interstitial nephritis, diabetic nephropathy, amyloidosis, polycystic kidney disease and renin-producing tumours.

In either case, renal hypertension can be produced by one of the following 3 inter-related pathogenetic mechanisms:
a) Activation of renin-angiotensin system
b) Sodium and water retention
c) Release of vasodepressor material

2. Endocrine hypertension A number of hormonal secretions may produce secondary hypertension as follows:

i) *Adrenal gland*—e.g. in primary aldosteronism, Cushing's syndrome, adrenal virilism and pheochromocytoma.

ii) *Parathyroid gland*—e.g. hypercalcaemia in hyperparathyroidism.

iii) *Oral contraceptives*—Oestrogen component in the oral contraceptives stimulates hepatic synthesis of renin substrate.

3. Coarctation of aorta Coarctation of the aorta causes systolic hypertension in the upper part of the body due to constriction itself. Diastolic hypertension results from changes in circulation.

4. Neurogenic Psychogenic, polyneuritis, increased intracranial pressure and section of spinal cord are all uncommon causes of secondary hypertension.

EFFECTS OF HYPERTENSION

Systemic hypertension causes major effects in three main organs—heart and its blood vessels, nervous system, and kidneys. An important and early clinical marker for renal injury from hypertension and risk factor for cardiovascular disease is *macroalbuminuria* (i.e. albuminuria > 150 mg/day or random urine albumin/creatinine ratio of >300 mg/gm creatinine), or *microalbuminuria* estimated by radioimmunoassay (i.e. microalbumin 30-300 mg/day or random urine microalbumin/creatinine ratio of 30-300 mg/gm creatinine).

BENIGN NEPHROSCLEROSIS

Benign nephrosclerosis is the term used to describe the kidney of benign phase of hypertension. Mild benign nephrosclerosis is the most common form of renal disease in persons over 60 years of age but its severity increases in the presence of hypertension and diabetes mellitus.

G/A Both the kidneys are affected equally and are reduced in size and weight, often weighing about 100 gm or less. The capsule is often adherent to the cortical surface. The surface of the kidney is finely granular and shows V-shaped areas of scarring.

M/E There are predominant vascular changes causing secondary parenchymal changes:

i) Vascular changes: Changes in blood vessels involve arterioles and arteries up to the size of arcuate arteries. There are 2 types of changes in these blood vessels:

a) *Hyaline arteriolosclerosis*

b) *Intimal thickening* due to proliferation of smooth muscle cells in the intima.

ii) **Parenchymal changes:** As a consequence of ischaemia, there is variable degree of atrophy of parenchyma. This includes: glomerular shrinkage, deposition of collagen in Bowman's space, periglomerular fibrosis, tubular atrophy and fine interstitial fibrosis.

CLINICAL FEATURES There is variable elevation of the blood pressure with headache, dizziness, palpitation and nervousness. Eye ground changes may be found but papilloedema is absent.

MALIGNANT NEPHROSCLEROSIS

Malignant nephrosclerosis is the form of renal disease that occurs in malignant or accelerated hypertension. Malignant nephrosclerosis is uncommon and usually occurs as a superimposed complication in 5% cases of pre-existing benign essential hypertension or in those having secondary hypertension with identifiable cause such as in chronic renal diseases.

G/A In a case of malignant hypertension superimposed on pre-existing benign nephrosclerosis, the kidneys are small in size, shrunken and reduced in weight and have finely granular surface. However, the kidneys of a patient who develops malignant hypertension in pure form are enlarged, oedematous and have petechial haemorrhages on the surface producing so called *'flea-bitten kidney'*. Cut surface shows red and yellow mottled appearance .

M/E Commonly, the changes are superimposed on benign nephrosclerosis.

i) **Vascular changes** These are more severe and involve the arterioles. The two characteristic vascular changes seen are:

a) *Necrotising arteriolitis*

b) *Hyperplastic intimal sclerosis* or *onion-skin proliferation*

ii) **Ischaemic changes** The effects of vascular narrowing on the parenchyma include tubular loss, fine interstitial fibrosis and foci of infarction necrosis.

CLINICAL FEATURES Headache, dizziness and impaired vision are commonly found. The presence of papilloedema distinguishes malignant from benign phase of hypertension. The urine frequently shows microscopic haematuria and proteinuria. Approximately 90% of patients die within one year from causes such as uraemia, congestive heart failure and cerebrovascular accidents.

THROMBOTIC MICROANGIOPATHY

Thrombotic renal disease encompasses a group of diseases having in common the formation of thrombi composed by platelets and fibrin in arterioles and glomeruli of the kidney and culminating clinically in acute renal failure. Causes of thrombotic microangiopathy of renal microvasculature are as under:

1. Infections
   (*E. coli, Shigella, Pseudomonas*)
2. Drugs
   (e.g. mitomycin, cisplatin, cyclosporine)
3. Autoimmune disease
   (scleroderma, SLE)
4. Thrombotic thrombocytopenic purpura
5. Haemolytic-uraemic syndrome
6. Pregnancy and pre-eclampsia
7. Malignant hypertension

The common clinical manifestations include microangiopathic haemolytic anaemia, thrombocytopenia, DIC, and eventually renal failure.

RENAL CORTICAL NECROSIS

Renal cortical necrosis is infarction of renal cortex varying from microscopic foci to a situation where most of the renal cortex is destroyed. The medulla, spared. The condition develops most commonly as an obstetrical emergency (e.g. in eclampsia, pre-eclampsia, premature separation of the placenta). Other causes include septic shock, poisoning, severe trauma etc.

The lesions may be focal, patchy or diffuse. The gross and microscopic characteristics of infarcts of cortex are present.

TUMOURS OF KIDNEY *(p. 680)*

Both benign and malignant tumours occur in the kidney, the latter being more common. These may arise from *renal tubules* (adenoma, adenocarcinoma), *embryonic tissue* (mesoblastic nephroma, Wilms' tumour), *mesenchymal tissue* (angiomyolipoma, medullary interstitial tumour) and from the *epithelium of the renal pelvis* (urothelial carcinoma). Besides these tumours, the kidney may be the site of the secondary tumours.

BENIGN TUMOURS

CORTICAL ADENOMA

Cortical tubular adenomas are more common than other benign renal neoplasms. They are frequently multiple and associated with chronic pyelonephritis or benign nephrosclerosis.

G/A These tumours may form tiny nodules up to 3 cm in diameter. They are encapsulated and white or yellow.

M/E They are composed of tubular cords or papillary structures projecting into cystic space. The cells of the adenoma are usually uniform, cuboidal with no atypicality or mitosis. However, size of the tumour rather than histologic criteria is considered more significant parameter to predict the behaviour of the tumour—those larger than 3 cm in diameter are potentially malignant and metastasising.

ONCOCYTOMA

Oncocytoma is a benign epithelial tumour arising from collecting ducts.
G/A The tumour is encapsulated and has variable size. Cut section is homogeneous and has characteristic mahogany-brown or tan colour.
M/E The tumour cells are plump with abundant, finely granular, acidophilic cytoplasm and round nuclei.

OTHER BENIGN TUMOURS

❖ *Angiomyolipoma* is a hamartoma of the kidney that contains differentiated tissue element derived from blood vessels, smooth muscle and fat.
❖ *Mesoblastic nephroma* is a congenital benign tumour.
❖ *Multicystic nephroma* is another uncommon tumour of early infancy.
❖ *Medullary interstitial cell tumour* is a tiny nodule in the medulla composed of fibroblast-like cells in hyalinised stroma.
❖ *Juxtaglomerular tumour or reninoma* is a rare tumour of renal cortex consisting of sheets of epithelioid cells with many small blood vessels.

MALIGNANT TUMOURS

The two most common primary malignant tumours of the kidney are *adenocarcinoma* and *Wilms' tumour*. A third malignant renal tumour is *urothelial carcinoma* occurring more commonly in the renal pelvis is described in the next section along with other tumours of the lower urinary tract.

ADENOCARCINOMA OF KIDNEY (SYNONYMS: RENAL CELL CARCINOMA, HYPERNEPHROMA, GRAWITZ TUMOUR)

This cancer comprises 70 to 80% of all renal cancers and occurs most commonly in 50 to 70 years of age with male preponderance (2:1).

ETIOLOGY AND PATHOGENESIS Various factors in the etiology of RCC are as under:

1. Tobacco Tobacco is the major risk factor for RCC, whether chewed or smoked and accounts for 20-30% cases of RCC.

2. Genetic factors Heredity and first-degree relatives of RCC are associated with higher risk. Although majority of cases of RCC are sporadic but about 5% cases are inherited. These cases have following associations:

i) *von Hippel-Lindau (VHL) disease:* It is an autosomal dominant cancer syndrome that includes: haemangioblastoma of the cerebellum, retinal angiomas, multiple RCC (clear cell type), pheochromocytoma and cysts in different organs.

ii) *Hereditary clear cell RCC:* These are cases of clear cell type RCC confined to the kidney without other manifestations of VHL but having autosomal dominant inheritance.

iii) *Papillary RCC:* This form of RCC is characterised by bilteral and multifocal cancer with papillary growth pattern.

iv) *Chromophobe RCC:* These cases have genetic defects in the form of multiple losses of whole chromosomes.

3. Cystic diseases of the kidneys Both hereditary and acquired cystic diseases of the kidney have increased risk of development of RCC.

4. Other risk factors These include:

i) Exposure to asbestos, heavy metals and petrochemical products.

ii) In women, obesity and oestrogen therapy.

iii) Analgesic nephropathy.

iv) Tuberous sclerosis.

CLASSIFICATION Based on cytogenetics of sporadic and familial tumours, RCC has been reclassified into clear cell, papillary, granular cell, chromophobe, sarcomatoid and collecting duct type.

G/A RCC commonly arises from the poles of the kidney as a solitary and unilateral tumour, more often in the upper pole. The tumour is generally large, golden yellow and circumscribed. Papillary tumours have grossly visible papillae and may be multifocal. About 1% RCC are bilateral. Cut section of the tumour commonly shows large areas of ischaemic necrosis, cystic change and foci of haemorrhages.

M/E The features of various types are as under:

1. *Clear cell type RCC (70%):* This is the most common pattern. The tumour cells have a variety of patterns: solid, trabecular and tubular, separated by delicate vasculature. Majority of clear cell tumours are well differentiated.

2. *Papillary type RCC (15%):* The tumour cells are arranged in papillary pattern over the fibrovascular stalks. The tumour cells are cuboidal with small round nuclei. Psammoma bodies may be seen.

3. *Granular cell type RCC (8%):* The tumour cells have abundant acidophilic cytoplasm. These tumours have more marked nuclear pleomorphism, hyper-chromatism and cellular atypia.

4. *Chromophobe type RCC (5%):* This type shows admixture of pale clear cells with perinuclear halo and acidophilic granular cells.

5. *Sarcomatoid type RCC (1.5%):* This is the most anaplastic and poorly differentiated form. The tumour is characterised by whorls of atypical spindle tumour cells.

6. *Collecting duct type RCC (0.5%):* This is a rare type that occurs in the medulla. It is composed of a single layer of cuboidal tumour cells arranged in tubular and papillary pattern.

CLINICAL FEATURES The classical clinical evidence for diagnosis of renal cell carcinoma is the triad of *gross haematuria, flank plain* and *palpable abdominal mass.* The most common presenting abnormality is haematuria that occurs in about 60% of cases. By the time the tumour is detected, it has spread to distant sites via haematogenous route to the lungs, brain and bone, and locally to the liver and perirenal lymph nodes.

Systemic symptoms of fatiguability, weight loss, cachexia and intermittent fever unassociated with evidence of infection are found in many cases at presentation. A number of paraneoplastic syndromes due to ectopic hormone production by the renal cell carcinoma have been described. These include *polycythaemia* (by erythropoietin), *hypercalcaemia* (by parathyroid hormone and prostaglandins), *hypertension* (by renin).

The **prognosis** in renal cell carcinoma depends upon the extent of tumour involvement at the time of diagnosis. Presence of metastases, renal vein invasion and higher nuclear grade of the tumour are some of the predictors of poor prognosis.

WILMS' TUMOUR (SYNONYM: NEPHROBLASTOMA)

Nephroblastoma or Wilms' tumour is an embryonic tumour derived from primitive renal epithelial and mesenchymal components. It is the most common abdominal malignant tumour of young children, seen most commonly between 1 to 6 years of age with equal sex incidence.

ETIOLOGY AND PATHOGENESIS Wilms' tumour has following etiologic associations:

1. A higher incidence has been seen in monozygotic *twins* and cases with family history.

2. Association of Wilms' tumour with some *other congenital anomalies* has been observed.

3. A few *other malignancies* are known to have higher incidence of Wilms' tumour. These include osteosarcoma, botryoid sarcoma, retinoblastoma, neuroblastoma etc.

G/A The tumour is usually quite large, spheroidal, replacing most of the kidney. It is generally solitary and unilateral but 5-10% cases may have bilateral tumour. On cut section, the tumour shows characteristic variegated appearance—soft, fishflesh-like grey-white to cream-yellow tumour with foci of necrosis and haemorrhages and grossly identifiable myxomatous or cartilaginous elements.

M/E Nephroblastoma shows mixture of primitive epithelial and mesenchymal elements. Most of the tumour consists of small, round to spindled, anaplastic, sarcomatoid tumour cells. In these areas, abortive tubules and poorly-formed glomerular structures are present. Mesenchymal elements such as smooth and skeletal muscle, cartilage and bone, fat cells and fibrous tissue, may be seen.

CLINICAL FEATURES The most common presenting feature is a palpable abdominal mass in a child. Other common abnormalities are haematuria, pain, fever and hypertension. The tumour rapidly spreads via blood, especially to lungs.

SECONDARY TUMOURS

Leukaemic infiltration of the kidneys is a common finding, particularly in chronic myeloid leukaemia. Kidney is a common site for blood-borne metastases from different primary sites, chiefly from cancers of the lungs, breast and stomach.

LOWER URINARY TRACT (p. 685)

NORMAL STRUCTURE

The lower urinary tract consists of *ureters, urinary bladder* and *urethra.*

URETERS These are tubular structures, 30 cm in length and half a centimeter in diameter, and extend from the renal pelvis (pelvi-ureteric junction) to the urinary bladder (vesico-ureteric junction).

M/E It is lined internally by transitional epithelium or urothelium similar to the lining of the renal pelvis above and bladder below.

URINARY BLADDER Besides *superior* surface (or dome), the bladder has *posterior surface (or base)* and two *lateral surfaces.* The *trigone* is at the base of the bladder and continues as *bladder neck.*

M/E The greater part of the bladder wall is made up of muscular layer (detrusor muscle) having 3 coats—internal, middle and external. The *trigone* muscle is derived from the prolongation of the longitudinal muscle layer of each ureter. The inner layer of bladder consists of urothelium 6-7 layers in thickness.

URETHRA It runs from the bladder up to the external meatus. The *male urethra* consists of 3 parts—prostatic, membranous and penile. It is lined in the prostatic part by urothelium but elsewhere by stratified columnar epithelium except near its orifice where the epithelium is stratified squamous. The *female urethra* is shorter and runs from the bladder parallel with the anterior wall of the vagina. The mucous membrane in female urethra is lined throughout by columnar epithelium except near the bladder where the epithelium is transitional.

CONGENITAL ANOMALIES (p. 685)

DOUBLE URETER This is a condition in which the entire ureter or only the upper part is duplicated. Double ureter is invariably associated with a double renal pelvis, *one* in the upper part and the *other* in the lower part of the kidney.

URETEROCELE Ureterocele is cystic dilatation of the terminal part of the ureter which lies within the bladder wall.

ECTOPIA VESICAE (EXSTROPHY) This is a rare condition owing to congenital developmental deficiency of anterior wall of the bladder and is associated with splitting of the overlying anterior abdominal wall. The condition in males is often associated with *epispadias* in which the urethra opens on the dorsal aspect of penis.

URACHAL ABNORMALITIES Rarely, there may be persistence of the urachus in which urine passes from the bladder to the umbilicus. Persistence of central portion gives rise to *urachal cyst* lined by transitional or squamous epithelium. Adenocarcinoma may develop in urachal cyst. Other abnormalities due to urachal remnants are patent urachus, urachal-umbilical sinus and vesico-urachal diverticulum.

INFLAMMATIONS (p. 685)

URETERITIS

Infection of the ureter is almost always secondary to pyelitis above, or cystitis below. Ureteritis is usually mild but repeated and longstanding infection may give rise to chronic ureteritis.

CYSTITIS

Inflammation of the urinary bladder is called cystitis. Cystitis may occur by spread of infection from upper urinary tract as seen following renal tuberculosis, or may spread from the urethra such as in instrumentation. The most common pathogenic organism in UTI is *E. coli,* followed in decreasing frequency by *Enterobacter, Klebsiella, Pseudomonas* and *Proteus.* Infection with *Candida albicans* may occur in the bladder in immunosuppressed patients. Besides bacterial and fungal organisms, parasitic infestations such as with *Schistosoma haematobium* is common in the Middle-East countries, particularly in Egypt. *Chlamydia* and *Mycoplasma* may occasionally cause cystitis. In addition, radiation, direct exposure to chemical irritant, foreign bodies and local trauma may all initiate cystitis.

Cystitis, like UTI, is more common in females than in males because of the shortness of urethra which is liable to faecal contamination and due to mechanical trauma during sexual intercourse. In males, prostatic obstruction is a frequent cause of cystitis. All forms of cystitis are clinically characterised by a *triad* of symptoms—*frequency* (repeated urination), *dysuria* (painful or burning micturition) and *low abdominal pain.* There may, however, be systemic manifestations of bacteraemia such as fever, chills and malaise.

MORPHOLOGIC FEATURES Cystitis may be acute or chronic.

ACUTE CYSTITIS *G/A* The bladder mucosa is red, swollen and haemorrhagic.

M/E This form of cystitis is characterised by intense neutrophilic exudate admixed with lymphocytes and macrophages.

CHRONIC CYSTITIS Repeated attacks of acute cystitis lead to chronic cystitis.

G/A The mucosal epithelium is thickened, red and granular with formation of polypoid masses.

M/E There is patchy ulceration of the mucosa with formation of granulation tissue in the regions of polypoid masses. Submucosa and muscular coat show fibrosis and infiltration by chronic inflammatory cells. A form of chronic cystitis characterised by formation of lymphoid follicles in the bladder mucosa is termed *cystitis follicularis*.

INTERSTITIAL CYSTITIS (HUNNER'S ULCER) This variant of cystitis occurs in middle-aged women. Cystoscopy often reveals a localised ulcer. The *etiology* of the condition is unknown but it is thought to be neurogenic in origin.

CYSTITIS CYSTICA As a result of long-standing chronic inflammation, there occurs a downward projection of epithelial nests known as *Brunn's nests* from the deeper layer of bladder mucosa.

MALAKOPLAKIA This is a rare condition most frequently found in the urinary bladder but can occur in the ureters, kidney, testis and prostate, and occasionally in the gut. The *etiology* of the condition is unknown but it probably results from persistence of chronic inflammation with defective phagocytic process by the macrophages.

G/A The lesions appear as soft, flat, yellowish, slightly raised plaques on the bladder mucosa.

M/E The plaques are composed of massive accumulation of foamy macrophages with occasional multinucleate giant cells and some lymphocytes. These macrophages have granular PAS-positive cytoplasm and some of them contain cytoplasmic laminated concretions of calcium phosphate called *Michaelis-Gutmann bodies*.

POLYPOID CYSTITIS Polypoid cystitis is characterised by papillary projections on the bladder mucosa due to submucosal oedema and can be confused with transitional cell carcinoma.

URETHRITIS

◈   **Gonococcal (gonorrhoeal) urethritis** is an acute suppurative condition caused by gonococci *(Neisseria gonorrhoeae)*.

◈   **Non-gonococcal urethritis** is more common and is most frequently caused by *E. coli*. The infection of urethra often accompanies cystitis in females and prostatitis in males.

TUMOURS *(p. 686)*

Majority of lower urinary tract tumours are epithelial. Both benign and malignant tumours occur; the latter being more common. About 90% of malignant tumours of the lower urinary tract occur in the urinary bladder, 8% in the renal pelvis and remaining 2% are seen in the urethra or ureters.

TUMOURS OF THE BLADDER

The tumours of urinary bladder are divided into epithelial and non-epithelial, the latter being uncommon. Thus, epithelial tumours are the main tumours, vast majority of which are of transitional cell type (urothelial) tumours.

More than 90% of bladder tumours arise from transitional epithelial (urothelium) lining of the bladder in continuity with the epithelial lining of the renal pelvis, ureters, and the major part of the urethra.

ETIOPATHOGENESIS Urothelial tumours in the urinary tract are typically multifocal and the pattern of disease becomes apparent over a period of years. A number of environmental and host factors are associated with increased risk of bladder cancer. These are as under:

1. *Smoking* Tobacco smoking is associated with 2 to 4 fold increased risk.

2. *Industrial occupations* Workers in industries that produce aniline dyes, rubber, plastic, textiles, and cable have high incidence of bladder cancer.

3. *Schistosomiasis* There is increased risk of bladder cancer, particularly squamous cell carcinoma, in patients having bilharzial infestation (*Schistosoma haematobium*) of the bladder.

4. *Dietary factors* Certain carcinogenic metabolites of tryptophan are excreted in urine of patients with bladder cancer.

5. *Local lesions* Ectopia vesicae (extrophied bladder), vesical diverticulum, leukoplakia of the bladder mucosa and urinary diversion in defunctionalised bladder.

6. *Drugs* Immunosuppressive therapy with cyclophosphamide and patients having analgesic-abuse (phenacetin-) nephropathy have high risk of developing bladder cancer.

7. *Prior irradiation* Patients who have received prior irradiation for some other pelvic cancers have higher risk of developing bladder cancer.

Multicentric nature of urothelial cancer and high rate of recurrence has led to the hypothesis that a *field effect* in the urothelium is responsible for this form of cancer.

G/A Urothelial tumours may be single or multiple. About 90% of the tumours are papillary (non-invasive or invasive), whereas the remaining 10% are flat indurated (non-invasive or invasive). Most common location in the bladder is lateral walls, followed by posterior wall and region of trigone.

M/E Most common epithelial tumours of the bladder are urothelial (90%); others are squamous cell, glandular, small cell and mixed.

UROTHELIAL (TRANSITIONAL CELL) TUMOURS The WHO and ISUP (International Society of Urologic Pathology), in 1998 have proposed consensus histologic criteria to categorise urothelial tumours into papillomas (exophytic, inverted), carcinoma in situ (CIS), papillary urothelial neoplasms of low malignant potential (PUNLMP), and urothelial carcinoma (low grade and high grade).

1. Urothelial papilloma Papillomas may occur singly or may be multiple. These may be exophytic or inverted.

Exophytic papillomas are generally small, less than 2 cm in diameter, having delicate papillae.

Inverted papillomas have an endophytic growth pattern and are benign tumours.

2. Carcinoma in situ (CIS) (Flat urothelial carcinoma) Carcinoma *in situ* is characterised by anaplastic malignant cells confined to layers superficial to basement membrane of the bladder mucosa.

3. Papillary urothelial neoplasms of low malignant potential (PUNLMP) These cases have many features similar to papillomas with additional features such as increase in the number of epithelial layers, having round to oval nuclei and diffuse nuclear enlargement. PUNLMP is unassociated with invasion and may have recurrences.

4. Papillary urothelial (Transitional cell) carcinoma Histologic criteria for categorising these tumours are based on *architecture, cytologic features and invasiveness*.

i) *Architecture* takes into consideration the type of papillae and relationship of cell layers with basement membrane as regards polarity.

ii) *Cytologic criteria* of neoplasm are the extent of resemblance with normal cells, crowding, variation in nuclear size, shape, chromatin, nucleoli (their presence and type), and mitotic figures.

iii) *Criteria for invasion* in papillary as well as non-papillary tumours are penetration of the basement membrane of bladder mucosa and presence or absence of invasion by neoplastic cells in the muscle.

Based on these salient features, the characteristics of two grades are as under:

Papillary urothelial carcinoma, low grade: These tumours show fused and branching papillary pattern but overall there is an orderly arrangement of layers of cells. These cells are cohesive and show mild variation in polarity, nuclear size, chromatin and shape (round to oval), and inconspicuous small and regular nucleoli.

Papillary urothelial carcinoma, high grade: High-grade tumours have increased thickness and have fused and branching papillae which show quite disorderly arrangement. The tumour cells show nuclear enlargement, moderate to marked variation in nuclear size, shape, hyperchromatism, and multiple prominent nucleoli.

Invasive urothelial carcinoma Any grade of papillary urothelial carcinoma may show invasion into lamina propria or further into muscularis propria (detrusor).

OTHER VARIANTS A few less common histologic types are as under:

Squamous cell carcinoma Squamous cell carcinoma comprises about 5% of the bladder carcinomas.

Adenocarcinoma Adenocarcinoma has association with exostrophy of the bladder with glandular metaplasia, or may arise from urachal rests, periurethral and periprostatic glands, or from cystitis cystica.

Small cell carcinoma This variant has morphologic resemblance with small cell carcinoma of the lung or other neuroendocrine carcinomas and has a worse outcome.

Mixed carcinoma Occasionally, combination of more than one histologic types are seen.

STAGING OF BLADDER CANCER The clinical behaviour and prognosis of bladder cancer can be assessed by the following simple staging system:
Stage 0: Carcinoma confined to the mucosa.
Stage A: Carcinoma invades the lamina propria but not the muscularis.
Stage B1: Carcinoma invades the superficial muscle layer.
Stage B2: Carcinoma invades the deep muscle layer.
Stage C: Carcinoma invades the perivesical tissues.
Stage D1: Carcinoma shows regional metastases.
Stage D2: Carcinoma shows distant metastases.

NON-EPITHELIAL BLADDER TUMOURS

Mesenchymal tumours of the bladder are less common and may be benign or malignant.

BENIGN Benign mesenchymal tumour of the bladder is uncommon but most common is leiomyoma. Other less common examples are neurofibroma, haemangioma and granular cell myoblastoma.

MALIGNANT Rhabdomyosarcoma is the most frequent malignant mesenchymal tumour. It exists in 2 forms:
◈ *Adult form* occurring in adults over 40 years of age and resembles the rhabdomyosarcoma of skeletal muscle.
◈ *Childhood form* occurring in infancy and childhood and appears as large polypoid, soft, fleshy, grapelike mass and is also called *sarcoma botryoides* or *embryonal rhabdomyosarcoma*. It is morphologically characterised by masses of embryonic mesenchyme consisting of masses of highly

pleomorphic stellate cells in myxomatous background. Similar tumours occur in the female genital tract.

TUMOURS OF RENAL PELVIS AND URETERS

Almost all the tumours of the renal pelvis and ureters are of epithelial origin. They are of the same types as are seen in the urinary bladder. However, tumours in the ureters are quite rare.

TUMOURS OF URETHRA

URETHRAL CARUNCLE Urethral caruncle is not uncommon. It is an inflammatory lesion present on external urethral meatus in elderly females.

G/A The caruncle appears as a solitary, 1 to 2 cm in diameter, pink or red mass, protruding from urethral meatus.

M/E The mass may be covered by squamous or transitional epithelium or there may be ulcerated surface. The underlying tissues show proliferating blood vessels, fibroblastic connective tissue and intense acute and chronic inflammatory infiltrate.

URETHRAL CARCINOMA Carcinoma of the urethra is uncommon. In most cases it occurs in the distal urethra near the external meatus and thus is commonly squamous cell carcinoma. Less often, there may be transitional cell carcinoma or adenocarcinoma arising from periurethral glands.

SELF ASSESSMENT

---

1. **Glomerular tuft contains capillaries forming following number of lobules:**
   - A. Four
   - B. Six
   - C. Eight
   - D. Ten

2. **Azotaemia results from elevation of following waste-products of protein metabolism <u>except</u>:**
   - A. Blood urea
   - B. Blood urea nitrogen
   - C. Serum uric acid
   - D. Serum creatinine

3. **In end-stage kidney disease, GFR is:**
   - A. 5% of normal
   - B. 10% of normal
   - C. 15% of normal
   - D. 20% of normal

4. **Infantile polycystic kidney disease has the following features <u>except</u>:**
   - A. It has autosomal recessive inheritance
   - B. It is invariably bilateral
   - C. The condition often manifests in adults
   - D. The condition is frequently associated with multiple hepatic cysts

5. **The most common features of nephritic syndrome include the following <u>except</u>:**
   - A. Heavy proteinuria
   - B. Hypertension
   - C. Microscopic haematuria
   - D. Oliguria

6. **The most common form of glomerulonephritis (GN) in adults is:**
   - A. Minimal change disease
   - B. Membranous GN
   - C. Membranoproliferative GN
   - D. Focal segmental GN

7. **The most frequent form of primary glomerular disease in children is:**
   - A. Minimal change disease
   - B. Acute glomerulonephritis
   - C. Membranous GN
   - D. Membranoproliferative GN

8. **Examples of immune complex GN include the following <u>except</u>:**
   - A. Acute GN
   - B. Membranous GN

C. Membranoproliferative GN
D. RPGN in Goodpasture's disease

9. **Classic example of anti-GBM disease is:**
   A. Minimal change disease   B. Acute GN
   C. Membranous GN   D. Goodpasture's disease

10. **Alternate pathway disease occurs in following forms of glomerular disease _except_:**
    A. Membranous GN
    B. Membranoproliferative GN
    C. Rapidly progressive GN
    D. IgA nephropathy

11. **Acute post-streptococcal GN is characterised by proteinuria of:**
    A. Non-selective
    B. Selective
    C. Albuminuria only
    D. Low molecular weight only

12. **The serum markers for RPGN are as follows _except_:**
    A. Serum C3 levels
    B. Anti-GBM antibody
    C. Anti-neutrophil cytoplasmic antibody (ANCA)
    D. Anti-endothelial cell antibody (AECA)

13. **In Goodpasture disease, the antigen is:**
    A. Collagen IV of basement membrane
    B. DNA
    C. Bacterial products
    D. Cationic proteins

14. **Children having minimal change disease have selective proteinuria because of:**
    A. Reduction of negative charge on GBM
    B. Extensive damage to the GBM
    C. Deposits of IgG and C3 on GBM
    D. Increased mesangial matrix in the glomeruli

15. **Majority of cases of membranous glomerulonephritis have following etiology:**
    A. SLE   B. Viral infections
    C. History of drugs   D. Idiopathic

16. **Basement membrane material in membranous glomerulonephritis appears as:**
    A. Dense deposits
    B. Spikes protruding from GBM
    C. Double-contoured
    D. Tram-track

17. **Membranoproliferative glomerulonephritis is characterised by lobular proliferation of:**
    A. Epithelial cells   B. Endothelial cells
    C. Mesangial cells   D. Leucocytes

18. **HIV infection commonly produces the following type of glomerular lesions:**
    A. Membranous GN
    B. Membranoproliferative GN
    C. Focal GN
    D. Focal segmental glomerulosclerosis

19. **The most common and most severe form of lupus nephritis shows the following lesions:**
    A. Mesangial lupus nephritis
    B. Focal segmental lupus nephritis
    C. Diffuse proliferative lupus nephritis
    D. Membranous lupus nephritis

20. **In diabetic nephropathy, the following lesions are specific for juvenile-onset diabetes:**
    A. Diffuse glomerulosclerosis
    B. Nodular glomerulosclerosis

C. Diabetic pyelonephritis

D. Armanni-Ebstein lesions

21. In ischaemic ATN, the following holds true **except**:
   A. There is dilatation of proximal and distal convoluted tubules
   B. There is disruption of tubular basement membrane
   C. There is diffuse tubular necrosis
   D. Tubular lumina contain casts

22. **The most common mechanism in pathogenesis of chronic pyelonephritis is:**
   A. Ascending infection
   B. Reflux nephropathy
   C. Obstructive nephropathy
   D. Haematogenous infection

23. **Nephrocalcinosis is characterised by deposition of calcium salt at the following locations except:**
   A. Basement membrane   B. Within mitochondria
   C. Lysosomes   D. Cytoplasm

24. **The causes of renal hypertension include the following except:**
   A. Fibromuscular dysplasia of renal artery
   B. Polyarteritis nodosa
   C. Sickle cell nephropathy
   D. Polycystic kidney disease

25. **Causes of flea-bitten kidney include the following except:**
   A. Acute post-streptococcal GN
   B. Rapidly progressive GN
   C. Haemolytic uraemic syndrome
   D. Benign nephrosclerosis

26. **The following type of renal calculi are radiolucent:**
   A. Calcium oxalate   B. Struvite
   C. Uric acid   D. Calcium phosphate

27. **The following type of renal calculi are infection-induced:**
   A. Calcium oxalate   B. Struvite
   C. Uric acid   D. Cystine

28. **In hereditary renal cell carcinoma (RCC), the following syndrome is implicated in carcinogenesis:**
   A. von Hippel-Lindau disease   B. Polycystic kidney disease
   C. Alport's syndrome   D. Fabry's disease

29. **Out of various histologic types of renal cell carcinoma, the following type has worst prognosis:**
   A. Clear cell type   B. Granular cell type
   C. Sarcomatoid type   D. Papillary type

30. **Malakoplakia of the urinary bladder is a form of:**
   A. Dysplasia   B. Metaplasia
   C. Papillary hyperplasia D. Chronic inflammation

31. **Schistosomiasis of the urinary bladder is implicated in the following type of bladder tumour:**
   A. Transitional cell carcinoma
   B. Squamous cell carcinoma
   C. Adenocarcinoma
   D. Adenoacanthoma

32. **Collapsing sclerosis is a feature of following type of primary glomerular disease:**
   A. Membranoproliferative GN
   B. IgA nephropathy
   C. Focal segmental glomerulosclerosis
   D. Focal glomerulonephritis

33. **Genetic basis of minimal change disease consists of mutation in:**
   A. Podocin   B. Nephrin
   C. *Alpha*-3 collagen   D. Fibrillin

34. **Pseudo-crescent formation is seen in:**
   A. Membranous glomerulonephritis
   B. Membranoproliferative glomerulonephritis

C. Focal segmental glomerulosclerosis
D. IgA nephropathy

35. All are classes of lupus nephritis except:
    A. Membranoproliferative lupus nephritis
    B. Mesangial lupus nephritis
    C. Focal segmental lupus nephritis
    D. Minimal lesions

36. Prehypertension is defined as blood pressure between:
    A. 110-120/75-80 mmHg
    B. 120-139/80-89 mmHg
    C. 130-149/90-95 mmHg
    D. 140-159/95-99 mmHg

37. Which of the following is a congenital benign tumour of kidney?
    A. Angiomyolipoma   B. Reninoma
    C. Multicystic nephroma   D. Mesoblastic nephroma

38. Which of the following is the histologic hallmark for the diagnosis of rapidly progressive glomerulonephritis?
    A. Crescents within the glomeruli
    B. Fibrinoid necrosis of the efferent arterioles
    C. Fibrin thrombi in the glomerular tuft
    D. Granular deposits in the subendothelium

KEY

1 = C	2 = C	3 = A	4 = C	5 = A
6 = B	7 = A	8 = D	9 = D	10 = A
11 = A	12 = D	13 = A	14 = A	15 = D
16 = B	17 = C	18 = D	19 = C	20 = B
21 = C	22 = B	23 = C	24 = C	25 = D
26 = C	27 = B	28 = A	29 = C	30 = D
31 = B	32 = C	33 = B	34 = C	35 = A
36 = B	37 = D	38 = A		

21

The Male Reproductive System and Prostate

TESTIS AND EPIDIDYMIS *(p. 691)*

NORMAL STRUCTURE

Contents of the scrotal sac include the testicle and epididymis along with lower end of the spermatic cord and the tunica vaginalis that forms the outer serous investing layer. The epididymis is attached to body of the testis posteriorly.

M/E The seminiferous tubules are formed of a lamellar connective tissue membrane and contain several layers of cells. In the adult, the cells lining the seminiferous tubules are of 2 types:

1. *Spermatogonia* or germ cells which produce spermatocytes (primary and secondary), spermatids and mature spermatozoa.

2. *Sertoli cells* which are larger and act as supportive cells to germ cells, produce mainly androgen (testosterone) and little oestrogen.

The fibrovascular stroma present between the seminiferous tubules contains varying number of *interstitial cells of Leydig.* Leydig cells have abundant cytoplasm containing lipid granules and elongated Reinke's crystals. These cells are the main source of testosterone and other androgenic hormones in males.

DEVELOPMENTAL DISORDERS *(p. 691)*

CRYPTORCHIDISM

Cryptorchidism or undescended testis is a condition in which the testicle is arrested at some point along its descent. Its incidence is about 0.2% in adult male population. In 70% of cases, the undescended testis lies in the inguinal ring, in 25% in the abdomen and, in the remaining 5%, it may be present at other sites along its descent from intra-abdominal location to the scrotal sac.

ETIOLOGY The exact etiology is not known in majority of cases. Following factors are implicated:

1. **Mechanical factors** e.g. short spermatic cord, narrow inguinal canal, adhesions to the peritoneum.

2. **Genetic factors** e.g. trisomy 13, maldevelopment of the scrotum or cremaster muscles.

3. **Hormonal factors** e.g. deficient androgenic secretions.

G/A The cryptorchid testis is small in size, firm and fibrotic.

M/E The changes begin to appear by 2 years of age.
1. *Seminiferous tubules:* There is progressive loss of germ cell elements so that the tubules may be lined by only spermatogonia and spermatids but foci of spermatogenesis are discernible in 10% of cases. The tubular basement membrane is thickened. Advanced cases show hyalinised tubules with a few Sertoli cells only, surrounded by prominent basement membrane.
2. *Interstitial stroma:* There is usually increase in the interstitial fibrovascular stroma and conspicuous presence of Leydig cells, seen singly or in small clusters.

CLINICAL FEATURES As such, cryptorchidism is completely asymptomatic and is discovered only on physical examination. Following significant adverse clinical outcome may result:

1. Sterility-infertility
2. Inguinal hernia
3. *Malignancy* Cryptorchid testis is at 30-50 times increased risk of developing testicular malignancy.

MALE INFERTILITY

The morphologic pattern of testicular atrophy described above for cryptorchidism can result from various other congenital or acquired causes of male infertility. These causes can be divided into 3 groups: pre-testicular, testicular and post-testicular.

A. PRE-TESTICULAR CAUSES

1. Hypopituitarism
2. Oestrogen excess
3. Glucocorticoid excess
4. *Other endocrine disorders* Hypothyroidism and diabetes mellitus.

B. TESTICULAR CAUSES

1. Agonadism
2. Cryptorchidism
3. Maturation arrest
4. Hypospermatogenesis
5. Sertoli cell-only syndrome
6. Klinefelter's syndrome
7. Mumps orchitis
8. Irradiation damage

C. POST-TESTICULAR CAUSES

1. Congenital block
2. Acquired block
3. Impaired sperm motility

INFLAMMATIONS *(p. 692)*

Inflammation of the testis is termed as orchitis and of epididymis is called as epididymitis; the latter being more common. A combination epididymo-orchitis may also occur.

NON-SPECIFIC EPIDIDYMITIS AND ORCHITIS

Non-specific epididymitis and orchitis, or their combination, may be acute or chronic. The common routes of spread of infection are via the vas deferens, or via lymphatic and haematogenous routes. Most frequently, the infection is caused by urethritis, cystitis, prostatitis and seminal vesiculitis. Other causes are mumps, smallpox, dengue fever, influenza, pneumonia and filariasis.

G/A In acute stage the testicle is firm, tense, swollen and congested. There may be multiple abscesses, especially in gonorrhoeal infection. In chronic cases, there is usually variable degree of atrophy and fibrosis.

M/E Acute orchitis and epididymitis are characterised by congestion, oedema and diffuse infiltration by neutrophils, lymphocytes, plasma cells and macrophages or formation of neutrophilic abscesses. Acute inflammation may resolve, or may progress to chronic form. In chronic epididymo-orchitis, there is focal or diffuse chronic inflammation, disappearance of seminiferous tubules, fibrous scarring and destruction of interstitial Leydig cells.

GRANULOMATOUS (AUTOIMMUNE) ORCHITIS

Non-tuberculous granulomatous orchitis is a peculiar type of unilateral, painless testicular enlargement in middle-aged men that may resemble a testicular tumour clinically. The exact etiology and pathogenesis of the condition are not known though an autoimmune basis is suspected.

G/A   The affected testis is enlarged with thickened tunica. Cut section of the testicle is greyish-white to tan-brown.

M/E   There are circumscribed non-caseating granulomas lying within the seminiferous tubules. These granulomas are composed of epithelioid cells, lymphocytes, plasma cells, some neutrophils and multinucleate giant cells. The origin of the epithelioid cells is from Sertoli cells lining the tubules.

TUBERCULOUS EPIDIDYMO-ORCHITIS

Tuberculosis invariably begins in the epididymis and spreads to involve the testis. Tuberculous epididymo-orchitis is generally secondary tuberculosis from elsewhere in the body.

G/A   Discrete, yellowish, caseous necrotic areas are seen.

M/E   Numerous tubercles which may coalesce to form large caseous mass are seen. Characteristics of typical tubercles such as epithelioid cells, peripheral mantle of lymphocytes, occasional multinucleate giant cells and central areas of caseation necrosis are seen. Numerous acid-fast bacilli can be demonstrated by Ziehl-Neelsen staining.

SPERMATIC GRANULOMA

Spermatic granuloma is the term used for development of inflammatory lesions due to invasion of spermatozoa into the stroma. Spermatic granuloma may develop due to trauma, inflammation and loss of ligature following vasectomy.

G/A   The sperm granuloma is a small nodule, 3 mm to 3 cm in diameter, firm, white to yellowish-brown.

M/E   It consists of a granuloma composed of histiocytes, epithelioid cells, lymphocytes and some neutrophils. Characteristically, the centre of spermatic granuloma contains spermatozoa and necrotic debris.

ELEPHANTIASIS

Elephantiasis is enormous thickening of the scrotal skin resembling the elephant's hide and results in enlargement of the scrotum. The condition results from filariasis in which the adult worm lives in the lymphatics, while the larvae travel in the blood. The most important variety of filaria is *Wuchereria bancrofti*. The condition is common in all tropical countries. The vector is generally the Culex mosquito.

G/A   The affected leg and scrotum are enormously thickened with enlargement of regional lymph nodes.

M/E   The changes begin with lymphatic obstruction by the adult worms. The worm in alive, dead or calcified form may be found in the dilated lymphatics or in the lymph nodes. Dead or calcified worm in lymphatics is usually followed by lymphangitis with intense infiltration by eosinophils.

MISCELLANEOUS LESIONS (p. 694)

TORSION OF TESTIS

Torsion of the testicle may occur either in a fully-descended testis or in an undescended testis. The latter is more common and more severe. It results from sudden cessation of venous drainage and arterial supply to the testis, usually following sudden muscular effort or physical trauma.

M/E   There may be coagulative necrosis of the testis and epididymis, or there may be haemorrhagic infarction.

VARICOCELE

Varicocele is the dilatation, elongation and tortuosity of the veins of the pampiniform plexus in the spermatic cord. It is of 2 types: primary (idiopathic) and secondary.

◈ **Primary or idiopathic form** is more frequent and is more common in young unmarried men. It is nearly always on the left side as the loaded rectum presses the left vein.

◈ **Secondary form** occurs due to pressure on the spermatic vein by enlarged liver, spleen or kidney.

HYDROCELE

A hydrocele is abnormal collection of serous fluid in the tunica vaginalis. It may be acute or chronic, congenital or acquired. The usual causes are trauma, systemic oedema such as in cardiac failure and renal disease, and as a complication of gonorrhoea, syphilis and tuberculosis.

The hydrocele fluid is generally clear and straw-coloured but may be slightly turbid or haemorrhagic. The wall of the hydrocele sac is composed of fibrous tissue infiltrated with lymphocytes and plasma cells.

HAEMATOCELE

Haematocele is haemorrhage into the sac of the tunica vaginalis. It may result from direct trauma, from injury to a vein by the needle, or from haemorrhagic diseases.

In recent haematocele, the blood coagulates and the wall is coated with ragged deposits of fibrin. In long-standing cases, the tunica vaginalis is thickened with dense fibrous tissue coated with brownish material due to old organised haemorrhage and occasionally may get partly calcified.

TESTICULAR TUMOURS *(p. 694)*

They have *trimodal* age distribution—a peak during infancy, another during late adolescence and early adulthood, and a third peak after 60 years of age.

CLASSIFICATION

The most widely accepted classification is the histogenetic classification proposed by the World Health Organisation. Based on this, all testicular tumours are divided into 3 groups: *germ cell tumours, sex cord-stromal tumours* and *mixed forms*. Vast majority of the testicular tumours (95%) arise from germ cells or their precursors in the seminiferous tubules, while less than 5% originate from sex cord-stromal components of the testis.

I. GERM CELL TUMOURS
1. Seminoma
2. Spermatocytic seminoma
3. Embryonal carcinoma
4. Yolk sac tumour (*Syn.* endodermal sinus tumour, orchioblastoma, infantile type embryonal carcinoma)
5. Polyembryoma
6. Choriocarcinoma
7. Teratomas
     (i) Mature
     (ii) Immature
     (iii) With malignant transformation
8. Mixed germ cell tumours

II. SEX CORD-STROMAL TUMOURS
1. Leydig cell tumour
2. Sertoli cell tumour (Androblastoma)
3. Granulosa cell tumour
4. Mixed forms

III. COMBINED GERM CELL-SEX CORD-STROMAL TUMOURS
     Gonadoblastoma

IV. OTHER TUMOURS
1. Malignant lymphoma (5%)
2. Rare tumours

From clinical point of view, germ cell tumours of the testis are categorised into 2 main groups—seminomatous and non-seminomatous which need to be distinguished.

ETIOLOGIC FACTORS

1. Cryptorchidism The probability of a germ cell tumour developing in an undescended testis is 30-50 times greater than in a normally-descended testis. However, surgical correction is still helpful since it is easier to detect the tumour in scrotal testis than in an abdominal or inguinal testis.

2. Other developmental disorders Dysgenetic gonads associated with endocrine abnormalities such as androgen insensitivity syndrome have higher incidence of development of germ cell tumours.

3. Genetic factors Genetic factors play a role in the development of germ cell tumours supported by the observation of high incidence in first-degree family members, twins and in white male populations.

4. Other factors A few less common factors are as under:

i) Orchitis A history of mumps or other forms of orchitis may be given by the patient with germ cell tumour.

ii) Trauma Many patients give a history of trauma prior to the development of the tumour but it is not certain how trauma initiates the neoplastic process.

iii) Carcinogens e.g. use of certain drugs (e.g. LSD, hormonal therapy for sterility, copper, zinc etc), exposure to radiation and endocrine abnormalities.

HISTOGENESIS

1. Developmental disorders Disorders such as cryptorchidism, gonadal dysgenesis and androgen insensitivity syndrome are high risk factors for development of testicular germ cell tumours.

2. Molecular genetic features Testicular germ cell tumours have been found to have several genetic abnormalities suggesting a common mole-cular pathogenesis of all germ cell tumours e.g.

i) Hyperdiploidy

ii) Isochromosome of short arm of chromosome 12.

iii) Deletion of long arm of chromosome 12 abbreviated.

iv) Telomerase activity.

v) Other mutations *p53, cyclin E* and *FAS* gene.

3. CIS/ITGCN A preinvasive stage of carcinoma *in situ* (CIS) termed *intratubular germ cell neoplasia (ITGCN)* generally precedes the development of most of the invasive testicular germ cell tumours in adults. CIS originates from spermatogenic elements.

4. 'Three hit' process Germ cells in seminiferous tubules undergo activation *('first hit')* before undergoing malignant transformation confined to seminiferous tubules (CIS) *('second hit')* and eventually into invasive stage by some epigenetic phenomena *('third hit')*.

CLINICAL FEATURES AND DIAGNOSIS

The usual presenting clinical symptoms of testicular tumours are gradual gonadal enlargement and a dragging sensation in the testis.

SPREAD Testicular tumours may spread by both lymphatic and haematogenous routes:

1. Lymphatic spread occurs to retroperitoneal para-aortic lymph nodes, mediastinal lymph nodes and supraclavicular lymph nodes.

2. Haematogenous spread primarily occurs to the lungs, liver, brain and bones.

TUMOUR MARKERS Two tumour markers widely used in the diagnosis, staging and monitoring the follow-up of patients with testicular tumours are: human chorionic gonadotropin (hCG) and alpha-foetoprotein (AFP). In addition, carcinoembryonic antigen (CEA), human placental lactogen (HPL), placental alkaline phosphatase, testosterone, oestrogen and luteinising hormone may also be elevated.

Stage I: tumour confined to the testis.

Stage II: distant spread confined to retroperitoneal lymph nodes below the diaphragm.

Stage III: distant metastases beyond the retroperitoneal lymph nodes.

Seminomas tend to remain localised to the testis (stage I) while non-seminomatous germ cell tumours more often present with advanced clinical disease (stage II and III). In general, seminomas have a better prognosis with 90% cure rate while the non-seminomatous tumours behave in a more aggressive manner and have poor prognosis.

GERM CELL TUMOURS

Testicular germ cell tumours are almost always malignant. Nearly half of them contain more than one histologic type. Besides their counterparts in the female gonads, germ cell tumours are also found at the extragonadal sites such as the retroperitoneum, mediastinum, base of the brain, coccyx etc.

INTRATUBULAR GERM CELL NEOPLASIA

The term intratubular germ cell neoplasia (ITGCN) is used to describe the preinvasive stage of germ cell tumours, notably intratubular seminoma and intratubular embryonal carcinoma. Others have used carcinoma *in situ* (CIS) stage of germ cell tumours as synonymous term.

CLASSIC SEMINOMA

Seminoma is the commonest malignant tumour of the testis and corresponds to dysgerminoma in the female. It constitutes about 45% of all germ cell tumours, and in another 15% comprises the major component of mixed germ cell tumour. Seminoma is divided into 2 main categories: classic and spermatocytic. Classic seminoma comprises about 95% of all seminomas and has a peak incidence in the 4th decade of life and is rare before puberty. Undescended testis harbours seminoma more frequently as compared to other germ cell tumours.

G/A The involved testis is enlarged up to 10 times its normal size but tends to maintain its normal contour since the tumour rarely invades the tunica. Cut section of the affected testis shows homogeneous, grey-white lobulated appearance.

M/E The tumour has following features:

1. Tumour cells The seminoma cells generally lie in cords, sheets or columns forming lobules. Typically, in a classic seminoma, the tumour cells are fairly uniform in size with clear cytoplasm and well-defined cell borders. The cytoplasm contains variable amount of glycogen that stains positively with PAS reaction. The nuclei are centrally located, large, hyperchromatic and usually contain 1-2 prominent nucleoli. Tumour giant cells may be present. About 10% of seminomas have increased mitotic activity and have aggressive behaviour and are categorised as *anaplastic seminomas.*

2. Stroma The stroma of seminoma is delicate fibrous tissue which divides the tumour into lobules. The stroma shows a characteristic lymphocytic infil-tration, indicative of immunologic response of the host to the tumour. About 20% of the tumours show granulomatous reaction in the stroma.

The *prognosis* of classic seminoma is better than other germ cell tumours. The tumour is highly radiosensitive.

SPERMATOCYTIC SEMINOMA

Spermatocytic seminoma is both clinically and morphologically a distinctive tumour from classic seminoma. It is an uncommon tumour having an inci-dence of about 5% of all germ cell tumours. Spermatocytic seminoma usually occurs in older patients, generally in 6th decade of life.

G/A Spermatocytic seminoma is homogeneous, larger, softer and more yellowish and gelatinous than the classic seminoma.

M/E The distinctive features are as under:

1. Tumour cells The tumour cells vary considerably in size from lymphocyte-like to huge mononucleate or multinucleate giant cells. The cells have eosinophilic cytoplasm devoid of glycogen. The nuclei of intermediate and large cells have filamentous pattern. Mitoses are often frequent.

2. Stroma The stroma lacks lymphocytic and granulomatous reaction seen in classic seminoma.

The *prognosis* of spermatocytic seminoma is excellent and better than classic seminoma since the tumour is slow-growing and rarely metastasises. The tumour is radiosensitive.

EMBRYONAL CARCINOMA

Pure embryonal carcinoma constitutes 30% of germ cell tumours but areas of embryonal carcinoma are present in 40% of various other germ cell tumours. These tumours are more common in 2nd to 3rd decades of life. They are more aggressive than the seminomas.

G/A Embryonal carcinoma is usually a small tumour in the testis. Cut surface of the tumour is grey-white, soft with areas of haemorrhages and necrosis.

M/E Following features are seen:
1.   The tumour cells are arranged in a variety of *patterns*—glandular, tubular, papillary and solid.
2.   The *tumour cells* are highly anaplastic carcinomatous cells having large size, indistinct cell borders, amphophilic cytoplasm and prominent hyperchromatic nuclei showing considerable variation in nuclear size. Mitotic figures and tumour giant cells are frequently present.
3.   The *stroma* may contain variable amount of primitive mesenchyme.

YOLK SAC TUMOUR (SYNONYMS: ENDODERMAL SINUS TUMOUR, ORCHIOBLASTOMA, INFANTILE EMBRYONAL CARCINOMA)

This characteristic tumour is the most common testicular tumour of infants and young children up to the age of 4 years. In adults, however, yolk sac tumour in pure form is rare but may be present as the major component in 40% of germ cell tumours. AFP levels are elevated in 100% cases of yolk sac tumours.

G/A The tumour is generally soft, yellow-white, mucoid with areas of necrosis and haemorrhages.

M/E It has following features:
1.   The tumour cells form a variety of *patterns*—loose reticular network, papillary, tubular and solid arrangement.
2.   The *tumour cells* are flattened to cuboid epithelial cells with clear vacuolated cytoplasm.
3.   The tumour cells may form distinctive perivascular structures resembling the yolk sac or endodermal sinuses of the rat placenta called *Schiller-Duval bodies.*
4.   There may be presence of both intracellular and extracellular PAS-positive *hyaline globules,* many of which contain AFP.

POLYEMBRYOMA

Polyembryoma is defined as a tumour composed predominantly of embryoid bodies. Embryoid bodies are structures containing a disc and cavities surrounded by loose mesenchyme simulating an embryo of about 2 weeks' gestation.

CHORIOCARCINOMA

Pure choriocarcinoma is a highly malignant tumour composed of elements consisting of syncytiotrophoblast and cytotrophoblast.

The patients are generally in their 2nd decade of life. The primary tumour is usually small and the patient may manifest initially with symptoms of metastasis. The serum and urinary levels of hCG are greatly elevated in 100% cases.

G/A The tumour is usually small and may appear as a soft, haemorrhagic and necrotic mass.

M/E Following characteristic features are seen:

i) *Syncytiotrophoblastic cells* are large with many irregular and bizarre nuclei and abundant eosinophilic vacuolated cytoplasm which stains positively for hCG. These cells often surround masses of cytotrophoblastic cells.

ii) *Cytotrophoblastic cells* are polyhedral cells which are more regular and have clear or eosinophilic cytoplasm with hyperchromatic nuclei.

TERATOMA

Teratomas are complex tumours composed of tissues derived from more than one of the three germ cell layers—endoderm, mesoderm and ectoderm. Testicular teratomas are more common in infants and children and constitute about 40% of testicular tumours in infants, whereas in adults they comprise 5% of all germ cell tumours. However, teratomas are found in combination with other germ cell tumours.

MORPHOLOGIC FEATURES Testicular teratomas are classified into 3 types:
1. Mature (differentiated) teratoma
2. Immature teratoma
3. Teratoma with malignant transformation.

G/A Most teratomas are large, grey-white masses enlarging the involved testis. Cut surface shows characteristic variegated appearance—grey-white solid areas, cystic and honey-combed areas, and foci of cartilage and bone. Dermoid tumours commonly seen in the ovaries are rare in testicular teratomas.

M/E Three categories of teratomas show different features:

1. Mature (differentiated) teratoma Mature teratoma is composed of disorderly mixture of a variety of well-differentiated structures such as cartilage, smooth muscle, intestinal and respiratory epithelium, mucus glands, cysts lined by squamous and transitional epithelium, neural tissue, fat and bone. It is believed that *all testicular teratomas in the adults are malignant.*

As mentioned earlier, dermoid cysts similar to those of the ovary are rare in the testis.

2. Immature teratoma Immature teratoma is composed of incompletely differentiated and primitive or embryonic tissues along with some mature elements. Primitive or embryonic tissue commonly present are poorly-formed cartilage, mesenchyme, neural tissues, abortive eye, intestinal and respiratory tissue elements etc. Mitoses are usually frequent.

3. Teratoma with malignant transformation This is an extremely rare form of teratoma in which one or more of the tissue elements show malignant transformation.

MIXED GERM CELL TUMOURS

About 60% of germ cell tumours have more than one of the above histologic types (except spermatocytic seminoma) and are called mixed germ cell tumours. The clinical behaviour of these tumours is worsened by inclusion of more aggressive tumour component in a less malignant tumour.

The most common combinations of mixed germ cell tumours are as under:
1. Teratoma, embryonal carcinoma, yolk sac tumour and syncytiotro-phoblast.
2. Embryonal carcinoma and teratoma (teratocarcinoma).
3. Seminoma and embryonal carcinoma.

Tumours arising from specialised gonadal stroma are classified on the basis of histogenesis. The biologic behaviour of these tumours generally cannot be determined on histological grounds alone but is related to clinical parameters and hormonal elaboration by these tumours.

LEYDIG (INTERSTITIAL) CELL TUMOUR

Leydig cell tumours are quite uncommon. They may occur at any age but are more frequent in the age group of 20 to 50 years. Characteristically, these cells secrete androgen, or both androgen and oestrogen, and rarely corticosteroids. Bilateral tumours may occur typically in congenital adrenogenital syndrome.

G/A The tumour appears as a small, well-demarcated and lobulated nodule. Cut surface is homogeneously yellowish or brown.

M/E The tumour is composed of sheets and cords of normal-looking Leydig cells. These cells contain abundant eosinophilic cytoplasm and Reinke's crystals and a small central nucleus.

SERTOLI CELL TUMOURS (ANDROBLASTOMA)

Sertoli cell tumours correspond to arrhenoblastoma of the ovary. They may occur at all ages but are more frequent in infants and children.

GRANULOSA CELL TUMOUR

This is an extremely rare tumour in the testis and resembles morphologically with its ovarian counterpart.

MIXED GERM CELL-SEX CORD STROMAL TUMOURS

GONADOBLASTOMA

Dysgenetic gonads and undescended testis are predisposed to develop such combined proliferations of germ cells and sex cord-stromal elements. The patients are commonly intersexuals, particularly phenotypic females.

OTHER TUMOURS

MALIGNANT LYMPHOMA

Malignant lymphomas comprises 5% of testicular malignancies and is the most common testicular tumour in the elderly. Bilaterality is seen in half the cases. Most common are large cell non-Hodgkin's lymphoma of B cell type.

PENIS *(p. 702)*

NORMAL STRUCTURE

The structure of penis consists of 3 masses of erectile tissue—two corpora cavernosa, one on each side dorsally, and the corpus spongiosum ventrally through which the urethra passes. The expanded free end of the corpus spongiosum forms the glans.

The lumen of the urethra in sectioned surface of the penis appears as an irregular cleft in the middle of the corpus spongiosum. In the prostatic part, it is lined by transitional epithelium, but elsewhere it is lined by columnar epithelium except near its orifice where stratified squamous epithelium lines it.

DEVELOPMENTAL AND INFLAMMATORY DISORDERS *(p. 702)*

PHIMOSIS

Phimosis is a condition in which the prepuce is too small to permit its normal retraction behind the glans. It may be congenital or acquired. *Congenital phimosis* is a developmental anomaly whereas *acquired phimosis* may result from inflammation, trauma or oedema leading to narrowing of preputial opening.

Paraphimosis is a condition in which the phimotic prepuce is forcibly retracted resulting in constriction over the glans penis and subsequent swelling.

HYPOSPADIAS AND EPISPADIAS

Hypospadias is a developmental defect of the urethra in which the urethral meatus fails to reach the end of the penis, but instead, opens on the ventral surface of the penis. Similar developmental defect with resultant urethral opening on the dorsal surface of the penis is termed *epispadias*.

BALANOPOSTHITIS

Balanoposthitis is the term used for non-specific inflammation of the inner surface of the prepuce *(balanitis)* and adjacent surface of the glans *(posthitis)*. It is caused by a variety of microorganisms such as staphylo-cocci, streptococci, coliform bacilli and gonococci.

BALANITIS XEROTICA OBLITERANS

Balanitis xerotica obliterans is a white atrophic lesion on the glans penis and the prepuce and is a counterpart of the *lichen sclerosus et atrophicus* in the vulva.

TUMOURS *(p. 702)*

BENIGN TUMOURS

CONDYLOMA ACUMINATUM

Condyloma acuminatum or anogenital wart is a benign tumour caused by human papilloma virus (HPV) types 6 and 11. The tumour may occur singly, or there may be conglomerated papillomas. A more extensive, soli-tary, exophytic and cauliflower-like warty mass is termed *giant condyloma or Buschke-Löwenstein tumour or verrucous carcinoma*.

G/A The tumour consists of solitary or multiple, warty, cauliflower-shaped lesions of variable size with exophytic growth pattern.

M/E The lesions are essentially like common warts (verruca vulgaris). The features include formation of papillary villi composed of connective tissue stroma and covered by squamous epithelium which shows hyperkeratosis, parakeratosis, and hyperplasia of prickle cell layer. Many of the prickle cells show clear vacuolisation of the cytoplasm *(koilocytosis)* indicative of HPV infection.

Giant condyloma shows upward as well as downward growth of the tumour but is otherwise histologically identical to condyloma acuminatum.

PREMALIGNANT LESIONS (CARCINOMA *IN SITU*)

BOWEN'S DISEASE

Bowen's disease is located on the shaft of the penis and the scrotum besides the sun-exposed areas of the skin.

M/E The changes are superficial to the dermo-epidermal border. The epithelial cells of the epidermis show hyperplasia, hyperkeratosis, para-keratosis and scattered bizarre dyskeratotic cells.

ERYTHROPLASIA OF QUEYRAT

The lesions of erythroplasia of Queyrat appear on the penile mucosa.

M/E The thickened and acanthotic epidermis shows variable degree of dysplasia.

The lesions of bowenoid papulosis appear on the penile shaft and adjacent genital skin.

M/E There is orderly maturation of epithelial cells in hyperplastic epidermis with scattered hyperchromatic nuclei and dysplastic cells.

MALIGNANT TUMOURS

SQUAMOUS CELL CARCINOMA

The incidence of penile carcinoma shows wide variation in different populations. In the United States, the overall incidence of penile cancer is less than 1% of all cancers in males but it is 3-4 times more common in blacks than in whites. Relationship of penile cancer with HPV has been well supported; high-risk HPV types 16 and 18 are strongly implicated and their DNA has been documented in the nuclei of malignant cells. In India, cancer of the penis is rare in Muslims who practice circumcision as a religious rite in infancy, whereas Hindus who are normally not circumcised have a higher incidence.

G/A The tumour is located, in decreasing frequency, on frenum, prepuce, glans and coronal sulcus. The tumour may be cauliflower-like and papillary, or flat and ulcerating.

M/E Squamous cell carcinoma of both fungating and ulcerating type is generally well differentiated to moderately-differentiated type which resembles in morphology to similar cancer elsewhere in the body.

PROSTATE (p. 703)

NORMAL STRUCTURE

The prostate gland in the normal adult weighs approximately 20 gm. It surrounds the commencement of the male urethra. At birth, the five lobes fuse to form 3 distinct lobes—two major lateral lobes and a small median lobe.

M/E The prostate is composed of tubular alveoli (acini) embedded in fibromuscular tissue mass. The glandular epithelium forms infoldings and consists of 2 layers—a basal layer of low cuboidal cells and an inner layer of mucus-secreting tall columnar cells. The alveoli are separated by thick fibromuscular septa containing abundant smooth muscle fibres.

Based on hormonal responsiveness, the prostate is divided into 2 separate parts:

1. *Inner periurethral female part* which is sensitive to oestrogen and androgen.
2. *Outer subcapsular true male part* which is sensitive to androgen.

PROSTATITIS (p. 704)

ACUTE PROSTATITIS

Acute focal or diffuse suppurative inflammation of the prostate is not uncommon. It occurs most commonly due to ascent of bacteria from the urethra, less often by descent from the upper urinary tract or bladder. The infection may occur spontaneously or may be a complication of urethral manipulation such as by catheterisation, cystoscopy, urethral dilatation and surgical procedures on the prostate.

G/A The prostate is enlarged, swollen and tense. Cut section shows multiple abscesses and foci of necrosis.

M/E The prostatic acini are dilated and filled with neutrophilic exudate. There may be diffuse acute inflammatory infiltrate.

Chronic prostatitis is more common and foci of chronic inflammation are frequently present in the prostate of men above 40 years of age.

Chronic prostatitis is of 2 types:

◈ **Chronic bacterial prostatitis** is caused in much the same way and by the same organisms as the acute prostatitis. It is generally a consequence of recurrent UTI.

◈ **Chronic abacterial prostatitis** is more common. There is no history of recurrent UTI and culture of urine and prostatic secretions is always negative, though leucocytosis is demonstrable in prostatic secretions.

G/A The prostate may be enlarged, fibrosed and shrunken.

M/E The diagnosis of chronic prostatitis is made by foci of lymphocytes, plasma cells, macrophages and neutrophils within the prostatic substance. Corpora amylacea, prostatic calculi and foci of squamous metaplasia in the prostatic acini may accompany inflammatory changes.

GRANULOMATOUS PROSTATITIS

Granulomatous prostatitis is a variety of chronic prostatitis, probably caused by leakage of prostatic secretions into the tissue, or could be of autoimmune origin.

NODULAR HYPERPLASIA *(p. 705)*

Non-neoplastic tumour-like enlargement of the prostate, commonly termed benign nodular hyperplasia (BNH) or benign enlargement of prostate (BEP), is a very common condition in men and considered by some as normal ageing process. It becomes increasingly more frequent above the age of 50 years and its incidence approaches 75-80% in men above 80 years.

ETIOLOGY A few etiologic factors such as *endocrinologic, racial, inflammation* and *arteriosclerosis* have been implicated but endocrine basis for hyperplasia has been more fully investigated. With advancing age, there is decline in the level of androgen and a corresponding rise of oestrogen in the males. The periurethral inner prostate which is primarily involved in BEP is responsive to the rising level of oestrogen, whereas the outer prostate which is mainly involved in the carcinoma is responsive to androgen.

G/A The enlarged prostate is nodular, smooth and firm and weighs 2-4 times its normal weight i.e. may weigh up to 40-80 gm. The appearance on cut section varies depending upon whether the hyperplasia is predominantly of the glandular or fibromuscular tissue.

M/E There is hyperplasia of all three tissue elements in varying proportions—glandular, fibrous and muscular:
◈ *Glandular hyperplasia* predominates in most cases and is identified by exaggerated intra-acinar papillary infoldings with delicate fibrovascular cores.
◈ *Fibromuscular hyperplasia* when present as dominant component appears as aggregates of spindle cells forming an appearance akin to fibromyoma of the uterus.

CLINICAL FEATURES Clinically, the symptomatic cases develop symptoms due to complications such as urethral obstruction and secondary effects on the bladder (e.g. hypertrophy, cystitis), ureter (e.g. hydroureter) and kidneys (e.g. hydronephrosis). The presenting features include frequency, nocturia, difficulty in micturition, pain, haematuria and sometimes, the patients present with acute retention of urine requiring immediate catheterisation.

CARCINOMA OF PROSTATE *(p. 706)*

Cancer of the prostate is the second most common form of cancer in males, followed in frequency by lung cancer. It is a disease of men above the age of

50 years and its prevalence increases with increasing age. It is common to classify carcinoma of the prostate into the following 4 types:

1. Latent carcinoma This is found unexpectedly as a small focus of carcinoma in the prostate during autopsy studies in men dying of other causes.

2. Incidental carcinoma About 15-20% of prostatectomies done for BEP reveal incidental carcinoma of the prostate.

3. Occult carcinoma This is the type in which the patient has no symptoms of prostatic carcinoma but shows evidence of metastases on clinical examination and investigations.

4. Clinical carcinoma Clinical prostatic carcinoma is the type detected by rectal examination and other investigations and confirmed by pathologic examination of biopsy of the prostate.

ETIOLOGY The cause of prostatic cancer remains obscure. However, a few factors have been suspected.

1. Endocrinologic factors Androgens are considered essential for development and maintenance of prostatic epithelium.
i) Orchiectomy causes arrest of metastatic prostatic cancer disease (testis being the main source of testosterone).
ii) Administration of oestrogen causes regression of prostatic carcinoma.
iii) Cancer of the prostate is extremely rare in eunuchs and in patients with Klinefelter's syndrome.
iv) Cancer of the prostate begins at the stage of life when androgen levels are high.

2. Racial and geographic influences There are some racial and geographic differences in the incidence of prostatic cancer. African Americans have a markedly higher incidence as compared to whites.

3. Environmental influences These include high dietary fat, and exposure to polycyclic aromatic hydrocarbons. Flavonoids, antioxidants and selenium may reduce the risk.

4. Nodular hyperplasia Approximately 15-20% of nodular hyperplastic prostates harbour carcinoma.

5. Heredity Men with prostatic cancer susceptibility gene, BRCA2, have 20-times increased risk of prostatic cancer.

HISTOGENESIS Histogenesis of prostatic adenocarcinoma has been documented as a multistep process arising from premalignant stage of *prostatic intraepithelial neoplasia (PIN)*. PIN refers to multiple foci of cytologically atypical luminal cells overlying diminished number of basal cells in prostatic ducts and is a forerunner of invasive prostatic carcinoma.

G/A The prostate may be enlarged, normal in size or smaller than normal. In 95% of cases, prostatic carcinoma is located in the peripheral zone, especially in the posterior lobe. The malignant prostate is firm and fibrous.

M/E 4 histologic types are described—adenocarcinoma, transitional cell carcinoma, squamous cell carcinoma and undifferentiated carcinoma. However, *adenocarcinoma* is the most common type found in 96% of cases.

The histologic characteristics of adenocarcinoma of the prostate are as under:

1 Architectural disturbance In contrast to convoluted appearance of the glands seen in normal and hyperplastic prostate, there is loss of intra-acinar papillary convolutions. The groups of acini are either closely packed in back-to-back arrangement without intervening stroma or are haphazardly distributed.

2. Stroma Normally, fibromuscular sling surrounds the acini, whereas malignant acini have little or no stroma between them.

3. Gland pattern Most frequently, the glands in well-differentiated prostatic adenocarcinoma are small or medium-sized, lined by a single layer of cuboidal or low columnar cells. Moderately-differentiated tumours have cribriform or fenestrated glandular appearance.

4. Tumour cells The outer basal layer seen in the normal or benign acini is lost. The tumour cells may be clear, dark and eosinophilic cells. The cells may show varying degree of anaplasia and nuclear atypia but is generally slight.

5. Invasion One of the important diagnostic features of malignancy in prostate is the early and frequent occurrence of invasion of intra-prostatic *perineural spaces.*

SPREAD The tumour spreads within the gland by direct extension, and to distant sites by blood and lymphatic route.

Direct spread Direct extension of the tumour occurs into the prostatic capsule and beyond. In late stage, the tumour may extend into the bladder neck, seminal vesicles, trigone and ureteral openings.

Metastases Distant spread occurs by both lymphatic and haematogenous routes. Haematogenous spread leads most often to characteristic osteoblastic *osseous metastases,* especially to pelvis, and lumbar spine; other sites of metastases are lungs, kidneys, breast and brain.

CLINICAL FEATURES AND DIAGNOSIS In symptomatic cases, clinical features are: urinary obstruction with dysuria, frequency, retention of urine, haematuria, and in 10% of cases pain in the back due to skeletal metastases. By the time symptoms appear, the carcinoma of prostate is usually palpable on digital rectal examination (DRE) as a hard and nodular gland fixed to the surrounding tissues.

Two biochemical serum *tumour markers* employed for diagnosis and monitoring the prognosis of prostatic carcinoma are as under:

1. Prostatic acid phosphatase (PAP) is secreted by prostatic epithelium. Elevation of serum level of PAP is found in cases of prostatic cancer which have extended beyond the capsule or have metastasised.

2. Prostate-specific antigen (PSA) can be detected by immunohistochemical method in the malignant prostatic epithelium as well as estimated in the serum. A reading between 4 and 10 ng/ml (normal 0-4 ng/ml) is highly suspicious (10% risk) but value above 10 is diagnostic of prostatic carcinoma. PSA assay is also helpful in distinguishing high-grade prostatic cancer from urothelial carcinoma, colonic carcinoma, lymphoma and prostatitis.

The diagnosis of prostatic carcinoma can be made by clinical, biochemical, radiologic, ultrasonographic, cytologic (FNA) and histopathologic methods (core biopsy, TUR specimen, or radical prostatectomy). However, for a definite diagnosis, triple approach is most commonly followed: i) DRE, ii) serum PSA determination, and iii) transrectal ultrasound (TRUS)-guided core needle biopsy.

HISTOLOGIC GRADING AND CLINICAL STAGING Clinical staging has good correlation with histologic grading and, thus, has a prognostic significance.

Gleason's histologic grading Mostofi's (WHO) histologic grading categorising prostate cancer into grade I (well-differentiated), grade II (moderately-differentiated) and grade III (poorly-differentiated) has largely been replaced with Gleason's microscopic *grading system* which is based on two features:
i) Degree of glandular differentiation and distribution.
ii) Growth pattern of the tumour in relation to the stroma.

TNM staging For clinical staging of prostate cancer, TNM system is considered international standard. This system of staging for prostate cancer takes into account cases with abnormal PSA and findings of DRE.

Treatment of prostatic carcinoma consists of surgery, radiotherapy and hormonal therapy. The hormonal dependence of prostate cancer consists of depriving the tumour cells of growth-promoting influence of testosterone. This can be achieved by bilateral orchiectomy followed by administration of oestrogen.

Systemic Pathology

1. In an undescended testis the risk of developing a testicular malignancy is increased to average of:
   A. 20 fold
   B. 25 fold
   C. 30 fold
   D. 35 fold
2. In an undescended testis, the following tumour develops most often:
   A. Seminoma
   B. Teratoma
   C. Choriocarcinoma
   D. Yolk sac tumour
3. Granulomatous orchitis is the term used for inflammation of testis due to following etiology:
   A. Tuberculosis
   B. Sarcoidosis
   C. Autoimmune
   D. Leprosy
4. The origin of epithelioid cells in autoimmune orchitis is from:
   A. Macrophages
   B. Sertoli cells
   C. Leydig cells
   D. Spermatogenic cells
5. Seminoma is a:
   A. Benign tumour
   B. Borderline tumour
   C. Malignant tumour
   D. Locally aggressive tumour
6. Sequential tumorigenesis in seminomatous tumours involves:
   A. Single hit
   B. Double hit
   C. Triple hit
   D. Multiple hits
7. Spermatocytic seminoma differs from classic seminoma in the following respects except:
   A. It occurs in older age (past 6th decade)
   B. Tumour cells are pleomorphic
   C. The stroma lacks lymphocytic infiltrate
   D. The tumour has worse prognosis
8. AFP levels are elevated in 100% cases of following type of germ cell tumour:
   A. Seminoma
   B. Embryonal carcinoma
   C. Yolk sac tumour
   D. Choriocarcinoma
9. All types of testicular teratomas in adults are:
   A. Benign tumours
   B. Borderline tumours
   C. Locally aggressive tumours
   D. Malignant tumours
10. The most common testicular tumour in the elderly is:
    A. Seminoma
    B. Teratoma
    C. Malignant lymphoma
    D. Leydig cell tumour
11. The following penile lesions are considered as in situ carcinoma except:
    A. Condyloma acuminatum
    B. Bowen's disease
    C. Erythroplasia of Queyrat
    D. Bowenoid papulosis
12. Prostatic hyperplasia affects most often:
    A. Peripheral prostate
    B. Periurethral prostate
    C. Capsule of prostate
    D. Entire prostate
13. Normally prostatic tissue responds to hormones as under:
    A. Periurethral prostate responds to oestrogen as well as androgen
    B. Outer prostate responds to androgen as well as oestrogen
    C. Periurethral prostate responds to rising level of oestrogen
    D. Outer prostate responds to rising level of oestrogen
14. Prostatic acid phosphatase (PAP) levels given below are diagnostic of prostatic carcinoma:
    A. 1-2 KA units
    B. 2-3 KA units
    C. 3-5 KA units
    D. 5-7 KA units
15. Metastasis to the following tissues occur early in prostatic carcinoma:
    A. Vertebrae
    B. Obturator lymph node
    C. Lungs
    D. Brain

16. Areas of intratubular germ cell neoplasia (ITGCN) are frequently found in seminiferous tubules adjacent to the following tumours **except**:
    - A. Seminoma
    - B. Spermatocytic seminoma
    - C. Embryonal carcinoma
    - D. Immature teratoma

17. Which of the following testicular tumour is most radiosensitive?
    - A. Seminoma
    - B. Embryonal carcinoma
    - C. Yolk sac tumour
    - D. Immature teratoma

18. Classic perivascular structures seen in yolk sac tumours are known as:
    - A. Schiller -Duval bodies
    - B. Call–Exner bodies
    - C. Michaelis-Guttmann bodies
    - D. Russel bodies

19. Latent prostatic carcinoma is:
    - A. Incidental carcinoma prostate found in prostatectomies done for BEH
    - B. Small focus of prostate carcinoma found during autopsy
    - C. Asymptomatic carcinoma of prostate presenting with metastasis on investigation
    - D. Prostatic carcinoma in-situ

20. Granulomatous prostatitis occurs due to:
    - A. Tuberculosis
    - B. Sarcoidosis
    - C. Autoimmune
    - D. Syphilis

KEY

1 = D	2 = A	3 = C	4 = B	5 = C
6 = C	7 = D	8 = C	9 = D	10 = C
11 = A	12 = B	13 = A	14 = D	15 = B
16 = B	17 = A	18 = A	19 = B	20 = C

22   The Female Genital Tract

VULVA *(p. 710)*

NORMAL STRUCTURE

The vulva consists of structures of ectodermal origin—labia majora, labia minora, mons pubis, clitoris, vestibule, hymen, Bartholin's glands and minor vestibular glands. The inner surface of labia majora, labia minora and vestibule are covered by stratified squamous epithelium. The clitoris is made up of vascular erectile tissue. Bartholin's or vulvovaginal glands are located one on each side of the mass of tissue forming labia majora.

MISCELLANEOUS CONDITIONS *(p. 710)*

BARTHOLIN'S CYST AND ABSCESS

Inflammation of Bartholin's vulvovaginal glands (Bartholin's adenitis) may occur due to bacterial infection, notably gonorrhoeal infection. Infection may be *acute* or *chronic*.

◆   **Acute Bartholin's adenitis** occurs from obstruction and dilatation of the duct by infection resulting in formation of a Bartholin's abscess.

M/E   Shows the usual appearance of acute suppurative inflammation with neutrophilic infiltration, hyperaemia, oedema and epithelial degeneration.

◆   **Chronic Bartholin's adenitis** results from a less virulent infection so that the process is slow and prolonged. Alternatively, the chronic process evolves from repeated attacks of less severe acute inflammation which may be short of abscess formation and resolves incompletely. In either case, the chronic inflammatory process terminates into fluid-filled Bartholin's cyst.

M/E   Shows variable lining of the cyst varying from the transitional epithelium of the normal duct to a flattened lining because of increased intracystic pressure. The cyst wall may show chronic inflammatory infiltrate and a few mucus-secreting acini.

NON-NEOPLASTIC EPITHELIAL DISORDERS

The older nomenclature vulvar dystrophy has been replaced by more descriptive and clinically relevant term, non-neoplastic epithelial disorders of vulval skin and mucosa of the vulva. The term is applied to chronic lesions of the vulva characterised clinically by white, plaque-like, pruritic mucosal thickenings and pathologically by disorders of epithelial growth. Clinicians often use the term *'leukoplakia'* for such white lesions.

Currently, non-neoplastic epithelial disorders of the skin of vulva includes following 2 lesions:

LICHEN SCLEROSUS

Lichen sclerosus may occur anywhere in the skin but is more common and more extensive in the vulva in post-menopausal women. The lesions may extend from vulva onto the perianal and perineal area. Clinically, the patient, usually a post-menopausal woman, complains of intense pruritus which may produce excoriation of the affected skin. Eventually, there is progressive shrinkage and atrophy resulting in narrowing of the introitus, clinically referred to as *kraurosis vulvae*.

M/E The features are:
1. Hyperkeratosis of the surface layer.
2. Thinning of the epidermis with disappearance of rete ridges.
3. Amorphous homogeneous degenerative change in the dermal collagen.
4. Chronic inflammatory infiltrate in the mid-dermis.
    Lichen sclerosus is *not* a premalignant lesion and responds favourably to topical treatment with androgens.

SQUAMOUS HYPERPLASIA

Squamous hyperplasia, or simply called keratosis, is characterised by white, thickened vulvar lesions which are usually itchy.

M/E The features are:
1. Hyperkeratosis.
2. Hyperplasia of squamous epithelium with elongation of rete ridges.
3. Increased mitotic activity of squamous layers but cytologically no atypia.
4. Chronic inflammatory infiltrate in the underlying dermis.
    Squamous hyperplasia is not a precancerous condition. However, a variant having marked acanthosis, parakeratosis and a verruciform architecture called *vulval acanthosis with altered differentiation (VAAD)*, does not have HPV association, but may be forerunner for HPV-negative vulvar cancer.

VULVAL TUMOURS *(p. 711)*

STROMAL POLYPS

Stromal (fibroepithelial) polyps or acrochordons may form in the vulva or vagina. There may be single or multiple polypoid masses.

M/E They are covered by an orderly stratified squamous epithelium. The stroma consists of loose fibrous and myxomatous connective tissue with some adipose tissue and blood vessels.

PAPILLARY HIDRADENOMA (HIDRADENOMA PAPILLIFERUM)

This is a benign tumour arising from apocrine sweat glands of the vulva. Most commonly, it is located in the labia or in the perianal region as a small sharply circumscribed nodule.

M/E The tumour lies in the dermis under a normal epidermis. The tumour consists of papillary structures composed of fibrovascular stalk and is covered by double layer of epithelial cells—a layer of flattened myoepithelial cells and an overlying layer of columnar cells.

CONDYLOMA ACUMINATUM

Condyloma acuminata or anogenital warts are benign papillary lesions of squamous epithelium which can be transmitted venereally to male sex partner. They may be solitary but more frequently are multiple forming soft warty masses. The common locations are the anus, perineum, vaginal wall, vulva and vagina. They are induced by human papilloma virus (HPV), particularly types 6 and 11.

M/E They are identical to their counterparts on male external genitalia. The features consist of a tree-like proliferation of stratified squamous epithelium, showing marked acanthosis, hyperkeratosis, parakeratosis, papillomatosis and perinuclear vacuolisation of epithelium called *koilocytosis,* indicative of HPV infection. The papillary projections consist of fibrovascular stoma.

EXTRA-MAMMARY PAGET'S DISEASE

Paget's disease of the vulva is a rare condition which has skin manifestations like those of Paget's disease of the nipple. The affected skin, most often on the labia majora, appears as map-like, red, scaly, elevated and indurated area.

M/E Extra-mammary Paget's disease is identified by the presence of large, pale, carcinoma cells lying singly or in small clusters within the epidermis and adnexal structures.

Unlike Paget's disease of the breast in which case there is always an underlying ductal carcinoma, extra-mammary Paget's disease is confined to the epidermis in most cases.

VULVAL INTRAEPITHELIAL NEOPLASIA AND INVASIVE CARCINOMA

Vulval intraepithelial neoplasia (VIN) and invasive squamous cell carcinoma are morphologically similar to those in the cervix and vagina. The etiologic role of certain viruses in carcinogenesis, particularly high-risk HPV types 16 and 18, in these sites is well documented. VIN is often multifocal within vulva and may be multicentric.

G/A VIN and vulval carcinoma in early stage is a 'white' lesion (leukoplakia) while later the area develops an exophytic or endophytic (ulcerative) growth pattern. The traditional VIN lesion, described as Bowen's disease of the vulva, is generally a slightly elevated, velvety, plaque lesion.

M/E Just as in cervix, VIN may also range from VIN I to VIN III, higher grade being also called Bowen's disease (*in situ* carcinoma). Vulvar cancer is squamous cell type with varying degree of anaplasia and depth of invasion depending upon the stage. HPV-positive tumours are more often poorly-differentiated squamous cell carcinoma while HPV-negative are well-differentiated keratinising type. *Verrucous carcinoma* is a rare variant which is a fungating tumour but is locally malignant.

VAGINA (p. 712)

NORMAL STRUCTURE

The vagina consists of a collapsed cylinder extending between vestibule externally and the cervix internally.

M/E The vaginal wall consists of 3 layers: an *outer* fibrous, a *middle* muscular and an *inner* epithelial. The epithelial layer consists of stratified squamous epithelium which undergoes cytologic changes under hormonal stimuli. Oestrogen increases its thickness such as during reproductive years, whereas the epithelium is thin in childhood, and atrophic after menopause when oestrogen stimulation is minimal.

VAGINITIS AND VULVOVAGINITIS (p. 712)

Since vulva and vagina are anatomically close to each other, often inflammation of one affects the other location. Certain other infections are quite common in the vulva and vagina as follows:
i)   Bacterial e.g. streptococci, staphylococci, *Escherichia coli, Haemophilus vaginalis.*
ii)   Fungal e.g. *Candida albicans.*
iii) Protozoal e.g. *Trichomonas vaginalis.*
iv)   Viral e.g. Herpes simplex.

The most common causes of vaginitis are *Candida* (moniliasis) and *Trichomonas* (trichomoniasis). The hyphae of *Candida* can be seen in the vaginal smears. Similarly, the protozoa, *Trichomonas,* can be identified in smears.

TUMOURS AND TUMOUR-LIKE CONDITIONS (p. 713)

Vaginal cysts such as Gartner's duct (Wolffian) cyst lined by glandular epithe-lium and vaginal inclusion cyst arising from inclusion of vaginal epithelium are more common benign vaginal tumours and tumour-like conditions.

CARCINOMA OF VAGINA

Primary carcinoma of the vagina is an uncommon tumour. Squamous cell dysplasia or vaginal intraepithelial neoplasia occur less frequently as compared to the cervix or vulva and can be detected by Pap smears. Invasive carcinoma of the vagina includes two main types:

1. **Squamous cell carcinoma** of vagina constitutes less than 2% of all gynaecologic malignancies and is similar in morphology as elsewhere in the female genital tract.

2. **Adenocarcinoma of the vagina** is much less frequent than squamous cell carcinoma of the vagina. It may be endometrioid or mucinous type.

EMBRYONAL RHABDOMYOSARCOMA (SARCOMA BOTRYOIDES)

This is an unusual and rare malignant tumour occurring in infants and children under 5 years of age. The common location is anterior vaginal wall. Similar tumours may occur in the urinary bladder, head and neck region (orbit, nasopharynx, middle ear, oral cavity) and biliary tract.

G/A The tumour is characterised by bulky and polypoid grape-like mass (*botryoides* = grape) that fills and projects out of the vagina.

M/E The features are as under:
1. Groups of round to fusiform tumour cells are characteristically lying underneath the vaginal epithelium, called *cambium layer* of tumour cells.
2. The central core of polypoid masses is composed of loose and myxoid stroma with many inflammatory cells.

The tumour invades extensively in the pelvis and metastasises to regional lymph nodes and distant sites such as to lungs and liver.

CERVIX (p. 713)

NORMAL STRUCTURE

The cervix consists of an *internal os* communicating with the endometrial cavity above, and an *external os* opening into the vagina below. *Ectocervix* (exocervix) or *portio vaginalis* is the part of the cervix exposed to the vagina and is lined by stratified squamous epithelium, whereas the endocervix is continuous with the endocervical canal and is lined by a single layer of tall columnar mucus-secreting epithelium. The junction of the ectocervix and endocervix—*junctional mucosa*, consists of gradual transition between squamous and columnar epithelia (squamo-columnar junction) and is clinically and pathologically significant landmark.

CERVICITIS (p. 713)

ACUTE CERVICITIS

Acute cervicitis is usually associated with puerperium or gonococcal infection. Other causes are primary chancre and infection with herpes simplex.

CHRONIC CERVICITIS

Chronic nonspecific cervicitis is encountered quite frequently and is the common cause of leucorrhoea. The most common organisms responsible for chronic cervicitis are the normal mixed vaginal flora that includes streptococci, enterococci (e.g. *E. coli*) and staphylococci. Factors predisposing to chronic cervicitis are sexual intercourse, trauma of childbirth, instrumentation and excess or deficiency of oestrogen.

G/A There is eversion of ectocervix with hyperaemia, oedema and granular surface. Nabothian (retention) cysts may be grossly visible from the surface as pearly grey vesicles.

M/E Chronic cervicitis is characterised by extensive subepithelial inflammatory infiltrate of lymphocytes, plasma cells, large mononuclear cells and a few neutrophils. There may be formation of lymphoid follicles termed *follicular cervicitis*. The surface epithelium may be normal, or may show squamous metaplasia.

Both benign and malignant tumours are common in the cervix. In addition, cervix is the site of 'shades of grey' lesions that include cervical dysplasia and carcinoma *in situ* (cervical intraepithelial neoplasia, CIN), currently termed squamous intraepithelial lesions (SIL).

CERVICAL POLYPS

Cervical polyps are localised benign proliferations of endocervical mucosa though they may protrude through the external os. They are found in 2-5% of adult women and produce irregular vaginal spotting.

G/A Cervical polyp is a small (up to 5 cm in size), bright red, fragile growth which is frequently pedunculated but may be sessile.

M/E Most cervical polyps are endocervical polyps and are covered with endocervical epithelium which may show squamous metaplasia. Less frequently, the covering is by squamous epithelium of the portio vaginalis. The stroma of the polyp is composed of loose and oedematous fibrous tissue with variable degree of inflammatory infiltrate.

MICROGLANDULAR HYPERPLASIA

Microglandular hyperplasia is a benign condition of the cervix in which there is closely packed proliferation of endocervical glands without intervening stroma. The condition is caused by progestrin stimulation such as during pregnancy, postpartum period and in women taking oral contraceptives.

SQUAMOUS INTRAEPITHELIAL LESION (SIL) (CERVICAL INTRAEPITHELIAL NEOPLASIA, CIN)

TERMINOLOGY

Presently, the terms dysplasia, CIN, carcinoma *in situ*, and SIL are used synonymously as follows:

DYSPLASIA The term 'dysplasia' (meaning 'bad moulding') has been commonly used for atypical cytologic changes in the layers of squamous epithelium, the changes being progressive. Depending upon the thickness of squamous epithelium involved by atypical cells, dysplasia is conventionally graded as *mild, moderate* and *severe*. Carcinoma *in situ* is the full-thickness involvement by atypical cells, or in other words carcinoma confined to layers above the basement membrane.

CIN An alternative classification is to group various grades of dysplasia and carcinoma *in situ* together into cervical intraepithelial neoplasia (CIN) which is similarly graded from grade I to III.

SIL Currently, the National Cancer Institute (NCI) of the US has proposed the *Bethesda System (TBS)* for reporting cervical and vaginal cytopathology. According to the Bethesda system, based on cytomorphologic features and HPV types implicated in their etiology, the three grades of CIN are readjusted into two grades of squamous intraepithelial lesions (SIL)—low-grade SIL (L-SIL) and high-grade SIL (H-SIL) as under:

◈ *L-SIL* corresponds to CIN-1 and is a flat condyloma, having koilocytic atypia, usually related to HPV 6 and 11 infection (i.e. includes mild dysplasia and HPV infection). About 10% cases of L-SIL may progress to H-SIL.

◈ *H-SIL* corresponds to CIN-2 and 3 and has abnormal pleomorphic atypical squamous cells. HPV 16 and 18 are implicated in the etiology of H-SIL (i.e. includes moderate dysplasia, severe dysplasia, and carcinoma *in situ*). Approximately, 10% cases of H-SIL may progress to invasive cervical cancer over a period of about two years.

The use of Pap smear followed by colposcopy-directed biopsy confirms the diagnosis which has helped greatly in instituting early effective therapy and thus has reduced the incidence of cervical cancer in many developed countries.

The biology of CIN/SIL and its relationship to invasive carcinoma of the cervix is well understood by epidemiologic, virologic, molecular, immunologic and ultrastructural studies.

1. Epidemiologic studies Based on epidemiology of large population of women with cervical cancer, several risk factors have been identified which include the following 4 most important factors:

i) Women having *early age of sexual activity.*

ii) Women having *multiple sexual partners.*

iii) Women with *persistent HPV infection* with high-risk types of oncogenic virus.

iv) *Potential role of high risk male* sexual partner such as promiscuous male having previous multiple sexual partners, having history of penile condyloma, or male who had previous spouse with cervical cancer.

　　In addition to the above factors, other epidemiologic observations reveal high incidence of cervical cancer in lower socioeconomic strata, in multiparous women, cigarette smoking women, users of oral contraceptives, HIV infection and immunosuppression, while a low incidence is noted in virgins and nuns.

2. Virologic studies Human papillomavirus (HPV) infection is strongly implicated in the etiology of cervical cancer.

i) *High-risk type* HPV, most commonly of types 16 and 18 (in 70% cases), and less often types 31, 33, 52 and 58, are present in 70-100% cases of cervical cancer.

ii) *Low-risk type* HPV types 6 and 11 are found most frequently in condylomas.

iii) *Mixed high and low risk types* of HPV may be found in dysplasias.

3. Molecular studies Immunohistochemical, cytogenetic and molecular studies have shown that low-risk HPV types do not integrate in the host cell genome, while high-risk HPV types are integrated into the nucleus of cervical epithelial cells. Upon integration, protein product of HPV-16 and 18, E7 and E6 proteins respectively, inactivate tumour suppressor genes, *p53* and *RB-1 gene,* thus permitting uncontrolled cellular proliferation.

4. Immunologic studies Circulating tumour specific antigens and antibodies are detected in patients of cervical cancer.

5. Ultrastructural studies The changes observed on ultrastructural studies of cells in CIN/SIL reveal increased mitochondria and free ribosomes, and depletion of normally accumulated glycogen in the surface cells. The latter change forms the basis of *Schiller's test* in which the suspected cervix is painted with solution of iodine and potassium iodide. The cancerous focus, if present, fails to stain because of lack of glycogen in the surface cells.

G/A No specific picture is associated with cellular atypia found in dysplasias or carcinoma *in situ* except that the changes begin at the squamocolumnar junction or transitional zone. The diagnosis can be suspected clinically on the basis of Schiller's test done on bedside.

M/E Distinction between various grades of CIN is quite subjective, but, in general dysplastic cells are distributed in the layers of squamous epithelium for varying thickness, and accordingly graded as mild, moderate and severe dysplasia, and carcinoma *in situ.*

◈　In *mild dysplasia (CIN-1),* the abnormal cells extend up to one-third thickness from the basal to the surface layer;

◈　In *moderate dysplasia (CIN-2)* up to two-thirds;

◈　In *severe dysplasia (CIN-3),* these cells extend from 75-90% thickness of epithelium; and

◈　In *carcinoma in situ* (included in *CIN-3),* the entire thickness from the basement membrane to the surface shows dysplastic cells.

　　The degree of atypicality in the exfoliated surface epithelial cells can be objectively graded on the basis of 3 principal features:

1. More severe nuclear dyskaryotic changes such as increased hyperchromasia and nuclear membrane folding.

2. Decreased cytoplasmic maturation i.e. less cytoplasm as the surface cells show less maturation.

3. In lower grades of dysplasia (CIN-1/L-SIL) predominantly superficial and intermediate cells are shed off whereas in severe dysplasia and in carcinoma *in situ* (CIN-3/H-SIL) the desquamated cells are mainly small, dark basal cells.

CERVICAL SCREENING AND THE BETHESDA SYSTEM

Naked eye visual inspection of the uterine cervix with either 5% acetic acid (VIA) or with Lugol's iodine (VILI) under intense illumination provide simple tests for early detection of cervical precancerous lesions and invasive cervical cancer. These tests have largely superseded the earlier Schiller's test due to their ease and low cost.

With introduction of effective Pap screening programme in developed countries, incidence of invasive cervical cancer has declined greatly. However, still worldwide cervical cancer remains third most common cancer in women, next to breast and lung cancer.

Cervical screening recommendations include annual cervical smear in all sexually active women having any risk factors listed above. However, if three consecutive Pap smears are negative in 'high-risk women' or satisfactory in 'low risk women', frequency of Pap screening is reduced. There is no upper age limit for cervical screening.

The broad principles of *the* **Bethesda system** (TBS) of cytologic evaluation are as under:

1. Pap smears are evaluated as regards *adequacy of specimen* i.e. satisfactory for evaluation, satisfactory but limited, or unsatisfactory for evaluation giving reason.

2. General diagnosis is given in the form of *normal or abnormal smear.*

3. *Descriptive diagnosis* is given in abnormal smears that includes: benign cellular changes, reactive cellular changes, and abnormalities of epithelial cells.

4. Cellular abnormalities include: *ASCUS* (atypical squamous cells of undetermined significance), *L-SIL* (mentioning HPV infection and CIN-1 present or not), *H-SIL* (stating CIN-2 or CIN-3) and *squamous cell carcinoma.*

INVASIVE CERVICAL CANCER

Invasive cervical cancer in about 80% of cases is epidermoid (squamous cell) carcinoma. The incidence of invasive carcinoma of the cervix has shown a declining trend in developed countries in the last half of the century due to increased use of Pap smear technique for early detection and diagnosis but the incidence remains high in developing countries with low living standards.

G/A Invasive cervical carcinoma may present 3 types of patterns: fungating, ulcerating and infiltrating.

M/E The following patterns are seen:

1. Epidermoid (Squamous cell) carcinoma This type comprises vast majority of invasive cervical carcinomas (about 70%).
◈ The most common pattern (70%) is moderately-differentiated non-keratinising large cell type and has better prognosis.
◈ Next in frequency (25%) is well-differentiated keratinising epidermoid carcinoma.
◈ Small cell undifferentiated carcinoma (neuroendocrine or oat cell carcinoma) is less common (5%) and has a poor prognosis.

2. Adenocarcinoma Adenocarcinomas comprise about 20-25% of cases.

3. Others The remaining 5% cases are a variety of other patterns such as adenosquamous carcinoma, verrucous carcinoma and undifferentiated carcinoma.

NORMAL STRUCTURE

The *myometrium* is the thick muscular wall of the uterus which is covered internally by uterine mucosa called the *endometrium*. The endometrium extends above the level of the internal os where it joins the endocervical epithelium. The myometrium is capable of marked alterations in its size, capacity and contractility during pregnancy and labour. The endometrium responds in a cyclic fashion to the ovarian hormones with resultant monthly menstruation and has remarkable regenerative capacity.

EFFECTS OF HORMONES (p. 720)

NORMAL CYCLIC CHANGES

The normal endometrial cycle begins with proliferative phase lasting for about 14 days under the influence of oestrogen, followed by ovulation on or around 14th day, and consequent secretory phase under the influence of progesterone. The cycle ends with endometrial shedding and the next cycle begins anew.

M/E Essentially, the endometrium consists of 3 structures: the endometrial lining epithelium, endometrial glands and stroma.

◈ **Epithelial lining** undergoes increase in its thickness from cuboidal to tall columnar appearance at ovulation and subsequently regresses.

◈ **Endometrial glands** with their lining provide most of the information on phase of the menstrual cycle. In the immediate postmenstrual period, the glands are straight and tubular, having columnar lining with basal nuclei. This phase is under the predominant influence of oestrogen and lasts for about 14 days and is called *proliferative phase*. The evidence of ovulation is taken from the appearance of convolutions in the glands and subnuclear vacuolation in the cells indicative of secretions. The secretory changes remain prominent for the next 7 days after ovulation for implantation of the ovum if it has been fertilised. Otherwise, the secretory activity wanes during the following 7 days with increased luminal secretions and a frayed and ragged luminal border of the cells lining the glands. This phase is under the predominant influence of progesterone and is called *secretory phase*.

◈ **Endometrial stroma** in the pre-ovulatory phase or proliferative phase is generally dense and compact, composed of oval to spindled cells. In the post-ovulatory phase or secretory phase, the stroma is loose and oedematous, composed of large, pale and polyhedral cells. The true *decidual reaction* of the stroma occurs if the pregnancy has taken place.

EFFECT OF OESTROGEN AND PROGESTERONE

Oestrogen produces the characteristic changes of proliferative phase at the time of menopause and in young women with anovulatory cycles as occurs in Stein-Leventhal syndrome. The therapeutic addition of progesterone produces secretory pattern in an oestrogen-primed endometrium. Oestrogen-progesterone combination hormonal therapy is employed for control of conception.

EFFECT OF PREGNANCY

The implantation of a fertilised ovum results in interruption of the endometrial cycle. The endometrial glands are enlarged with abundant glandular secretions and the stromal cells become more plump, polygonal with increased cytoplasm termed *decidual reaction*. About 25% cases of uterine or extrauterine pregnancy show hyperactive secretory state called *Arias-Stella reaction*.

EFFECT OF MENOPAUSE

The onset of menopause is heralded with hormonal transition and consequent varying morphologic changes in the endometrium. Most commonly, the *senile endometrium,* as it is generally called, is thin and atrophic with inactive glands and fibrous stroma. However, some of the glands may show cystic dilatation.

DYSFUNCTIONAL UTERINE BLEEDING (DUB)

Dysfunctional uterine bleeding (DUB) may be defined as excessive bleeding occurring during or between menstrual periods without a causative uterine lesion such as tumour, polyp, infection, hyperplasia, trauma, blood dyscrasia or pregnancy. The causes for *anovulation* at different ages are as follows:

1. In *pre-puberty:* precocious puberty of hypothalamic, pituitary or ovarian origin.

2. In *adolescence:* anovulatory cycles at the onset of menstruation.

3. In *reproductive age:* complications of pregnancy, endometrial hyperplasia, carcinoma, polyps, leiomyomas and adenomyosis.

4. At *premenopause:* anovulatory cycles, irregular shedding, endometrial hyperplasia, carcinoma and polyps.

5. At *perimenopause:* endometrial hyperplasia, carcinoma, polyps and senile atrophy.

ENDOMETRITIS AND MYOMETRITIS *(p. 721)*

Inflammatory involvement of the endometrium and myometrium are uncommon clinical problems; myometritis is seen less frequently than endometritis and occurs in continuation with endometrial infections. Endometritis and myometritis may be acute or chronic.

M/E In *acute endometritis and myometritis,* there is progressive infiltration of the endometrium, myometrium and parametrium by polymorphs and marked oedema. *Chronic nonspecific endometritis and myometritis* are characterised by infiltration of plasma cells alongwith lymphocytes and macrophages. *Tuberculous endometritis* is almost always associated with tuberculous salpingitis and shows small caseating granulomas.

ADENOMYOSIS *(p. 721)*

Adenomyosis is defined as abnormal distribution of histologically benign endometrial tissue within the myometrium alongwith myometrial hypertrophy. The term *adenomyoma* is used for actually circumscribed mass made up of endometrium and smooth muscle tissue. Pathogenesis of the condition remains unexplained. The possible underlying cause of the invasiveness and increased proliferation of the endometrium into the myometrium appears to be either a metaplasia or oestrogenic stimulation due to endocrine dysfunction of the ovary.

G/A The uterus may be slightly or markedly enlarged. On cut section, there is diffuse thickness of the uterine wall with presence of coarsely trabecular, ill-defined areas of haemorrhages.

M/E The diagnosis is based on the finding of normal, benign endometrial islands composed of glands as well as stroma deep within the muscular layer. The minimum distance between the endometrial islands within the myometrium and the basal endometrium should be one low-power microscopic field (2-3 mm) for making the diagnosis.

ENDOMETRIOSIS *(p. 722)*

Endometriosis refers to the presence of endometrial glands and stroma in abnormal locations outside the uterus.

The chief locations where the abnormal endometrial development may occur are as follows (in descending order of frequency): ovaries, uterine ligaments, rectovaginal septum, pelvic peritoneum, laparotomy scars, and infrequently in the umbilicus, vagina, vulva, appendix and hernial sacs.

The **histogenesis** of endometriosis has been a debatable matter for years. Currently, however, the following 3 theories of its histogenesis are described:

1. *Transplantation or regurgitation theory* is based on the assumption that ectopic endometrial tissue is transplanted from the uterus to an abnormal location by way of fallopian tubes.

2. *Metaplastic theory* suggests that ectopic endometrium develops *in situ* from local tissues by metaplasia of the coelomic epithelium.

3. *Vascular or lymphatic dissemination* explains the development of endometrial tissue at extrapelvic sites by these routes.

G/A Typically, the foci of endometriosis appear as blue or brownish-black underneath the surface of the sites mentioned. Ovarian involvement is often bilateral. Larger cysts, 3-5 cm in diameter, filled with old dark brown blood form *'chocolate cysts'* of the ovary.

M/E The diagnosis is simple and rests on identification of foci of endometrial glands and stroma, old or new haemorrhages, haemosiderin-laden macrophages and surrounding zone of inflammation and fibrosis.

ENDOMETRIAL HYPERPLASIAS (p. 723)

Endometrial hyperplasia is characterised by exaggerated proliferation of glandular and stromal tissues. It is commonly associated with prolonged, profuse and irregular uterine bleeding in a menopausal or postmenopausal woman. Hyperplasia results from prolonged oestrogenic stimulation unopposed with any progestational activity. Endometrial hyperplasia is clinically significant due to the presence of cellular atypia which is closely linked to endometrial carcinoma.

The following classification of endometrial hyperplasias is widely employed by most gynaecologic pathologists:

1. Simple hyperplasia without atypia (Cystic glandular hyperplasia).
2. Complex hyperplasia without atypia (Complex non-atypical hyperplasia).
3. Complex hyperplasia with atypia (Complex atypical hyperplasia).

SIMPLE HYPERPLASIA WITHOUT ATYPIA (CYSTIC GLANDULAR HYPERPLASIA) Commonly termed cystic glandular hyperplasia (CGH), this form of endometrial hyperplasia is characterised by the presence of varying-sized glands, many of which are large and cystically dilated and are lined by atrophic epithelium. Mitoses are scanty and there is no atypia. The stroma between the glands is sparsely cellular and oedematous.

There is minimal risk (<1%) of adenocarcinoma developing in cystic hyperplasia.

COMPLEX HYPERPLASIA WITHOUT ATYPIA (COMPLEX NON-ATYPICAL HYPERPLASIA) This type of hyperplasia shows distinct proliferative pattern. The glands are increased in number, exhibit variation in size and are irregular in shape. The glands are lined by multiple layers of tall columnar epithelial cells with large nuclei which have not lost basal polarity and there is no significant atypia. The glandular epithelium at places is thrown into papillary infolds or out-pouchings into adjacent stroma i.e. there is crowding and complexity of glands without cellular atypia. The stroma is generally dense, cellular and compact.

The malignant potential of complex hyperplasia in the absence of cytologic atypia is 3%.

COMPLEX HYPERPLASIA WITH ATYPIA (COMPLEX ATYPICAL HYPERPLASIA) Complex hyperplasia with atypia is distinguished from complex non-atypical hyperplasia by the presence of 'atypical cells' in the hyperplastic epithelium. The extent of cellular atypia may be mild, moderate or severe. The cytologic features present in these cells include loss of polarity, large size, irregular and hyperchromatic nuclei, prominent nucleoli, and altered nucleocytoplasmic ratio.

About 20-25% cases of untreated atypical hyperplasia progress to carcinoma.

TUMOURS OF ENDOMETRIUM AND MYOMETRIUM (p. 723)

Tumours arising from endometrium and myometrium may be benign or malignant. They may originate from different tissues as under:

◈ *Endometrial glands*—endometrial polyps, endometrial carcinoma.
◈ *Endometrial stroma*—stromal nodules, stromal sarcoma.
◈ *Smooth muscle of the myometrium*—leiomyoma, leiomyosarcoma.
◈ *Mullerian mesoderm*—mixed mesodermal or mullerian tumours.

ENDOMETRIAL POLYPS

'Uterine polyp' is clinical term used for a polypoid growth projecting into the uterine lumen and may be composed of benign lesions or malignant polypoid tumours. The most common variety, however, is the one having the structure like that of endometrium and is termed *endometrial or mucus polyp*. They are more common in the perimenopausal age group.

G/A Endometrial polyps may be single or multiple, usually sessile and small (0.5 to 3 cm in diameter) but occasionally they are large and pedunculated.

M/E They are essentially made up of mixture of endometrial glands and stroma. The histologic pattern of the endometrial tissue in the polyp may resemble either functioning endometrium or hyperplastic endometrium of cystic hyperplasia type, the latter being more common.

ENDOMETRIAL CARCINOMA

Carcinoma of the endometrium, commonly called uterine cancer, is the most common pelvic malignancy in females in the United States and Eastern Europe but is uncommon in Asia where cervical cancer continues to be the leading cancer in women. Increased frequency of endometrial carcinoma in these countries may be due to longevity of women's life to develop this cancer of older females. The most important presenting complaint is abnormal bleeding in postmenopausal woman or excessive flow in the premenopausal years.

ETIOLOGY Following factors are implicated:
1. Chronic unopposed oestrogen excess
2. Obesity
3. Diabetes mellitus
4. Hypertension
5. Nulliparous state
6. Heredity.
      There are irrefutable evidences of *relationship of endometrial carcinoma with prolonged oestrogenic stimulation* as under:
i) Endometrial carcinoma has association with endometrial hyperplasia in which there is unopposed chronic hyperoestrogenism.
ii) In postmenopausal years when endometrial carcinoma occurs characteristically, there is excessive synthesis of oestrogen in the body from adrenal as well as from ovarian sources.
iii) Women having oestrogen-secreting tumours (e.g. granulosa cell tumour) have increased risk.
iv) Patients receiving prolonged exogenous oestrogen therapy.
v) Women of breast cancer receiving tamoxifen for prolonged period.
vi) Prolonged administration of oestrogen to laboratory animals can produce endometrial hyperplasia and carcinoma.
vii) Women with gonadal agenesis rarely develop endometrial carcinoma.

PATHOGENESIS At molecular level, it is explained as under:
◈ Endometrial hyperplasia is a forerunner of endometrioid cancer is supported by mutated *PTEN* gene (located on chromosome 10) seen in 20% cases of complex hyperplasia.
◈ Papillary serous endometrial carcinoma is seen in a background of atrophic endometrium and is associated with mutation in *p53* tumour suppressor gene.
◈ Higher incidence in hereditary non-polyposis colon cancer (HNPCC) syndrome (having simultaneous cancers of the colon and endometrioid adenocarcinoma) and in Cowden syndrome.

G/A Endometrial carcinoma may have 2 patterns—localised *polypoid tumour,* or a *diffuse tumour;* the latter being more common. The tumour protrudes into the endometrial cavity as irregular, friable and grey-tan mass. Extension of the growth into the myometrium may be identified.

M/E Most endometrial carcinomas are adenocarcinomas, commonly termed *endometrioid adenocarcinomas.* Depending upon the pattern of glands and individual cell changes, these may be well-differentiated, moderately-differentiated or poorly-differentiated.

◈ **Papillary serous carcinoma** of the endometrium resembling its ovarian counterpart is distinct since it occurs in the background of atrophic endometrium and is more aggressive.

◈ **Uncommon histologic variants** of endometrial carcinoma are: adenocarcinoma with squamous metaplasia (adenoacanthoma), adenosquamous carcinoma (when both components are frankly malignant), clear cell carcinoma, mucinous adenocarcinoma and papillary serous carcinoma.

LEIOMYOMA

Leiomyomas or fibromyomas, commonly called *fibroids* by the gynaecologists, are the most common uterine tumours of smooth muscle origin, often admixed with variable amount of fibrous tissue component. About 20% of women above the age of 30 years harbour uterine myomas of varying size. Malignant transformation occurs in less than 0.5% of leiomyomas. Symptomatic cases may produce abnormal uterine bleeding, pain, symptoms due to compression of surrounding structures and infertility.

MORPHOLOGIC FEATURES Leiomyomas are most frequently located in the uterus where they may occur within the myometrium (*intramural or interstitial*), the serosa (*subserosal*), or just underneath the endometrium (*submucosal*).

G/A Irrespective of their location, leiomyomas are often multiple, circumscribed, firm, nodular, grey-white masses of variable size. On cut section, they exhibit characteristic whorled pattern.

M/E They are essentially composed of 2 tissue elements—whorled bundles of smooth muscle cells admixed with variable amount of connective tissue. The smooth muscle cells are uniform in size and shape with abundant cytoplasm and central oval nuclei.

Cellular leiomyoma has preponderance of smooth muscle elements and may superficially resemble leiomyosarcoma but is distinguished from it by the absence of mitoses.

The pathologic appearance may be altered by secondary changes in the leiomyomas; these include: hyaline degeneration, cystic degeneration, infarction, calcification, infection and suppuration, necrosis, fatty change, and rarely, sarcomatous change.

LEIOMYOSARCOMA

Leiomyosarcoma is an uncommon malignant tumour as compared to its rather common benign counterpart. The incidence of malignancy in pre-existing leiomyoma is less than 0.5% but primary uterine sarcoma is less common than that which arises in the leiomyoma. The peak age incidence is seen in 4th to 6th decades of life.

G/A The tumour may form a diffuse, bulky, soft and fleshy mass, or a polypoid mass projecting into lumen.

M/E Though there are usually some areas showing whorled arrangement of spindle-shaped smooth muscle cells having large and hyperchromatic nuclei, the hallmark of diagnosis and prognosis is the number of mitoses per high power field (HPF). The essential diagnostic criteria are: more than 10 mitoses per 10 HPF with or without cellular atypia, or 5-10 mitoses per 10 HPF with cellular atypia. More the number of mitoses per 10 HPF, worse is the prognosis.

NORMAL STRUCTURE

The fallopian tube or oviducts are paired structures, each extending from superior angle of the uterus laterally to the region of the ovaries and running in the superior border of the broad ligaments forming mesosalpinx. Each tube is 7-14 cm long and is divided into 4 parts—*interstitial portion* in the uterine cornual wall; narrow *isthmic portion;* wider *ampullary region;* and funnel-like distal *infundibulum*. The infundibulum is fringed by fimbriae.

M/E The wall of tube has 4 coats—*serous* forming the peritoneal covering, *subserous* consisting of fibrovascular tissue, *muscular* composed of longitudinal and circular smooth muscle layers, and *tubal mucosa* having 3 types of cells namely: ciliated, columnar and dark intercalated cells.

INFLAMMATIONS *(p. 728)*

SALPINGITIS AND PELVIC INFLAMMATORY DISEASE

Pelvic inflammatory disease (PID) by definition is a clinical syndrome characterised by signs and symptoms of ascending infection beginning in the vulva or vagina and spreading through the entire genital tract. Although ascending route of infection is the most common mode of spread, PID may occur following abortion and puerperium, with use of intrauterine contraceptive devices, or from local intra-abdominal infections such as appendicitis with peritonitis. In addition, haematogenous spread may occur, though this route is more important in the pathogenesis of tuberculosis.

Patients generally complain of lower abdominal and pelvic pain which is often bilateral, dysmenorrhoea, menstrual abnormalities and fever with tachycardia. Long-standing chronic PID may lead to infertility and adhesions between small intestine and pelvic organs.

G/A The fallopian tubes are invariably involved bilaterally. The distal end is blocked by inflammatory exudate and the lumina are dilated. There may be formation of loculated tubo-ovarian abscess involving the tube, ovary, broad ligament and adjacent part of uterus.

M/E The appearance varies with duration:
1. The process begins with *acute salpingitis* characterised by oedema and intense acute inflammatory infiltrate of neutrophils involving the tubal mucosa as well as wall.
2. The purulent process may extend to involve tube as well as ovary causing salpingo-oophoritis and forming *tubo-ovarian abscess.*
3. The escape of purulent exudate into the peritoneal cavity produces *pelvic peritonitis* and *pelvic abscess.*
4. *Pyosalpinx* is distension of the fallopian tube with pus due to occluded fimbrial end.
5. End-result of pyosalpinx after resorption of the purulent exudate is *hydrosalpinx* in which the tube is thin-walled, dilated and filled with clear watery fluid.
6. Acute salpingitis may resolve with treatment but some cases pass into *chronic salpingitis* with infiltrate of polymorphs, lymphocytes and plasma cells and fibrosis.

TUBERCULOUS SALPINGITIS

Tuberculous salpingitis is almost always secondary to focus elsewhere in the body. The tubercle bacilli reach the tube, most commonly by haematogenous route, generally from the lungs, but occasionally from the urinary tract or abdominal cavity. Tubal tuberculosis is always present when there is tuberculosis of other female genital organs such as of endometrium, cervix and lower genital tract. Concomitant involvement of endometrium is present in about 80% cases. It affects more commonly young women in their active reproductive life and the most common complaint is infertility.

G/A The tube is dilated and contains purulent exudate though the fimbrial end is generally patent. The tubal peritoneum as well as the peritoneum in general is studded with yellowish tubercles.

M/E Typical caseating granulomas and chronic inflammation are identified in the tubal serosa, muscularis and mucosa.

ECTOPIC TUBAL PREGNANCY *(p. 729)*

The term ectopic tubal pregnancy is used for implantation of a fertilised ovum in the tube. Though ectopic pregnancy may rarely occur in the uterine horn, cornu, ovary and abdominal cavity, tubal pregnancy is by far the most common form of ectopic gestation. Several factors which predispose to ectopic tubal pregnancy are: PID, previous tubal surgery, use of IUCD and congenital anomalies of the female genital tract. Ectopic tubal pregnancy is a potentially hazardous problem because of rupture which is followed by intraperitoneal haemorrhage.

TUMOURS AND TUMOUR-LIKE LESIONS *(p. 729)*

Tumours in the fallopian tubes are rare. Relatively more common are tumour-like conditions such as hydatids of Morgagni or parovarian cysts which are unilocular, thin-walled cysts hanging from the tubal fimbriae. Rare tumours include adenomatoid tumours, leiomyomas, teratomas, adenocarcinomas and choriocarcinoma all of which are similar in morphology to such tumours elsewhere in the body.

OVARIES *(p. 729)*

NORMAL STRUCTURE

The ovaries are paired bean-shaped organs hanging from either tube by a mesentery called the mesovarium, the lateral suspensory ligament and the ovarian ligament. Each ovary measures 2.5-5 cm in length, 1.5-3 cm in breadth and 0.7-1.5 cm in width and weighs 4-8 gm.

M/E The ovarian structure consists of covering by coelomic epithelium, outer cortex and inner medulla.

Coelomic epithelium The surface of the ovary is covered by a single layer of cuboidal epithelial cells.

Cortex During active reproductive life, the cortex is broad and constitutes the predominant component of the ovary. The cortex contains numerous ovarian follicles and their derivative structures. Each follicle consists of a central *germ cell ovum* surrounded by specialised gonadal stroma. This stroma consists of *granulosa cells* encircling the ovum, and concentrically-arranged plump spindle-shaped *theca cells*.

Medulla The ovarian medulla is primarily made up of connective tissue fibres, smooth muscle cells and numerous blood vessels, lymphatics and nerves. In addition, the medulla may also contain clusters of hilus cell (or hilar-Leydig cells) which may have androgenic role in contrast to oestrogenic role of the ovarian cortex.

NON-NEOPLASTIC CYSTS *(p. 729)*

FOLLICULAR AND LUTEAL CYSTS

Normally follicles and corpus luteum do not exceed a diameter of 2 cm. When their diameter is greater than 3 cm, they are termed as cysts.

◈ **Follicular cysts** are frequently multiple, filled with clear serous fluid and may attain a diameter upto 8 cm. When large, they produce clinical symptoms.

M/E They are lined by granulosa cells. Occasionally, however, there may be difficulty in distinguishing between a large cyst of coelomic epithelial origin (*serous cyst*) lined by flattened epithelial cells and a cyst of follicular origin. Such cases are appropriately designated as *'simple cysts'*.

◈ **Luteal cysts** are formed by rupture and sealing of corpus haemorrhagicum. The wall of these cysts is composed of yellowish luteal tissue (*lutein* = yellow pigment).

M/E Luteal cysts are commonly lined by luteinised granulosa cells.

POLYCYSTIC OVARY DISEASE (STEIN-LEVENTHAL SYNDROME)

Polycystic ovary syndrome (PCOS) is a syndrome characterised by oligomenorrhoea, anovulation, infertility, hirsutism and obesity in young women having bilaterally enlarged and cystic ovaries. The principal biochemical abnormalities in most patients are excessive production of androgens, and low levels of pituitary follicle stimulating hormone (FSH). Current concept of pathogenesis of PCOS is the unbalanced release of FSH and LH by the pituitary. A hereditary basis for the syndrome has been suggested in some cases.

G/A The ovaries are usually involved bilaterally and are at least twice the size of the normal ovary. They are grey-white in colour and studded with multiple small (0.5-1.5 cm in diameter) bluish cysts just beneath the cortex. The medullary stroma is abundant, solid and grey.

M/E The outer cortex is thick and fibrous. The subcortical cysts are lined by prominent luteinised theca cells and represent follicles in various stages of maturation but there is no evidence of corpus luteum.

OVARIAN TUMOURS (p. 730)

The ovary is third most common site of primary malignancy in the female genital tract, preceded only by endometrial and cervical cancer. Both benign and malignant tumours occur in the ovaries.

ETIOPATHOGENESIS

Unlike the two other female genital cancers (cervix and endometrium), not much is known about the etiology of ovarian tumours. However, a few risk factors have been identified as under:

1. **Nulliparity** There is higher incidence of ovarian cancer in unmarried women and married women with low or no parity.

2. **Heredity** About 10% cases of ovarian cancer occur in women with family history of ovarian or breast cancer. Women with hereditary breast-ovarian cancer susceptibility have mutation in tumour suppressor *BRCA* genes. Interestingly, men in such families have an increased risk of prostate cancer.

3. **Complex genetic syndromes** Besides the above two main factors, several complex genetic syndromes are associated with ovarian tumours:
i) Lynch syndrome
ii) Peutz-Jeghers syndrome
iii) Gonadal dysgenesis
iv) Nevoid basal cell carcinoma.

CLINICAL FEATURES AND CLASSIFICATION

In general, benign ovarian tumours are more common, particularly in young women between the age of 20 and 40 years, and account for 80% of all ovarian neoplasms. Malignant tumours may be primary or metastatic, ovary being a common site for receiving metastases from various other cancers.

A simplified classification proposed by the WHO with minor modifications has been widely adopted. According to this classification, ovarian tumours arise from normally-occurring cellular components of the ovary. Five major groups have been described:

I. TUMOURS OF SURFACE EPITHELIUM (COMMON EPITHELIAL TUMOURS) (60-70%)
A. Serous tumours
  1. Serous cystadenoma

  2. Borderline serous tumour
  3. Serous cystadenocarcinoma
B. Mucinous tumours
  1. Mucinous cystadenoma
  2. Borderline mucinous tumour
  3. Mucinous cystadenocarcinoma
C. Endometrioid tumours
D. Clear cell (mesonephroid) tumours
E. Brenner tumours

II. GERM CELL TUMOURS (15-20%)
A. Teratomas
  1. Benign (mature, adult) teratoma
   • Benign cystic teratoma (dermoid cyst)
   • Benign solid teratoma
  2. Malignant (immature) teratoma
  3. Monodermal or specialised teratoma
   • Struma ovarii
   • Carcinoid tumour
B. Dysgerminoma
C. Endodermal sinus (yolk sac) tumour
D. Choriocarcinoma
E. Others (embryonal carcinoma, polyembryoma, mixed germ cell tumours)

III. SEX CORD-STROMAL TUMOURS (5-10%)
A. Granulosa-theca cell tumours
  1. Granulosa cell tumour
  2. Thecoma
  3. Fibroma
B. Sertoli-Leydig cell tumours (Androblastoma, arrhenoblastoma)
C. Gynandroblastoma

IV. MISCELLANEOUS TUMOURS
A. Lipid cell tumours
B. Gonadoblastoma

V. METASTATIC TUMOURS (5%)
A. Krukenberg tumour
B. Others

I. TUMOURS OF SURFACE EPITHELIUM (COMMON EPITHELIAL TUMOURS)

Tumours derived from the surface (coelomic) epithelium called common epithelial tumours form the largest group of ovarian tumours. This group constitutes about 60-70% of all ovarian neoplasms and 90% of malignant ovarian tumours. The common epithelial tumours are of 3 major types—*serous, mucinous* and *endometrioid,* though mixtures of these epithelia may occur in the same tumour.

  Depending upon the aggressiveness, the surface epithelial tumours are divided into 3 groups: *clearly benign, clearly malignant,* and *borderline* (or *atypical proliferating* or *low-grade) malignant tumours.* In general, the criteria for diagnosis of these 3 grades of aggressiveness are as follows:

1. Clearly benign tumours are lined by a single layer of well-oriented columnar epithelium. Papillary projections, if present, are covered by the same type of epithelium without any invasion into fibrovascular stromal stalk.

2. Clearly malignant tumours have anaplastic epithelial component, multilayering, loss of basal polarity and unquestionable stromal invasion. The prognosis of these tumours is very poor.

3. Borderline (atypical proliferating) tumours or tumours with low malignant potential have some morphological features of malignancy, apparent detachment of cellular clusters from their site of origin and essential absence of stromal invasion. This group has a much better prognosis than frankly malignant tumours of the ovary.

Serous tumours comprise the largest group constituting about 50% of all surface ovarian tumours and 40% of malignant ovarian tumours. About 60% of serous tumours are benign, 15% borderline and 25% malignant. Serous tumours occur most commonly in 2nd to 5th decades of life, the malignant forms being more frequent in later life.

Histogenesis of the serous tumours is by metaplasia from the surface (coelomic) epithelium or mesothelium which differentiates along tubal-type of epithelium.

G/A Benign, borderline and malignant serous tumours are large (above 5 cm in diameter) and spherical masses. Small masses are generally unilocular while the larger serous cysts are multiloculated similar to the mucinous variety, or may have one large loculus and many daughter loculi in its wall. These serous variants contain serous fluid rather than the viscid fluid of mucinous tumours. *Malignant serous tumours* may have solid areas in the cystic mass. Exophytic as well as intracystic papillary projections may be present in all grades of serous tumours but are more frequent in malignant tumours termed papillary serous cystadenocarcinomas.

M/E The features are as under:

1. Serous cystadenoma is characteristically lined by properly-oriented low columnar epithelium which is sometimes ciliated resembling tubal epithelium. Microscopic papillae may be found.

2. Borderline (atypical proliferating) serous tumour usually has stratification (2-3 layers) of benign serous type of epithelium. There is detachment of cell clusters from their site of origin and moderate features of malignancy but there is absence of stromal invasion.

3. Serous cystadenocarcinoma has multilayered malignant cells which show loss of polarity, presence of solid sheets of anaplastic epithelial cells and definite evidence of stromal invasion. Papillae formations are more frequent in malignant variety and may be associated with psammoma bodies.

MUCINOUS TUMOURS

Mucinous tumours are somewhat less common than serous tumours and constitute about 30% of all ovarian tumours. In mucinous tumours associated with mucinous ascites (i.e. *pseudomyxoma peritonei*), it is important to assess the state of appendix because mucinous tumours of ovary and appendix are clearly linked. As compared with serous tumours, mucinous tumours are more commonly unilateral. Benign mucinous tumours occur bilaterally in 5% of cases while vast majority of bilateral borderline and malignant mucinous tumours are metastatic to the ovaries. Bilateral mucinous adenocarcinoma of the ovary is invariably metastatic deposits to the ovary.

Histogenesis of mucinous tumours, in line with that of serous tumours, is by metaplasia from the coelomic epithelium that differentiates along endocervical type or intestinal type of mucosa.

G/A Mucinous tumours are much larger than serous tumours. They are smooth-surfaced cysts with characteristic multiloculations containing thick and viscid gelatinous fluid. Benign tumours generally have thin wall and septa dividing the loculi are also thin and often translucent, but malignant varieties usually have thickened areas.

M/E The features are as under:

1. Mucinous cystadenoma is lined by a single layer of these cells having basal nuclei and apical mucinous vacuoles. There is very little tendency to papillary proliferation of the epithelium.

2. Borderline (atypical proliferating) mucinous tumour is identified by the same histologic criteria as for borderline serous tumour i.e. stratification (usually 2-3 cell thick) of typical epithelium without stromal invasion.

3. Mucinous cystadenocarcinoma likewise is characterised by piling up of malignant epithelium, at places forming solid sheets, papillary formation, adenomatous pattern and infiltration into stroma with or without pools of mucin.

ENDOMETRIOID TUMOURS

Endometrioid tumours comprise about 5% of all ovarian tumours. Most of them are malignant accounting for about 20% of all ovarian cancers. They are called endometrioid carcinomas because of the close resemblance of histologic pattern to that of uterine endometrioid adenocarcinoma.

Histogenesis of these tumours in majority of cases is believed to be from ovarian coelomic epithelium differentiating towards endometrial type of epithelium.

G/A These tumours are partly solid and partly cystic and may have foci of haemorrhages, especially in benign variety.

M/E The endometrioid adenocarcinoma is distinguished from serous and mucinous carcinomas by typical glandular pattern that closely resembles that of uterine endometrioid adenocarcinoma.

CLEAR CELL (MESONEPHROID) TUMOURS

Clear cell (mesonephroid) tumours are almost always malignant and comprise about 5% of all ovarian cancers. They are termed clear cell or mesonephroid carcinomas because of the close histologic resemblance to renal adenocarcinoma.

G/A These tumours are large, usually unilateral, partly solid and partly cystic.

M/E Clear cell or mesonephroid carcinoma is characterised by tubules, glands, papillae, cysts and solid sheets of tumour cells resembling cells of renal adenocarcinoma.

BRENNER TUMOUR

Brenner tumours are uncommon and comprise about 2% of all ovarian tumours. They are characteristically solid ovarian tumours. Most Brenner tumours are benign. Rarely, borderline form is encountered called *proliferating Brenner tumour* while the one with carcinomatous change is termed *malignant Brenner tumour*.

Histogenesis of the tumour is from coelomic epithelium by metaplastic transformation into transitional epithelium (urothelium).

G/A Brenner tumour is typically solid, yellow-grey, firm mass of variable size.

M/E Brenner tumour consists of nests, masses and columns of epithelial cells, scattered in fibrous stroma of the ovary. These epithelial cells resemble urothelial cells which are ovoid in shape, having clear cytoplasm, vesicular nuclei with characteristic nuclear groove called 'coffee-bean' nuclei.

II. GERM CELL TUMOURS

Ovarian germ cell tumours arising from germ cells which produce the female gametes account for about 15-20% of all ovarian neoplasms. Nearly 95% of them are benign and occur chiefly in young females, vast majority of them being benign cystic teratomas (dermoid cysts). Most germ cell tumours of the ovaries have their counterparts in the testis. But their frequency differs from one site to the other. For instance, benign cystic teratoma or dermoid cyst so common in ovaries is extremely rare in the testis.

TERATOMAS

Teratomas are tumours composed of different types of tissues derived from the three germ cell layers—ectoderm, mesoderm and endoderm, in varying combinations. Cytogenetic studies have revealed that these tumours arise from a single germ cell (ovum) after its first meiotic division.

Teratomas are divided into 3 types:

MATURE (BENIGN) TERATOMA Vast majority of ovarian teratomas are benign and cystic and have the predominant ectodermal elements, often termed clinically as *dermoid cyst*. Infrequently, mature teratoma may be solid and benign and has to be distinguished from immature or malignant teratoma. Benign cystic teratomas are more frequent in young women during their active reproductive life.

G/A Benign cystic teratoma or dermoid cyst is characteristically a unilocular cyst, 10-15 cm in diameter, usually lined by the skin and hence its name. On sectioning, the cyst is filled with paste-like sebaceous secretions and desquamated keratin admixed with masses of hair. Generally, in one area of the cyst wall, a solid prominence is seen (Rokitansky's protuberance) where tissue elements such as tooth, bone, cartilage and various other odd tissues are present.

M/E The most prominent feature is the lining of the cyst wall by stratified squamous epithelium and its adnexal structures such as sebaceous glands, sweat glands and hair follicles. Though ectodermal derivatives are most prominent features, tissues of mesodermal and endodermal origin are also commonly present.

IMMATURE (MALIGNANT) TERATOMA Immature or malignant teratomas of the ovary are rare and account for approximately 0.2% of all ovarian tumours. They are predominantly solid tumours. They are more common in prepubertal adolescents and young women under 20 years of age.

G/A Malignant teratoma is a unilateral solid mass which on cut section shows characteristic variegated appearance revealing areas of haemorrhages, necrosis, tiny cysts and heterogeneous admixture of various tissue elements.

M/E Parts of the tumour may show mature tissues, while most of it is composed of immature tissues having an embryonic appearance. Immature tissue elements may differentiate towards cartilage, bone, glandular structures, neural tissue etc, and are distributed in spindle-shaped myxoid or undifferentiated sarcoma cells. An important factor in grading and determining the prognosis of immature teratoma is the relative amount of immature neural tissue.

MONODERMAL (SPECIALISED) TERATOMA Monodermal or highly specialised teratomas are rare and include 2 important examples.

◈ **Struma ovarii** It is a teratoma composed exclusively of thyroid tissue, recognisable grossly as well as microscopically. Most often, the tumour has the appearance of a follicular adenoma of the thyroid.

◈ **Carcinoid tumour** This is an ovarian teratoma arising from argentaffin cells of intestinal epithelium in the teratoma.

◈ **Struma-carcinoid** This is a rare combination of struma ovarii and ovarian carcinoid.

DYSGERMINOMA

Dysgerminoma is an ovarian counterpart of seminoma of the testes. Dysgerminomas comprise about 2% of all ovarian cancers. They occur most commonly in 2nd to 3rd decades. All dysgerminomas are malignant and are extremely radiosensitive.

G/A Dysgerminoma is a solid mass of variable size. Cut section of the tumour is grey-white to pink, lobulated, soft and fleshy with foci of haemorrhages and necrosis.

M/E Their structure is similar to that of seminoma of the testis. The tumour cells are arranged in diffuse sheets, islands and cords separated by scanty fibrous stroma. The tumour cells are uniform in appearance and large, with vesicular nuclei and clear cytoplasm rich in glycogen. The fibrous stroma generally contains lymphocytic infiltrate and sometimes may have sarcoid-like granulomas.

ENDODERMAL SINUS (YOLK SAC) TUMOUR

Endodermal sinus tumour or yolk sac tumour is the second most common germ cell tumour occurring most frequently in children and young women. More often, endodermal sinus tumour is found in combination with other germ cell tumours rather than in pure form. The tumour is rich in alphafetoprotein (AFP) and α-1-antitrypsin.

G/A The tumour is generally solid with areas of cystic degeneration.

M/E Like its testicular counterpart, the endodermal sinus tumour is characterised by the presence of papillary projections having a central blood vessel with perivascular layer of anaplastic embryonal germ cells. Such structures resemble the endodermal sinuses of the rat placenta (Schiller-Duval body) from which the tumour derives its name. It is common to find intracellular and extracelluar PAS-positive hyaline globules which are composed of AFP.

CHORIOCARCINOMA

Choriocarcinoma in females is of 2 types—*gestational and non-gestational*. Gestational choriocarcinoma of placental origin is more common. The patients are usually young girls under the age of 20 years.

M/E Ovarian choriocarcinoma is identical to gestational choriocarcinoma. Ovarian choriocarcinoma is more malignant than that of placental origin and disseminates widely via bloodstream to the lungs, liver, bone, brain and kidneys. The marker for both types of choriocarcinoma is hCG.

III. SEX CORD-STROMAL TUMOURS

GRANULOSA-THECA CELL TUMOURS

Granulosa-theca cell tumours comprise about 5% of all ovarian tumours. The group includes: pure granulosa cell tumours, pure thecomas, combination of granulosa-theca cell tumours and fibromas.

GRANULOSA CELL TUMOUR Pure granulosa cell tumours may occur at all ages. These tumours invade locally but occasionally may have more aggressive and malignant behaviour. Recurrences after surgical removal are common. Most granulosa cell tumours secrete oestrogen.

G/A Granulosa cell tumour is a small, solid, partly cystic and usually unilateral tumour. Cut section of solid areas is yellowish-brown.

M/E The granulosa cells are arranged in a variety of patterns including micro- and macrofollicular, trabecular, bands and diffuse sheets. The micro-follicular pattern is characterised by the presence of characteristic rosette-like structures, Call-Exner bodies, having central rounded pink mass surrounded by a circular row of granulosa cells.

THECOMA Pure thecomas are almost always benign. They occur more frequently in postmenopausal women. Thecomas are typically oestrogenic.

G/A Thecoma is a solid and firm mass, 5-10 cm in diameter. Cut section is yellowish.

M/E Thecoma consists of spindle-shaped theca cells of the ovary admixed with variable amount of hyalinised collagen. The cytoplasm of theca cells is lipid-rich and vacuolated which reacts with lipid stains.

GRANULOSA-THECA CELL TUMOUR Mixture of both granulosa and theca cell elements in the same ovarian tumour is seen in some cases with elaboration of oestrogen.

FIBROMA Fibromas of the ovary are more common and account for about 5% of all ovarian tumours. These tumours are hormonally inert but some of them are associated with pleural effusion and benign ascites termed Meig's syndrome.

G/A These tumours are large, firm and fibrous, usually unilateral masses.

M/E They are composed of spindle-shaped well-differentiated fibroblasts and collagen. Sometimes, combination of fibroma and thecoma is present called fibrothecoma.

SERTOLI-LEYDIG CELL TUMOURS (ANDROBLASTOMA, ARRHENOBLASTOMA)

Tumours containing Sertoli and Leydig cells in varying degree of maturation comprise Sertoli-Leydig cell tumours, also called androblastomas or arrhenoblastomas.

G/A Sertoli-Leydig cell tumour resembles a granulosa-theca cell tumour.

M/E Three histologic types are distinguished:
1. *Well-differentiated* androblastoma composed almost entirely of Sertoli cells or Leydig cells forming well-defined tubules.
2. *Tumours with intermediate differentiation* have a biphasic pattern with formation of solid sheets in which abortive tubules are present.
3. *Poorly-differentiated or sarcomatoid variety* is composed of spindle cells resembling sarcoma with interspersed scanty Leydig cells.

GYNANDROBLASTOMA

Gynandroblastoma is an extremely rare tumour in which there is combination of patterns of both granulosa-theca cell tumour and Sertoli-Leydig cell tumour. The term gynandroblastoma stands for combination of female *(gyn)* and male *(andro)*.

IV. MISCELLANEOUS TUMOURS

LIPID CELL TUMOURS There is a small group of ovarian tumours that appears as soft yellow or yellow-brown nodules which on histologic examination are composed of large lipid-laden cells. The examples of these tumours are: hilus cell tumours, adrenal rest tumours and luteomas. These tumours elaborate steroid hormones.

GONADOBLASTOMA This is a rare tumour occurring exclusively in dysgenetic gonads, more often in phenotypic females and in hermaphrodites. Dysfunctions include virilism, amenorrhoea and abnormal external genitalia.

V. METASTATIC TUMOURS

About 10% of ovarian cancers are secondary carcinomas. Metastasis may occur by lymphatic or haematogenous route but direct extension from adjacent organs (e.g. uterus, fallopian tube and sigmoid colon) too occurs frequently. Bilaterality of the tumour is the most helpful clue to diagnosis of metastatic tumour. Most common primary sites from where metastases to the ovaries are encountered are: carcinomas of the breast, genital tract, gastrointestinal tract (e.g. stomach, colon appendix, pancreas, biliary tract) and haematopoietic malignancies.

KRUKENBERG TUMOUR

Krukenberg tumour is a distinctive bilateral tumour metastatic to the ovaries by transcoelomic spread. The tumour is generally secondary to a gastric carcinoma but other primary sites where signet ring carcinomas occur (e.g. colon, appendix and breast) may also produce Krukenberg tumour in the ovary.

G/A Krukenberg tumour forms moderately large, rounded or kidney-shaped, firm, multinodular masses in both ovaries. Cut section shows grey-white to yellow, firm, fleshy tumour and may have areas of haemorrhage and necrosis.

M/E It is characterised by the presence of mucin-filled signet ring cells which may lie singly or in clusters. It is accompanied by cellular proliferation of ovarian stroma in a storiform pattern.

NORMAL STRUCTURE

At term, the normal placenta is blue red, rounded, flattened and discoid organ 15-20 cm in diameter and 2-4 cm thick. It weighs 400-600 gm or about one-sixth the weight of the newborn. The umbilical cord is about 50 cm long and contains two umbilical arteries and one umbilical vein attached at the foetal surface. The placenta is derived from both maternal and foetal tissues. The *maternal portion* of the placenta has irregular grooves dividing it into cotyledons which are composed of sheets of decidua basalis and remnants of blood vessels. The *foetal portion* of the placenta is composed of numerous functional units called chorionic villi and comprise the major part of placenta at term. The villi consist of a loose fibrovascular stromal core and a few phagocytic (Höffbauer's) cells. The villous core is covered by an inner layer of cytotrophoblast and outer layer of syncytiotrophoblast.

HYDATIDIFORM MOLE *(p. 741)*

The word 'hydatidiform' means *drop of water* and 'mole' for a *shapeless mass*. Hydatidiform mole is defined as an abnormal placenta characterised by 2 features:

i) Enlarged, oedematous and hydropic change of the chorionic villi which become vesicular.

ii) Variable amount of circumferential trophoblastic proliferation.

Most workers consider hydatidiform mole as a benign tumour of placental tissue with potential for developing into choriocarcinoma, while some authors have described mole as a degenerative lesion though capable of neoplastic change. The incidence of molar pregnancy is high in teenagers and in older women.

Hydatidiform mole may be non-invasive or invasive. Two types of non-invasive moles are distinguished.

◈ **Complete (classic) mole** by cytogenetic studies has been shown to be derived from the father (androgenesis) and has 46, XX or rarely 46, XY chromosomal pattern. Complete mole bears relationship to choriocarcinoma.

◈ **Partial mole** is mostly triploid (i.e. 69,XXY or 69,XXX) and rarely tetraploid. Partial mole rarely develops into choriocarcinoma.

Clinically, the condition appears in 4th-5th month of gestation and is characterised by increase in uterine size, vaginal bleeding and often with symptoms of toxaemia. Frequently, there is history of passage of grape-like masses per vaginum.

The single most significant *investigation* forming the mainstay of management is the serial determination of β-hCG which is elevated more in both blood and urine as compared with the levels in normal pregnancy. About 10% of patients with complete mole develop into invasive moles and 2.5% into choriocarcinoma.

COMPLETE (CLASSIC) MOLE *G/A* The uterus is enlarged and characteristically filled with grape-like vesicles up to 3 cm in diameter. The vesicles contain clear watery fluid. Rarely, a macerated foetus may be found.

M/E The features are quite typical:

i) Large, round, oedematous and acellular villi due to hydropic degeneration forming central cisterns.

ii) Decreased vascularity of villous stroma.

iii) Trophoblastic proliferation in the form of masses and sheets of both cytotrophoblast and syncytiotrophoblast, generally circumferential around the villi.

PARTIAL MOLE *G/A* The uterus is generally smaller than expected and contains some cystic villi, while part of the placenta appears normal. A foetus with multiple malformations is often present.

M/E Some of the villi show oedematous change while others are normal or even fibrotic. Trophoblastic proliferation is usually slight and focal.

INVASIVE (DESTRUCTIVE) MOLE (CHORIOADENOMA DESTRUENS)

G/A Invasive mole shows invasion of the molar tissue into the uterine wall which may be a source of haemorrhage.

M/E The lesion is benign and identical to classic mole but has potential for haemorrhage. It is always associated with persistent elevation of β-hCG levels.

CHORIOCARCINOMA *(p. 742)*

Gestational choriocarcinoma is a highly malignant and widely metastasising tumour of trophoblast. Approximately 50% of cases occur following hydatidiform mole, 25% following spontaneous abortion, 20% after an otherwise normal pregnancy, and 5% develop in an ectopic pregnancy.

Clinically, the most common complaint is vaginal bleeding following a normal or abnormal pregnancy. Occasionally, the patients present with metastases in the brain or lungs. The diagnosis is confirmed by demonstration of persistently high levels of β-hCG in the plasma and urine. Widespread haematogenous metastases are early and frequent in choriocarcinoma if not treated; these are found chiefly in the lungs, vagina, brain, liver and kidneys.

G/A The tumour appears as haemorrhagic, soft and fleshy mass. Sometimes, the tumour may be small, often like a blood clot, in the uterus.

M/E The characteristic features are:
i) Absence of identifiable villi.
ii) Masses and columns of highly anaplastic and bizarre cytotrophoblast and syncytiotrophoblast cells which are intermixed.
iii) Invariable presence of haemorrhages and necrosis.
iv) Invasion of the underlying myometrium and other structures, blood vessels and lymphatics.

Gestational choriocarcinoma and its metastases respond very well to chemotherapy while non-gestational choriocarcinoma is quite resistant to therapy and has worse prognosis. Death from choriocarcinoma is generally due to fatal haemorrhage in the CNS or lungs or from pulmonary insufficiency.

SELF ASSESSMENT

1. **The following vulval lesion can progress to vulval carcinoma:**
   A. Stromal polyp
   B. Papillary hidradenoma
   C. Squamous hyperplasia
   D. Lichen sclerosus
2. **High risk HPV types implicated in cervical intraepithelial lesions are:**
   A. 6 and 11
   B. 5 and 8
   C. 16 and 18
   D. 19 and 22
3. **The most common histologic type of cervical cancer is:**
   A. Well-differentiated keratinising squamous cell carcinoma
   B. Moderately-differentiated non-keratinising squamous cell carcinoma
   C. Small cell undifferentiated carcinoma
   D. Adenocarcinoma
4. **Arias-Stella reaction occurs in:**
   A. Ectopic tubal gestation only
   B. All ectopic gestations
   C. Uterine gestation
   D. Uterine as well as ectopic gestations
5. **Chocolate cyst of the ovary is:**
   A. Haemorrhagic corpus luteum
   B. Ruptured luteal cyst
   C. Endometriotic cyst
   D. Ruptured follicular cyst
6. **The malignant potential of atypical hyperplasia is:**
   A. About 5%
   B. About 25%
   C. About 50%
   D. About 75%
7. **Peak incidence of endometrial adenocarcinoma is in:**
   A. Reproductive years
   B. Premenopausal years
   C. Perimenopausal years
   D. Postmenopausal years

8. **The commonest site for endometriosis is:**
   - A. Hernial sacs
   - B. Vulva
   - C. Ovaries
   - D. Vagina
9. **Bilaterality of following ovarian tumours is most common:**
   - A. Benign serous tumours
   - B. Malignant serous tumours
   - C. Benign mucinous tumours
   - D. Brenner tumour
10. **The most common germ cell tumour of the ovary is:**
    - A. Dysgerminoma
    - B. Benign teratoma
    - C. Immature teratoma
    - D. Endodermal sinus tumour
11. **The most aggressive ovarian germ cell tumour is:**
    - A. Malignant teratoma
    - B. Embryonal carcinoma
    - C. Endodermal sinus tumour
    - D. Dysgerminoma
12. **Granulosa cell tumour is associated with following except:**
    - A. Endometrial hyperplasia
    - B. Endometrial adenocarcinoma
    - C. Endometrioid tumour
    - D. Fibrocystic change in breast
13. **Krukenberg tumour is bilateral metastatic tumour from the following primary sites except:**
    - A. Stomach
    - B. Colon
    - C. Breast
    - D. Endometrium
14. **The following trophoblastic tumour does not respond to chemotherapy:**
    - A. Complete mole
    - B. Invasive mole
    - C. Gestational choriocarcinoma
    - D. Ovarian choriocarcinoma
15. **Identifiable chorionic villi are present in the following tumours except:**
    - A. Complete mole
    - B. Partial mole
    - C. Invasive mole
    - D. Gestational choriocarcinoma
16. **According to the Bethesda system, the squamous intraepithelial lesions for the grades of cervical cytology are:**
    - A. Two
    - B. Three
    - C. Four
    - D. Five
17. **In the etiology of condyloma acuminatum, the most commonly implicated HPV types are:**
    - A. Types 1,2
    - B. Types 6, 11
    - C. Types 2,3,9
    - D. Types 16,18
18. **Protein product of HPV 16 is:**
    - A. E2
    - B. E5
    - C. E6
    - D. E7
19. **Upper age limit for cervical screening is:**
    - A. 50 years
    - B. 55 years
    - C. 60 years
    - D. None
20. **Characteristic mutation seen in endometrioid carcinoma is:**
    - A. PTEN
    - B. p53
    - C. Rb
    - D. K-ras
21. **Genetic syndrome associated with increased risk of ovarian cancer includes all except:**
    - A. Lynch syndrome
    - B. Peutz-Jegher's syndrome
    - C. Nevoid basal cell carcinoma
    - D. Turcot's syndrome
22. **Pick the odd one out:**
    - A. Sertoli-Leydig cell tumour
    - B. Androblastoma
    - C. Arrhenoblastoma
    - D. Gonadoblastoma

23. **A 60 years old woman reports to physician for progressive fatigue, loss of appetite and malaise for the last 2 months. An upper GI endoscopy reveals an ulcerative mass located along the lesser curvature. CT scan of the abdomen shows bilateral ovarian masses. Which of the following condition this patient is most likely to have?**
   A. Ampullary carcinoma
   B. Krukenberg tumour
   C. Serous adenocarcinoma of the ovary
   D. Endometrioid carcinoma of the uterine body

24. **Pap smear of a 30 years old woman is found to have atypical cells suggestive of HPV infection. Which of the following abnormalities describes the characteristic cytologic feature caused by HPV infection in Pap smear?**
   A. Acanthosis
   B. Parakeratosis
   C. Hyperkeratosis
   D. Koilocytosis

KEY

1 = C	2 = C	3 = B	4 = D	5 = C
6 = B	7 = D	8 = C	9 = B	10 = B
11 = B	12 = C	13 = D	14 = D	15 = D
16 = A	17 = B	18 = D	19 = D	20 = A
21 = D	22 = D	23 = B	24 = D	

23 The Breast

NORMAL STRUCTURE

Microanatomy of the breast reveals 2 types of tissue components: *epithelial* and *stromal*. In a fully-developed non-lactating female breast, the epithelial component comprises less than 10% of the total volume but is more significant pathologically since majority of lesions pertain to this portion of the breast.

EPITHELIAL COMPONENT The epithelial component of the breast consists of 2 major parts: terminal duct-lobular unit (TDLU) which performs the main secretory function during lactation, and large duct system which performs the function of collection and drainage of secretions; both are interconnected to each other.

The entire ductal-lobular epithelial system has bilayered lining: the inner epithelium with secretory and absorptive function, and an outer supporting myoepithelial lining, both having characteristic ultrastructure and immunoreactivity. The inner epithelium stains positive for epithelial membrane antigen (EMA) and lactalbumin while the myoepithelium is positive for smooth muscle actin (SMA) and S-100.

STROMAL COMPONENT The supportive stroma of the breast consists of variable amount of loose connective tissue and adipose tissue during different stages of reproductive life. The stromal tissue of the breast is present at 2 locations: intralobular and interlobular stroma.

NON-NEOPLASTIC CONDITIONS (p. 746)

INFLAMMATIONS (p. 746)

ACUTE MASTITIS AND BREAST ABSCESS

Acute pyogenic infection of the breast occurs chiefly during the first few weeks of lactation and sometimes by eczema of the nipples. Bacteria such as staphylococci and streptococci gain entry into the breast by development of cracks and fissures in the nipple. Initially a localised area of acute inflammation is produced which, if not effectively treated, may cause single or multiple breast abscesses.

GRANULOMATOUS MASTITIS

Although chronic non-specific mastitis is uncommon, chronic granulomatous inflammation in the breast may occur as a result of the following:

1. *Systemic non-infectious granulomatous disease* e.g. as part of systemic sarcoidosis, Wegener's granulomatosis.

2. *Infections* e.g. tuberculosis which is not so uncommon in developing countries like India and may be misdiagnosed clinically as breast cancer owing to axillary nodal involvement. Tubercle bacilli reach the breast by haematogenous, lymphatic or direct spread, usually from the lungs or pleura. Pathologically, typical caseating tubercles with discharging sinuses through the surface of the breast are found.

3. *Silicone breast implants* implanted on breast cancer patients after mastectomy or as breast augmentation cosmetic surgery may rupture or silicone may slowly leak into surrounding breast tissue.

4. *Idiopathic granulomatous mastitis* is an uncommon form of reaction around lobules and ducts in the absence of any known etiology. Exact

pathogenesis is not known but probably it is a form of hypersensitivity reaction to luminal secretion of the breast epithelium during lactation.

MAMMARY DUCT ECTASIA (PLASMA CELL MASTITIS)

Mammary duct ectasia is a condition in which one or more of the larger ducts of the breast are dilated and filled with inspissated secretions. These are associated with periductal and interstitial chronic inflammatory changes. Duct ectasia affects women in their 4th to 7th decades of life. The etiology of the condition remains unknown but it appears to begin with periductal inflammation followed by destruction of the elastic tissue to cause ectasia and periductal fibrosis.

G/A The condition appears as a single, poorly-defined indurated area in the breast with ropiness on the surface. Cut section shows dilated ducts containing cheesy inspissated secretions.

M/E The features are as under:
1. Dilated ducts with either necrotic or atrophic lining by flattened epithelium and lumen containing granular, amorphous, pink debris and foam cells.
2. Periductal and interstitial chronic inflammation, chiefly lymphocytes, histiocytes with multinucleate histiocytic giant cells. Sometimes, plasma cells are present in impressive numbers and the condition is then termed *plasma cell mastitis*.
3. Occasionally, there may be obliteration of the ducts by fibrous tissue and varying amount of inflammation and is termed *obliterative mastitis*.

FAT NECROSIS

Focal fat necrosis of an obese and pendulous breast followed by an inflammatory reaction is generally initiated by trauma. The condition presents as a well-defined mass with indurated appearance.

G/A The excised lump has central pale cystic area of necrosis.

M/E There is disruption of the regular pattern of lipocytes with formation of lipid-filled spaces surrounded by neutrophils, lymphocytes, plasma cells and histiocytes having foamy cytoplasm and frequent foreign body giant cell formation.

GALACTOCELE

A galactocele is cystic dilatation of one or more ducts occurring during lactation. The mammary duct is obstructed and dilated to form a thin-walled cyst filled with milky fluid.

FIBROCYSTIC CHANGE *(p. 746)*

Fibrocystic change is the most common benign breast condition producing vague 'lumpy' breast rather than palpable lump in the breast. Its incidence has been reported to range from 10-20% in adult women, most often between 3rd and 5th decades of life, with dramatic decline in its incidence after menopause suggesting the role of oestrogen in its pathogenesis.

As such, fibrocystic change of the female breast is a histologic entity characterised by following features:
i) Cystic dilatation of terminal ducts.
ii) Relative increase in inter- and intralobular fibrous tissue.
iii) Variable degree of epithelial proliferation in the terminal ducts.

It is important to identify the spectrum of histologic features by core needle biopsy or cytologic findings by FNAC in fibrocystic changes since only some subset of changes has an increased risk of development of breast cancer. Presently, the spectrum of histologic changes is divided into two clinicopathologically relevant groups:

A. NONPROLIFERATIVE FIBROCYSTIC CHANGES: SIMPLE FIBROCYSTIC CHANGE

Simple fibrocystic change most commonly includes 2 features—formation of cysts of varying size, and increase in fibrous stroma.

G/A The cysts are rarely solitary but are usually multifocal and bilateral. They vary from microcysts to 5-6 cm in diameter. The usual large cyst is rounded, translucent with bluish colour prior to opening (blue-dome cyst).

M/E Following 2 features are seen:

1. Cyst formation The cyst lining shows a variety of appearances. Often, the epithelium is flattened or atrophic. Frequently, there is apocrine change or apocrine metaplasia in the lining of the cyst resembling the cells of apocrine sweat glands.

2. Fibrosis There is increased fibrous stroma surrounding the cysts and variable degree of stromal lymphocytic infiltrate.

B. PROLIFERATIVE FIBROCYSTIC CHANGES: EPITHELIAL HYPERPLASIA AND SCLEROSING ADENOSIS

Proliferative fibrocystic change in the breasts includes 2 entities: epithelial hyperplasia and sclerosing adenosis.

EPITHELIAL HYPERPLASIA Epithelial hyperplasia or epitheliosis is defined as increase in the layers of epithelial cells over the basement membrane to three or more layers in the ducts *(ductal hyperplasia)* or lobules *(lobular hyperplasia)*. The latter condition, lobular hyperplasia, must be distinguished from adenosis (discussed separately) in which there is increase in the number of ductules or acini without any change in the number or type of cells lining them.

M/E Epithelial hyperplasia is characterised by epithelial proliferation to more than its normal double layer. In general, ductal hyperplasia is termed as *epithelial hyperplasia of usual type* and may show various grades of epithelial proliferations (mild, moderate and atypical) as under, while *lobular hyperplasia* involving the ductules or acini is always atypical.

1. Mild hyperplasia of ductal epithelium consists of at least three layers of cells above the basement membrane, present focally or evenly throughout the duct.

2. Moderate and florid hyperplasia of ductal type is associated with tendency to fill the ductal lumen with proliferated epithelium. Such epithelial proliferations into the lumina of ducts may be focal, forming papillary epithelial projections called *ductal papillomatosis,* or may be more extensive, termed *florid papillomatosis,* or may fill the ductal lumen leaving only small fenestrations in it.

3. Of all the ductal hyperplasias, **atypical ductal hyperplasia** is more ominous and has to be distinguished from intraductal carcinoma. The proliferated epithelial cells in the atypical ductal hyperplasia partially fill the duct lumen and produce irregular microglandular spaces or *cribriform pattern.*

4. Atypical lobular hyperplasia is closely related to lobular carcinoma *in situ* but differs from the latter in having cytologically atypical cells only in half of the ductules or acini.

SCLEROSING ADENOSIS Sclerosing adenosis is benign proliferation of small ductules or acini and intralobular fibrosis. The lesion may be present as diffusely scattered microscopic foci in the breast parenchyma, or may form an isolated palpable mass.

G/A The lesion may be coexistent with other components of fibrocystic disease, or may form an isolated mass which has hard cartilage-like consistency, resembling an infiltrating carcinoma.

M/E There is proliferation of ductules or acini and fibrous stromal overgrowth. The histologic appearance may superficially resemble infiltrating carcinoma but differs from the latter in having maintained lobular pattern.

PROGNOSTIC SIGNIFICANCE

1. *Simple fibrocystic change* or *nonproliferative fibrocystic changes* of fibrosis and cyst formation do not carry any increased risk of developing invasive breast cancer.

2. Identification of *general proliferative fibrocystic changes* are associated with 1.5 to 2 times increased risk for development of invasive breast cancer.

3. *Multifocal and bilateral proliferative changes* in the breast pose increased risk to both the breasts equally.

4. Within the group of proliferative fibrocystic changes, *atypical hyperplasia* in particular, carries 4 to 5 times increased risk to develop invasive breast cancer later. This risk is further more if there is a history of breast cancer in the family.

GYNAECOMASTIA (HYPERTROPHY OF MALE BREAST) (p. 748)

Unilateral or bilateral enlargement of the male breast is known as gynaecomastia. Since the male breast does not contain secretory lobules, the enlargement is mainly due to proliferation of ducts and increased periductal stroma. Gynaecomastia occurs in response to hormonal stimulation, mainly oestrogen. Such excessive oestrogenic activity in males is seen in young boys between 13 and 17 years of age *(pubertal gynaecomastia),* in men over 50 years *(senescent gynaecomastia).*

G/A One or both the male breasts are enlarged having smooth glistening white tissue.

M/E There are 2 main features:
1. Proliferation of branching ducts which display epithelial hyperplasia with formation of papillary projections at places.
2. Increased fibrous stroma with, myxoid appearance.

BREAST TUMOURS (p. 748)

FIBROADENOMA

Fibroadenoma or adenofibroma is a benign tumour of fibrous and epithelial elements. It is the most common benign tumour of the female breast. Though it can occur at any age during reproductive life, most patients are between 15 to 30 years of age. Clinically, fibroadenoma generally appears as a solitary, discrete, freely mobile nodule within the breast.

G/A Typical fibroadenoma is a small (2-4 cm diameter), solitary, well-encapsulated, spherical or discoid mass. The cut surface is firm, grey-white, slightly myxoid and may show slit-like spaces formed by compressed ducts. Less commonly, a fibroadenoma may be fairly large in size, up to 15 cm in diameter, and is called *giant fibroadenoma* but lacks the histologic features of cystosarcoma phyllodes.

M/E Fibrous tissue comprises most of a fibroadenoma. The arrangements between fibrous overgrowth and ducts may produce two types of patterns which may coexist in the same tumour.
◈ **Intracanalicular pattern** is one in which the stroma compresses the ducts so that they are reduced to slit-like clefts lined by ductal epithelium or may appear as cords of epithelial elements surrounding masses of fibrous stroma.
◈ **Pericanalicular pattern** is characterised by encircling masses of fibrous stroma around the patent or dilated ducts.

VARIANTS A few morphologic variants of fibroadenomas have been described:
1. Occasionally, the fibrous tissue element in the tumour is scanty, and the tumour is instead predominantly composed of closely-packed ductular or acinar proliferation and is termed *tubular adenoma.*
2. If an adenoma is composed of acini with secretory activity, it is called *lactating adenoma* seen during pregnancy or lactation.
3. *Juvenile fibroadenoma* is an uncommon variant of fibroadenoma which is larger and rapidly growing mass seen in adolescent girls but fortunately does not recur after excision.

PHYLLODES TUMOUR (CYSTOSARCOMA PHYLLODES) (p. 749)

Cystosarcoma phyllodes was the nomenclature given by Müller in 1838 to an uncommon bulky breast tumour with leaf-like gross appearance *(phyllodes*=leaf-like) having an aggressive clinical behaviour. Most patients are between 30 to 70 years of age. Local recurrences are much more frequent than metastases.

G/A The tumour is generally large, 10-15 cm in diameter, round to oval, bosselated, and less fully encapsulated than a fibroadenoma. The cut surface is grey-white with cystic cavities, areas of haemorrhages, necrosis and degenerative changes.

M/E The phyllodes tumour is composed of an extremely hypercellular stroma, accompanied by benign ductal structures. Thus, phyllodes tumour resembles fibroadenoma except for marked stromal overgrowth. The histologic criteria considered to distinguish benign, borderline and malignant categories of phyllodes tumour are based on following cellular features of stroma:

i) frequency of mitoses;
ii) cellular atypia;
iii) cellularity; and
iv) infiltrative margins.

About 20% of phyllodes tumours are histologically malignant and less than half of them may metastasise.

INTRADUCTAL PAPILLOMA *(p. 749)*

Intraductal papilloma is a benign papillary tumour occurring most commonly in a lactiferous duct or lactiferous sinus near the nipple. Clinically, it produces serous or serosanguineous nipple discharge. It is most common in 3rd and 4th decades of life.

G/A Intraductal papilloma is usually solitary, small, less than 1 cm in diameter, commonly located in the major mammary ducts close to the nipple. Less commonly, there are multiple papillomatosis which are more frequently related to a papillary carcinoma.

M/E An intraductal papilloma is characterised by multiple papillae having well-developed fibrovascular stalks attached to the ductal wall and covered by benign cuboidal epithelial cells supported by myoepithelial cells.

CARCINOMA OF THE BREAST *(p. 750)*

Cancer of the female breast is among the commonest of human cancers throughout the world. Its incidence varies in different countries. In the United States, carcinoma of the breast constitutes about 25% of all cancers in females. However, there has been some decline in mortality from the breast cancer in recent years in developed countries due to both early diagnosis and modern therapy.

Currently, emphasis is on early diagnosis by *triple technique*: palpation, mammography, and fine needle aspiration cytology (FNAC). Additional techniques such as stereotactic biopsy and frozen section are immensely valuable to the surgeon for immediate pathological diagnosis in doubtful cases.

RISK (EPIDEMIOLOGIC) FACTORS

1. **Geographic and racial factors** The incidence of breast cancer is about 4-6 times higher in developed countries (North America, North Europe, Australia), intermediate in Southern European and Latin American countries, and low in developing countries of Asia and Africa, with the notable exception of Japan.

2. **Family history** First-degree relatives (mother, sister, daughter) of women with breast cancer have 2 to 6-fold higher risk of development of breast cancer.

3. **Menstrual and obstetric history** Total length of menstrual life is directly related to increased risk.

4. **Fibrocystic change** Fibrocystic change, particularly when associated with atypical epithelial hyperplasia, has about 5-fold higher risk of developing breast cancer subsequently.

5. **Miscellaneous factors** These include:
i) Consumption of large amounts of animal fats, high calorie foods.
ii) Cigarette smoking.
iii) Alcohol consumption.
iv) Breast augmentation surgery.
v) High breast density.
vi) Exposure to ionising radiation during breast developement.

ETIOPATHOGENESIS

Overall, two major etiologic factors in pathogenesis of breast cancer are: hormonal and genetic.

1. HORMONAL FACTORS Breast cancer is a hormone-dependent disease. There is sufficient evidence to suggest that excess endogenous oestrogen or exogenously administered oestrogen for prolonged duration is an important factor in the development of breast cancer. Evidences in support of relationship of increased risk with oestrogen excess are as follows:

i) Women with prolonged reproductive life, with menarche setting in at an early age and menopause relatively late.
ii) Unmarried and nulliparous women than in married and multiparous women.
iii) Women with first childbirth at a late age (over 30 years).
iv) Lactation and breastfeeding reduces the risk.
v) Bilateral oophorectomy reduces the risk.
vi) Functioning ovarian tumours (e.g. granulosa cell tumour) which elaborate oestrogen are associated with increased incidence of breast cancer.
vii) Hormone replacement therapy (HRT) administered to postmenopausal women may result in increased risk of breast cancer.
viii) Long-term use of oral contraceptives containing balanced oestrogen-progesterone preparations do not pose increased risk.
ix) Men who have been treated with oestrogen for prostatic cancer have increased risk of developing cancer of the male breast.

2. GENETIC FACTORS About 10% breast cancers have been found to have inherited mutations. These mutations include the following.
a) *BRCA1* mutation
b) *BRCA 2 gene* mutation
   In *BRCA1* as well as *BRCA2*, both copies of the genes (homozygous state) must be inactivated for development of breast cancer.
c) *Mutation in p53 tumour suppressor gene*

GENERAL FEATURES AND CLASSIFICATION

Anatomically, upper outer quadrant is the site of tumour in half the breast cancers; followed in frequency by central portion, and equally in the remaining both lower and the upper inner quadrant.

Carcinoma of the breast arises from the ductal epithelium in 90% cases while the remaining 10% originate from the lobular epithelium. For variable period of time, the tumour cells remain confined within the ducts or lobules (non-invasive carcinoma) before they invade the breast stroma (invasive carcinoma). While only 2 types of *non-invasive carcinoma* have been described—intraductal carcinoma and lobular carcinoma *in situ*, there is a great variety of histological patterns of *invasive carcinoma breast* which have clinical correlations and prognostic implications as follows.

A. NON-INVASIVE *(IN SITU)* CARCINOMA
   1. Intraductal carcinoma
   2. Lobular carcinoma *in situ*
B. INVASIVE CARCINOMA
   1. Infiltrating (invasive) duct carcinoma-NOS (not otherwise specified) (80%)
   2. Infiltrating (invasive) lobular carcinoma (10%)
   3. Tubular (cribriform) carcinoma (6%)
   4. Medullary carcinoma (2%)

5. Colloid (mucinous) carcinoma (2%)
6. Other types: Papillary carcinoma, adenoid cystic (invasive cribriform) carcinoma, secretory (juvenile) carcinoma, inflammatory carcinoma, metaplastic carcinoma

C. PAGET'S DISEASE OF THE NIPPLE.

A. NON-INVASIVE *(IN SITU)* BREAST CARCINOMA

INTRADUCTAL CARCINOMA

Carcinoma *in situ* confined within the larger mammary ducts is called intraductal carcinoma. The tumour initially begins with atypical hyperplasia of ductal epithelium followed by filling of the duct with tumour cells. Clinically, it produces a palpable mass in 30-75% of cases and presence of nipple discharge in about 30% patients.

G/A The tumour may vary from a small poorly-defined focus to 3-5 cm diameter mass. On cut section, the involved area shows cystically dilated ducts containing cheesy necrotic material *(in comedo pattern),* or the intraductal tumour may be polypoid and friable resembling intraductal papilloma *(in papillary pattern).*

M/E The proliferating tumour cells within the ductal lumina may have 4 types of patterns in different combinations.
i) *Solid pattern* is characterised by filling and plugging of the ductal lumina with tumour cells.
ii) *Comedo pattern* is centrally placed necrotic debris surrounded by neoplastic cells in the duct.
iii) *Papillary pattern* has formation of intraductal papillary projections of tumour cells which lack a fibrovascular stalk so as to distinguish it from intra-ductal papilloma.
iv) *Cribriform pattern* is recognised by neat punched out fenestrations in the intraductal tumour.

LOBULAR CARCINOMA IN SITU

Lobular carcinoma *in situ* is not a palpable or grossly visible tumour. Patients of *in situ* lobular carcinoma treated with excisional biopsy alone develop invasive cancer of the ipsilateral breast in about 25% cases in 10 years as in intraductal carcinoma but, in addition, have a much higher incidence of developing a contralateral breast cancer (30%).

G/A No visible tumour is identified.

M/E *In situ* lobular carcinoma is characterised by filling up of terminal ducts and ductules or acini by rather uniform cells which are loosely cohesive and have small, rounded nuclei with indistinct cytoplasmic margins.

B. INVASIVE BREAST CARCINOMA

INFILTRATING (INVASIVE) DUCT CARCINOMA-NOS

Infiltrating duct carcinoma-NOS *(not otherwise specified)* is the classic breast cancer and is the most common histologic pattern accounting for 80% cases of breast cancer. Clinically, majority of infiltrating duct carcinomas have a hard consistency due to dense collagenous stroma (scirrhous carcinoma).

G/A The tumour is irregular, 1-5 cm in diameter, hard cartilage-like mass that cuts with a grating sound. The sectioned surface of the tumour is grey-white to yellowish with chalky streaks and often extends irregularly into the surrounding fat.

M/E As the name NOS suggests, the tumour is different from other special types in lacking a regular and uniform pattern throughout the lesion. A variety of histologic features commonly present are as under.
i) Anaplastic tumour cells forming solid nests, cords, poorly-formed glandular structures and some intraductal foci.
ii) Infiltration by these patterns of tumour cells into diffuse fibrous stroma and fat.

iii)   Invasion into perivascular and perineural spaces as well as lymphatic and vascular invasion.

INFILTRATING (INVASIVE) LOBULAR CARCINOMA

Invasive lobular carcinoma comprises about 10% of all breast cancers. This peculiar morphologic form differs from other invasive cancers in being more frequently bilateral; and within the same breast, it may have multicentric origin.

G/A   The appearance varies from a well-defined scirrhous mass to a poorly-defined area of induration that may remain undetected by inspection as well as on palpation.

M/E   There are 2 distinct features:

i)   **Pattern**   A characteristic single file (Indian file) linear arrangement of stromal infiltration by the tumour cells with very little tendency to gland formation is seen.

ii)   **Tumour cytology**   Individual tumour cells resemble cells of *in situ* lobular carcinoma. They are round and regular with very little pleomorphism and infrequent mitoses.

TUBULAR CARCINOMA

Tubular carcinoma comprises about 6% cases of invasive ductal carcinoma and has more favourable prognosis. These tumours are generally small (~1 cm diameter) ill-defined and gritty nodules.

M/E   The tumour is highly well-differentiated having following characteristics:
i) Pattern   The tumour is almost exclusively composed of tubules having angulated shape.
ii) Tumour cells   The tumour cells are regular and form a single layer in well-defined tubules.
iii) Stroma   Tubules are quite evenly distributed in dense fibrous stroma.

MEDULLARY CARCINOMA

Medullary carcinoma is a variant of ductal carcinoma and comprises about 2% of all breast cancers. The tumour has a significantly better prognosis than the usual infiltrating duct carcinoma, probably due to good host immune response in the form of lymphoid infiltrate in the tumour stroma.

G/A   The tumour is characterised by a large, well-circumscribed, rounded mass that is typically soft and fleshy or brain-like and hence the alternative name of 'encephaloid carcinoma'. Cut section shows areas of haemorrhages and necrosis.

M/E   Medullary carcinoma is characterised by 2 distinct features.

i)   **Tumour cells**   Sheets of large, pleomorphic tumour cells with abundant cytoplasm, large vesicular nuclei and many bizarre and atypical mitoses are diffusely spread in the scanty stroma.

ii)   **Stroma**   The loose connective tissue stroma is scanty and usually has a prominent lymphoid component as aggregates and infiltrate.

COLLOID (MUCINOUS) CARCINOMA

This pattern of breast cancer is seen in about 2% cases, occurs more frequently in older women and is slow-growing. Colloid carcinoma has better prognosis than the usual infiltrating duct carcinoma.

G/A   The tumour is usually a soft and gelatinous mass with well-demarcated borders.

M/E   Colloid carcinoma contains large amount of extracellular epithelial mucin and acini filled with mucin. Cuboidal to tall columnar tumour cells, some showing mucus vacuolation, are seen floating in large lakes of mucin.

1. Papillary carcinoma It is a rare variety of infiltrating duct carcinoma in which the stromal invasion is in the form of papillary structures.

2. Adenoid cystic carcinoma Adenoid cystic or invasive cribriform carcinoma is a unique histologic pattern of breast cancer in which there is stromal invasion by islands of cells having characteristic cribriform (fenestrated) appearance. The tumour has an excellent prognosis.

3. Secretory (Juvenile) carcinoma This pattern is found more frequently in children and young girls and has a better prognosis.

4. Inflammatory carcinoma Inflammatory carcinoma of the breast is a clinical entity and does not constitute a histological type. The term has been used for breast cancers in which there is redness, oedema, tenderness and rapid enlargement.

5. Metaplastic carcinoma Rarely, invasive ductal carcinomas, besides epithelial elements, may have various components of metaplastic alterations such as squamous metaplasia, cartilaginous and osseous metaplasia, or their combinations.

C. PAGET'S DISEASE OF THE NIPPLE

Paget's disease of the nipple is an eczematoid lesion of the nipple, often associated with an invasive or non-invasive ductal carcinoma of the underlying breast. The nipple bears a crusted, scaly and eczematoid lesion with a palpable subareolar mass in about half the cases. Most of the patients with palpable mass are found to have infiltrating duct carcinoma, while those with no palpable breast lump are usually subsequently found to have intraductal carcinoma.

G/A The skin of the nipple and areola is crusted, fissured and ulcerated with oozing of serosanguineous fluid from the erosions.

M/E The skin lesion is characterised by the presence of Paget's cells singly or in small clusters in the epidermis. These cells are larger than the epidermal cells, spherical, having hyperchromatic nuclei with cytoplasmic halo that stains positively with mucicarmine. In addition, the underlying breast contains invasive or non-invasive duct carcinoma which shows no obvious direct invasion of the skin of nipple.

GRADING, STAGING AND PROGNOSIS

Histologic grading and clinical staging of breast cancer determines the management and clinical course in these patients.

A. HISTOLOGIC GRADING The breast cancers are subdivided into various histologic grades depending upon the following parameters:

1. Histologic type of tumour Various microscopic types of breast cancer can be subdivided into 3 histologic grades:

i) *Non-metastasising*—Intraductal and lobular carcinoma *in situ*.

ii) *Less commonly metastasising*—Medullary, colloid, papillary, tubular, adenoid cystic (invasive cribriform), and secretory (juvenile) carcinomas.

iii) *Commonly metastasising*—Infiltrating duct, invasive lobular, and inflammatory carcinomas.

2. Microscopic grade Widely used system for microscopic grading of breast carcinoma is Nottingham modification of the Bloom-Richardson system. It is based on 3 features: i) tubule formation; ii) nuclear pleomorphism; and iii) mitotic count.

3. Tumour size There is generally an inverse relationship between diameter of primary breast cancer at the time of mastectomy and long-term survival.

4. Axillary lymph node metastasis More the number of regional lymph nodes involved, worse is the survival rate. Involvement of the lymph nodes from proximal to distal axilla (i.e. *level I*—superficial axilla, to *level III*—deep axilla) is directly correlated with the survival rate. In this regards, identification and dissection of sentinel lymph node followed by its histopathologic examination has attained immense prognostic value.

5. Oestrogen and progesterone receptors (ER/PR) Oestrogen is known to promote the breast cancer. Presence or absence of hormone receptors on the tumour cells can help in predicting the response of breast cancer to endocrine therapy. Accordingly, patients with high levels of ER and PR on breast tumour cells have a slightly better prognosis.

6. HER2/neu overexpression *HER2/neu* (also called *erbB2*), An individual having overexpression of *HER2/neu* by tumour cells is likely to respond to higher dose of herceptin therapy but is not related to other forms of chemotherapy.

7. DNA content Tumour cell subpopulations with aneuploid DNA content as evaluated by mitotic markers (e.g. *Ki-67*) or by flow cytometry have a worse prognosis than purely diploid tumours.

B. CLINICAL STAGING The American Joint Committee (AJC) on cancer staging has modified the TNM (primary *T*umour, *N*odal, and distant *M*etastasis) staging proposed by UICC (Union International for Control of Cancer).

Spread of breast cancer to axillary lymph nodes occurs early. Later, however, distant spread by lymphatic route to internal mammary lymphatics, mediastinal lymph nodes, supraclavicular lymph nodes, pleural lymph nodes and pleural lymphatics may occur. Common sites for haematogenous metastatic spread from breast cancer are the lungs, liver, bones, adrenals, brain and ovaries.

C. PROGNOSTIC FACTORS IN BREAST CANCER These prognostic factors are divided into following 3 groups:

1. Potentially pre-malignant lesions These conditions are as under:
i) *Atypical ductal hyperplasia* is associated with 4-5 times increased risk.
ii) *Clinging carcinoma* is a related lesion in the duct.
iii) *Fibroadenoma* is a long-term risk factor (after over 20 years).

2. Breast carcinoma *in situ* Following factors act as determinants:
i) *Ductal carcinoma in situ* (comedo and non-comedo subtypes) is diagnosed on the basis of three histologic features—nuclear grade, nuclear morphology and necrosis, while *lobular neoplasia* includes full spectrum of changes of lobular carcinoma *in situ* and atypical lobular hyperplasia.
ii) *Breast conservative therapy* is used more frequently nowadays in carcinoma *in situ* which requires consideration of three factors for management: *margins, extent of disease,* and *biological markers.*

3. Invasive breast cancer These can be broadly divided into 3 groups:
1. routine histopathology criteria;
2. hormone receptor status; and
3. biological indicators.
Overall, taking the most important parameter of node-positive or node-negative breast cancer, the prognosis varies— localised form of breast cancer without axillary lymph node involvement has a survival rate of 84% while survival rate falls to 56% with nodal metastases.

4. Molecular classification More recently, based on gene profiling of breast cancer by microarray, a molecular classification has been proposed. It takes into consideration patterns of gene expression by the breast cancer which may be one of the four types: luminal type A or B, *HER2/neu* type, basal-like type, and normal breast-like type. Out of all these, basal-like type has worst prognosis while luminal type A responds well to endocrine therapy and has good prognosis.

1. **Mammary duct ectasia is characterised by the following features <u>except</u>:**
   A. It affects women in 2nd to 3rd decade of life
   B. There are dilated ducts containing inspissated secretions
   C. There is periductal chronic inflammation
   D. There may be presence of multinucleate giant cells

2. **Out of the various epithelial hyperplasias in breast the most ominous is:**
   A. Papillary ductal hyperplasia
   B. Florid ductal papillomatosis
   C. Lobular hyperplasia
   D. Epithelial hyperplasia of usual type

3. **Tubular adenoma of breast is mainly composed of:**
   A. Closely-packed ductules
   B. Ductal epithelial hyperplasia
   C. Lobular hyperplasia
   D. Lactational hyperplasia

4. **Phyllodes tumour is distinguished from fibroadenoma by having:**
   A. More ductal hyperplasia
   B. Compressed ducts
   C. More cellular stroma
   D. More lobular hyperplasia

5. **Intraductal papilloma occurs most often in the following region:**
   A. Collecting ducts
   B. Lactiferous ducts
   C. Terminal ducts
   D. Acini

6. **Lobular carcinoma *in situ* has the following features <u>except</u>:**
   A. A palpable lump is generally present
   B. After excision, about 25% cases develop ipsilateral invasive cancer in 10 years
   C. There is a higher incidence of bilaterality
   D. The tumour cells are rather uniform and cohesive

7. **The following type of carcinoma of the breast is characterised by 'Indian file' pattern of tumour cells:**
   A. Infiltrating duct carcinoma
   B. Invasive lobular carcinoma
   C. Medullary carcinoma
   D. Tubular carcinoma

8. **The following type of breast carcinoma is seen in children:**
   A. Papillary carcinoma
   B. Adenoid cystic carcinoma
   C. Secretory carcinoma
   D. Metaplastic carcinoma

9. **Paget's cells in Paget's disease of the breast are malignant cells of following type:**
   A. Squamous cell carcinoma
   B. Basal cell carcinoma
   C. Melanoma
   D. Adenocarcinoma

10. **Patients of breast cancer having high levels of oestrogen receptors imply:**
    A. Patient has an anaplastic breast cancer
    B. Anti-oestrogen therapy will be helpful
    C. Patient has an oestrogen-secreting ovarian tumour
    D. Patient is likely to have poor prognosis

11. **Men who have mutated *BRCA 1* have increased risk of following cancer:**
    A. Male breast
    B. Germ cell tumours of testis
    C. Sex-cord-stromal tumour of testis
    D. Carcinoma of prostate

12. **What percentage of phyllodes tumours are malignant:**
    A. 10%
    B. 20%
    C. 30%
    D. 40%

13. **All are genetic mutations seen in breast cancer <u>except</u>:**
    A. BRCA-1　　　　　　　　　B. p53
    C. PTEN　　　　　　　　　　D. Rb

14. **All are true about medullary carcinoma breast <u>except</u>:**
    A. Worse prognosis than IDC
    B. Prominent lymphoid infiltrate
    C. Bizarre and atypical mitosis
    D. Soft and fleshy consistency

15. **Which of the following feature is <u>not</u> used in modified Bloom-Richardson grading system for breast cancer?**
    A. Tubule formation　　　　　B. Nuclear pleomorphosis
    C. Mitotic count　　　　　　　D. Tumour necrosis

16. **HER2/neu overexpression in breast cancer:**
    A. Is a bad prognostic marker
    B. Responds to herceptin therapy
    C. Responds to tamoxifen
    D. Is a serum marker for breast cancer

17. **A 60 years old woman complains of itching and scaling of the right breast nipple area, which on biopsy is confirmed as Paget's disease. On further work-up, a 2 cm in diameter palpable mass is noted under the skin of the nipple. Which of the following is likely to be an association?**
    A. Infiltrating ductal carcinoma
    B. Lobular carcinoma in situ
    C. Invasive lobular carcinoma
    D. Intraductal papilloma

18. **Which of the following is the most common location for extra-mammary Paget disease?**
    A. Uterus　　　　　　　　　　B. Cervix
    C. Vulva　　　　　　　　　　　D. Penis

KEY

1 = A	2 = C	3 = A	4 = C	5 = B
6 = A	7 = B	8 = C	9 = D	10 = B
11 = D	12 = B	13 = D	14 = A	15 = D
16 = B	17 = A	18 = C		

NORMAL STRUCTURE

The histology of normal skin shows some variation in different parts of the body. In general, it is composed of 2 layers, the epidermis and the dermis, which are separated by an irregular border. Cone-shaped dermal papillae extend upward into the epidermis forming peg-like *rete ridges* of the epidermis.

EPIDERMIS The epidermis is composed of the following 5 layers from base to the surface:
1. Basal cell layer (stratum germinatum)
2. Prickle cell layer (Stratum spinosum, Stratum malpighii)
3. Granular cell layer (Stratum granulosum)
4. Stratum lucidum
5. Horny layer (Stratum corneum)

Intraepidermal nerve endings are present in the form of *Merkel cells* which are touch receptors.

DERMIS The dermis consists of 2 parts—the superficial *pars papillaris* or *papillary dermis,* and the deeper *pars reticularis* or *reticular dermis.* The dermis is composed of fibrocollagenic tissue containing blood vessels, lymphatics and nerves. The specialised nerve endings present at some sites perform specific functions.

Besides these structures, the dermis contains cutaneous appendages or adnexal structures. These are sweat glands, sebaceous glands, hair follicles, arrectores pilorum and nails:

1.   SWEAT GLANDS   These are of 2 types—eccrine and apocrine.

i)   Eccrine glands   They are present all over the skin but are most numerous on the palms, soles and axillae.

ii)   Apocrine glands   Apocrine glands are encountered in some areas only—in the axillae, in the anogenital region, in the external ear as modified glands called ceruminous glands, in the eyelids as Moll's glands, and in the breast as mammary glands.

2.   SEBACEOUS (HOLOCRINE) GLANDS   Sebaceous glands are found everywhere on the skin except on the palms and soles.

3.   HAIR   The hair grows from the bottom of the follicle. It has, therefore, an intracutaneous portion present in the hair follicle and the shaft.

4.   ARRECTORES PILORI   These are small bundles of smooth muscle attached to each hair follicle.

5.   NAILS   The nails are thickenings of the deeper part of the stratum corneum that develop at specially modified portion of the skin called nail bed.

HISTOPATHOLOGIC TERMS

Acanthosis   Thickening of the epidermis due to hyperplasia of stratum malpighii.

Acantholysis   Loss of cohesion between epidermal cells with formation of intraepidermal space containing oedema fluid and detached epithelial cells.

Dyskeratosis   Abnormal development of epidermal cells resulting in rounded cells devoid of their prickles and having pyknotic nuclei.

Dyskeratosis is a feature of premalignant and malignant lesions and is rarely seen in benign conditions.

Hyperkeratosis Thickening of the horny layer.

Parakeratosis Abnormal keratinisation of the cells so that the horny layer contains nucleated keratinocytes rather than the normal non-nucleate keratin layer.

Spongiosis Intercellular oedema of the epidermis which may progress to vesicle formation in the epidermis.

Pigment incontinence Loss of melanin pigment from damaged basal cell layer so that the pigment accumulates in the melanophages in the dermis.

DERMATOSES *(p. 760)*

Dermatosis is a common term used for any skin disorder.

I. GENETIC DERMATOSES *(p. 760)*

1. ICHTHYOSIS Two important forms of ichthyosis are—
◈ **Ichthyosis vulgaris** is an autosomal dominant disorder. It is more common and appears a few months after birth as scaly lesions on the extensor surfaces of the extremities.
◈ **Sex-linked ichthyosis** is a sex-(X) linked recessive disorder. It begins shortly after birth and affects extensor as well as flexor surfaces but palms and hands are spared.

2. KERATOSIS PALMARIS *ET PLANTARIS* The condition occurs as both autosomal dominant and autosomal recessive forms. It mainly affects the palms and soles as localised or diffuse lesions.

3. XERODERMA PIGMENTOSUM This is an autosomal recessive disorder in which sun-exposed skin is more vulnerable to damage. The condition results from decreased ability to repair the sunlight-induced damage to DNA. Patients of xeroderma pigmentosum are more prone to develop various skin cancers like squamous cell carcinoma, basal cell carcinoma and melanocarcinoma.

M/E The changes include hyperkeratosis, thinning and atrophy of stratum malpighii, chronic inflammatory cell infiltrate in the dermis and irregular accumulation of melanin in the basal cell layer.

4. DARIER'S DISEASE (KERATOSIS FOLLICULARIS) The condition is either transmitted as autosomal dominant disorder or as a mutation. In typical cases, there is extensive papular eruption.

M/E The characteristic changes are hyperkeratosis, papillomatosis and dyskeratosis. Dyskeratosis results in the formation of *'corps ronds'* and *'grains'* and there is appearance of suprabasal clefts containing acantholytic cells. The dermis often shows chronic inflammatory cell infiltrate.

5. URTICARIA PIGMENTOSA Urticaria pigmentosa may occur as congenital form or may appear without any family history in the adolescents. Clinically, the condition presents as extensive pigmented macules.

M/E The epidermis is normal except for an increase in melanin pigmentation in the basal cell layer. The characteristic feature is the presence of numerous mast cells in the dermis.

6. ATAXIA TELANGIECTASIA An autosomal recessive disorder, ataxia appears in infancy, while telangiectasia appears in childhood. The lesions are located on the conjunctivae, cheeks, ears and neck.

M/E The papillary dermis shows numerous dilated blood vessels.

II. NON-INFECTIOUS INFLAMMATORY DERMATOSES *(p. 761)*

1. DERMATITIS (ECZEMA) The pathologic term dermatitis is synonymous with the clinical term eczema. Both refer to inflammatory response to a variety of agents acting on the skin from outside or from within the body such as chemicals and drugs, hypersensitivity to various antigens and haptens etc. Accordingly, clinical types such as contact dermatitis, atopic dermatitis, drug-induced dermatitis, photo-eczematous dermatitis and primary irritant dermatitis are described. However, irrespective of the clinical type of dermatitis, the histopathologic picture is similar.

M/E Dermatitis reaction may be acute, subacute or chronic:

◈ **Acute dermatitis** is characterised by considerable spongiosis (intercellular oedema) that may lead to formation of intraepidermal vesicles or bullae. The vesicles and bullae as well as the oedematous epidermis are permeated by acute inflammatory cells.

◈ **Subacute dermatitis** may follow acute dermatitis. Spongiosis and vesicles are smaller than in acute dermatitis. The epidermis shows moderate acanthosis and varying degree of parakeratosis in the horny layer with formation of surface crusts containing degenerated leucocytes, bacteria and fibrin. The dermis contains perivascular mononuclear infiltrate.

◈ **Chronic dermatitis** shows hyperkeratosis, parakeratosis and acanthosis with elongation of the rete ridges and broadened dermal papillae. The upper dermis shows perivascular chronic inflammatory infiltrate and fibrosis.

2. URTICARIA Urticaria or hives is the presence of transient, recurrent, pruritic wheals (i.e. raised erythematous areas of oedema). Hereditary angioneurotic oedema is an uncommon variant of urticaria in which there is recurrent oedema not only on the skin but also on the oral, laryngeal and gastrointestinal mucosa.

M/E There is dermal oedema and a perivascular mononuclear infiltrate. There is localised mast cell degranulation by sensitisation with specific IgE antibodies but no increase in dermal mast cells.

3. MILIARIA Miliaria is a condition in which there is cutaneous retention of sweat due to obstruction of sweat ducts. There are 2 types of miliaria:

◈ **Miliaria crystallina** occurs when there is obstruction of sweat duct within the stratum corneum. It occurs in areas of the skin exposed to sun or may occur during a febrile illness.

◈ **Miliaria rubra** occurs when there is obstruction of sweat ducts within the deeper layers of the epidermis. It is seen more often in areas of skin covered by clothes following profuse sweating and the lesions are itchy.

4. PANNICULITIS (ERYTHEMA NODOSUM AND ERYTHEMA INDURATUM) Panniculitis is inflammation of the subcutaneous fat. Panniculitis may be acute or chronic. Generally, panniculitis appears as nodular lesions, predominantly on the lower legs. The following types of panniculitis are described:

◈ **Erythema nodosum,** acute or chronic, is the most common form. The lesions consist of tender red nodules, 1-5 cm in diameter, seen more often on the anterior surface of the lower legs.

◈ **Erythema induratum** is a less common variety. The lesions are chronic, painless, slightly tender, recurrent and found on the calves of lower legs.

M/E The early lesions show necrotising vasculitis involving the blood vessels in the deep dermis and subcutis. In chronic stage, there is inflammatory infiltrate consisting of lymphocytes, histiocytes and multinucleate giant cells. The infiltrate is located in the septa separating the lobules of fat.

5. ACNE VULGARIS Acne vulgaris is a very common chronic inflammatory dermatosis found predominantly in adolescents in both sexes. The lesions are seen more commonly on the face, upper chest and upper back. The appearance of lesions around puberty is related to physiologic hormonal variations. The condition affects the hair follicle, the opening of which is blocked by keratin material resulting in formation of *comedones*.

M/E A comedone consists of keratinised cells, sebum and bacteria. The hair follicle containing a comedone is surrounded by lymphocytic infiltrate in papular acne, and neutrophilic infiltrate in pustular acne.

1.   **IMPETIGO**   Impetigo is a common superficial bacterial infection caused by staphylococci and streptococci. The lesions appear as vesico-pustules which may rupture and are followed by characteristic yellowish crusts.

M/E   The characteristic feature is the subcorneal pustule which is a collection of neutrophils under the stratum corneum. Often, a few acantholytic cells and gram-positive bacteria are found within the pustule. The upper dermis contains severe inflammatory reaction composed of neutrophils and lymphoid cells.

2.   **VERRUCAE (WARTS)**   Verrucae or warts are common viral lesions of the skin. They are caused by human papillomaviruses (HPV) that belong to papovirus group, a type of DNA oncogenic virus. More than 100 HPV types have been identified. But it must be appreciated that various types of HPVs produce not only different morphologic lesions but also have variable oncogenic potential. Depending upon the clinical appearance and location, they are classified into different types described below.

i)   **Verruca vulgaris** is the most common human wart, commonly caused by HPV-1 and 2. Occurring more commonly on the dorsal surfaces of hands and fingers.

ii)   **Verruca plana** on the other hand, is flat or slightly elevated wart, common on the face and dorsal surface of hands and is usually associated with HPV-10.

iii)   **Verruca planatairs or plantar warts** occur on the sole of the foot and is caused by HPV-1.

iv)   **Epidermodysplasia verruciformis** resembles verruca plana but differs by having familial occurrence with autosomal recessive inheritance. Epidermodysplasia verruciformis is of special clinical significance as it may undergo malignant change.

v)   **Condyloma acuminatum or venereal wart or anogenital wart** occurs on the penis, on the vulva and around the anus. They are commonly caused by HPV-6. The lesions appear as soft, papillary, cauliflower-like mass that may grow fairly large in size (giant condyloma acuminata).

M/E   Prototype of verruca is common viral wart having following features:
i)   Papillomatosis (papillary folds).
ii)   Acanthosis (hyperplasia of stratum malpighii) containing foci of vacuolated cells in the upper stratum malpighii.
iii)   Hyperkaratosis with parakeratosis.
iv)   Clumped keratohyaline granules in the granular cells in the valleys between adjacent papillae.
v)   Elongation of rete ridges with their lower tips bent inwards.
vi)   Virus-infected epidermal cells contain prominent vacuolation (koilo-cytosis) and keratohyaline granules of intracytoplasmic keratin aggregates.

3.   **MOLLUSCUM CONTAGIOSUM**   Molluscum contagiosum is a common self-limiting contagious lesion caused by a poxvirus which is a DNA virus. Clinically, the lesions are often multiple, discrete, waxy, papules, about 5 mm in diameter and are seen more frequently on the face and trunk.

M/E   Typical lesion consists of sharply circumscribed cup-like epidermal lesion growing down into the dermis. The proliferating epidermal cells contain the pathognomonic intracytoplasmic eosinophilic inclusion bodies called *molluscum bodies*. These bodies contain numerous viral particles.

4.   **VIRAL EXANTHEMATA**   Viral exanthemata are a group of contagious conditions in which the epidermal cells are destroyed by replicating viruses causing eruption or rash. There are predominantly two groups of viruses which may cause exanthem. These are: the *poxvirus group* (e.g. smallpox or variola, cowpox or vaccinia), and the *herpesvirus group* (e.g. chickenpox or varicella, herpes zoster or shingles, herpes simplex).

      Variola (smallpox) has been globally eradicated since 1978. The route of infection is via upper respiratory tract or mouth followed by viraemia and characteristic skin lesions. **Vaccinia (cowpox)** is primarily a disease of the teats and udders of cows but humans are infected by milking the infected animals. **Varicella (chickenpox)** and **herpes zoster (shingles)** are both caused by a common virus, varicella-zoster virus. **Herpes simplex,** caused by HSV-1, and another related herpetic infection, **herpes genitalis,** caused by HSV-2, are characterised by transmission by direct physical contact and prolonged latency.

M/E The characteristic feature of viral exanthemata is the formation of intra-epidermal vesicles or bullae due to cytopathic effects of viruses. In the early stage, there is proliferation of epidermal cells and formation of multinucleate giant cells. This is followed by intracellular oedema and ballooning degeneration that progresses on to rupture of the cells with eventual formation of vesicles or bullae.

5. SUPERFICIAL MYCOSES Superficial fungal infections of the skin are localised to stratum corneum. These include some of the common dermatophytes such as *Trichophyton rubrum* and *Pityrosporum*. Clinically, these fungal infections are labelled according to the region involved. These are as follows:

i) **Tinea capitis** occurring on the scalp, especially in children.

ii) **Tinea barbae** affecting the region of beard in adult males.

iii) **Tinea corporis** involving the body surface at all ages.

iv) **Tinea cruris** occurs most frequently in the region of groin in obese men, especially in hot weather.

v) **Tinea pedis** or 'athlete foot' is located in the web spaces between the toes.

vi) **Onychomycosis** shows disintegration of the nail substance.

vii) **Tinea versicolor** caused by *Malassezia furfur* generally affects the upper trunk.

M/E Fungal hyphae (or mycelia) and arthrospores of dermatophytes are present in the stratum corneum of skin, nails or hair. Hyphae may be septate or nonseptate. Special stains can be used to demonstrate the fungi. These are: *periodic acid-Schiff (PAS) reaction* which stains the fungi deep pink to red, and Grocott's *methenamine silver nitrate method* that stains fungi black.

IV. GRANULOMATOUS DISEASES *(p. 765)*

1. LUPUS VULGARIS The lesions of lupus vulgaris, the prototype of skin tuberculosis, are found most commonly on the head and neck, especially skin of the nose. They are yellowish-brown to reddish-brown tiny nodules (apple-jelly nodules).

M/E The nodules consist of well-defined tubercles lying in the upper dermis. They consist of accumulation of epithelioid cells surrounded by lymphoid cells. Caseation necrosis may be slight or absent. Langhans' and foreign body type of giant cells are often present. Tubercle bacilli are present in very small numbers that are hard to demonstrate by acid-fast staining.

2. CUTANEOUS SARCOIDOSIS Sarcoidosis is a systemic granulomatous disease of unknown etiology. The lesions appear in the lungs, skin, eyes, nose and lymph nodes. Cutaneous manifestations appear as presenting feature in about a quarter of patients and include erythema nodosum, or brown-red jelly-like papules or plaques with central clearing.

M/E Characteristic feature is the presence of non-caseating epithelioid cell granulomas having Langhans giant cells but having paucity of lymphocytes, also called 'naked granulomas'. Fibrinoid necrosis and presence of intracellular inclusions such as asteroid bodies are some other features which may be seen.

3. GRANULOMA ANNULARE The lesions of granuloma annulare are often numerous. The condition appears to have correlation with diabetes mellitus.

M/E The centre of the lesion shows a well-demarcated focus of complete collagen degeneration. These foci are surrounded by an infiltrate composed largely of histiocytes and some mononuclear inflammatory cells forming a palisade arrangement and are therefore also referred to as palisading granulomas.

V. CONNECTIVE TISSUE DERMATOSES (p. 765)

1. LUPUS ERYTHEMATOSUS Two types of lupus erythematosus are recognised—a chronic form, *discoid lupus erythematosus (DLE)* which is confined to the skin; and a systemic form, *systemic lupus erythematosus (SLE)* that has widespread visceral vascular lesions. The discoid variety is more common which is generally benign, while systemic form may be fatal, usually from renal involvement. The diagnosis is made on the basis of clinical, serologic and pathologic changes. The characteristic cutaneous lesions in DLE consist of well-defined erythematous discoid patches associated with scaling and atrophy and often limited to the face.

M/E The important features are:
i) Hyperkeratosis with keratotic plugging.
ii) Thinning and flattening of rete malpighii.
iii) Hydropic degeneration of basal layer.
iv) Patchy lymphoid infiltrate around cutaneous adnexal structures.
v) Upper dermis showing oedema, vasodilatation and extravasation of red cells.

Direct immunofluorescence reveals granular deposits of immunoglobulins, most commonly IgG and IgM, and components of complement on the basement membrane of the affected skin in both DLE and SLE. High serum titres of antinuclear antibodies and demonstration of LE cells are other notable features, especially in SLE.

2. SYSTEMIC SCLEROSIS (SCLERODERMA) Two types of systemic sclerosis or scleroderma are identified: a localised form called *morphea,* and a generalised form called *progressive systemic sclerosis.* A variant of progressive systemic sclerosis is *CREST syndrome.* (C = calcinosis, R = Raynaud's phenomenon, E = esophageal dismotility, S = sclerodactyly and T = telangiectasia). Morphea consists of lesions limited to the skin and subcutaneous tissue, while progressive systemic sclerosis consists of extensive involvement of the skin and the subcutaneous tissue and has visceral lesions too.

M/E There is thickening of the dermal collagen extending into the subcutaneous tissue. There is pronounced chronic inflammatory infiltrate in the affected area. The epidermis is often thin, devoid of rete ridges and adnexal structures, and there is hyalinised thickening of the walls of dermal arterioles and capillaries. Subcutaneous calcification may develop.

3. LICHEN SCLEROSUS *ET ATROPHICUS* This condition involves genital skin most frequently and is often the only site of involvement. It occurs in both sexes, more commonly in women than in men. It is termed *kraurosis vulvae* in women while the counterpart in men is referred to as *balanitis xerotica obliterans.*

M/E The characteristic features are:
i) Hyperkeratosis with follicular plugging.
ii) Thinning and atrophy of the epidermis.
iii) Hydropic degeneration of the basal layer.
iv) Upper dermis showing oedema and hyaline appearance of collagen.
v) Inflammatory infiltrate in mid-dermis.

VI. NON-INFECTIOUS BULLOUS DERMATOSES (p. 766)

1. PEMPHIGUS Pemphigus is an autoimmune bullous disease of the skin and mucosa which has 4 clinical and pathologic variants.

All forms of pemphigus have acantholysis as common histologic feature. Sera from these patients contain IgG antibodies to cement substance of skin and mucosa.

i) **Pemphigus vulgaris** is the most common type characterised by the development of flaccid bullae on the skin and oral mucosa. These bullae break easily leaving behind denuded surface.

M/E The bullae are suprabasal in location so that the basal layer remains attached to dermis like a row of tombstones. The bullous cavity contains serum and acantholytic epidermal cells.

ii) **Pemphigus vegetans** is an uncommon variant consisting of early lesions resembling pemphigus vulgaris.

M/E There is considerable acanthosis and papillomatosis. Intraepidermal abscesses composed almost entirely of eosinophils are diagnostic of pemphigus vegetans.

iii) **Pemphigus foliaceous** is characterised by quite superficial bullae which leave shallow zones of erythema and crust.

M/E Superficial subcorneal bullae are found which contain acantholytic epidermal cells.

iv) **Pemphigus erythematosus** is an early form of pemphigus foliaceous. The distribution of clinical lesions is similar to lupus erythematosus involving face.

M/E The picture is identical to that of pemphigus foliaceous.

2. **PEMPHIGOID** This is a form of bullous disease affecting skin or the mucous membranes. Three variants have been described—*localised form* occurring on the lower extremities; *vesicular form* consisting of small tense blisters; and *vegetating form* having verrucous vegetations found mainly in the axillae and groins.

M/E The characteristic distinguishing feature from pemphigus is the subepidermal location of the non-acantholytic bullae. With passage of time, there is some epidermal regeneration from the periphery at the floor of the bulla. The bullous cavity contains fibrin network and many mononuclear inflammatory cells and many eosinophils. Dermal changes seen in inflammatory bullae consist of infiltrate of mononuclear cells, a few eosinophils and neutrophils.

3. **DERMATITIS HERPETIFORMIS** Dermatitis herpetiformis is a form of chronic, pruritic, vesicular dermatosis. The lesions are found more commonly in males in 3rd to 4th decades of life. The disease has an association with gluten-sensitive enteropathy (coeliac disease). Both dermatitis herpetiformis and gluten-sensitive enteropathy respond to a gluten-free diet.

M/E The early lesions of dermatitis herpetiformis consist of neutrophilic micro-abscesses at the tips of papillae, producing separation or blister between the papillary dermis and the epidermis. The older blisters contain fair number of eosinophils causing confusion with bullous pemphigoid. Direct immunofluorescence shows granular deposits of IgA at the papillary tips in dermatitis herpetiformis.

4. **ERYTHEMA MULTIFORME** This is an acute, self-limiting but recurrent dermatosis. The condition occurs due to hypersensitivity to certain infections and drugs, and in many cases, it is idiopathic. As the name suggests, the lesions are *multiform* such as macular, papular, vesicular and bullous. Quite often, the lesions have symmetric involvement of the extremities. *Stevens-Johnson syndrome* is a severe, at times fatal, form of involvement of skin and mucous membranes of the mouth, conjunctivae, genital and perianal area.

M/E The features are as under:
i) *Early lesions* show oedema and lymphocytic infiltrate at the dermo-epidermal junction. The superficial dermis shows perivascular lymphocytic infiltrate.
ii) *Later stage* is associated with migration of lymphocytes upwards into the epidermis resulting in epidermal necrosis and blister formation.

1.   PSORIASIS   Psoriasis is a chronic inflammatory dermatosis that affects about 2% of the population. It usually appears first between the age of 15 and 30 years. As the scales are removed by gentle scrapping, fine bleeding points appear termed *Auspitz sign*. Commonly involved sites are the scalp, upper back, sacral region and extensor surfaces of the extremities, especially the knees and elbows.

M/E Fully-developed lesions show:

i)   Acanthosis with regular downgrowth of rete ridges to almost the same dermal level with thickening of their lower portion.

ii)   Elongation and oedema of the dermal papillae with broadening of their tips.

iii)   Suprapapillary thinning of stratum malpighii.

iv)   Absence of granular cell layer.

v)   Prominent parakeratosis.

vi)   Presence of Munro microabscesses in the parakeratotic horny layer is diagnostic of psoriasis.

2.   LICHEN PLANUS   Lichen planus is a chronic dermatosis characterised clinically by irregular, violaceous, shining, flat-topped, pruritic papules. The lesions are distributed symmetrically with sites of predilection being flexor surfaces of the wrists, forearms, legs and external genitalia. Buccal mucosa is also involved in many cases of lichen planus.

M/E The characteristic features are:

i)   Marked hyperkeratosis.

ii)   Focal hypergranulosis.

iii)   Irregular acanthosis with elongated saw-toothed rete ridges.

iv)   Liquefactive degeneration of the basal layer.

v)   A band-like dermal infiltrate of mononuclear cells, sharply demarcated at its lower border and closely hugging the basal layer.

VIII. METABOLIC DISEASES OF SKIN (p. 769)

Skin is involved in a variety of systemic metabolic derangements. The examples include the following:

1.   Amyloidosis (primary as well as secondary).
2.   Lipoid proteinosis is rare.
3.   Porphyria of various types.
4.   Calcinosis cutis
5.   Gout due to urate deposits or tophi.
6.   Ochronosis due to alkaptonuria.
7.   Mucinosis seen in myxoedema.
8.   Idiopathic haemochromatosis with skin pigmentation.

CALCINOSIS CUTIS   There are four types of calcification in the skin:

i)   **Metastatic calcinosis cutis** develops due to hypercalcaemia or hyper-phosphataemia.

ii)   **Dystrophic calcinosis cutis** results when there is deposition of calcium salts at damaged tissue.

iii)   **Idiopathic calcinosis cutis** resembles dystrophic type but is not associated with any underlying disease. A special manifestation of idiopathic calcinosis cutis is *tumoral calcinosis* in which there are large subcutaneous calcified masses, often accompanied by foreign body giant cell reaction. Calcium may discharge from the surface of the lesion. *Idiopathic calcinosis of the scrotum* consists of multiple asymptomatic nodules of the scrotal skin.

iv)   **Subepidermal calcified nodule** or *cutaneous calculus* is a single raised hard calcified nodule in the upper dermis.

TUMOURS AND TUMOUR-LIKE LESIONS (p. 770)

The skin is the largest organ of the body. Tumours and tumour-like lesions may arise from different components of the skin such as surface epidermis, epidermal appendages and dermal tissues. Each of these tissues may give rise to benign and malignant tumours as well as tumour-like lesions. Another group of tumours have their origin from elsewhere in the body but are cellular migrants to the skin.

I. TUMOURS AND CYSTS OF THE EPIDERMIS (p. 771)

A. BENIGN TUMOURS

1. SQUAMOUS PAPILLOMA Squamous papilloma is a benign epithelial tumour of the skin. Though considered by many authors to include common viral warts (verrucae) and condyloma acuminata, true squamous papillomas differ from these viral lesions. If these 'viral tumours' are excluded, squamous papilloma is a rare tumour.

M/E Squamous papillomas are characterised by hyperkeratosis, acanthosis with elongation of rete ridges and papillomatosis.

2. SEBORRHEIC KERATOSIS Seborrheic keratosis is a very common lesion in middle-aged adults. There may be only one lesion, but more often these are many. The common locations are trunk and face.

M/E The pathognomonic feature is a sharply-demarcated exophytic tumour overlying a straight line from the normal epidermis at one end of the tumour to the normal epidermis at the other end. The other features are papillomatosis, hyperkeratosis and acanthosis as seen in squamous cell papillomas.

3. FIBROEPITHELIAL POLYPS Also known by other names such as 'skin tags', 'acrochordons' and 'soft fibromas', these are the most common cutaneous lesions. They are often multiple, soft, small (a few mm in size), bag-like tumours commonly seen on the neck, trunk and axillae.

M/E The tumours are composed of loosely-arranged fibrovascular cores with overlying hyperplastic epidermis.

B. EPITHELIAL CYSTS

1. EPIDERMAL CYST These intradermal or subcutaneous cysts, commonly called sebaceous cysts, are common and may occur spontaneously or due to implantation of the epidermis into the dermis or subcutis (implantation cysts). Most frequent sites are the skin of face, scalp, neck and trunk.

M/E Epidermal cysts have a cyst wall composed of true epidermis with laminated layers of keratin. Rupture of the cyst may incite foreign body giant cell inflammatory reaction in the wall.

2. PILAR (TRICHILEMMAL, SEBACEOUS) CYST These cysts clinically resemble epidermal cysts but occur more frequently on the scalp and are less common than the epidermal cysts.

M/E The cyst wall is composed of palisading squamous epithelial cells having abruptly keratinised layer without an intervening granular cell layer. These squamous cells undergo degeneration towards the cyst cavity.

3. DERMOID CYST These are subcutaneous cysts often present since birth. Dermoid cysts are more common on the face, along the lines of embryonic closure.

M/E The cyst wall contains epidermis as well as appendages such as hair follicles, sebaceous glands and sweat glands.

4. STEATOCYSTOMA MULTIPLEX This is an inherited autosomal dominant disorder having multiple cystic nodules, 1-3 cm in size. They are more common in the axillae, sternum and arms.

M/E The cyst walls are composed of several layers of epithelial cells and contain lobules of sebaceous glands in the cyst wall.

C. PRE-MALIGNANT LESIONS

1. SOLAR KERATOSIS (ACTINIC KERATOSIS, SENILE KERATOSIS) Solar (sun-induced) or actinic (induced by a variety of rays) keratoses are multiple lesions occurring in sun-exposed areas of the skin in fair-skinned elderly people. Similar lesions may be induced by exposure to ionising radiation, hydrocarbons and arsenicals. The condition is considered to be a forerunner of invasive squamous cell and/or basal cell carcinoma.

M/E The features are:
i) Considerable hyperkeratosis.
ii) Marked acanthosis.
iii) Dyskeratosis and dysplasia of the epidermal cells showing features such as hyperchromatism, loss of polarity, pleomorphism and increased number of mitotic figures.
iv) Non-specific chronic inflammatory cell infiltrate in the upper dermis.

2. BOWEN'S DISEASE Bowen's disease is also a carcinoma *in situ* of the entire epidermis but differs from solar keratosis in having solitary lesion often that may occur on sun-exposed as well as sun-unexposed skin. The condition may occur anywhere on the skin but is found more often on the trunk, buttocks and extremities.

M/E The lesions show:
i) Marked hyperkeratosis.
ii) Pronounced parakeratosis.
iii) Marked epidermal hyperplasia with disappearance of dermal papillae.
iv) Scattered bizarre dyskeratotic cells distributed throughout the epidermis.

3. XERODERMA PIGMENTOSUM This condition is a hypersensitivity of the skin to sunlight that is determined by a recessive gene. The disorder may lead to multiple malignancies of the skin such as basal cell carcinoma, squamous cell carcinoma and malignant melanoma.

D. MALIGNANT TUMOURS

1. SQUAMOUS CELL CARCINOMA Two important factors in the pathogenesis of squmaous cell carcinoma are: *prolonged sun exposure* and *immunosuppression*. In such cases, DNA damage is induced followed by *p53* mutation and other events leading to dysregulation of signaling pathway. Various predisposing conditions include the following:
i) Xeroderma pigmentosum
ii) Epidermodysplasia verruciformis induced by HPV
iii) Solar keratosis
iv) Chronic inflammatory conditions e.g. chronic ulcers and draining osteomyelitis
v) Old burn scars (Marjolin's ulcers)
vi) Chemical burns
vii) Psoriasis
viii) HIV infection
ix) Ionising radiation
x) Industrial carcinogens (coal tars, oils etc)
xi) In the case of cancer of oral cavity, chewing betel nuts and tobacco.

Cancer of scrotal skin in chimney-sweeps was the first cancer in which an occupational carcinogen (soot) was implicated. *'Kangari cancer'* of the skin of inner side of thigh and lower abdomen common in natives of Kashmir is another example of skin cancer due to chronic irritation (*Kangari* is an earthenware pot containing glowing charcoal embers used by Kashmiris close to their abdomen to keep them warm).

Squamous cell carcinoma may arise on any part of the skin and mucous membranes lined by squamous epithelium. Most common locations are the face, pinna of the ears, back of hands and mucocutaneous junctions such as on the lips, anal canal and glans penis.

G/A It shows one of the following 2 patterns:
i) More commonly, an *ulcerated growth* with elevated and indurated margin is seen.
ii) Less often, a raised *fungating or polypoid verrucous* lesion without ulceration is found.

M/E It is characterised by following features:

i) There is irregular downward proliferation of epidermal cells into the dermis.

ii) Depending upon the grade of malignancy, the masses of epidermal cells show atypical features such as variation in cell size and shape, nuclear hyperchromatism, absence of intercellular bridges, individual cell keratinisation and occurrence of atypical mitotic figures.

iii) Better-differentiated squamous carcinomas have whorled arrangement of malignant squamous cells forming horn pearls. The centres of these horn pearls may contain laminated, keratin material.

iv) *Verrucous carcinoma* (Ackerman tumour) is a low-grade variant located most commonly in oral cavity.

It is customary with pathologists to label squamous cell carcinomas with descriptive terms such as: well-differentiated, moderately-differentiated, undifferentiated, keratinising, non-keratinising, spindle cell type etc.

2. BASAL CELL CARCINOMA (RODENT ULCER) Typically, the basal cell carcinoma is a locally invasive, slow-growing tumour of middle-aged that rarely metastasises. It occurs exclusively on hairy skin, the most common location (90%) being the face, usually above a line from the lobe of the ear to the corner of the mouth.

Following conditions predispose an individual to develop basal cell carcinoma:

i) Light-skinned people who have little melanin.

ii) Prolonged exposure to strong sunlight like in those living in Australia and New Zealand.

iii) Inherited defect in DNA repair mechanism in xeroderma pigmentosum.

iv) *Nevoid basal cell carcinoma syndrome* It is an autosomal dominant condition in which multiple basal cell carcinomas appear at a young age (under 20 years).

G/A The most common pattern is a nodulo-ulcerative basal cell carcinoma in which a slow-growing small nodule undergoes central ulceration with pearly, rolled margins. The tumour enlarges in size by burrowing and by destroying the tissues locally like a rodent and hence the name 'rodent ulcer'.

M/E The most characteristic feature is the proliferation of basaloid cells (resembling basal layer of epidermis). A variety of patterns of these cells may be seen: solid masses, masses of pigmented cells, strands and nests of tumour cells in morphea pattern, keratotic masses, cystic change with sebaceous differentiation, and adenoid pattern with apocrine or eccrine differentiation.

3. METATYPICAL CARCINOMA (BASOSQUAMOUS CELL CARCI-NOMA) Metatypical or basosquamous cell carcinoma is the term used for a tumour in which the cell type and arrangement of cells cause difficulty in deciding between basal cell carcinoma and squamous cell carcinoma.

II. ADNEXAL (APPENDAGEAL) TUMOURS (p. 776)

A. TUMOURS OF HAIR FOLLICLE

1. TRICHOEPITHELIOMA (BROOKE'S TUMOUR) This tumour may occur as a solitary lesion or as multiple inherited lesions, predominantly on the face, scalp and neck.

M/E The tumour is often circumscribed. The most characteristic histologic feature is the presence of multiple horn cysts having keratinised centre and surrounded by basophilic cells resembling basal cells. These horn cysts simulate abortive pilar structures which are interconnected by epithelial tracts.

2. PILOMATRICOMA (CALCIFYING EPITHELIOMA OF MALHERBE) Pilomatricoma usually occurs as a solitary lesion, more often on the face and upper extremities. It may be seen at any age.

M/E The circumscribed tumour is located in deeper dermis and subcutis. The masses of tumour cells embedded in cellular stroma characteristically consist of 2 types of cells: the *peripheral basophilic cells* resembling hair matrix cells, and the *inner shadow cells* having central unstained shadow in place of the lost nucleus.

B. TUMOURS OF SEBACEOUS GLANDS

1.   NAEVUS SEBACEUS   Naevus sebaceus of Jadassohn occurs mainly on the scalp or face as a solitary lesion that may be present at birth. Initially, the lesion appears as a hairless plaque, but later it becomes verrucous and nodular.

M/E   Naevus sebaceus is characterised by hyperplasia of immature sebaceous glands and pilar structures. The overlying epidermis shows papillary acanthosis.

2.   SEBACEOUS ADENOMA   Sebaceous adenoma occurs in middle-aged persons, most commonly on the face.

M/E   It is sharply demarcated from the surrounding tissue. The tumour is composed of irregular lobules of incompletely differentiated sebaceous glands.

3.   SEBACEOUS CARCINOMA   Sebaceous carcinoma is a rare tumour that may occur anywhere in the body except the palms and soles.

M/E   The tumour is composed of variable-sized lobules of poorly-differentiated cells containing some sebaceous cells. The tumour cells show marked cytologic atypia such as pleomorphism and hyperchromasia.

C.   TUMOURS OF SWEAT GLANDS

1.   ECCRINE TUMOURS   Depending upon the portion of eccrine sweat gland from which the tumour takes origin, the eccrine tumours are of 3 types:
i)   arising from intraepidermal portion of the duct e.g. eccrine poroma;
ii)   arising from intradermal portion of the duct e.g. hidradenoma; and
iii) arising from secretory coils e.g. eccrine spiradenoma.

◈   **Eccrine poroma**   This tumour arises from intraepidermal portion of the sweat gland duct. The tumour is found more commonly on the sole and hands.

M/E   It consists of tumour cells arising from the lower portion of the epidermis and extending downward into dermis as broad anastomosing bands.

◈   **Eccrine hidradenoma**   Hidradenoma originates from the intradermal portion of the eccrine sweat duct. The tumour may occur anywhere in the body.

M/E   Hidradenoma consists of solid masses and cords of tumour cells which may have an occasional duct-like structure containing mucin.

◈   **Eccrine spiradenoma**   This is found as a solitary, painful, circumscribed nodule in the dermis.

M/E   The tumour consists of lobules which are surrounded by a thin capsule. The tumour lobules contain 2 types of epithelial cells like in the secretory coils of the eccrine sweat gland. Peripheral cells are small with dark nuclei, while the centre of lobules contains large cells with pale nuclei.

2.   APOCRINE TUMOURS   Two common examples are papillary hidradenoma and cylindroma.

◈   **Papillary hidradenoma**   Papillary hidradenoma or hidradenoma papilliferum is usually located as a small lesion commonly in women in the skin of the anogenital area.

M/E   It is a circumscribed tumour in the dermis under a normal epidermis. Papillary hidradenoma represents an adenoma with apocrine differentiation and containing papillary, tubular and cystic structures.

◈   **Cylindroma**   Also called as 'turban tumour' due to its common location on the scalp, cylindroma may occur as both solitary and multiple lesions.

M/E The tumour is composed of irregular islands of tumour cells creating a pattern resembling jigsaw puzzle. The islands are surrounded by a hyaline sheath. The tumour cells comprising the islands consist of 2 types of epithelial cells: *peripheral small cells* with dark nuclei, and *inner large cells* with light staining nuclei.

3. SWEAT GLAND CARCINOMA Rarely, the eccrine and apocrine gland tumours described above may turn malignant.

III. MELANOCYTIC TUMOURS *(p. 777)*

Melanocytic tumours may arise from one of the three cell types: naevus cells, epidermal melanocytes and dermal melanocytes.

◈ Benign tumours originating from *naevus cells* are called naevocellular naevi.

◈ The examples of benign tumours *arising from epidermal melanocytes* are lentigo, freckles, pigmentation associated with Albright's syndrome and *café-au-lait* spots of neurofibromatosis.

◈ Benign tumours *derived from dermal melanocytes* are Mongolian spots, naevi of Ota and of Ito and the blue naevus.

◈ *Malignant melanoma* is the malignant counterpart of melanocytic tumours.

The important examples amongst these are described below.

1. NAEVOCELLULAR NAEVI Pigmented naevi or moles are extremely common lesions on the skin of most individuals. They are often flat or slightly elevated lesions; rarely they may be papillomatous or pedunculated.

M/E Irrespective of the histologic types, all naevocellular naevi are composed of 'naevus cells' which are actually identical to melanocytes but differ from melanocytes in being arranged in clusters or nests. Naevus cells are cuboidal or oval in shape with homogeneous cytoplasm and contain large round or oval nucleus. Melanin pigment is abundant in the naevus cells present in the lower epidermis and upper dermis, but the cells in the mid-dermis and lower dermis hardly contain any melanin.

The important *histological variants* of naevi are as under:

i) Lentigo is the replacement of the basal layer of the epidermis by melanocytes.

ii) Junctional naevus is the one in which the naevus cells lie at the epidermal-dermal junction.

iii) Compound naevus is the commonest type of pigmented naevus. These lesions, in addition to the junctional activity as in junctional naevi, show nests of naevus cells in the dermis to a variable depth.

iv) Intradermal naevus shows slight or no junctional activity. The lesion is mainly located in the upper dermis as nests and cords of naevus cells.

v) Spindle cell (epithelioid) naevus or juvenile melanoma is a compound naevus with junctional activity. The naevus cells are, however, elongated and epithelioid in appearance which may or may not contain melanin.

vi) Blue naevus is characterised by dendritic spindle naevus cells rather than the usual rounded or cuboidal naevus cells.

vii) Dysplastic naevi are certain atypical naevi which have increased risk of progression to malignant melanoma. These lesions are larger than the usual acquired naevi, are often multiple, and appear as flat macules to slightly elevated plaques with irregular borders and variable pigmentation.

2. MALIGNANT MELANOMA Malignant melanoma or melanocarcinoma arising from melanocytes is one of the most rapidly spreading malignant tumour of the skin that can occur at all ages. The etiology is unknown but there is role of excessive exposure of white skin to sunlight e.g. higher incidence in New Zealand and Australia where sun exposure in high. Besides the skin, melanomas may occur at various other sites such as oral and anogenital mucosa, oesophagus, conjunctiva, orbit and leptomeninges.

Some high risk factors associated with increased incidence of malignant melanoma are as under:

i) Persistent change in appearance of a mole.

ii)   Presence of pre-existing naevus (especially dysplastic naevus).
iii)   Family history of melanoma in a patient of atypical mole.
iii)   Higher age of the patient.
iv)   More than 50 moles 2 mm or more in diameter.

Malignant melanoma can be differentiated from benign pigmented lesions by subtle features; the dermatologists term this as ABCD of melanoma (acronym for Asymmetry, Border irregularity, Colour change and Diameter >6 mm).

G/A Depending upon the clinical course and prognosis, cutaneous malignant melanomas are of the following 5 types:

i) Lentigo maligna melanoma This often develops from a pre-existing lentigo. It is essentially a malignant melanoma *in situ*. It is slow-growing and has good prognosis.

ii) Superficial spreading melanoma This is a slightly elevated lesion with variegated colour and ulcerated surface. It often develops from a superficial spreading melanoma *in situ* in 5 to 7 years. The prognosis is worse than for lentigo maligna melanoma.

iii) Acral lentigenous melanoma This occurs more commonly on the soles, palms and mucosal surfaces. The prognosis is worse than that of superficial spreading melanoma.

iv) Nodular melanoma This often appears as an elevated and deeply pigmented nodule that grows rapidly and undergoes ulceration. This variant carries the worst prognosis.

v) Desmoplastic melanoma In this variant, the tumour has a fibrotic stroma, neural invasion and frequent local recurrences.

M/E Irrespective of the type, following features are seen:

i) Origin The malignant melanoma, whether arising from a pre-existing naevus or starting *de novo,* has marked junctional activity at the epidermo-dermal junction and grows downward into the dermis.

ii) Tumour cells The malignant melanoma cells are usually larger than the naevus cells. They may be epithelioid or spindle-shaped, the former being more common. The tumour cells have amphophilic cytoplasm and large, pleomorphic nuclei with conspicuous nucleoli. These tumour cells may be arranged in various patterns such as solid masses, sheets, island, alveoli etc.

iii) Melanin Melanin pigment may be present (melanotic) or absent (amelanotic melanoma) without any prognostic influence. The pigment, if present, tends to be in the form of uniform fine granules. Immuno-histochemically, melanoma cells are positive for HMB-45 (most specific), S-100 and Melan-A.

iv) Inflammatory infiltrate Some amount of inflammatory infiltrate is present in the invasive melanomas.

STAGING AND PROGNOSIS Depending upon the depth of invasion into the dermis, *Clark* has described following 5 levels:
Level I: Malignant melanoma cells confined to the epidermis and its appendages.
Level II: Extension into the papillary dermis.
Level III: Extension of tumour cells upto the interface between papillary and reticular dermis.
Level IV: Invasion of reticular dermis.
Level V: Invasion of the subcutaneous fat.

The prognosis for patients with malignant melanoma depends upon the stage at presentation. AJCC staging for melanoma takes into account the microscopic depth of invasion of the primary tumour, ulceration, nodal metastasis and presence of metastatic disease in internal sites. Metastatic spread of malignant melanoma is very common and takes place via lymphatics to the regional lymph nodes and through blood to distant sites like lungs, liver, brain, spinal cord, and adrenals. Just as in breast cancer, sentinel lymph node biopsy is quite helpful in evaluation of regional nodal status.

533

Chapter 24

The Skin

IV. TUMOURS OF THE DERMIS *(p. 779)*

1. DERMATOFIBROMA AND MALIGNANT FIBROUS HISTIOCYTOMA

These soft tissue tumours are composed of cells having mixed features of fibroblasts, myofibroblasts, histiocytes and primitive mesenchymal cells. The tumours appear at any age but are more common in advanced age. The commonest sites are the lower and upper extremities, followed in decreasing frequency, by abdominal cavity and retroperitoneum. The benign variant is also known by various synonyms like dermatofibroma, histiocytoma, sclerosing haemangioma, fibroxanthoma and xanthogranuloma. Benign histiocytomas are often small but malignant fibrous histiocytomas may be of enormous size. They are circumscribed but unencapsulated.

M/E The tumours are composed of spindle-shaped fibrohistiocytoid cells which are characteristically arranged in cartwheel or storiform pattern. The benign variety contains uniform spindle-shaped cells with admixture of numerous foamy histiocytes. The malignant fibrous histiocytoma shows pleomorphic tumour cells and some multinucleate giant cells in a stroma that may show myxoid change and inflammatory infiltrate.

2. DERMATOFIBROSARCOMA PROTUBERANS

This is a low-grade fibrosarcoma that rarely metastasises but is locally recurrent. The tumour usually forms a solid nodule, within the dermis and subcutaneous fat, protruding the epidermis outwards.

M/E The tumour is very cellular and is composed of uniform fibroblasts arranged in a cartwheel or storiform pattern. A few mitoses are often present. The overlying epidermis is generally thin and stretched and may be ulcerated.

3. XANTHOMAS

These are solitary or multiple tumour-like lesions, often associated with high levels of serum cholesterol and phospholipids. Many of the cases result from familial hyperlipidaemia.

M/E Xanthomas are composed of dermal collections of benign-appearing foamy histiocytes. Multinucleate tumour giant cells surrounded by lipid-laden cytoplasm are often present.

V. CELLULAR MIGRANT TUMOURS *(p. 780)*

There are some tumours which have their precursor cells elsewhere in the body, but are cellular immigrants to the skin. The examples are Langerhans' cell histiocytosis, mycosis fungoides, mastocytosis, lymphomas and leukaemias.

MYCOSIS FUNGOIDES (CUTANEOUS T-CELL LYMPHOMA) AND SEZARY SYNDROME Mycosis fungoides or cutaneous T-cell lymphoma (CTCL) is the commonest form of lymphoma in the skin having an indolent course but in advanced stage, mycosis fungoides may disseminate to the lymph nodes and other organs. Clinically, mycosis fungoides may manifest in 3 stages:

i) **Premycotic stage** in which the lesions are erythematous, red-brown, scaly and pruritic, resembling eczema or psoriasis.

ii) **Infiltrative stage** has slightly elevated, bluish-red, firm plaques.

iii) **Fungoid (Tumour) stage** is characterised by red-brown nodules of tumour which often undergo ulceration.

The etiology of mycosis fungoides or CTCL has been found to be the same as for adult T cell lymphoma-leukaemia syndrome which is human T cell-leukaemia virus-I (HTLV-1).

Sézary syndrome is a variant of CTCL, often due to dissemination of underlying CTCL to the blood and infiltration into the skin causing generalised erythroderma, lymphadenopathy and hepatosplenomegaly.

534 *M/E* The condition has following features:

i) Initially, lower portion of the epidermis contains hyperchromatic enlarged lymphocytes. In about half the cases, there is formation of intraepidermal clusters of atypical lymphoid cells forming *Darier-Pautrier's microabscesses*.

ii) Later, there are band-like sharply demarcated aggregates of polymorphous cellular infiltrate in the dermis including atypical lymphoid cells (Sézary-Lutzner cells) and multinucleated cells.

iii) The individual mycosis cells are malignant T lymphocytes which have hyperchromatic and cerebriform nuclei and express CD4 and HLA-DR antigen.

Besides CTCL, other forms of cutaneous lymphomas are adult T cell leukaemia-lymphoma (ATLL), anaplastic large cell lymphoma (ALCL), lymphomatoid papulosis and cutaneous B cell lymphoma.

SELF ASSESSMENT

1. **Molluscum contagiosum is caused by:**
   A. Papilloma virus
   B. Herpes virus
   C. Pox virus
   D. EB virus

2. **Xeroderma pigmentosum is characterised by the following features <u>except</u>:**
   A. Autosomal recessive inheritance
   B. Inability to repair sunlight-induced damage to DNA
   C. Proneness to develop various skin cancers
   D. Irregular accumulation of melanin in the basal layer

3. **The etiologic agent implicated in epidermodysplasia verruciformis is:**
   A. Herpes virus (HSV)
   B. Pox virus
   C. EB virus
   D. Papilloma virus (HPV)

4. **Herpesviruses cause the following exanthemata <u>except</u>:**
   A. Herpes simplex
   B. Herpes zoster
   C. Vaccinia
   D. Varicella

5. **The following bullous dermatosis is associated with coeliac disease:**
   A. Pemphigus vulgaris
   B. Pemphigoid
   C. Erythema multiforme
   D. Dermatitis herpetiformis

6. **Psoriasis has the following features <u>except</u>:**
   A. Acanthosis with thickened lower portion
   B. Suprapapillary thinning of epidermis
   C. Prominent granular cell layer
   D. Munro abscesses in parakeratotic layer

7. **Lichen planus is characterised by the following features <u>except</u>:**
   A. Marked hyperkeratosis
   B. Acanthosis with elongated saw-toothed lower border
   C. Band-like dermal infiltrate of inflammatory cells
   D. Intact basal cell layer

8. **The following conditions are premalignant <u>except</u>:**
   A. Solar keratosis
   B. Seborrheic keratosis
   C. Bowen's disease
   D. Xeroderma pigmentosum

9. **The following tumour is commonly non-metastasising:**
   A. Squamous cells carcinoma
   B. Basal cell carcinoma
   C. Melanoma
   D. Sweat gland carcinoma

10. **Papillary hidradenoma occurs most commonly in the following region:**
    A. Scalp
    B. Back
    C. Anogenital region
    D. Extremities

11. **The following type of naevi most often progress to malignant melanoma:**
    A. Compound naevus
    B. Blue naevus
    C. Dysplastic naevus
    D. Epithelioid naevus

12. **The following type of malignant melanoma has worse prognosis:**
    A. Nodular melanoma
    B. Superficial spreading melanoma

    C. Acral lentiginous melanoma
    D. Lentigo maligna melanoma

13. **Darier-Pautrier's abscess is composed of the following cells:**
    A. Neutrophils   **B.** Macrophages
    C. Plasma cells   **D.** Atypical lymphoid cells

14. **The following HPV types are implicated in the etiology of verruca vulgaris:**
    A. Types 1, 2   **B.** Types 6, 11
    C. Types 2, 3   **D.** Types 16, 18

15. **High risk factor for malignant melanoma include the following except:**
    A. Change in appearance
    B. Higher age of the patient
    C. More than 50 or more moles 2 mm or more in diameter
    D. Uniform pigmentation

16. **All are types of calcification in the skin except:**
    A. Metastatic calcinosis cutis
    B. Dystrophic calcinosis cutis
    C. Secondary calcinosis cutis
    D. Subepidermal calcified nodule

17. **Metatypical carcinoma is:**
    A. Basosquamous carcinoma   **B.** Rodent ulcer
    C. Sebaceous carcinoma   **D.** Sweat gland carcinoma

18. **Familial cases of malignant melanoma show germ line mutations in:**
    A. p53   **B.** Rb
    C. CDKN2A   **D.** C-myc

19. **All are immunohistochemical stains for melanoma except:**
    A. HMB-45   **B.** S-100
    C. Melan-A   **D.** SMA

20. **Which of the following is true about the behaviour of dermato-fibrosarcoma protuberans?**
    A. Rare metastasis, rare recurrence
    B. Rare metastasis, locally recurrent
    C. Frequent metastasis and recurrence
    D. No metastasis or recurrence

KEY

1 = C	2 = D	3 = D	4 = C	5 = D
6 = C	7 = D	8 = B	9 = B	10 = C
11 = C	12 = A	13 = D	14 = A	15 = D
16 = C	17 = A	18 = C	19 = D	20 = B

BASIC CONCEPT OF ENDOCRINES (p. 782)

The development, structure and functions of human body are governed and maintained by 2 mutually interlinked systems—*the endocrine system* and *the nervous system*; a third system combining features of both these systems is appropriately called *neuroendocrine system*.

NEUROENDOCRINE SYSTEM (p. 782)

This system forms a link between endocrine glands and nervous system. The cells of this system elaborate polypeptide hormones; owing to these biochemical properties, it has also been called as *APUD cell system* (acronym for *A*mine *P*recursor *U*ptake and *D*ecarboxylation properties). Cells comprising this system are as under:

1.   *Neuroendocrine cells* which are present in the gastric and intestinal mucosa and elaborate peptide hormones.
2.   *Neuroganglia cells* lie in the ganglia cells in the sympathetic chain and elaborate amines.
3.   *Adrenal medulla* elaborates epinephrine and norepinephrine.
4.   *Parafollicular C cells* of the thyroid secrete calcitonin.
5.   *Islets of Langerhans* in the pancreas (included in both endocrine and neuroendocrine systems) secrete insulin.
6.   *Isolated cells in the left atrium* of the heart secrete atrial natriuretic (salt-losing) peptide hormone.

THE ENDOCRINE SYSTEM (p. 782)

Anatomically, the endocrine system consists of 6 distinct organs: pituitary, adrenals, thyroid, parathyroids, gonads, and pancreatic islets; the last one is included in neuroendocrine system also.

Broadly speaking, human hormones are further divided into 5 major classes which are further grouped under two headings depending upon their site of interactions on the target cell receptors (whether cell membrane or nuclear receptor):

Group I: Those interacting with cell-surface membrane receptors:
1.   *Amino acid derivatives:* thyroid hormone, catecholamines.
2.   *Small neuropeptides:* gonadotropin-releasing hormone (GnRH), thyrotropin-releasing hormone (TRH), somatostatin, vasopressin.

Group II: Those interacting with intracellular nuclear receptors:
3.   *Large proteins:* insulin, luteinising hormone (LH), parathormone hormone.
4.   *Steroid hormones:* cortisol, estrogen.
5.   *Vitamin derivatives:* retinol (vitamin A) and vitamin D.
     Major functions of hormones are as under:
i)   *Growth and differentiation of cells:* by pituitary hormones, thyroid, parathyroid, steroid hormones.
ii) *Maintenance of homeostasis:* by thyroid (by regulating BMR), parathormone, mineralocorticoids, vasopressin, insulin.
iii) *Reproduction:* sexual development and activity, pregnancy, foetal development, menopause etc.

A basic feature of all endocrine glands is the existence of both negative and positive **feedback control system** that *stimulates* or *regulates* hormone production in a way that levels remain within the normal range. The stimulatory or regulatory action by endocrine hormonal secretions may follow paracrine or autocrine pathways:

◈ *Paracrine regulation* means that the stimulatory/regulatory factors are released by one type of cells but act on another adjacent cell of the system.

◈ *Autocrine regulation* refers to action of the factor on the same cell that produced it.

In general, pathologic processes affecting endocrine glands with resultant hormonal abnormalities may occur from following processes:

Hyperfunction This results from excess of hormone secreting tissues e.g. hyperplasia, tumours (adenoma, carcinoma), ectopic hormone production, excessive stimulation from inflammation (often autoimmune), infections, iatrogenic (drugs-induced, hormonal administration).

Hypofunction Deficiency of hormones occurs from destruction of hormone-forming tissues from inflammation (often autoimmune), infections, iatrogenic (e.g. surgical removal, radiation damage), developmental defects (e.g. Turner's syndrome, hypoplasia), enzyme deficiency, haemorrhage and infarction (e.g. Sheehan's syndrome), nutritional deficiency (e.g. iodine deficiency).

Hormone resistance There may be adequate or excessive production of a hormone but there is peripheral resistance, often from inherited mutations in receptors (e.g. defect in membrane receptors, nuclear receptors or receptor for signal transduction).

PITUITARY GLAND (p. 784)

NORMAL STRUCTURE

ANATOMY The pituitary gland or hypophysis in an adult weighs about 500 mg and is slightly heavier in females. It is situated at the base of the brain in a hollow called *sella turcica* formed out of the sphenoid bone. The gland is composed of 2 major anatomic divisions: anterior lobe (adenohypophysis) and posterior lobe (neurohypophysis).

◈ The **anterior lobe or adenohypophysis** is an ectodermal derivative formed from Rathke's pouch which is an upward diverticulum from the primitive buccal cavity.

◈ The **posterior lobe or neurohypophysis** is a downgrowth from the primitive neural tissue.

HISTOLOGY AND FUNCTIONS The histology and functions of the anterior and posterior lobes of the pituitary gland are quite distinct.

A. ANTERIOR LOBE (ADENOHYPOPHYSIS) It is composed of round to polygonal epithelial cells arranged in cords and islands having fibrovascular stroma. These epithelial cells, depending upon their staining characteristics and functions, are divided into 3 types, each of which performs separate functions:

1. Chromophil cells with acidophilic granules The acidophils are further of 2 types:
i) *Somatotrophs (GH cells)* which produce growth hormone (GH).
ii) *Lactotrophs (PRL cells)* which produce prolactin (PRL).

2. Chromophil cells with basophilic granules These cells constitute about 10% of the anterior lobe. The chromatophils include 3 types of cells:
i) *Gonadotrophs (FSH-LH cells)* which are the source of the FSH and LH or interstitial cell stimulating hormone (ICSH).
ii) *Thyrotrophs (TSH cells)* are the cells producing TSH.
iii) *Corticotrophs (ACTH-MSH cells)* produce ACTH, melanocyte stimulating hormone (MSH), β-lipoprotein and β-endorphin.

3. Chromophobe cells without visible granules These cells comprise the remainder 50% of the adenohypophysis. These cells by light microscopy contain no visible granules.

B. POSTERIOR LOBE (NEUROHYPOPHYSIS) The neurohypophysis is composed mainly of interlacing nerve fibres in which are scattered specialised glial cells called *pituicytes*. These nerve fibres on electron microscopy contain granules of neurosecretory material made up of 2 octapeptides.

1. ADH It causes reabsorption of water from the renal tubules and is essential for maintenance of osmolality of the plasma. Its deficiency results in diabetes insipidus characterised by uncontrolled diuresis and polydipsia.

2. Oxytocin It causes contraction of mammary myoepithelial cells resulting in ejection of milk from the lactating breast and causes contraction of myometrium of the uterus at term.

HYPERPITUITARISM (p. 784)

A. HYPERFUNCTION OF ANTERIOR PITUITARY

Three common syndromes of adenohypophyseal hyperfunction are as under:

GIGANTISM AND ACROMEGALY Both these clinical syndromes result from sustained excess of growth hormone (GH), most commonly by somatotroph (GH-secreting) adenoma.

Gigantism When GH excess occurs prior to epiphyseal closure, gigantism is produced. Gigantism, therefore, occurs in prepubertal boys and girls and is much less frequent than acromegaly. The main clinical feature in gigantism is the excessive and proportionate growth of the child.

Acromegaly Acromegaly results when there is overproduction of GH in adults following cessation of bone growth and is more common than gigantism. There is enlargement of hands and feet, coarseness of facial features with increase in soft tissues, prominent supraorbital ridges and a more prominent lower jaw which when clenched results in protrusion of the lower teeth in front of upper teeth.

PROLACTINAEMIA Prolactinaemia is lactotroph (PRL-secreting) pituitary adenoma, also called prolactinoma having excessive production of prolactin. Occasionally, hyperprolactinaemia results from hypothalamic inhibition of PRL secretion by certain drugs (e.g. chlorpromazine, reserpine and methyl-dopa).

CUSHING'S SYNDROME Pituitary-dependent Cushing's syndrome results from ACTH excess. Most frequently, it is caused by corticotroph (ACTH-secreting) adenoma.

B. HYPERFUNCTION OF POSTERIOR PITUITARY AND HYPOTHALAMUS

INAPPROPRIATE RELEASE OF ADH Inappropriate release of ADH results in its excessive secretion which manifests clinically by passage of concentrated urine due to increased reabsorption of water and loss of sodium in the urine, consequent hyponatraemia, haemodilution and expansion of intra- and extracellular fluid volume.

PRECOCIOUS PUBERTY A tumour in the region of hypothalamus or the pineal gland may result in premature release of gonadotropins causing the onset of pubertal changes prior to the age of 9 years.

HYPOPITUITARISM (p. 785)

A. HYPOFUNCTION OF ANTERIOR PITUITARY

Adenohypophyseal hypofunction is invariably due to destruction of the anterior lobe of more than 75% because the anterior pituitary possesses a large functional reserve. This may result from anterior pituitary lesions or pressure and destruction from adjacent lesions.

PANHYPOPITUITARISM The classical clinical condition of major anterior pituitary insufficiency is called panhypopituitarism.

Sheehan's syndrome and Simmond's disease Pituitary insufficiency occurring due to postpartum pituitary (Sheehan's) necrosis is called Sheehan's syndrome, whereas occurrence of similar process without preceding pregnancy as well as its occurrence in males is termed Simmond's disease.

The first *clinical manifestation* of Sheehan's syndrome is failure of lactation following delivery which is due to deficiency of prolactin. Subsequently, other symptoms develop.

M/E Sheehan's syndrome during early stage shows ischaemic necrosis and haemorrhage in the anterior pituitary, while later necrotic tissue is replaced by fibrous tissue.

Empty-sella syndrome Empty-sella syndrome is characterised by the appearance of an empty sella and features of panhypopituitarism.

PITUITARY DWARFISM Severe deficiency of GH in children before growth is completed results in retarded growth and pituitary dwarfism. Most commonly, isolated GH deficiency is the result of an inherited autosomal recessive disorder.

B. HYPOFUNCTION OF POSTERIOR PITUITARY AND HYPOTHALAMUS

DIABETES INSIPIDUS Deficient secretion of ADH causes diabetes insipidus. The causes of ADH deficiency are: inflammatory and neoplastic lesions of the hypothalamo-hypophyseal axis, destruction of neurohypophysis due to surgery, radiation, head injury, and lastly, are those cases where no definite cause is known and are labelled as idiopathic. The main features of diabetes insipidus are excretion of a very large volume of dilute urine of low specific gravity (below 1.010), polyuria and polydipsia.

PITUITARY TUMOURS *(p. 786)*

All pituitary tumours, whether benign or malignant, cause symptoms by following 2 ways:

1. Pressure effects These are caused by expansion of the lesion resulting in destruction of the surrounding glandular tissue by pressure atrophy.

2. Hormonal effects Depending upon their cell types, pituitary adenomas produce excess of pituitary hormones and the corresponding clinical syndromes of hyperpituitarism.

PITUITARY ADENOMAS

Adenomas are the most common pituitary tumours. They are conventionally classified according to their H & E staining characteristics of granules into acidophil, basophil and chromophobe adenomas. As a result of advances in the ultrastructural and immunocytochemical studies, a functional classification of pituitary adenoma has emerged.

G/A Pituitary adenomas range in size from small foci of less than 10 mm in size (termed microadenoma) to large adenomas several centimeters in diameter (> 1 cm called macroadenomas). They are spherical, soft and encapsulated.

M/E By light microscopy of H & E stained sections, an adenoma is composed predominantly of one of the normal cell types of the anterior pituitary i.e. acidophil, basophil or chromophobe cells. These cells may have following 3 types of patterns:
1. Diffuse pattern
2. Sinusoidal pattern
3. Papillary pattern.

Functionally, most common pituitary adenomas, in decreasing order of frequency, are: lactotroph (PRL-secreting) adenoma, somatotroph (GH-secreting) adenoma and corticotroph (ACTH-secreting) adenoma. Infrequently, mixed somatotroph-lactotroph (GH-PRL-secreting) adenoma, gonadotroph (FSH-LH-secreting) adenomas and null-cell (endocrinologically inactive) adenomas or oncocytoma are found.

Pituitary adenomas occur in the age group of 3rd to 6th decade of life. They are mostly sporadiac. Less than 5% are familial having germline mutation in *MEN1* gene. The latter cases occur as a part of multiple endocrine neoplasia type I (MEN-I) in which pituitary adenoma is associated with adenomas of pancreatic islets and parathyroids.

CRANIOPHARYNGIOMA

Craniopharyngioma is a benign tumour arising from remnants of Rathke's pouch. It has 2 peaks of occurrence: children and young adults in 1st to 2nd decade and then in adults past 6th decade. The tumour, though benign, compresses as well as invades the adjacent structures extensively.

G/A The tumour is encapsulated, adherent to surrounding structures and is typically cystic, reddish-grey mass. The fluid in the cystic cavity typically has colour and consistency of machinery oil.

M/E Craniopharyngioma closely resembles ameloblastoma of the jaw. There are 2 distinct histologic features:
1. Stratified squamous epithelium frequently lining a cyst and containing loose stellate cells in the centre.
2. Solid ameloblastic areas.

ADRENAL GLAND (p. 787)

NORMAL STRUCTURE

ANATOMY The adrenal glands lie at the upper pole of each kidney. Each gland weighs approximately 4 gm in the adult but in children the adrenals are proportionately larger. On sectioning, the adrenal is composed of 2 distinct parts: an outer yellow-brown *cortex* and an inner grey *medulla*.

HISTOLOGY AND PHYSIOLOGY Microscopically and functionally, cortex and medulla are quite distinct.

ADRENAL CORTEX It is composed of 3 layers:
1. Zona glomerulosa
2. Zona fasciculata
3. Zona reticularis.

The synthesis of glucocorticoids and adrenal androgens is under the control of ACTH from hypothalamus-anterior pituitary. In turn, ACTH release is under the control of a hypothalamic releasing factor called corticotropin-releasing factor.

ADRENAL MEDULLA The adrenal medulla is a component of the dispersed neuroendocrine system derived from primitive neuroectoderm; the other components of this system being *paraganglia* distributed in the vagi, paravertebral and visceral autonomic ganglia. The cells comprising this system are neuroendocrine cells, the major function of which is synthesis and secretion of catecholamines (epinephrine and norepinephrine).

ADRENOCORTICAL HYPERFUNCTION (HYPERADRENALISM) (p. 788)

Hypersecretion of each of the three types of corticosteroids elaborated by the adrenal cortex causes distinct corresponding hyperadrenal clinical syndromes:

CUSHING'S SYNDROME (CHRONIC HYPERCORTISOLISM)

Cushing's syndrome is caused by excessive production of cortisol of whatever cause.

ETIOPATHOGENESIS There are 4 major etiologic types of Cushing's syndrome.

1. Pituitary Cushing's syndrome About 60-70% cases of Cushing's syndrome are caused by excessive secretion of ACTH due to a lesion in the pituitary gland, most commonly a corticotroph adenoma or multiple corticotroph microadenomas.

2. Adrenal Cushing's syndrome Approximately 20-25% cases of Cushing's syndrome are caused by disease in one or both the adrenal glands.

3. Ectopic Cushing's syndrome About 10-15% cases of Cushing's syndrome have an origin in ectopic ACTH elaboration by non-endocrine tumours. Most often, the tumour is small cell carcinoma of the lung.

4. Iatrogenic Cushing's syndrome Prolonged therapeutic administration of high doses of glucocorticoids or ACTH may result in Cushing's syndrome.

CLINICAL FEATURES Cushing's syndrome occurs more often in patients between the age of 20-40 years with three times higher frequency in women than in men. The severity of the syndrome varies considerably, but in general the following features characterise a case of Cushing's syndrome:
1. Central or truncal obesity
2. Increased protein breakdown
3. Systemic hypertension
4. Impaired glucose tolerance and diabetes mellitus
5. Amenorrhoea, hirsutism and infertility in many women.
6. Insomnia, depression, confusion and psychosis.

CONN'S SYNDROME (PRIMARY HYPERALDOSTERONISM)

This is an uncommon syndrome occurring due to overproduction of aldosterone, the potent salt-retaining hormone.

ETIOPATHOGENESIS It results from following adrenocortical diseases:
1. Adrenocortical adenoma, producing aldosterone.
2. Bilateral adrenal hyperplasia, especially in children.
3. Rarely, adrenal carcinoma.
◈ *Primary hyperaldosteronism* from any of the above causes is associated with low plasma renin levels.
◈ *Secondary hyperaldosteronism,* on the contrary, occurs in response to high plasma renin level due to overproduction of renin by the kidneys such as in renal ischaemia, reninoma or oedema.

CLINICAL FEATURES Conn's syndrome is more frequent in adult females. Its principal features are as under:
1. Hypertension
2. Hypokalaemia
3. Retention of sodium and water
4. Polyuria and polydipsia.

ADRENOGENITAL SYNDROME (ADRENAL VIRILISM)

Adrenal cortex secretes a smaller amount of sex steroids than the gonads.

ETIOPATHOGENESIS Hypersecretion of sex steroids, mainly androgens, may occur in children or in adults:
◈ *In children,* it is due to congenital adrenal hyperplasia in which there is congenital deficiency of a specific enzyme.
◈ *In adults,* it is caused by an adrenocortical adenoma or a carcinoma. Cushing's syndrome is often present as well.

CLINICAL FEATURES The clinical features depend upon the age and sex of the patient.
◈ *In children,* there is distortion of the external genitalia in girls, and precocious puberty in boys.
◈ *In adults,* the features in females show virilisation (e.g. hirsutism, oligomenorrhoea, deepening of voice, hypertrophy of the clitoris); and in males may rarely cause feminisation.

ADRENOCORTICAL INSUFFICIENCY (HYPOADRENALISM) (p. 789)

Adrenocortical insufficiency may result from deficient synthesis of cortical steroids from the adrenal cortex or may be secondary to ACTH deficiency. Three types of adrenocortical hypofunction are distinguished as under.

Primary adrenal hypofunction occurs due to defect in the adrenal glands and normal pituitary function. It may develop in 2 ways:

A. Primary Acute Adrenocortical Insufficiency (Adrenal Crisis)

Sudden loss of adrenocortical function may result in an acute condition called *adrenal crisis*.

ETIOPATHOGENESIS Causes of acute insufficiency are as under:
1. Bilateral adrenalectomy e.g. in the treatment of cortical hyperfunction, hypertension and in selected cases of breast cancer.
2. Septicaemia e.g. in endotoxic shock and meningococcal infection producing grossly haemorrhagic and necrotic adrenal cortex termed adrenal apoplexy.
3. Rapid withdrawal of steroids.
4. Any form of acute stress in a case of chronic insufficiency i.e. in Addison's disease.

CLINICAL FEATURES These are:
1. Deficiency of mineralocorticoids (i.e. aldosterone deficiency) result in salt deficiency, hyperkalaemia and dehydration.
2. Deficiency of glucocorticoids (i.e. cortisol deficiency) leads to hypoglycaemia, increased insulin sensitivity and vomitings.

B. Primary Chronic Adrenocortical Insufficiency (Addison's Disease)

Progressive chronic destruction of more than 90% of adrenal cortex on both sides results in an uncommon clinical condition called Addison's disease.

ETIOPATHOGENESIS Any condition which causes marked chronic adrenal destruction may produce Addison's disease. These include: tuberculosis, autoimmune or idiopathic adrenalitis, histoplasmosis, amyloidosis, metastatic cancer, sarcoidosis and haemochromatosis. However, currently the first two causes—tuberculosis and autoimmune chronic destruction of adrenal glands, are implicated in majority of cases of Addison's disease.

CLINICAL FEATURES These develop slowly:
1. Asthenia i.e. progressive weakness, weight loss and lethargy as the cardinal symptoms.
2. Hyperpigmentation, initially most marked on exposed areas, but later involves unexposed parts and mucous membranes as well.
3. Arterial hypotension.
4. Vague upper gastrointestinal symptoms such as mild loss of appetite, nausea, vomiting and upper abdominal pain.
5. Lack of androgen causing loss of hair in women.
6. Episodes of hypoglycaemia.
7. Biochemical changes include reduced GFR, acidosis, hyperkalaemia and low levels of serum sodium, chloride and bicarbonate.

SECONDARY ADRENOCORTICAL INSUFFICIENCY

Adrenocortical insufficiency resulting from deficiency of ACTH is called secondary adrenocortical insufficiency.

ETIOPATHOGENESIS ACTH deficiency may appear in 2 settings :
1. *Selective ACTH deficiency* due to prolonged administration of high doses of glucocorticoids.
2. *Panhypopituitarism* due to hypothalamus-pituitary diseases.

CLINICAL FEATURES These are those of Addison's disease except following:
1. These cases lack hyperpigmentation because of suppressed production of melanocyte-stimulating hormone (MSH) from the pituitary.
2. Plasma ACTH levels are low-to-absent in secondary insufficiency but are elevated in Addison's disease.
3. Aldosterone levels are normal due to stimulation by renin.

Isolated deficiency of aldosterone with normal cortisol level may occur in association with reduced renin secretion.

ETIOPATHOGENESIS Causes of hyporeninism are:
1. Congenital defect due to deficiency of an enzyme required for its synthesis.
2. Prolonged administration of heparin.
3. Certain diseases of the brain.
4. Excision of an aldosterone-secreting tumour.

CLINICAL FEATURES The patients of isolated hypoaldosteronism are adults with mild renal failure and diabetes mellitus. The predominant features are hyperkalaemia and metabolic acidosis.

TUMOURS OF ADRENAL GLANDS (p. 790)

Primary tumours of the adrenal glands are uncommon and include distinct adrenocortical tumours and medullary tumours.

ADRENOCORTICAL TUMOURS

CORTICAL ADENOMA

The commonest cortical tumour is adenoma. They are indistinguishable from hyperplastic nodules except that lesions smaller than 2 cm diameter are labelled *hyperplastic nodules*. A cortical adenoma is a benign and slow-growing tumour. It is usually small and nonfunctional.

G/A An adenoma is usually a small (2–5 cm), solitary, spherical and encapsulated tumour which is well-delineated from the surrounding normal adrenal gland. Cut section is typically bright yellow.

M/E The tumour cells are arranged in trabeculae and generally resemble the cells of zona fasciculata.

CORTICAL CARCINOMA

Carcinoma of the adrenal cortex is an uncommon tumour occurring mostly in adults. It invades locally as well as spreads to distant sites.

G/A An adrenal carcinoma is generally large, spherical and well-demarcated tumour. On cut section, it is predominantly yellow with intermixed areas of haemorrhages, necrosis and calcification.

M/E The cortical carcinoma may vary from well-differentiated to anaplastic growth.

MEDULLARY TUMOURS

The most significant lesions of the adrenal medulla are neoplasms. These include the following:
1. *Benign tumours*: These are less common and include pheochromocytoma and myelolipoma.
2. *Tumours arising from embryonic nerve cells*: These are more common and include neuroblastoma and ganglioneuroma.

PHEOCHROMOCYTOMA (CHROMAFFIN TUMOUR)

Pheochromocytoma is a tumour arising from pheochromocytes (i.e. chromaffin cells) of the adrenal medulla. Its name is derived from its characteristic *dark brown black* appearance of this tumour caused by chromaffin oxidation of catecholamines. The extra-adrenal pheochromocytomas arising from other paraganglia are preferably called *paragangliomas,* named along with the anatomic site of origin.

Pheochromocytoma may occur at any age but most patients are 20-60 years old. Most pheochromocytomas are slow-growing and benign but about 10% of the tumours are malignant, invasive and metastasising. These tumours are commonly sporadic but 10% are associated with familial syndromes of multiple endocrine neoplasia (MEN) having bilaterality and association with medullary carcinoma of the thyroid, hyperparathyroidism, pituitary adenoma, mucosal neuromas and von Recklinghausen's neurofibromatosis in varying combinations. Thus, the traditional "10% rule" for pheochromocytoma is 10% familial, 10% malignant, 10% extra-adrenal.

The *clinical features* of pheochromocytoma are predominantly due to secretion of catecholamines, both epinephrine and norepinephrine. The most common feature is hypertension.

G/A The tumour is soft, spherical, may be quite variable in size and weight, and well-demarcated from the adjacent adrenal gland. On cut section, the tumour is grey to dusky brown with areas of haemorrhages, necrosis, calcification and cystic change. On immersing the tumour in dichromate fixative, it turns brown-black due to oxidation of catecholamines in the tumour and hence the name chromaffin tumour.

M/E The tumour has following characteristics:
1. The tumour cells are arranged characteristically as well-defined nests (also termed as zellballen pattern) separated by abundant fibrovascular stroma.
2. Other arrangements are as solid columns, sheets, trabeculae or clumps.
3. The tumour cells are large, polyhedral and pleomorphic with abundant granular amphophilic or basophilic cytoplasm and vesicular nuclei.
4. The tumour cells of pheochromocytoma stain positively with neuroendocrine substances such as neuron-specific enolase (NSE) and chromogranin.

MYELOLIPOMA

Myelolipoma is an uncommon benign adrenal medullary tumour, sometimes found incidentally at autopsy. Less often, it may produce symptoms due to excessive hormone elaboration.

G/A A myelolipoma is usually a small tumour, measuring 0.2-2 cm in diameter.

M/E It consists of well-differentiated adipose tissue in which is scattered clumps of haematopoietic cells are seen.

NEUROBLASTOMA

Neuroblastoma, also called as sympathicoblastoma, is a common malignant tumour of neural crest cells, occurring most commonly in children under 5 years of age. Vast majority of cases occur within the abdomen (in the adrenal medulla and paravertebral autonomic ganglia) and rarely in the cerebral hemisphere.

The *clinical manifestations* of neuroblastoma are related to its rapid local growth, metastatic spread or development of hormonal syndrome. Local symptoms include abdominal distension, fever, weight loss and malaise. Foci of calcification may be observed on radiologic examination of the abdomen. Metastatic spread occurs early and widely through haematogenous as well as lymphatic routes and involves bones (especially skull), liver, lungs and regional lymph nodes. Neuroblastoma produces variable amounts of catecholamines and its metabolites such as vanillyl mandelic acid (VMA) and homovanillic acid (HVA), which can be detected in the 24-hour urine.

G/A The tumour is generally large, soft and lobulated mass with extensive areas of necrosis and haemorrhages. Cut surface of the tumour is grey white and may reveal minute foci of calcification.

M/E It has following features:
1. The tumour cells are small, round and oval, slightly larger than lymphocytes, and have scanty and poorly-defined cytoplasm and hyperchromatic nuclei.
2. They are generally arranged in irregular sheets separated by fibrovascular stroma.

settes). The central fibrillar material stains positively by silver impregnation methods indicating their nature as young nerve fibrils.

4. The tumour cells stain positively with immunohistochemical markers such as neuron-specific enolase (NSE), neurofilaments (NF) and chromo-granin.

Prognosis of neuroblastoma depends upon a few variables; favourable prognostic features are as under:

i) *Age* of child below 2 years.

ii) Extra-abdominal *location* of the tumour than abdominal masses.

iii) *Tumour histology* with schwannian or ganglionic differentiation.

iv) *Patients in clinical stage* I (confined to the organ of origin) or stage II (tumour extending in continuity beyond the organ of origin but not crossing the midline).

GANGLIONEUROMA

A ganglioneuroma is a mature, benign and uncommon tumour occurring in adults. It is derived from ganglion cells, most often in the posterior mediastinum, and uncommonly in other peripheral ganglia and brain.

G/A The tumour is spherical, firm and encapsulated.

M/E It contains large number of well-formed ganglionic nerve cells scattered in fibrillar stroma and myelinated and non-myelinated nerve fibres.

EXTRA-ADRENAL PARAGANGLIOMA (CHEMODECTOMA)

Parasympathetic paraganglia located in extra-adrenal sites such as the carotid bodies, vagus, jugulotympanic and aorticosympathetic (pre-aortic) paraganglia may produce neoplasms, collectively termed *paragangliomas* with the anatomic site of origin e.g. carotid body paraganglioma, intravagal paraganglioma, jugulotympanic paraganglioma etc. These tumours are also called chemodectomas because of their responsiveness to chemoreceptors.

THYROID GLAND *(p. 792)*

NORMAL STRUCTURE

The thyroid gland in an adult weighs 15-40 gm and is composed of two lateral lobes connected in the midline by a broad isthmus which may have a pyramidal lobe extending upwards.

M/E The thyroid is composed of lobules of colloid-filled spherical follicles or acini. The lobules are enclosed by fibrovascular septa. The follicles are the main functional units of the thyroid. They are lined by cuboidal epithelium with numerous fine microvilli extending into the follicular colloid that contains the glycoprotein, *thyroglobulin*. Calcitonin-secreting C-cells or parafollicular cells are dispersed within the follicles.

FUNCTIONS The major function of the thyroid gland is to maintain a high rate of metabolism which is done by means of iodine-containing thyroid hormones, thyroxine (T_4) and tri-iodothyronine (T_3).

The *synthesis and release* of the two main circulating thyroid hormones, T_3 and T_4 are regulated by hypophyseal thyroid-stimulating hormone (TSH) and involves the following steps:

1. **Iodine trapping** by thyroidal cells involves absorbing of iodine from the blood and concentrating it more than twenty-fold.

2. **Oxidation** of the iodide takes place within the cells by a thyroid peroxidase.

3. **Iodination** occurs next, at the microvilli level between the oxidised iodine and the tyrosine residues of thyroglobulin so as to form mono-iodotyrosine (MIT) and di-iodotyrosine (DIT).

4. **Coupling** of MIT and DIT in the presence of thyroid peroxidase forms tri-iodothyronine (T_3) and thyroxine (T_4).

A number of *thyroid function tests* are currently available. These include the following:

i) Determination of serum levels of T_3, T_4 by radioimmunoassay (RIA).

ii) TSH and TRH determination.

iii) Determination of calcitonin secreted by parafollicular C cells.

iv) Estimation of thyroglobulin secreted by thyroid follicular cells.

v) Assessment of thyroid activity by its ability to uptake radioactive iodine (RAIU).

vi) Assessment whether thyroid lesion is a nonfunctioning ('cold nodule') or hyperactive mass ('hot nodule').

FUNCTIONAL DISORDERS *(p. 793)*

HYPERTHYROIDISM (THYROTOXICOSIS)

Hyperthyroidism, also called thyrotoxicosis, is a hypermetabolic clinical and biochemical state caused by excess production of thyroid hormones. The condition is more frequent in females and is associated with rise in both T_3 and T_4 levels in blood, though the increase in T_3 is generally greater than that of T_4.

ETIOPATHOGENESIS Hyperthyroidism may be caused by many diseases but three most common causes are: Graves' disease (diffuse toxic goitre), toxic multinodular goitre and a toxic adenoma.

CLINICAL FEATURES Patients with hyperthyroidism have a slow and insidious onset, varying in severity from case to case. The usual symptoms are emotional instability, nervousness, palpitation, fatigue, weight loss in spite of good appetite, heat intolerance, perspiration, menstrual disturbances and fine tremors of the outstretched hands. Cardiac manifestations in the form of tachycardia, palpitations and cardiomegaly are invariably present in hyperthyroidism. The skin of these patients is warm, moist and flushed.

HYPOTHYROIDISM

Hypothyroidism is a hypometabolic clinical state resulting from inadequate production of thyroid hormones for prolonged periods, or rarely, from resistance of the peripheral tissues to the effects of thyroid hormones. The clinical manifestations of hypothyroidism, depending upon the age at onset of disorder, are divided into 2 forms:

1. *Cretinism* or *congenital hypothyroidism* is the development of severe hypothyroidism during infancy and childhood.

2. *Myxoedema* is the adulthood hypothyroidism.

CRETINISM

A cretin is a child with severe hypothyroidism present at birth or developing within first two years of postnatal life. This is the period when brain development is taking place; in the absence of treatment the child is both physically and mentally retarded.

ETIOPATHOGENESIS The causes are as under:

1. *Developmental anomalies* e.g. thyroid agenesis and ectopic thyroid.

2. *Genetic defect* in thyroid hormone synthesis e.g. defect in iodine trapping, oxidation, iodination, coupling and thyroglobulin synthesis.

3. *Foetal exposure* to iodides and antithyroid drugs.

4. *Endemic cretinism* in regions with endemic goitre due to dietary lack of iodine.

CLINICAL FEATURES The clinical manifestations usually become evident within a few weeks to months of birth. The presenting features of a cretin are: slow to thrive, poor feeding, constipation, dry scaly skin, hoarse cry and bradycardia. As the child ages, clinical picture of fully-developed cretinism emerges characterised by impaired skeletal growth and consequent dwarfism.

Characteristic laboratory findings include a rise in TSH level and fall in T_3 and T_4 levels.

The adult-onset severe hypothyroidism causes myxoedema. The term myxoedema connotes non-pitting oedema due to accumulation of hydrophilic mucopolysaccharides in the ground substance of dermis and other tissues.

ETIOPATHOGENESIS Causes of myxoedema are:
1. Ablation of the thyroid by surgery or radiation.
2. Autoimmune (lymphocytic) thyroiditis (termed primary idiopathic myxoedema).
3. Endemic or sporadic goitre.
4. Hypothalamic-pituitary lesions.
5. Thyroid cancer.
6. Prolonged administration of antithyroid drugs.
7. Mild developmental anomalies and dyshormonogenesis.

CLINICAL FEATURES The onset of myxoedema is slow and a fully-developed clinical syndrome may appear after several years of hypothyroidism. The striking features are cold intolerance, mental and physical lethargy, constipation, slowing of speech and intellectual function, puffiness of face, loss of hair and altered texture of the skin.

The laboratory diagnosis in myxoedema is made by low serum T_3 and T_4 levels and markedly elevated TSH levels.

THYROIDITIS (p. 794)

Inflammation of the thyroid, thyroiditis, is more often due to non-infectious causes and is classified on the basis of onset and duration of disease into acute, subacute and chronic.

HASHIMOTO'S (AUTOIMMUNE, CHRONIC LYMPHOCYTIC) THYROIDITIS

Hashimoto's thyroiditis, also called diffuse lymphocytic thyroiditis, struma lymphomatosa or goitrous autoimmune thyroiditis, is characterised by 3 principal features:
1. Diffuse goitrous enlargement of the thyroid.
2. Lymphocytic infiltration of the thyroid gland.
3. Occurrence of thyroid autoantibodies.

Hashimoto's thyroiditis occurs more frequently between the age of 30 and 50 years and shows an approximately ten-fold preponderance among females. Hashimoto's thyroiditis is the most common cause of *goitrous hypothyroidism* in regions where iodine supplies are *adequate*. Regions where iodine intake is more have higher incidence of Hashimoto's thyroiditis e.g. in Japan and the United States.

ETIOPATHOGENESIS Autoimmune pathogenesis of Hashimoto's thyroiditis is explained by the following observations:

1. Other autoimmune disease association Like in many autoimmune diseases, Hashimoto's disease has been found in association with other autoimmune diseases such as Graves' disease, SLE, Sjögren's syndrome, rheumatoid arthritis, pernicious anaemia and Type 1 diabetes mellitus.

2. Immune destruction of thyroid cells An association of cytotoxic lymphocyte-associated antigen 4 *(CTLA4)*, a T cell regulatory gene, with autoimmune phenomenon in Hashimoto's disease has been reported. There is initial activation of CD4+ T helper cells, which then induce infiltration of CD8+ T cytotoxic cells in the thyroid parenchyma.

3. Detection of autoantibodies The following autoantibodies against different thyroid cell antigens are detected:
i) Thyroid microsomal autoantibodies (against the microsomes of the follicular cells).
ii) Thyroglobulin autoantibodies.
iii) TSH receptor autoantibodies.

4. Inhibitory TSH-receptor antibodies TSH-receptor antibody seen on the surface of thyroid cells in Hashimoto's thyroiditis is inhibitory to TSH, producing hypothyroidism. Similar antibody is observed in Graves' disease where it causes hyperthyroidism. It appears that TSH-receptor antibody may act both to depress or stimulate the thyroid cells to produce hypo- or hyper-thyroidism respectively.

5. Genetic basis   The disease has higher incidence in first-degree relatives of affected patients. Hashimoto's thyroiditis is seen more often with HLA-DR3 and HLA-DR5 subtypes.

G/A   The *classic form* is characterised by diffuse, symmetric, firm and rubbery enlargement of the thyroid which may weigh 100-300 gm. Sectioned surface of the thyroid is fleshly with accentuation of normal lobulations but with retained normal shape of the gland. The *fibrosing variant* has a firm, enlarged thyroid with compression of the surrounding tissues.

M/E   The classic form shows following features:
1.   There is extensive infiltration of the gland by lymphocytes, plasma cells, immunoblasts and macrophages, with formation of lymphoid follicles having germinal centres.
2.   There is decreased number of thyroid follicles which are generally atrophic and are often devoid of colloid.
3.   The follicular epithelial cells are transformed into their degenerated state termed Hurthle cells (also called Askanazy cells, or oxyphil cells, or oncocytes).
4.   There is slight fibrous thickening of the septa separating the thyroid lobules.
5.   The less common *fibrosing variant* of Hashimoto's thyroiditis shows considerable fibrous replacement of thyroid parenchyma and a less prominent lymphoid infiltrate.

CLINICAL FEATURES   The presenting feature of Hashimoto's thyroiditis is a painless, firm and moderate goitrous enlargement of the thyroid gland, usually associated with hypothyroidism, in a middle-aged woman. At this stage, serum T_3 and T_4 levels are decreased and RAIU is also reduced. A few cases, however, develop hyperthyroidism, termed *hashitoxicosis*, further substantiating the similarities in the autoimmune phenomena between Hashimoto's thyroiditis and Graves' thyrotoxicosis.

SUBACUTE GRANULOMATOUS (DE QUERVAIN'S) THYROIDITIS

Granulomatous thyroiditis, also called de Quervain's or subacute, or giant cell thyroiditis, is a distinctive form of self-limited inflammation of the thyroid gland. Etiology of the condition is not known but clinical features of a prodromal phase and preceding respiratory infection suggest a possible viral etiology. The disease is more common in young and middle-aged women and may present clinically with painful moderate thyroid enlargement with fever, features of hyperthyroidism in the early phase of the disease, and hypothyroidism if the damage to the thyroid gland is extensive.

G/A   There is moderate enlargement of the gland which is often asymmetric or focal. The cut surface of the involved area is firm and yellowish-white.

M/E   The features vary according to the stage:
❖   *Initially,* there is acute inflammatory destruction of the thyroid parenchyma and formation of microabscesses.
❖   *Later,* the more characteristic feature of granulomatous appearance is produced. These granulomas consist of central colloid material surrounded by histiocytes and scattered multinucleate giant cells.
❖   More *advanced* cases may show fibroblastic proliferation.

RIEDEL'S THYROIDITIS

Riedel's thyroiditis, also called Riedel's struma or invasive fibrous thyroiditis, is a rare chronic disease characterised by stony-hard thyroid that is densely adherent to the adjacent structures in the neck. The condition is clinically significant due to compressive clinical features (e.g. dysphagia, dyspnoea, recurrent laryngeal nerve paralysis and stridor) and resemblance with thyroid cancer. The etiology is unknown but possibly Riedel's thyroiditis is a part of *multifocal idiopathic fibrosclerosis*.

G/A   The thyroid gland is usually contracted, stony-hard, asymmetric and firmly adherent to the adjacent structures. Cut section is hard and devoid of lobulations.

M/E   There is extensive fibrocollagenous replacement, marked atrophy of the thyroid parenchyma, focally scattered lymphocytic infiltration and invasion of the adjacent muscle tissue by the process.

GRAVES' DISEASE (DIFFUSE TOXIC GOITRE) *(p. 796)*

Graves' disease, also known as Basedow's disease, primary hyperplasia, exophthalmic goitre, and diffuse toxic goitre, is characterised by a triad of features:
1.   Hyperthyroidism (thyrotoxicosis)
2.   Diffuse thyroid enlargement
3.   Ophthalmopathy.
    The disease is more frequent between the age of 30 and 40 years and has five-fold increased prevalence among females.

ETIOPATHOGENESIS   Graves' disease is an autoimmune disease and, there are many immunologic similarities between this condition and Hashimoto's thyroiditis.

1.   Genetic factor association   Like in Hashimoto's thyroiditis. Graves' disease too has genetic predisposition. A familial occurrence has been observed.

2.   Autoimmune disease association   Graves' disease may be found in association with other organ-specific autoimmune diseases.

3.   Other factors   Besides these two factors, Graves' disease has higher prevalence in women (7 to 10 times), and association with emotional stress and smoking.

4.   Autoantibodies   These are:
i)   Thyroid-stimulating immunoglobulin (TSI)
ii)   Thyroid growth-stimulating immunoglobulins (TGI)
iii)   TSH-binding inhibitor immunoglobulins (TBII)
    However, it is not quite clear what stimulates B cells to form these autoantibodies in Graves' disease. Possibly, intrathyroidal CD4+ helper T cells are responsible for stimulating B cells to secrete autoantibodies.

G/A   The thyroid is moderately, diffusely and symmetrically enlarged and may weigh up to 70-90 gm. On cut section, the thyroid parenchyma is typically homogeneous, red-brown and meaty and lacks the normal translucency.

M/E   Following features are found:
1.   There is considerable epithelial hyperplasia and hypertrophy as seen by increased height of the follicular lining cells and formation of papillary infoldings of piled up epithelium into the lumina of follicles which are small.
2.   The colloid is markedly diminished and is lightly staining, watery and finely vacuolated.
3.   The stroma shows increased vascularity and accumulation of lymphoid cells.

CLINICAL FEATURES   Graves' disease generally develops slowly and insidiously.
◈   Patients are usually young women who present with symmetric, moderate *enlargement of the thyroid gland* with features of thyrotoxicosis, ophthalmopathy and dermatopathy.
◈   *Ocular abnormalities* are lid lag, upper lid retraction, stare, weakness of eye muscles and proptosis. In extreme cases, the lids can no longer close and may produce corneal injuries and ulcerations.
◈   *Dermatopathy* in Graves' disease most often consists of pretibial (localised) myxoedema in the form of firm plaques.

GOITRE *(p. 797)*

The term goitre is defined as thyroid enlargement caused by compensatory hyperplasia and hypertrophy of the follicular epithelium in response to thyroid hormone deficiency. Though at some stages there may be hypo- or hyperthyroidism. Two morphologic forms of goitre are distinguished:

A. Diffuse goitre (simple nontoxic goitre or colloid goitre).

B. Nodular goitre (multinodular goitre or adenomatous goitre).

PATHOGENESIS OF GOITRE

The pathogenetic mechanisms of both forms of goitre can be considered together since nodular goitre is generally regarded as the end-stage of long-standing simple goitre. The fundamental defect is deficient production of thyroid hormones due to various etiologic factors, but most common is *dietary lack of iodine*. Deficient thyroid hormone production causes excessive TSH stimulation which leads to hyperplasia of follicular epithelium as well as formation of new thyroid follicles. Cyclical hyperplastic stage followed by involution stage completes the picture of *simple goitre*.

DIFFUSE GOITRE (SIMPLE NON-TOXIC GOITRE, COLLOID GOITRE)

Diffuse, nontoxic simple or colloid goitre is the name given to diffuse enlargement of the thyroid gland, unaccompanied by hyperthyroidism.

ETIOLOGY Epidemiologically, goitre occurs in 2 forms:

Endemic goitre Prevalence of goitre in a geographic area in more than 10% of the population is termed endemic goitre. Such endemic areas are several high mountainous regions far from the sea where iodine content of drinking water and food is low such as in the regions of the Himalayas, the Alps and the Ande.

Goitrogens are substances which interfere with the synthesis of thyroid hormones. These substances are drugs used in the treatment of hyperthyroidism and certain items of food such as cabbage, cauliflower, turnips and cassava roots.

Sporadic (non-endemic) goitre Non-endemic or sporadic simple goitre is less common than the endemic variety. A number of causal influences have been attributed.

i) Suboptimal iodine intake in conditions of increased demand as in puberty and pregnancy.

ii) Genetic factors.

iii) Dietary goitrogenes.

iv) Hereditary defect in thyroid hormone synthesis and transport (dyshormonogenesis).

v) Inborn errors of iodine metabolism.

G/A The enlargement of the thyroid gland in simple goitre is moderate (weighing up to 100-150 gm), symmetric and diffuse. Cut surface is gelatinous and translucent brown.

M/E Two stages are seen:

1. *Hyperplastic stage* is the early stage and is characterised by tall columnar follicular epithelium showing papillary infoldings and formation of small new follicles.

2. *Involution stage* generally follows hyperplastic stage after variable period of time. This stage is characterised by large follicles distended by colloid and lined by flattened follicular epithelium.

NODULAR GOITRE (MULTINODULAR GOITRE, ADENOMATOUS GOITRE)

Nodular goitre is regarded as the end-stage of long-standing simple goitre. It is characterised by most extreme degree of tumour-like enlargement of the thyroid gland and characteristic nodularity. The enlargement of the gland may be sufficient to not only cause cosmetic disfigurement, but in many cases may cause dysphagia and choking due to compression of oesophagus and trachea.

ETIOLOGY Etiologic factors implicated in endemic and non-endemic or sporadic variety of simple goitre are involved in the etiology of nodular goitre too. Possibly, epithelial hyperplasia, generation of new follicles, and irregular accumulation of colloid in the follicles—all contribute to produce increased tension and stress in the thyroid gland causing rupture of follicles and vessels. This is followed by haemorrhages, cystic change, scarring and sometimes calcification, resulting in development of nodular pattern.

G/A The thyroid in nodular goitre shows asymmetric and extreme enlargement, weighing 100-500 gm or even more. The *five* cardinal macroscopic features are as under:
1. Nodularity with poor encapsulation
2. Fibrous scarring
3. Haemorrhages
4. Focal calcification
5. Cystic degeneration.
    Cut surface generally shows multinodularity but occasionally there may be only one or two nodules which are poorly-circumscribed.

M/E The same heterogenicity as seen on gross is seen:
1. Partial or incomplete encapsulation of nodules.
2. The follicles varying from small to large and lined by flat to high epithelium. A few may show macropapillary formation.
3. Areas of haemorrhages, haemosiderin-laden macrophages and cholesterol crystals.
4. Fibrous scarring with foci of calcification.
5. Micro-macrocystic change.

THYROID TUMOURS *(p. 800)*

FOLLICULAR ADENOMA

Follicular adenoma is the most common benign thyroid tumour occurring more frequently in adult women. Clinically, it appears as a solitary nodule which can be found in approximately 1% of the population. Besides the follicular adenoma, other conditions which may produce clinically apparent solitary nodule in the thyroid are a dominant nodule of nodular goitre and thyroid carcinoma.

G/A The follicular adenoma is characterised by *four* features so as to distinguish it from a nodule of nodular goitre:
1. solitary nodule;
2. complete encapsulation;
3. clearly distinct architecture inside and outside the capsule; and
4. compression of the thyroid parenchyma outside the capsule.
    Usually, an adenoma is small (up to 3 cm in diameter) and spherical. On cut section, the adenoma is grey-white to red-brown, less colloidal than the surrounding thyroid parenchyma.

M/E The tumour shows complete fibrous encapsulation. The tumour cells are benign follicular epithelial cells lining follicles of various sizes. These cells may also form trabecular, solid and cord patterns with little follicle formation. Accordingly, the following 6 types of growth patterns are distinguished.
1. *Microfollicular (foetal) adenoma* consists of small follicles containing little or no colloid and separated by abundant loose stroma.
2. *Normofollicular (simple) adenoma* has closely packed follicles like that of normal thyroid gland.
3. *Macrofollicular (colloid) adenoma* contains large follicles of varying size and distended with colloid.
4. *Trabecular (embryonal) adenoma* resembles embryonal thyroid and consists of closely packed solid or trabecular pattern of epithelial cells.
5. *Hurthle cell (oxyphilic) adenoma* is an uncommon variant composed of solid trabeculae of large cells having abundant granular oxyphilic cytoplasm and vesicular nuclei.
6. *Atypical adenoma* is the term used for a follicular adenoma which has more pronounced cellular proliferation so that features may be considered indicative of malignancy such as pleomorphism, increased mitoses and nuclear atypia.

Approximately 95% of all primary thyroid cancers are carcinomas. Primary lymphomas of the thyroid comprise less than 5% of thyroid cancers and majority of them possibly evolve from autoimmune (lymphocytic) thyroiditis.

In line with most other thyroid lesions, most carcinomas of the thyroid too have female preponderance and are twice more common in women.

Carcinoma of the thyroid gland has 4 major morphologic types with distinctly different clinical behaviour and variable prevalence.

ETIOPATHOGENESIS Most important environmental factor implicated in the etiology of thyroid cancer is external radiation, and to some extent, there is role of TSH receptors and iodine excess.

1. External radiation The single most important environmental factor associated with increased risk of developing thyroid carcinoma after many years of exposure to external radiation of high dose.

2. Iodine excess and TSH In regions where endemic goitre is widespread, addition of iodine to diet has resulted in increase in incidence of papillary cancer.

3. Genetic basis Familial clustering of thyroid cancer has been observed, especially in medullary carcinoma. Molecular studies reveal that thyroid carcinoma is a multistep process:

i) *Papillary thyroid carcinoma*: Mutation in *RET* gene (gene over-expression) located on chromosome 10q is seen in about 20% cases of papillary thyroid carcinoma.

ii) *Follicular thyroid carcinoma*: About 50% cases of follicular thyroid carcinoma have mutation in *RAS* family of oncogenes that includes *HRAS, NRAS* and *KRAS*.

iii) *Medullary thyroid carcinoma:* Medullary thyroid carcinoma arises from parafollicular C-cells in the thyroid. Point mutation in *RET*-protooncogene is seen in both familial (MEN2) as well as sporadic cases of medullary thyroid carcinoma.

iv) *Anaplastic thyroid carcinoma:* This tumour either arises from further dedifferentiation of differentiated papillary or follicular thyroid carcinoma, or by inactivating point mutation in *p53* tumour suppressor gene or by mutation in gene coding for β-catenin pathway.

PAPILLARY THYROID CARCINOMA

Papillary carcinoma is the most common type of thyroid carcinoma, comprising 75-85% of cases. It can occur at all ages including children and young adults but the incidence is higher with advancing age. The tumour is found about three times more frequently in females than in males.

Involvement of the regional lymph nodes is common but distant metastases to organs are rare. *'Lateral aberrant thyroid'* is the term used for occurrence of thyroid tissue in the lateral cervical lymph node, which in most patients represents a well-differentiated metastasis of an occult papillary carcinoma of the thyroid.

G/A Papillary carcinoma may range from microscopic foci to nodules upto 10 cm in diameter and is generally poorly delineated. Cut surface of the tumour is greyish-white, hard and scar-like.

M/E The following features are present:

1. Papillary pattern Papillae composed of fibrovascular stalk and covered by single layer of tumour cells is the predominant feature.

2. Tumour cells The tumour cells have characteristic nuclear features due to dispersed nuclear chromatin imparting it *ground glass or optically clear appearance* and clear or oxyphilic cytoplasm.

3. Invasion The tumour cells invade the capsule and intrathyroid lymphatics but invasion of blood vessels is rare.

4. Psammoma bodies Half of papillary carcinomas show typical small, concentric, calcified spherules called psammoma bodies in the stroma.

The prognosis of papillary carcinoma is good.

FOLLICULAR THYROID CARCINOMA

Follicular carcinoma is the other common type of thyroid cancer, next only to papillary carcinoma and comprises about 10-20% of all thyroid carcinomas. It is more common in middle and old age and has preponderance in females (female-male ratio 2.5:1). In contrast to papillary carcinoma, follicular carcinoma has a positive correlation with endemic goitre but the role of external radiation in its etiology is unclear.

Follicular carcinoma presents clinically either as a solitary nodule or as an irregular, firm and nodular thyroid enlargement. Distant metastases by haematogenous route are common, especially to the lungs and bones.

G/A Follicular carcinoma may be either in the form of a solitary adenoma-like circumscribed nodule or as an obvious cancerous irregular thyroid enlargement. The cut surface of the tumour is grey-white with areas of haemorrhages, necrosis and cyst formation and may extend to involve adjacent structures.

M/E The following features are present:

1. **Follicular pattern** Follicular carcinoma, like follicular adenoma, is composed of follicles of various sizes and may show trabecular or solid pattern. The tumour cells have hyperchromatic nuclei and the cytoplasm resembles that of normal follicular cells.

2. **Vascular invasion and direct extension** Vascular invasion and direct extension to involve the adjacent structures (e.g. into the capsule) are significant features but lymphatic invasion is rare.

The prognosis of follicular carcinoma is between that of papillary and undifferentiated carcinoma.

MEDULLARY THYROID CARCINOMA

Medullary carcinoma is a less frequent type derived from parafollicular or C-cells present in the thyroid and comprises about 5% of thyroid carcinomas. It is equally common in men and women.

1. **Familial occurrence** Most cases of medullary carcinoma occur sporadically, but about 10% have a genetic background with point mutation in *RET*-protooncogene located on chromosome 10q. The familial form of medullary carcinoma has association with pheochromocytoma and parathyroid adenoma (multiple endocrine neoplasia, MEN II A), or with pheochromocytoma and multiple mucosal neuromas (MEN II B).

2. **Secretion of calcitonin and other peptides** Like normal C-cells, tumour cells of medullary carcinoma secrete calcitonin, the hypocalcaemic hormone. In addition, the tumour may also elaborate prostaglandins, histaminase, somatostatin, vasoactive intestinal peptide (VIP) and ACTH.

3. **Amyloid stroma** Most medullary carcinomas have amyloid deposits in the stroma which stains positively with usual amyloid stains such as Congo red.

G/A The tumour may either appear as a unilateral solitary nodule *(sporadic form)*, or have bilateral and multicentric involvement *(familial form)*. Cut surface of tumour in both forms shows well-defined tumour areas which are firm to hard, grey-white to yellow-brown with areas of haemorrhages and necrosis.

M/E The features are as under:

1. **Tumour cells** Like other neuroendocrine tumours (e.g. carcinoid, islet cell tumour, paraganglioma etc.), medullary carcinoma of the thyroid too has a well-defined organoid pattern, forming nests of tumour cells separated by fibrovascular septa. Sometimes, the tumour cells may be arranged in sheets, ribbons pseudopapillae or small follicles.

2. **Amyloid stroma** The tumour cells are separated by amyloid stroma derived from altered calcitonin which can be demonstrated by immunostain for calcitonin. The staining properties of amyloid are similar to that seen in systemic amyloidosis and may have areas of irregular calcification but without regular laminations seen in psammoma bodies.

3. C-cell hyperplasia Familial cases generally have C-cell hyperplasia as a precursor lesion but not in sporadic cases.

Most medullary carcinomas are slow-growing. Regional lymph node metastases may occur but distant organ metastases are infrequent. The prognosis is better in familial form than in the sporadic form.

ANAPLASTIC CARCINOMA

Undifferentiated or anaplastic carcinoma of the thyroid comprises less than 5% of all thyroid cancers and is one of the most malignant tumour in humans. The tumour is predominantly found in old age (7th-8th decades) and is slightly more common in females than in males (female-male ratio 1.5:1). The tumour is widely aggressive and rapidly growing.

G/A The tumour is generally large and irregular, often invading the adjacent strap muscles of the neck and other structures in the vicinity of the thyroid. Cut surface of the tumour is white and firm with areas of necrosis and haemorrhages.

M/E There are 3 histologic variants:

1. Small cell carcinoma This type of tumour is composed of closely packed small cells having hyperchromatic nuclei and numerous mitoses. This variant closely resembles malignant lymphoma.

2. Spindle cell carcinoma These tumours are composed of spindle cells resembling sarcoma. Some tumours may contain obvious sarcomatous component such as areas of osteosarcoma, chondrosarcoma or rhabdomyosarcoma.

3. Giant cell carcinoma This type is composed of highly anaplastic giant cells showing numerous atypical mitoses, bizarre and lobed nuclei and some assuming spindle shapes.

The prognosis is poor.

PARATHYROID GLANDS (p. 806)

NORMAL STRUCTURE

ANATOMY The parathyroid glands are usually 4 in number: the *superior pair* derived from the 4th branchial pouch and *inferior pair* from the 3rd branchial pouch of primitive foregut. In the adults, each gland is an oval, yellowish-brown, flattened body, weighing 35-45 mg.

M/E Parathyroid glands are composed of solid sheets and cords of parenchymal cells and variable amount of stromal fat. The parenchymal cells are of 3 types: *chief cells, oxyphil cells* and *water-clear cells.*

The major *function* of the parathyroid hormone, in conjunction with calcitonin and vitamin D, is to regulate serum calcium levels and metabolism of bone. The role of parathyroid hormone in regulating calcium metabolism in the body is at the following 3 levels:

1. Parathyroid hormone *stimulates osteoclastic activity* and results in resorption of bone and release of calcium. Calcitonin released by C-cells, on the other hand, opposes parathyroid hormone by preventing resorption of bone and lowering serum calcium level.

2. Parathyroid hormone acts *directly on renal tubular epithelial cells* and increases renal reabsorption of calcium and inhibits reabsorption of phosphate; calcitonin enhances renal excretion of phosphate.

3. Parathyroid hormone increases renal production of the *most active metabolite of vitamin D*, i.e. 1, 25-dihydrocholecalciferol, which in turn increases calcium absorption from the small intestine.

HYPERPARATHYROIDISM (p. 806)

PRIMARY HYPERPARATHYROIDISM

Primary hyperparathyroidism is not uncommon and occurs more commonly with increasing age. It is especially likely to occur in women near the time of menopause.

ETIOLOGY   Common causes are as under:
1.   Most commonly, parathyroid adenomas in approximately 80% cases.
2.   Carcinoma of the parathyroid glands in 2-3% patients.
3.   Primary hyperplasia in about 15% cases (usually chief cell hyperplasia).
Also included above are the familial cases of multiple endocrine neoplasia (MEN) syndromes where parathyroid adenoma or primary hyperplasia is one of the components.

CLINICAL FEATURES   Biochemical changes are:
i)   Elevated levels of parathyroid hormone
ii)   Hypercalcaemia
iii) Hypophosphataemia
iv)   Hypercalciuria
Clinical presentation of individuals with primary hyperparathyroidism may be in a variety of ways:
1.   Most commonly, *nephrolithiasis* and or/*nephrocalcinosis*.
2.   *Metastatic calcification*, especially in the blood vessels, kidneys, lungs, stomach, eyes and other tissues.
3.   *Generalised osteitis fibrosa cystica* due to osteoclastic resorption of bone and its replacement by connective tissue.
4.   *Neuropsychiatric disturbances* such as depression, anxiety, psychosis and coma.
5.   *Hypertension* is found in about half the cases.

SECONDARY HYPERPARATHYROIDISM

Secondary hyperparathyroidism occurs due to increased parathyroid hormone elaboration secondary to a disease elsewhere in the body. Hypocalcaemia stimulates compensatory hyperplasia of the parathyroid glands and causes secondary hyperparathyroidism.

ETIOLOGY   Important causes are:
1.   *Chronic renal insufficiency* resulting in retention of phosphate and impaired intestinal absorption of calcium.
2.   *Vitamin D deficiency* and consequent rickets and osteomalacia may cause parathyroid hyperfunction.
3.   *Intestinal malabsorption syndromes* causing deficiency of calcium and vitamin D.

CLINICAL FEATURES   The main biochemical abnormality in secondary hyperparathyroidism is mild hypocalcaemia, in striking contrast to hypercalcaemia in primary hyperparathyroidism. The patients with secondary hyperparathyroidism have signs and symptoms of the disease which caused it.

TERTIARY HYPERPARATHYROIDISM

Tertiary hyperparathyroidism is a complication of secondary hyperparathyroidism in which the hyperfunction persists in spite of removal of the cause of secondary hyperplasia. Possibly, a hyperplastic nodule in the parathyroid gland develops which becomes partially autonomous and continues to secrete large quantities of parathyroid hormone without regard to the needs of the body.

HYPOPARATHYROIDISM *(p. 807)*

PRIMARY HYPOPARATHYROIDISM

Primary hypoparathyroidism is caused by disease of the parathyroid glands. Most common causes of primary hypoparathyroidism are: surgical procedures involving thyroid, parathyroid, or radical neck dissection for cancer.

CLINICAL FEATURES   The main biochemical dysfunctions in primary hypoparathyroidism are hypocalcaemia, hyperphosphataemia and hypocalciuria. The clinical manifestations of these abnormalities are as under:

1. Increased neuromuscular irritability and tetany
2. Calcification of the lens and cataract formation
3. Abnormalities in cardiac conduction
4. Disorders of the CNS due to intracranial calcification
5. Abnormalities of the teeth.

PSEUDO-HYPOPARATHYROIDISM

In pseudo-hypoparathyroidism, the tissues fail to respond to parathyroid hormone though parathyroid glands are usually normal. It is a rare inherited condition with an autosomal dominant character. The patients are generally females and are characterised by signs and symptoms of hypoparathyroidism and other clinical features like short stature, short metacarpals and meta-tarsals, flat nose, round face and multiple exostoses.

PSEUDOPSEUDO-HYPOPARATHYROIDISM

Pseudopseudo-hypoparathyroidism is another rare familial disorder in which all the clinical features of pseudo-hypoparathyroidism are present except that these patients have no hypocalcaemia or hyperphosphataemia and the tissues respond normally to parathyroid hormone.

PARATHYROID TUMOURS (p. 808)

PARATHYROID ADENOMA

The commonest tumour of the parathyroid glands is an adenoma. It may occur at any age and in either sex but is found more frequently in adult life. Most adenomas are first brought to attention because of excessive secretion of parathyroid hormone causing features of hyperparathyroidism as described above.

G/A A parathyroid adenoma is small (less than 5 cm diameter) encapsulated, yellowish-brown, ovoid nodule and weighing up to 5 gm or more.

M/E Majority of adenomas are predominantly composed of chief cells arranged in sheets or cords. Oxyphil cells and water-clear cells may be found intermingled in varying proportions.

PARATHYROID CARCINOMA

Carcinoma of the parathyroid is rare and produces manifestations of hyperparathyroidism which is often more pronounced. Carcinoma tends to be irregular in shape and is adherent to the adjacent tissues. Most para-thyroid carcinomas are well-differentiated.

ENDOCRINE PANCREAS (p. 808)

The human pancreas, though anatomically a single organ, histologically and functionally, has 2 distinct parts—the exocrine and endocrine. The discussion here is focused on the endocrine pancreas and its two main disorders: *diabetes mellitus* and *islet cell tumours*.

NORMAL STRUCTURE

The endocrine pancreas consists of microscopic collections of cells called islets of Langerhans found scattered within the pancreatic lobules, as well as individual endocrine cells found in duct epithelium and among the acini. The total weight of endocrine pancreas in the adult, however, does not exceed 1-1.5 gm (total weight of pancreas 60-100 gm). Ultrastructurally and immunohistochemically, 4 *major* and 2 *minor* types of islet cells are distinguished, each type having its distinct secretory product and function.

A. Major cell types:

1. *Beta (β) or B cells* comprise about 70% of islet cells and secrete insulin, the defective response or deficient synthesis of which causes diabetes mellitus.

2. *Alpha (α) or A cells* comprise 20% of islet cells and secrete glucagon which induces hyperglycaemia.

3. *Delta (δ) or D cells* comprise 5-10% of islet cells and secrete somatostatin which suppresses both insulin and glucagon release.

4. *Pancreatic polypeptide (PP) cells or F cells* comprise 1-2% of islet cells and secrete pancreatic polypeptide having some gastrointestinal effects.

B. Minor cell types:

1. *D1 cells* elaborate vasoactive intestinal peptide (VIP) which induces glycogenolysis and hyperglycaemia and causes secretory diarrhoea by stimulation of gastrointestinal fluid secretion.

2. *Enterochromaffin cells* synthesise serotonin which in pancreatic tumours may induce carcinoid syndrome.

DIABETES MELLITUS (p. 808)

DEFINITION AND EPIDEMIOLOGY

As per the WHO, diabetes mellitus (DM) is defined as a hetrogeneous metabolic disorder characterised by common feature of chronic hyperglycaemia with disturbance of carbohydrate, fat and protein metabolism. At this point, it is also important to understand another related term, *metabolic syndrome* (also called syndrome X or insulin resistance syndrome), consisting of a combination of metabolic abnormalities which increase the risk to develop diabetes mellitus and cardiovascular disease. Major features of metabolic syndrome are central obesity, hypertriglyceridaemia, low LDL cholesterol, hyperglycaemia and hypertension.

CLASSIFICATION AND ETIOLOGY

The older classification systems dividing DM into primary (idiopathic) and secondary types, juvenile-onset and maturity onset types, and insulin-dependent (IDDM) and non-insulin dependent (NIDDM) types, have become obsolete and undergone major revision due to extensive understanding of etiology and pathogenesis of DM in recent times.

Current classification of DM based on etiology divides it into two broad categories—type 1 and type 2; besides there are a few uncommon specific etiologic types, and gestational DM. American Diabetes Association (2007) has identified risk factors for type 2 DM as under:

1. Family history of type 2 DM
2. Obesity
3. Habitual physical inactivity
4. Race and ethnicity (Blacks, Asians, Pacific Islanders)
5. Previous identification of impaired fasting glucose or impaired glucose tolerance
6. History of gestational DM or delivery of baby heavier than 4 kg
7. Hypertension
8. Dyslipidaemia (HDL level < 35 mg/dl or triglycerides > 250 mg/dl)
9. Polycystic ovary disease and acanthosis nigricans
10. History of vascular disease

TYPE 1 DM It constitutes about 10% cases of DM. It was previously termed as juvenile-onset diabetes (JOD) due to its occurrence in younger age, and was called insulin-dependent DM (IDDM). However, in the new classification, neither age nor insulin-dependence are considered as absolute criteria. Instead, based on underlying etiology, type 1 DM is further divided into 2 subtypes:

Subtype 1A (immune-mediated) DM characterised by autoimmune destruction of β-cells which usually leads to insulin deficiency.

Subtype 1B (idiopathic) DM characterised by insulin deficiency with tendency to develop ketosis but these patients are negative for autoimmune markers.

TYPE 2 DM This type comprises about 80% cases of DM. It was previously called maturity-onset diabetes, or non-insulin dependent diabetes mellitus (NIDDM) of obese and non-obese type.

Although type 2 DM predominantly affects older individuals, it is now known that it also occurs in obese adolescent children. Moreover, many type 2 DM patients also require insulin therapy to control hyperglycaemia or to prevent ketosis and thus are not truly non-insulin dependent contrary to its older nomenclature.

OTHER SPECIFIC ETIOLOGIC TYPES OF DM Besides the two main types, about 10% cases of DM have a known specific etiologic defect. One important subtype in this group is *maturity-onset diabetes of the young (MODY)* which has autosomal dominant inheritance, early onset of hyperglycaemia and impaired insulin secretion.

GESTATIONAL DM About 4% pregnant women develop DM due to metabolic changes during pregnancy. Although they revert back to normal glycaemia after delivery, these women are prone to develop DM later in their life.

PATHOGENESIS

Depending upon etiology of DM, hyperglycaemia may result from:
- ◈ Reduced insulin secretion
- ◈ Decreased glucose use by the body
- ◈ Increased glucose production.

Pathogenesis of two main types of DM and its complications is distinct and is discussed in relation to normal insulin metabolism.

NORMAL INSULIN METABOLISM *The major stimulus for both synthesis and release of insulin is glucose.*

Synthesis Insulin is synthesised in the β-cells of pancreatic islets of Langerhans:

i) It is initially formed as *pre-proinsulin* which is single-chain 86-amino acid precursor polypeptide.

ii) Subsequent proteolysis removes the amino terminal signal peptide, forming *proinsulin*.

iii) Further cleavage of proinsulin gives rise to *A (21 amino acids) and B (30 amino acids) chains* of insulin, linked together by connecting segment called *C-peptide*, all of which are stored in the secretory granules in the β-cells.

Release Glucose is the key regulator of insulin secretion from β-cells by a series of steps:

i) Hyperglycaemia (glucose level more than 70 mg/dl or above 3.9 mmol/L) stimulates transport into β-cells of a *glucose transporter, GLUT2*.

ii) An islet transcription factor, *glucokinase,* causes glucose phosphorylation, and thus acts as a step for controlled release of glucose-regulated insulin secretion.

iii) Metabolism of glucose to glucose-6-phosphate by glycolysis generates *ATP*.

iv) Generation of ATP *alters the ion channel activity* on the membrane.

Action Half of insulin secreted from β-cells into portal vein is degraded in the liver while the remaining half enters the systemic circulation for action on the target cells:

i) Insulin from circulation binds to its receptor on the target cells. *Insulin receptor has intrinsic tyrosine kinase activity.*

ii) This, in turn, activates post-receptor intracellular signalling pathway molecules, *insulin receptor substrates (IRS) 1 and 2 proteins*, which initiate sequence of phosphorylation and dephosphorylation reactions.

iii) These reactions on the target cells are responsible for the main *mitogenic and anabolic actions of insulin*—glycogen synthesis, glucose transport, protein synthesis, lipogenesis.

PATHOGENESIS OF TYPE 1 DM *The basic phenomenon in type 1 DM is destruction of β-cell mass, usually leading to absolute insulin deficiency.* While type 1B DM remains idiopathic, pathogenesis of type 1A DM is immune-mediated and has been extensively studied. Currently, pathogenesis of type 1A DM is explained on the basis of 3 mutually-interlinked mechanisms.

1. **Genetic susceptibility** Following features support it:
i)   It has been observed in *identical twins* that if one twin has type 1A DM, there is about 50% chance of the second twin developing it.
ii)   About half the cases with genetic predisposition to type 1A DM have the *susceptibility gene* located in the HLA region.

2. **Autoimmunity** Following immunologic abnormalities are seen:
i)   Presence of *islet cell antibodies* against GAD (glutamic acid decarboxylase), insulin etc.
ii)   Occurrence of lymphocytic infiltrate in and around the pancreatic islets termed *insulitis.*
iii) *Selective destruction of β-cells.*
iv)   Role of *T cell-mediated autoimmunity.*
v)   Association of type 1A DM with *other autoimmune diseases* in about 10-20% cases.
vi)   Remission of type 1A DM in response to immunosuppressive therapy such as administration of cyclosporin A.

3. **Environmental factors** These include:
i)   *Certain viral infections* preceding the onset of disease.
ii)   *Experimental induction* of type 1A DM with certain chemicals has been possible e.g. alloxan, streptozotocin and pentamidine.
iii) *Geographic and seasonal variations* in its incidence.
iv)   Possible relationship of early exposure to *bovine milk proteins.*

KEY POINTS Pathogenesis of type 1A DM .can be summed up by interlinking the above three factors as under:
1.   At birth, individuals with *genetic susceptibility* to this disorder have normal β-cell mass.
2.   β-cells act as autoantigens and activate CD4+ T lymphocytes, bringing about immune destruction of pancreatic β-cells by *autoimmune phenomena* and takes months to years. Clinical features of diabetes manifest after more than 80% of β-cell mass has been destroyed.
3.   The trigger for autoimmune process appears to be some *infectious or environmental factor* which specifically targets β-cells.

PATHOGENESIS OF TYPE 2 DM The basic metabolic defect in type 2 DM is either a delayed insulin secretion relative to glucose load *(impaired insulin secretion),* or the peripheral tissues are unable to respond to insulin *(insulin resistance).*

1. **Genetic factors** Genetic component has a stronger basis for type 2 DM than type 1A DM.
i)   There is approximately 80% chance of developing diabetes in the other *identical twin* if one twin has the disease.
ii)   A person with one parent having type 2 DM is at an increased risk of getting diabetes.

2. **Constitutional factors** Certain environmental factors such as obesity, hypertension, and level of physical activity play contributory role and modulate the phenotyping of the disease.

3. **Insulin resistance** Obesity, in particular, is strongly associated with insulin resistance and hence type 2 DM. Mechanism of hyperglycaemia in these cases is explained as under:
i)   Resistance to action of insulin *impairs glucose utilisation* and hence hyperglycaemia.
ii)   There is *increased hepatic synthesis* of glucose.
iii) *Hyperglycaemia in obesity* is related to high levels of free fatty acids and cytokines affect peripheral tissue sensitivity to respond to insulin.

4. **Impaired insulin secretion** Insulin release and resistance are interlinked:
i) Early in the course of disease, in response to insulin resistance there is compensatory increased secretion of insulin *(hyperinsulinaemia)* in an attempt to maintain normal blood glucose level.

ii) Eventually, however, there is *failure of β-cell function* to secrete adequate insulin, although there is some secretion of insulin i.e. cases of type 2 DM have mild to moderate deficiency of insulin.

5. Increased hepatic glucose synthesis One of the normal roles played by insulin is to promote hepatic storage of glucose as glycogen and suppress gluconeogenesis. In type 2 DM, there is increased hepatic synthesis of glucose which contributes to hyperglycaemia in these cases.

KEY POINTS In essence, hyperglycaemia in type 2 DM is not due to destruction of β-cells but is instead a failure of β-cells to meet the requirement of insulin in the body. Its pathogenesis can be summed up by interlinking the above factors as under:
1. Type 2 DM is a more *complex multifactorial disease.*
2. There is greater role of *genetic defect and heredity.*
3. Two main mechanisms for hyperglycaemia in type 2 DM—*insulin resistance and impaired insulin secretion*, are interlinked.
4. While *obesity* plays a role in pathogenesis of insulin resistance, impaired insulin secretion may be from many constitutional factors.
5. *Increased hepatic synthesis of glucose* in initial period of disease contributes to hyperglycaemia.

MORPHOLOGIC FEATURES IN PANCREATIC ISLETS
The changes are more distinctive in type 1 DM:

1. Insulitis:
◈ **In type 1 DM,** characteristically, in early stage there is lymphocytic infiltrate, mainly by T cells, in the islets.
◈ **In type 2 DM,** there is no significant leucocytic infiltrate in the islets but there is variable degree of fibrous tissue in the islets.

2. Islet cell mass:
◈ **In type 1 DM,** as the disease becomes chronic there is progressive depletion of β-cell mass.
◈ **In type 2 DM,** β-cell mass is either normal or mildly reduced.

3. Amyloidosis:
◈ **In type 1 DM,** deposits of amyloid around islets are absent.
◈ **In type 2 DM,** characteristically chronic long-standing cases show deposition of amyloid material, amylin, around the capillaries of the islets.
◈ **β-cell degranulation:**
◈ **In type 1 DM,** EM shows degranulation of remaining β-cells of islets.
◈ **In type 2 DM,** no such change is observed.

CLINICAL FEATURES

Type 1 DM:
i) Patients of type 1 DM usually manifest at early age, generally below the age of 35.
ii) The onset of symptoms is often abrupt.
iii) At presentation, these patients have polyuria, polydipsia and polyphagia.
iv) The patients are not obese but have generally progressive loss of weight.
v) These patients are prone to develop metabolic complications such as ketoacidosis and hypoglycaemic episodes.

Type 2 DM:
i) This form of diabetes generally manifests in middle life or beyond, usually above the age of 40.
ii) The onset of symptoms in type 2 DM is slow and insidious.
iii) Generally, the patient is asymptomatic when the diagnosis is made on the basis of glucosuria or hyperglycaemia during physical examination, or may present with polyuria and polydipsia.
iv) The patients are frequently obese and have unexplained weakness and loss of weight.
v) Metabolic complications such as ketoacidosis are infrequent.

It is now known that in both type 1 and 2 DM, *severity and chronicity of hyperglycaemia* forms the main pathogenetic mechanism for 'microvascular complications' (e.g. retinopathy, nephropathy, neuropathy); therefore control of blood glucose level constitutes the mainstay of treatment for minimising development of these complications. Longstanding cases of type 2 DM, however, in addition, frequently develop 'macrovascular complications' (e.g. atherosclerosis, coronary artery disease, peripheral vascular disease, cerebrovascular disease) which are more difficult to explain on the basis of hyperglycaemia alone.

The following biochemical mechanisms have been proposed to explain the development of complications of diabetes mellitus:

1. **Non-enzymatic protein glycosylation** The free amino group of various body proteins binds by non-enzymatic mechanism to glucose; this process is called *glycosylation* and is directly proportionate to the severity of hyperglycaemia.

2. **Polyol pathway mechanism** This mechanism is responsible for producing lesions in the aorta, lens of the eye, kidney and peripheral nerves. These tissues have an enzyme, aldose reductase, that reacts with glucose to form sorbitol and fructose in the cells of the hyperglycaemic patient.

These polyols result in disturbed processing of normal intermediary metabolites leading to complications of diabetes.

3. **Excessive oxygen free radicals** In hyperglycaemia, there is increased production of reactive oxygen free radicals from mitochondrial oxidative phosphorylation which may damage various target cells in diabetes.

COMPLICATIONS OF DIABETES

As a consequence of hyperglycaemia of diabetes, every tissue and organ of the body undergoes biochemical and structural alterations which account for the major complications in diabetics which may be *acute metabolic* or *chronic systemic*.

Both types of diabetes mellitus may develop complications which are broadly divided into 2 major groups:

I. ACUTE METABOLIC COMPLICATIONS Metabolic complications develop acutely.

1. **Diabetic ketoacidosis (DKA)** Ketoacidosis is almost exclusively a complication of type 1 DM. Clinically, the condition is characterised by anorexia, nausea, vomitings, deep and fast breathing, mental confusion and coma. Most patients of ketoacidosis recover.

2. **Hyperosmolar hyperglycaemic nonketotic coma (HHS)** Hyperosmolar hyperglycaemic nonketotic coma is usually a complication of type 2 DM. Blood sugar is extremely high and plasma osmolality is high. Thrombotic and bleeding complications are frequent due to high viscosity of blood. The mortality rate in hyperosmolar nonketotic coma is high.

3. **Hypoglycaemia** Hypoglycaemic episode may develop in patients of type 1 DM. It may result from excessive administration of insulin, missing a meal, or due to stress.

II. LATE SYSTEMIC COMPLICATIONS A number of systemic complications may develop after a period of 15-20 years in either type of diabetes.

1. **Atherosclerosis** Diabetes mellitus of both type 1 and type 2 accelerates the development of atherosclerosis. Consequently, atherosclerotic lesions appear earlier than in the general population, are more extensive, and are more often associated with complicated plaques such as ulceration, calcification and thrombosis.

The possible ill-effects of accelerated atherosclerosis in diabetes are early onset of coronary artery disease, silent myocardial infarction, cerebral stroke and gangrene of the toes and feet. Gangrene of the lower extremities is 100 times more common in diabetics than in non-diabetics.

2. Diabetic microangiopathy Microangiopathy of diabetes is characterised by basement membrane thickening of small blood vessels and capillaries of different organs and tissues such as the skin, skeletal muscle, eye and kidney.

3. Diabetic nephropathy Renal involvement is a common complication and a leading cause of death in diabetes. Four types of lesions are described in diabetic nephropathy:

i) *Diabetic glomerulosclerosis* which includes diffuse and nodular lesions of glomerulosclerosis.

ii) *Vascular lesions* that include hyaline arteriolosclerosis of afferent and efferent arterioles and atheromas of renal arteries.

iii) *Diabetic pyelonephritis* and *necrotising renal papillitis*.

iv) *Tubular lesions* or *Armanni-Ebstein lesion*.

4. Diabetic neuropathy Diabetic neuropathy may affect all parts of the nervous system but symmetric peripheral neuropathy is most characteristic. The basic pathologic changes are segmental demyelination.

5. Diabetic retinopathy Diabetic retinopathy is a leading cause of blindness. There are 2 types of lesions involving retinal vessels: *background* and *proliferative*.

6. Infections Diabetics have enhanced susceptibility to various infections such as tuberculosis, pneumonias, pyelonephritis, otitis, carbuncles and diabetic ulcers. This could be due to various factors such as impaired leucocyte functions, reduced cellular immunity, poor blood supply due to vascular involvement and hyperglycaemia *per se*.

DIAGNOSIS OF DIABETES

Hyperglycaemia remains the fundamental basis for the diagnosis of diabetes mellitus. In *symptomatic cases,* the diagnosis is not a problem and can be confirmed by finding glucosuria and a random plasma glucose concentration above 200 mg/dl.

◈ The severity of clinical symptoms of polyuria and polydipsia is directly related to the degree of hyperglycaemia.

◈ In *asymptomatic cases,* when there is persistently elevated fasting plasma glucose level, diagnosis again poses no difficulty.

◈ The problem arises in asymptomatic patients who have normal fasting glucose level in the plasma but are suspected to have diabetes on other grounds and are thus subjected to oral glucose tolerance test (GTT). The American Diabetes Association (2007) has recommended definite diagnostic criteria for early diagnosis of diabetes mellitus as under:

PLASMA GLUCOSE VALUE	DIAGNOSIS
FASTING (FOR > 8 HOURS) VALUE	
Below 100 mg/dl (< 5.6 mmol/L)	Normal fasting value
100-125 mg/dl (5.6-6.9 mmol/L)	Impaired fasting glucose (IFG)
126 mg/dl (7.0 mmol/L) or more	Diabetes mellitus
TWO-HOUR AFTER 75 GM ORAL GLUCOSE LOAD	
< 140 mg/dl (< 7.8 mmol/L)	Normal post-prandial GTT
140-199 mg/dl (7.8-11.1 mmol/L)	Impaired post-prandial glucose tolerance (IGT)
200 mg/dl (11.1 mmol/L) or more	Diabetes mellitus
RANDOM VALUE	
200 mg/dl (11.1 mmol/L) or more in a symptomatic patient	Diabetes mellitus

diabetes mellitus:

URINE TESTING Urine tests are cheap and convenient but the diagnosis of diabetes cannot be based on urine testing alone since there may be false-positives and false-negatives. They can be used in population screening surveys. Urine is tested for the presence of glucose and ketones.

. **Glucosuria** *Benedict's qualitative test* detects any reducing substance in the urine and is not specific for glucose. More sensitive and glucose specific test is *dipstick* method based on enzyme-coated paper strip which turns purple when dipped in urine containing glucose.

◆ *Renal glucosuria*: After diabetes, the next most common cause of glucosuria is the reduced renal threshold for glucose. In such cases although the blood glucose level is below 180 mg/dl (i.e. below normal renal threshold for glucose) but glucose still appears regularly and consistently in the urine due to lowered renal threshold.

Renal glucosuria is a benign condition unrelated to diabetes and runs in families and may occur temporarily in pregnancy without symptoms of diabetes.

◆ *Alimentary (lag storage) glucosuria*: A rapid and transitory rise in blood glucose level above the normal renal threshold may occur in some individuals after a meal. During this period, glucosuria is present. This type of response to meal is called 'lag storage curve' or more appropriately 'alimentary glucosuria'. A characteristic feature is that unusually high blood glucose level returns to normal 2 hours after meal.

. **Ketonuria** Tests for ketone bodies in the urine are required for assessing the severity of diabetes and not for diagnosis of diabetes.

I. **SINGLE BLOOD SUGAR ESTIMATION** For diagnosis of diabetes, blood sugar determinations are absolutely necessary. Whole blood or plasma may be used but *whole blood values are 15% lower than plasma values.*

A grossly elevated single determination of plasma glucose may be sufficient to make the diagnosis of diabetes. A *fasting plasma glucose value above 126 mg/dl (≥7 mmol/L) is certainly indicative of diabetes.* In other cases, oral GTT is performed.

II. **SCREENING BY FASTING GLUCOSE TEST** Fasting plasma glucose determination is a screening test for DM type 2.

V. **ORAL GLUCOSE TOLERANCE TEST** Oral GTT is performed principally for patients with borderline fasting plasma glucose value (i.e. between 100 and 140 mg/dl). A fasting blood sugar sample is first drawn. Then 75 gm of glucose dissolved in 300 ml of water is given. Blood and urine specimen are collected at half-hourly intervals for at least 2 hours. Blood or plasma glucose content is measured and urine is tested for glucosuria.

◆ Normal cut off value for fasting blood glucose level is considered as 100 mg/dl.

◆ Cases with fasting blood glucose value in range of 100-125 mg/dl are considered as *impaired fasting glucose tolerance (IGT);* these cases are at increased risk of developing diabetes later and therefore kept under observation for repeating the test. During pregnancy, however, a case of IGT is treated as a diabetic.

◆ Individuals with fasting value of plasma glucose higher than 126 mg/dl and 2-hour value after 75 gm oral glucose higher than 200 mg/dl are labelled as *diabetics*.

◆ In symptomatic case, the random blood glucose value above 200 mg/dl is diagnosed as diabetes mellitus.

V. **OTHER TESTS** A few other tests are sometimes performed in specific conditions in diabetics and for research purposes:

1. **Glycosylated haemoglobin (HbA$_{1C}$)** Measurement of blood glucose level in diabetics suffers from variation due to dietary intake of the previous day. Long-term objective assessment of degree of glycaemic control is better monitored by measurement of glycosylated haemoglobin (HbA$_{1C}$). This is because the non-enzymatic glycosylation of haemoglobin takes place over 90-120 days, lifespan of red blood cells. HbA$_{1C}$ assay, therefore, gives an estimate of diabetic control and compliance for the preceding 3-4 months.

2. **Glycated albumin** This is used to monitor degree of hyperglycaemia during previous 1-2 weeks when HbA$_{1C}$ can not be used.

3. **Extended GTT** The oral GTT is extended to 3-4 hours for appearance of symptoms of hyperglycaemia.

4. **Intravenous GTT** This test is performed in persons who have intestinal malabsorption or in postgastrectomy cases.

5. **Cortisone-primed GTT** This provocative test is a useful investigative aid in cases of potential diabetics.

6. **Insulin assay** Plasma insulin can be measured by radioimmunoassay and ELISA technique.

7. **Proinsulin assay** Proinsulin is included in immunoassay of insulin.

8. **C-peptide assay** This test is even more sensitive than insulin assay because its levels are not affected by insulin therapy.

9. **Islet autoantibodies** Glutamic acid decarboxylase and islet cell cytoplasmic antibodies may be used as a marker for type 1 DM.

10. **Screening for diabetes-associated complications** Screening tests are done for DM-associated complications e.g. microalbuniuria, dyslipidaemia, thyroid dysfunction etc.

ISLET CELL TUMOURS *(p. 818)*

INSULINOMA (β-CELL TUMOUR)

Insulinomas or beta (β)-cell tumours are the most common islet cell tumours. The neoplastic β-cells secrete insulin into the blood stream which remains unaffected by normal regulatory mechanisms. This results in characteristic attacks of hypoglycaemia with blood glucose level falling to 50 mg/dl or below, high plasma insulin level (hyperinsulinism) and high insulin-glucose ratio.

G/A Insulinoma is usually solitary and well-encapsulated tumour which may vary in size from 0.5 to 10 cm. Rarely, they are multiple.

M/E The tumour is composed of cords and sheets of well-differentiated β-cells which do not differ from normal cells.

GASTRINOMA (G-CELL TUMOUR, ZOLLINGER-ELLISON SYNDROME)

Zollinger and Ellison described diagnostic triad consisting of the following:
i) Fulminant peptic ulcer disease
ii) Gastric acid hypersecretion
iii) Presence of non-β pancreatic islet cell tumour.

Such non-β pancreatic islet cell tumour is the source of gastrin producing hypergastrinaemia and hence named gastrinoma.

MORPHOLOGIC FEATURES Majority of gastrinomas occur in the wall of the duodenum. They may be benign or malignant. Gastrinomas are associated with peptic ulcers. About one-third of patients have multiple endocrine neoplasia.

MISCELLANEOUS ENDOCRINE TUMOURS *(p. 819)*

MULTIPLE ENDOCRINE NEOPLASIA (MEN) SYNDROMES

Multiple adenomas and hyperplasias of different endocrine organs are a group of genetic disorders which produce heterogeneous clinical features called multiple endocrine neoplasia (MEN) syndromes.

1. **MEN type 1 syndrome (Wermer's syndrome)** includes adenomas of the parathyroid glands, pancreatic islets and pituitary. The syndrome is

inherited as an autosomal dominant trait. There is 50% chance of transmitting the predisposing gene, *MEN 1* (or *menin*) gene, to the child of an affected person. MEN 1 is characterised by the following features:

1. *Parathyroid:* Hyperplasia or adenoma; hyperparathyroidism is the most common (90%) clinical manifestation.

2. *Pancreatic islet cells:* Hyperplasia or adenoma seen in 80% cases; frequently with Zollinger-Ellison syndrome.

3. *Pituitary:* Hyperplasia or adenoma in 65% cases; manifest as acromegaly or hypopituitarism.

4. *Adrenal cortex:* Uncommonly involved by adenoma or pheochromocytoma.

5. *Thyroid:* Less commonly involved by adenoma or hyperplasia.

2. MEN type 2 syndrome (Sipple's syndrome) is characterised by medullary carcinoma thyroid and pheochromocytoma. Genetic abnormality in these cases is mutation in *RET* gene in almost all cases. MEN 2 has two major syndromes:

❖ **MEN type 2A** is the combination of medullary carcinoma thyroid, pheochromocytoma and hyperparathyroidism. MEN type 2A has further *three subvariants*:

i) MEN 2A with familial medullary carcinoma thyroid

ii) MEN 2A with cutaneous lichen amyloidosis

iii) MEN 2A with Hirschsprung's disease.

❖ **MEN type 2B** the combination of medullary carcinoma thyroid, pheochromocytoma, mucosal neuromas, intestinal ganglioneuromatosis, and marfanoid features.

3. Mixed syndromes include a variety of endocrine neoplastic combinations which are distinct from those in MEN type 1 and type 2. A few examples are as under:

i) von Hippel-Lindau syndrome from mutation in *VHL* gene is association of CNS tumours, renal cell carcinoma, pheochromocytoma and islet cell tumours.

ii) Type 1 neurofibromatosis from inactivation of neurofibromin protein and activation of *RAS* gene, is associated with MEN type 1 or type 2 features.

POLYGLANDULAR AUTOIMMUNE (PGA) SYNDROMES

Immunologic syndromes affecting two or more endocrine glands and some non-endocrine immune disturbances produce syndromic presentation termed polyglandular autoimmune (PGA) syndromes. PGA syndromes are of two types:

❖ PGA type I occurring in children is characterised by mucocutaneous candidiasis, hypoparathyroidism, and adrenal insufficiency.

❖ PGA type II (Schmidt syndrome) presents in adults and commonly comprises of adrenal insufficiency, autoimmune thyroiditis, and type 1 diabetes mellitus.

SELF ASSESSMENT

---

1. **Hyperfunction of anterior pituitary in pre-pubertal children generally results in:**
   A. Acromegaly
   B. Gigantism
   C. Hyperprolactinaemia
   D. Cushing's syndrome

2. **Excessive secretion of ADH from posterior pituitary results from the following conditions except:**
   A. Oat cell carcinoma
   B. Carcinoma pancreas
   C. Pituitary adenoma
   D. Thymoma

3. **Hypofunction of anterior pituitary results in the following except:**
   A. Sheehan's syndrome
   B. Diabetes insipidus
   C. Pituitary dwarfism
   D. Empty-sella syndrome

4. **The most common form of pituitary adenoma is:**
   - A. Somatotroph
   - B. Lactotroph
   - C. Gonadotroph
   - D. Corticotroph

5. **Craniopharyngioma arises from:**
   - A. Arachnoid cap cells
   - B. Lining epithelium of pharynx
   - C. Chromophil cells
   - D. Remnants of Rathke's pouch

6. **Cushing's syndrome due to ectopic elaboration of cortisol occurs in the following conditions <u>except</u>:**
   - A. Oat cell carcinoma lung
   - B. Adrenal cortical adenoma
   - C. Malignant thymoma
   - D. Pancreatic carcinoma

7. **Main causes of Addison's disease include the following <u>except</u>:**
   - A. Tuberculosis
   - B. Amyloidosis
   - C. Adrenal cortical adenoma
   - D. Autoimmune diseases

8. **Pheochromocytoma has the following features <u>except</u>:**
   - A. It is generally a benign tumour of adrenal medulla
   - B. Hypertension is generally presenting feature
   - C. It arises from embryonal nerve cells
   - D. 24 hours urinary measurement of catecholamines is diagnostic

9. **Neuroblastoma has the following features <u>except</u>:**
   - A. It arises from primitive nerve cells
   - B. It is a common malignant tumour in children under 5 years of age
   - C. The tumour spreads by haematogenous route early
   - D. The tumour cells are highly pleomorphic and large

10. **Common causes of myxoedema are as under <u>except</u>:**
    - A. Follicular adenoma
    - B. Ablation of thyroid by surgery
    - C. Thyroid cancer
    - D. Autoimmune thyroiditis

11. **There is higher incidence of lymphoma of the thyroid in the following condition:**
    - A. Graves' disease
    - B. Hashimoto's thyroiditis
    - C. Nodular goitre
    - D. Riedel's thyroiditis

12. **There is considerable depletion of colloid in the follicles in the following thyroid disease:**
    - A. Graves' disease
    - B. Hashimoto's thyroiditis
    - C. Nodular goitre
    - D. Follicular adenoma

13. **Nodular goitre is characterised by the following features <u>except</u>:**
    - A. Iodine deficiency plays role in etiology
    - B. There is repeated hyperplasia and involution
    - C. There is deficient thyroid hormone production
    - D. There is decreased TSH stimulation

14. **Role of external radiation in etiology of thyroid cancer is maximum in:**
    - A. Papillary carcinoma
    - B. Follicular carcinoma
    - C. Medullary carcinoma
    - D. Anaplastic carcinoma

15. **Haematogenous spread is rare and exceptional in following thyroid cancer:**
    - A. Follicular carcinoma
    - B. Medullary carcinoma
    - C. Papillary carcinoma
    - D. Anaplastic carcinoma

16. **Male: female ratio is equal in the following thyroid cancer:**
    - A. Papillary carcinoma
    - B. Follicular carcinoma
    - C. Medullary carcinoma
    - D. Anaplastic carcinoma

17. **The following thyroid cancer is a neuroendocrine tumour:**
    - A. Papillary carcinoma
    - B. Follicular carcinoma
    - C. Medullary carcinoma
    - D. Anaplastic carcinoma

18. **Following thyroid cancer has the past prognosis:**
    - A. Anaplastic carcinoma
    - B. Medullary carcinoma
    - C. Papillary carcinoma
    - D. Follicular carcinoma

19. **Secondary hyperparathyroidism secondary to disease elsewhere in the body causes:**
    - A. Hypercalcaemia
    - B. Hypocalcaemia
    - C. Normocalcaemia
    - D. Normal parathormone levels

20. **Islets of Langerhans are concentrated in the pancreas in the following zone:**
    A. Head
    B. Body
    C. Tail
    D. Uncinate process

21. **The following holds true for type 1 diabetes except:**
    A. There is association with HLA-DR 3 and HLA-DR 4
    B. There is autoimmune disease association
    C. There is more than 90% concordance for monozygotic twins to develop diabetes
    D. Viral infection may precede type I diabetes

22. **The following are correct statements for type 2 diabetes (NIDDM) except:**
    A. It is more than common than IDDM
    B. These patients are generally obese
    C. There is role of insulin resistance
    D. There is presence of 'insulitis'

23. **The following complication is almost exclusive for type 1 diabetes mellitus (IDDM):**
    A. Hyperosmolar nonketotic coma
    B. Diabetic ketoacidosis
    C. Atherosclerosis
    D. Diabetic nephropathy

24. **Renal glucosuria is characterised by:**
    A. Elevation of fasting blood glucose level
    B. Elevation of blood glucose at 1 hour after meal
    C. Elevation of blood glucose at 2 hours after meal
    D. Normal blood glucose level during entire GTT

25. **Long-term assessment of diabetes is provided by the following investigation:**
    A. Whole blood glucose estimation
    B. Plasma glucose estimation
    C. Capillary method of glucose estimation
    D. Glycosylated haemoglobin

26. **Hypoglycaemia (blood glucose 50 mg/dl or lower) is a characteristic finding in:**
    A. Gastrinoma
    B. Insulinoma
    C. Glucagonoma
    D. VIPoma

27. **Lateral aberrant thyroid is the term used for the following:**
    A. Ectopic normal thyroid tissue in lateral cervical region
    B. Abnormal thyroid tissue at unusual site
    C. Metastatic deposits in cervical lymph node from papillary carcinoma thyroid
    D. Metastatic deposits in cervical lymph node from gastric carcinoma

28. **Following pathologic finding is invariably present in pancreas in type 2 diabetes mellitus:**
    A. Insulitis
    B. Depleted islet cell mass
    C. B-cell degranulation
    D. Amyloidosis of islets

29. **Which of the following chromophil cells of the anterior pituitary have acidophilic granules:**
    A. GH cells
    B. FSH-LH cells
    C. TSH cells
    D. ACTH-MSH cells

30. **Sheehan's syndrome is:**
    A. Irradiation damage of pituitary gland
    B. Scarred pituitary adenoma
    C. Post partum pituitary necrosis
    D. Surgical removal of pituitary gland

31. **Conn's syndrome is:**
    A. Chronic hypercortisolism
    B. Adrenogenital syndrome
    C. Secondary hyperaldosteronism
    D. Primary hyperaldosteronism

32. **Pick the odd one out:**
    A. Papillary thyroid carcinoma—*RET* gene
    B. Follicular thyroid carcinoma—*PAX-8-PPARγ1* gene
    C. Medullary thyroid carcinoma—*K-RAS* gene
    D. Anaplastic thyroid carcinoma—*p53* gene

33. **Amyloidosis is seen in which type of diabetes:**
    A. Type I DM
    B. Type II DM
    C. Gestational diabetes
    D. MODY

34. **A 44 years old woman presents with worsening episodes of light-headedness and dizziness which get some relief on quickly eating some biscuits. Her laboratory investigations show low blood glucose level and increased serum insulin level. Which of the following is the most likely diagnosis?**
    A. Carcinoid tumour
    B. Thyrotoxicosis
    C. Pituitary adenoma
    D. Islet cell adenoma

35. **A 28 years old man has a nodule in the middle of his neck. On examination, the nodule is 3.5 cm diameter in the thyroid gland. The lesion is removed surgically, and histologic sections reveal groups of poorly differentiated tumour cells and areas of amyloid stroma. The familial form of this type of malignancy is associated with abnormalities of which of the following protooncogenes?**
    A. *PAX*
    B. *MYC*
    C. *RET*
    D. *SIS*

36. **A 25 years old man diagnosed as a case of pheochromocytoma has recurrent symptoms. Which of the following substance is most likely to be elevated in 24-hour urinary determination?**
    A. Vanillylmandelic acid
    B. Hydroxy-indole-acetic acid
    C. Homogentisic acid
    D. Methylmalonic acid

37. **Which of the following organs have tumours in patients with MEN type 1?**
    A. Adrenal, thyroid and parathyroid
    B. Kidneys, adrenal, and liver
    C. Pituitary, parathyroid, and pancreas
    D. Parathyroid, pineal, and pancreas

KEY

1 = B	2 = C	3 = B	4 = B	5 = D
6 = B	7 = C	8 = C	9 = D	10 = A
11 = B	12 = A	13 = D	14 = A	15 = C
16 = C	17 = C	18 = C	19 = B	20 = C
21 = C	22 = D	23 = B	24 = D	25 = D
26 = B	27 = C	28 = D	29 = A	30 = C
31 = D	32 = C	33 = B	34 = D	35 = C
36 = A	37 = C			

26   The Musculoskeletal System

NORMAL STRUCTURE OF BONE

◈   **Cortical or compact bone** comprises 80% of the skeleton and is the dense outer shell responsible for structural rigidity.

◈   **Trabecular or cancellous bone** composes 20% of the skeleton and has trabeculae traversing the marrow space.

M/E   Bone consists of large quantities of extracellular osteoid matrix which is loaded with calcium hydroxyapatite and relatively small number of bone cells which are of 3 main types:

1.   Osteoblasts   Osteoblasts are uninucleate cells found abundantly along the new bone-forming surfaces. They synthesise bone matrix. The serum levels of bone-related *alkaline phosphatase* (other being hepatic alkaline phosphatase) is a marker for osteoblastic activity.

2.   Osteocytes   Osteocytes are those osteoblasts which get incorporated into the bone matrix during its synthesis. Osteocytes are found within small spaces called lacunae lying in the bone matrix.

◈   *Woven bone* is immature and is rapidly deposited. It contains large number of closely-packed osteocytes and consists of irregular interlacing pattern of collagen fibre bundles in bone matrix.

◈   *Lamellar bone* differs from woven bone in having smaller and less numerous osteocytes and fine and parallel or lamellar sheets of collagen fibres. Lamellar bone usually replaces woven bone or pre-existing cartilage.

3.   Osteoclasts   Osteoclasts are large multinucleate cells of mononuclear-macrophage origin and are responsible for bone resorption. The osteoclastic activity is determined by bone-related serum *acid phosphatase* levels (other being prostatic acid phosphatase).

4.   Osteoid matrix   The osteoid matrix of bone consists of 90-95% of collagen type I and comprises nearly half of total body's collagen. Virtually whole of body's hydroxyproline and hydroxylysine reside in the bone.

BONE FORMATION AND RESORPTION   Bone is not a static tissue but its formation and resorption are taking place during period of growth as well as in adult life. Bone deposition is the result of osteoblasts while bone resorption is the function of osteoclasts. Bone formation may take place directly from collagen called *membranous ossification* seen in certain flat bones, or may occur through an intermediate stage of cartilage termed *endochondral ossification* found in metaphysis of long bones. Osteoblastic formation and osteoclastic resorption continue to take place into adult life in a balanced way termed *bone modelling*.

NORMAL STRUCTURE OF CARTILAGE

Unlike bone, the cartilage lacks blood vessels, lymphatics and nerves. It may have focal areas of calcification. Cartilage consists of 2 components:

Cartilage matrix   Like bone, cartilage too consists of organic and inorganic material. Inorganic material of cartilage is calcium hydroxyapatite similar to that in bone matrix but the organic material of the cartilage is distinct from the bone. It consists of very high content of water (80%) and remaining 20% consists of type II collagen and proteoglycans.

Chondrocytes Primitive mesenchymal cells which form bone cells from chondroblasts which give rise to chondrocytes.

Depending upon location and structural composition, cartilage is of 3 types:

1. *Hyaline cartilage* is the basic cartilaginous tissue comprising articular cartilage of joints, cartilage in the growth plates of developing bones.

2. *Fibrocartilage* is a hyaline cartilage that contains more abundant type II collagen fibres.

3. *Elastic cartilage* is hyaline cartilage that contains abundant elastin.

INFECTION, NECROSIS, FRACTURE HEALING *(p. 822)*

OSTEOMYELITIS

An infection of the bone is termed osteomyelitis (myelo = marrow). A number of systemic infectious diseases may spread to the bone such as enteric fever, actinomycosis, mycetoma (madura foot), syphilis, tuberculosis and brucellosis.

PYOGENIC OSTEOMYELITIS

Pyogenic or suppurative osteomyelitis is usually caused by bacterial infection and rarely by fungi.

Bacterial osteomyelitis may be a complication at all ages in patients with compound fractures, surgical procedures involving prosthesis or implants, gangrene of a limb in diabetics, debilitation and immunosuppression.

Though any etiologic agent may cause osteomyelitis, *Staphylococcus aureus* is implicated in a vast majority of cases. Less frequently, other organisms such as streptococci, *Escherichia coli, Pseudomonas, Klebsiella* and anaerobes are involved.

Clinically, the child with acute haematogenous osteomyelitis has painful and tender limb. Fever, malaise and leucocytosis generally accompany the bony lesion. Radiologic examination confirms the bony destruction.

MORPHOLOGIC FEATURES Depending upon the duration, osteomyelitis may be *acute, subacute* or *chronic.* The basic pathologic changes in any stage of osteomyelitis are: suppuration, ischaemic necrosis, healing by fibrosis and bony repair. The **sequence of pathologic changes** is as under:

1. The infection begins in the metaphyseal end of the *marrow cavity* which is largely occupied by *pus.*

2. Spread of infection along the marrow cavity, into the endosteum, and into the haversian and Volkmann's canal, causing *periosteitis.*

3. The infection may reach the subperiosteal space forming *subperiosteal abscesses.*

4. Combination of suppuration and impaired blood supply to the cortical bone results in erosion, thinning and infarction necrosis of the cortex called *sequestrum.*

5. With passage of time, there is formation of new bone beneath the periosteum present over the infected bone. This forms an encasing sheath around the necrosed bone and is known as *involucrum.*

6. Occasionally, acute osteomyelitis may be contained to a localised area and walled off by fibrous tissue and granulation tissue. This is termed *Brodie's abscess.*

7. In *vertebral pyogenic osteomyelitis,* infection begins from the disc (discitis) and spreads to involve the vertebral bodies.

COMPLICATIONS Osteomyelitis may develop following complications:

1. Septicaemia.

2. Acute bacterial arthritis.

3. Pathologic fractures.

4. Development of squamous cell carcinoma in long-standing cases.

5. Secondary amyloidosis in long-standing cases.

6. Vertebral osteomyelitis may cause vertebral collapse with paravertebral abscess, epidural abscess, cord compression and neurologic deficits.

TUBERCULOUS OSTEOMYELITIS

Tuberculous osteomyelitis, though rare in developed countries, continues to be a common condition in under-developed and developing countries of the world. The tubercle bacilli, *M. tuberculosis,* reach the bone marrow and synovium most commonly by haematogenous dissemination from infection elsewhere, usually from the lungs.

MORPHOLOGIC FEATURES The bone lesions in tuberculosis consist of central caseation necrosis surrounded by tuberculous granulation tissue and fragments of necrotic bone. The tuberculous lesions appear as a focus of bone destruction and replacement of the affected tissue by caseous material and formation of multiple discharging sinuses through the soft tissues and skin. Involvement of joint spaces and intervertebral disc are frequent. Tuberculosis of the spine, *Pott's disease,* often commences in the vertebral body and may be associated with compression fractures and destruction of intervertebral discs, producing permanent damage and paraplegia.

AVASCULAR NECROSIS (OSTEONECROSIS)

Avascular necrosis of the bones or osteonecrosis results from ischaemia. It is a relatively common condition.

ETIOPATHOGENESIS   Some of the common causes are:
1.   Fracture or dislocation
2.   Sickle cell disease
3.   Corticosteroid administration
4.   Radiation therapy
5.   Chronic alcoholism
6.   Idiopathic

MORPHOLOGIC FEATURES   There are pathological fractures of the involved bone due to infarcts. Most common sites are the ones where the disruption in blood supply is at end-arterial circulation. The infarcts mainly involve the medulla of the long bone in the diaphysis.

G/A   The lesional area shows a wedge-shaped area of infarction in the subchondral bone under the convex surface of the joint.

M/E   The infracted medulla shows saponified marrow fat. The overlying cartilage and the cortex of the long bones are relatively unaffected.

DISORDERS OF BONE GROWTH AND DEVELOPMENT *(p. 825)*

A number of abnormalities of the skeleton are due to disordered bone growth and development and are collectively termed *skeletal dysplasias.*
◈   *Local defects* involve a single bone or a group of bones such as: absence or presence in diminished form, fused with neighbouring bones (e.g. syndactyly), and formation of extra bones (e.g. supernumerary ribs).
◈   However, more importantly, skeletal dysplasias include *systemic disorders* involving particular epiphyseal growth plate. These include: achondroplasia (disorder of chondroblasts), osteogenesis imperfecta (disorder of osteoblasts), osteopetrosis (disorder of osteoclasts) and foetal rickets (disorder of mineralisation).

ACHONDROPLASIA

Achondroplasia is an autosomal dominant genetic abnormality. There is selective interference with normal endochondral ossification at the level of epiphyseal cartilaginous growth plates of long bones.

OSTEOGENESIS IMPERFECTA

Osteogenesis imperfecta is an autosomal dominant or recessive disorder of synthesis of type I collagen that constitutes 90-95% of bone matrix. The disorder, thus, involves not only the skeleton but other extra-skeletal tissues as well containing type I collagen such as sclera, eyes, joints, ligaments, teeth and skin. The skeletal manifestations of osteogenesis imperfecta are due to defective osteoblasts which normally synthesise type I collagen. This results in thin or non-existent cortices and irregular trabeculae *(too little bone)* so that the bones are very fragile and liable to multiple fractures.

OSTEOPETROSIS

Osteopetrosis, also called *marble bone disease,* is an autosomal dominant or recessive disorder of increased skeletal mass or osteosclerosis caused by a hereditary defect in osteoclast function. The condition may appear in 2 forms: autosomal recessive (malignant infantile form) and autosomal dominant (benign adult form). Failure of normal osteoclast function of bone resorption coupled with continued bone formation and endochondral ossification results in net overgrowth of calcified dense bone *(too much bone)* which occupies most of the available marrow space.

METABOLIC AND ENDOCRINE BONE DISEASES *(p. 826)*

A large number of metabolic and endocrine disorders produce generalised skeletal disorders. These include the following:

1. **Osteoporosis**—Resulting from quantitative reduction in otherwise normal bone.

2. **Osteomalacia and rickets**—Characterised by qualitative abnormality in the form of impaired bone mineralisation due to deficiency of vitamin D in adults and children respectively.

3. **Scurvy**—Caused by deficiency of vitamin C resulting in subperiosteal haemorrhages.

4. **Hyperparathyroidism**—Leading to osteitis fibrosa cystica.

5. **Pituitary dysfunctions**—Hyperpituitarism causing gigantism and acromegaly and hypopituitarism resulting in dwarfism.

6. **Thyroid dysfunctions**—Hyperthyroidism causing osteoporosis and hypothyroidism leading to cretinism.

7. **Renal osteodystrophy**—Occurring in chronic renal failure and resulting in features of osteitis fibrosa cystica, osteomalacia and areas of osteosclerosis.

8. **Skeletal fluorosis**—Occurring due to excess of sodium fluoride content in the soil and water in an area.

OSTEOPOROSIS

Osteoporosis or osteopenia is a common clinical syndrome involving multiple bones in which there is quantitative reduction of bone tissue mass but the bone tissue mass is otherwise normal. This reduction in bone mass results in fragile skeleton associated with increased risk of fractures and consequent pain and deformity. The condition is particularly common in elderly people and more frequent in postmenopausal women. The condition may remain asymptomatic or may cause only backache. However, more extensive involvement is associated with fractures, particularly of distal radius, femoral neck and vertebral bodies.

Many non-invasive techniques are now available for measurement of bone mass e.g. DEXA and SEXA scans, quantitative CT and ultrasound.

PATHOGENESIS Osteoporosis is conventionally classified into 2 major groups:

◈ **Primary osteoporosis** results primarily from osteopenia without an underlying disease or medication. Primary osteoporosis is further subdivided into 2 types: *idiopathic type* found in the young and juveniles and is less frequent, and *involutional type* seen in postmenopausal women and ageing individuals and is more common. A number of risk factors have been attributed to cause this imbalance between bone resorption and bone formation.

1. Genetic factors
2. Sex
3. Reduced physical activity

4.   Deficiency of sex hormones
5.   Combined deficiency of calcitonin and oestrogen
6.   Hyperparathyroidism
7.   Deficiency of vitamin D
8.   Local factors

◈   **Secondary osteoporosis** is attributed to a number of factors and conditions (e.g. immobilisation, chronic anaemia, acromegaly, hepatic disease, hyperparathyroidism, hypogonadism, thyrotoxicosis and starvation), or as an effect of medication (e.g. hypercortisonism, administration of anticonvulsant drugs and large dose of heparin).

Most commonly encountered osteoporotic fractures are: vertebral crush fracture, femoral neck fracture and wrist fracture. There is enlargement of the medullary cavity and thinning of the cortex.

M/E   Osteoporosis may be active or inactive type.
◈   **Active osteoporosis** is characterised by increased bone resorption and formation i.e. *accelerated turnover.*
◈   **Inactive osteoporosis** has the features of minimal bone formation and reduced resorptive activity i.e. *reduced turnover.*

OSTEITIS FIBROSA CYSTICA

Hyperparathyroidism of primary or secondary type results in oversecretion of parathyroid hormone which causes increased osteoclastic resorption of the bone. Severe and prolonged hyperparathyroidism results in osteitis fibrosa cystica. The lesion is generally induced as a manifestation of primary hyperparathyroidism, and less frequently, as a result of secondary hyperparathyroidism such as in chronic renal failure (renal osteodystrophy).

The chief biochemical abnormality of excessive parathyroid hormone is hypercalcaemia, hypophosphataemia and hypercalciuria.

G/A   There are focal areas of erosion of cortical bone and loss of lamina dura at the roots of teeth.

M/E   The following sequential changes appear over a period of time:
i)   Earliest change is *demineralisation* and *increased bone resorption* beginning at the subperiosteal and endosteal surface of the cortex and then spreading to the trabecular bone.
ii)   There is replacement of bone and bone marrow by fibrosis coupled with increased number of bizarre osteoclasts at the surfaces of moth-eaten trabeculae and cortex *(osteitis fibrosa).*
iii)   As a result of increased resorption, microfractures and microhaemorrhages occur in the marrow cavity leading to development of cysts *(osteitis fibrosa cystica).*
iv)   Haemosiderin-laden macrophages and multinucleate giant cells appear at the areas of haemorrhages producing an appearance termed *'brown tumour'* or *'reparative giant cell granuloma of hyperparathyroidism'* requiring differentiation from giant cell tumour or osteoclastoma.

RENAL OSTEODYSTROPHY (METABOLIC BONE DISEASE)

Renal osteodystrophy is a loosely used term that encompasses a number of skeletal abnormalities appearing in cases of chronic kidney disease and in patients treated by dialysis for several years. Renal osteodystrophy is more common in children than in adults.

PATHOGENESIS   Renal osteodystrophy involves two main events:

1.   **Hyperphosphataemia**   In CRF, there is impaired renal excretion of phosphate, causing phosphate retention and hyperphosphataemia. Hyperphosphataemia, in turn, causes hypocalcaemia which is responsible for secondary hyperparathyroidism.

2.   **Hypocalcaemia**   It may result from following:
◈   Due to renal dysfunction, there is decreased conversion of vitamin D metabolite 25(OH) cholecalciferol to its active form 1,25 $(OH)_2$ cholecalciferol.
◈   Reduced intestinal absorption of calcium.

3. Parathormone secretion Hypocalcaemia stimulates secretion of parathormone, eventually leading to secondary hyperparathyroidism.

4. Metabolic acidosis As a result of decreased renal function, acidosis sets in which may cause osteoporosis and bone decalcification.

5. Calcium phosphorus product > 70 When the product of biochemical value of calcium and phosphate is higher than 70, metastatic calcification may occur at extraosseous sites.

6. Dialysis-related metabolic bone disease Long-term dialysis employing use of aluminium-containing dialysate is currently considered to be a major cause of metabolic bone lesions.

M/E The following skeletal lesions can be identified in renal osteodystrophy:
1. *Mixed osteomalacia-osteitis fibrosa* is the most common manifestation of renal osteodystrophy resulting from disordered vitamin D metabolism and secondary hyperparathyroidism.
2. *Pure osteitis fibrosa* results from metabolic complications of secondary hyperparathyroidism.
3. *Pure osteomalacia* of renal osteodystrophy is attributed to aluminium toxicity.
4. *Renal rickets* resembling the changes seen in children with nutritional rickets with widened osteoid seams may occur.
5. *Osteosclerosis* is characterised by enhanced bone density in the upper and lower margins of vertebrae.
6. *Metastatic calcification* is seen at extraosseous sites such as in medium-sized blood vessels, periarticular tissues, myocardium, eyes, lungs and gastric mucosa.

SKELETAL FLUOROSIS

Fluorosis of bones occurs due to high sodium fluoride content in soil and water consumed by people in some geographic areas and is termed endemic fluorosis. Such endemic regions exist in some tropical and subtropical areas; in India it exists in some parts of Punjab and Andhra Pradesh. The condition affects farmers who consume drinking water from wells.

PATHOGENESIS In fluorosis, fluoride replaces calcium as the mineral in the bone and gets deposited without any regulatory control. This results in heavily mineralised bones which are thicker and denser but are otherwise weak and deformed (just as in osteopetrosis).

G/A The long bones and vertebrae develop nodular swellings which are present both inside the bones and on the surface.

M/E These nodules are composed of heavily mineralised irregular osteoid admixed with fluoride which requires confirmation chemically.

PAGET'S DISEASE OF BONE (OSTEITIS DEFORMANS) (p. 828)

Paget's disease of bone is an osteolytic and osteosclerotic bone disease of uncertain etiology involving one (monostotic) or more bones (polyostotic). The condition affects predominantly males over the age of 50 years.
1. There has been some evidence that osteitis deformans is a form of *slow-virus infection* by paramyxovirus (e.g. respiratory syncytial virus, measles) in osteoclasts.
2. Autosomal dominant inheritance and *genetic susceptibility* have been proposed on the basis of observation of 7-10 fold higher prevalence of disease in first-degree relatives.

Clinically, the *monostotic form* of the disease may remain asymptomatic and the lesion is discovered incidentally or on radiologic examination. *Polyostotic form,* however, is more widespread and may produce pain, fractures, skeletal deformities, and occasionally, sarcomatous transformation.

MORPHOLOGIC FEATURES Monostotic Paget's disease involves most frequently: tibia, pelvis, femur, skull and vertebra, while the order of

Three sequential stages are identified in Paget's disease:

1. Initial osteolytic stage: This stage is characterised by areas of osteoclastic resorption produced by increased number of large osteoclasts.

2. Mixed osteolytic-osteoblastic stage: In this stage, there is imbalance between osteoblastic laying down of new bone and osteoclastic resorption so that mineralisation of the newly-laid matrix lags behind, resulting in development of characteristic *mosaic pattern* or *jigsaw puzzle appearance* of osteoid seams or cement lines.

3. Quiscent osteosclerotic stage: After many years, excessive bone formation results and thus the bone becomes more compact and dense producing osteosclerosis.

TUMOUR-LIKE LESIONS OF BONE *(p. 829)*

FIBROUS DYSPLASIA

It is a benign condition, possibly of developmental origin, characterised by the presence of localised area of replacement of bone by fibrous connective tissue with a characteristic whorled pattern and containing trabeculae of woven bone. Radiologically, the typical focus of fibrous dysplasia has well-demarcated ground-glass appearance.

Three types of fibrous dysplasia are distinguished—

◈ **Monostotic fibrous dysplasia** Monostotic fibrous dysplasia affects a solitary bone and is the most common type, comprising about 70% of all cases. The condition affects either sex and most patients are between 20 and 30 years of age. The bones most often affected, in descending order of frequency, are: ribs, craniofacial bones (especially maxilla), femur, tibia and humerus. The condition generally remains asymptomatic and is discovered incidentally, but infrequently may produce tumour-like enlargement of the affected bone.

◈ **Polyostotic fibrous dysplasia** Polyostotic form of fibrous dysplasia affecting several bones constitutes about 25% of all cases. Both sexes are affected equally but the lesions appear at a relatively earlier age than the monostotic form. Most frequently affected bones are: craniofacial, ribs, vertebrae and long bones of the limbs.

◈ **Albright syndrome** Also called McCune-Albright syndrome, this is a form of polyostotic fibrous dysplasia associated with endocrine dysfunctions and accounts for less than 5% of all cases. The syndrome is characterised by polyostotic bone lesions, skin pigmentation *(café-au-lait* macular spots) and sexual precocity, and infrequently other endocrinopathies.

G/A The lesions appear as sharply-demarcated, localised defects measuring 2-5 cm in diameter, present within the cancellous bone, having thin and smooth overlying cortex. The epiphyseal cartilages are generally spared in the monostotic form but involved in the polyostotic form of disease.

M/E The lesions of fibrous dysplasia have characteristic benign-looking fibroblastic tissue arranged in a loose, whorled pattern in which there are irregular and curved trabeculae of woven (non-lamellar) bone in the form fish-hook appearance or Chinese letter shapes. Characteristically, there are no osteoblasts rimming the trabeculae of the bone, suggesting a maturation defect in the bone.

FIBROUS CORTICAL DEFECT (METAPHYSEAL FIBROUS DEFECT, NON-OSSIFYING FIBROMA)

Fibrous cortical defect or metaphyseal fibrous defect is a rather common benign tumour-like lesion occurring in the metaphyseal cortex of long bones in children. Most commonly involved bones are upper or lower end of tibia or lower end of femur. The lesion is generally solitary but rarely there may be multiple and bilaterally symmetrical defects. Radiologically, the lesion is eccentrically located in the metaphysis and has a sharply-delimited border.

G/A The lesion is generally small, less than 4 cm in diameter, granular and brown. Larger lesion (5-10 cm) occurring usually in response to trauma is referred to as *non-ossifying fibroma*.

M/E Fibrous cortical defect consists of cellular masses of fibrous tissue showing storiform pattern. There are numerous multinucleate osteoclast-like giant cells, haemosiderin-laden macrophages and foamy cells; hence the lesion is also termed histiocytic xanthogranuloma or fibrous xanthoma of bone.

SOLITARY (SIMPLE, UNICAMERAL) BONE CYST

Solitary, simple or unicameral bone cyst is a benign condition occurring in children and adolescents, most frequently located in the metaphyses at the upper end of humerus and femur. Possibly, the lesion arises due to local disorder of bone growth and development.

G/A Simple cyst of the bone is generally unilocular with smooth inner surface. The cavity is filled with clear fluid.

M/E The cyst wall consists of thin collagenous tissue having scattered osteoclast giant cells and newly formed reactive bony trabeculae.

ANEURYSMAL BONE CYST

Aneurysmal bone cyst, true to its name, is an expanding osteolytic lesion filled with blood *(aneurysm* = dilatation, distension). The condition is seen more commonly in young patients under 30 years of age. Most frequently involved bones are shafts of metaphyses of long bones or the vertebral column. The radiographic appearance shows characteristic ballooned-out expansile lesion underneath the periosteum.

M/E The cyst consists of blood-filled aneurysmal spaces of variable size, some of which are endothelium-lined. The spaces are separated by connective tissue septa containing osteoid tissue, numerous osteoclast-like multinucleate giant cells and trabeculae of bone. The condition has to be distinguished histologically from giant cell tumour or osteoclastoma and telangiectatic osteosarcoma.

TUMOURS OF BONE AND CARTILAGE *(p. 831)*

Bone and cartilage tumours, commonly called together as bone tumours, are comparatively infrequent but they are clinically quite significant since some of them are highly malignant. Bone tumours may be primary or metastatic.

It may be mentioned here that the diagnosis of any bone lesion is established by a combination of clinical, radiological and pathological examination, supplemented by biochemical and haematological investigations wherever necessary.

BONE-FORMING (OSTEOBLASTIC) TUMOURS

OSTEOMA

An osteoma is a rare benign, slow-growing lesion, regarded by some as a hamartoma rather than a true neoplasm. Osteoma is almost exclusively restricted to flat bones of the skull and face. It may grow into paranasal sinuses or protrude into the orbit.

M/E The lesion is composed of well-differentiated mature lamellar bony trabeculae separated by fibrovascular tissue.

OSTEOID OSTEOMA AND OSTEOBLASTOMA

Osteoid osteoma and osteoblastoma (or giant osteoid osteoma) are closely related benign tumours occurring in children and young adults. Osteoid osteoma is more common than osteoblastoma. There are no clear-cut histologic criteria to distinguish the two. The distinction between them is based on clinical features, size and radiographic appearance.

◈ **Osteoid osteoma** is small (usually less than 1 cm) tumour located in the cortex of a long bone, associated characteristically with noctural pain. The tumour is clearly demarcated having surrounding zone of reactive bone formation which radiographically appears as a small radiolucent central focus or nidus surrounded by dense sclerotic bone.

◈ **Osteoblastoma,** on the other hand, is larger in size (usually more than 1 cm), painless, located in the medulla, commonly in the vertebrae, ribs, ilium and long bones, and there is absence of reactive bone formation.

M/E The distinction between osteoid osteoma and osteoblastoma is not obvious. In either case, the lesion consists of trabeculae of osteoid, rimmed by osteoblasts and separated by highly vascularised connective tissue stroma.

OSTEOSARCOMA

Osteosarcoma or osteogenic sarcoma is the most common primary malignant tumour of the bone. The tumour is characterised by *formation of osteoid or bone, or both, directly by sarcoma cells*. Depending upon their locations within the bone, osteosarcomas are classified into 2 main categories: central (medullary or classic) and surface (parosteal and periosteal).

CENTRAL (MEDULLARY) OSTEOSARCOMA This is the more common and classic type and is generally referred to as 'osteosarcoma' if not specified. The tumour occurs in young patients between the age of 10 and 20 years. Males are affected more frequently than females. The tumour arises in the metaphysis of long bones. Most common sites, in descending order of frequency, are: the lower end of femur and upper end of tibia (i.e. around knee joint about 60%); the upper end of humerus (10%); pelvis and the upper end of femur (i.e. around hip joint about 15%); and less often in jaw bones, vertebrae and skull.

Based upon the pathogenesis, osteosarcoma is divided into 2 types:
◈ *Primary osteosarcoma* is more common and occurs in the absence of any known underlying disease. Its etiology is unknown. Cases of hereditary retinoblastoma have a very high prevalence risk of development of osteosarcoma implicating *RB* gene in their pathogenesis.
◈ *Secondary osteosarcoma,* on the other hand, develops following pre-existing bone disease e.g. Paget's disease of bone, fibrous dysplasia, multiple osteochondromas, chronic osteomyelitis, infarcts and fractures of bone. The tumour has a more aggressive behaviour than the primary osteosarcoma.

Medullary osteosarcoma is a highly malignant tumour. The tumour arises centrally in the metaphysis, extends longitudinally for variable distance into the medullary cavity, expands laterally on either side breaking through the cortex and lifting the periosteum. If radiographic appearance is quite distinctive: characteristic *'sunburst pattern'* due to osteogenesis within the tumour and presence of *Codman's triangle* formed at the angle between the elevated periosteum and underlying surface of the cortex.

Clinically, the usual osteosarcoma presents with pain, tenderness and an obvious swelling of affected extremity. Serum alkaline phosphatase level is generally raised but calcium and phosphorus levels are normal. The tumour metastasises rapidly and widely to distant sites by haematogenous route and disseminates commonly to the lungs, other bones, brain and various other sites.

G/A The tumour appears as a grey-white, bulky mass at the metaphyseal end of a long bone of the extremity. The articular end of the bone is generally uninvolved in initial stage. Codman's triangle, though identified radiologically, may be obvious on macroscopic examination. Cut surface of the tumour is grey-white with areas of haemorrhages and necrotic bone.

M/E The tumour shows following features:
1. **Sarcoma cells** The tumour cells of osteosarcomas are undifferentiated mesenchymal stromal cells which show marked pleomorphism and polymorphism i.e. variation in size as well as shape.

2. Osteogenesis The anaplastic sarcoma cells form osteoid matrix and bone directly; this is found interspersed in the areas of tumour cells.

VARIANTS A few histologic variants of the classic osteosarcoma have been described:

1. Telangiectatic osteosarcoma The tumour in this variant presents with pathological fractures. The tumour has large, cavernous, dilated vascular channels. This variant has a more aggressive course.

2. Small cell osteosarcoma This variant has small, uniform tumour cells just like the tumour cells of Ewing's sarcoma or lymphoma but osteogensis by these tumour cells is the distinguishing feature.

3. Fibrohistiocytic osteosarcoma This variant resembles malignant fibrous histiocytoma but having osteogenesis by the tumour cells.

4. Anaplastic osteosarcoma In this variant, the tumour has so marked anaplasia that it may resemble any other type of pleomorphic sarcoma and is identified by the presence of osteoid formed directly by the tumour cells.

5. Well-differentiated osteosarcoma Rarely a well-differentiated variant having minimal cytologic atypia resembling parosteal osteosarcoma may be seen.

SURFACE OSTEOSARCOMA About 5% of osteosarcomas occur on the surface of bone and are slow-growing tumours compared to medullary osteosarcomas. Surface osteosarcoma includes 2 variants:

Parosteal or juxtacortical osteosarcoma is an uncommon form of slow-growing osteosarcoma having its origin from the metaphysis on the external surface of the bone (*parosteal* or *juxtacortical* means outer to cortex). The tumour occurs in older age group (3rd to 4th decade), has no sex predilection and is slow growing. Its common locations are metaphysis of long bones.

G/A The tumour is lobulated and circumscribed, calcified mass in the subperiosteal location.

M/E The features which characterise the usual osteosarcoma (sarcomatous stroma and production of neoplastic osteoid and bone) are present, but the tumour shows a high degree of structural differentiation.

Periosteal osteosarcoma is a rarer form of osteosarcoma than parosteal type and arises between the cortex and the overlying periosteum. Its common location is the diaphysis of the tibia or the femur. It occurs in young adults (average age 25 years).

M/E Periosteal osteosarcoma has cartilaginous differentiation and higher degree of anaplasia than that seen in parosteal osteosarcoma but lower grade than conventional osteosarcoma i.e. it is an intermediate grade sarcoma.

CARTILAGE-FORMING (CHONDROBLASTIC) TUMOURS

OSTEOCARTILAGINOUS EXOSTOSES (OSTEOCHONDROMAS)

Osteocartilaginous exostoses or osteochondromas are the commonest of benign cartilage-forming lesions. It may occur as a *'solitary sporadic exostosis'* or there may be *'multiple hereditary exostoses'*.

Exostoses arise from metaphyses of long bones as exophytic lesions, most commonly lower femur and upper tibia (i.e. around knee) and upper humerus but may also be found in other bones such as the scapula or ilium. They are discovered most commonly in late childhood or adolescence and are more frequent in males.

G/A Osteochondromas have a broad or narrow base (i.e. may be either sessile or pedunculated) which is continuous with the cortical bone. They protrude exophytically as mushroom-shaped, cartilage-capped lesions enclosing well-formed cortical bone and marrow.

M/E They are composed of outer cap composed of mature cartilage resembling epiphyseal cartilage and the inner mature lamellar bone and bone marrow.

ENCHONDROMA

Enchondroma is the term used for the benign cartilage-forming tumour that develops centrally within the interior of the affected bone, while chondroma refers to the peripheral development of lesion similar to osteochondromas. Enchondromas may occur singly or they may be multiple, forming a non-hereditary disorder called *enchondromatosis* or *Ollier's disease.*

Most common locations for enchondromas are short tubular bones of the hands and feet.

G/A The enchondroma is lobulated, bluish-grey, translucent, cartilaginous mass lying within the medullary cavity.

M/E The tumour has characteristic lobulated appearance. The lobules are composed of normal adult hyaline cartilage separated by vascularised fibrous stroma. Foci of calcification may be evident within the tumour.

CHONDROBLASTOMA

Chondroblastoma is a relatively rare benign tumour arising from the epiphysis of long bones adjacent to the epiphyseal cartilage plate. Most commonly affected bones are upper tibia and lower femur (i.e. about knee) and upper humerus. The tumour usually occurs in patients under 20 years of age with male preponderance (male-female ratio 2:1). The radiographic appearance is of a sharply-circumscribed, lytic lesion with multiple small foci of calcification.

G/A Chondroblastoma is a well-defined mass, up to 5 cm in diameter, lying in the epiphysis. Cut surface reveals a soft chondroid tumour with foci of haemorrhages, necrosis and calcification.

M/E The tumour is highly cellular and is composed of small, round to polygonal mononuclear cells resembling chondroblasts and has multi-nucleate osteoclast-like giant cells.

CHONDROMYXOID FIBROMA

Chondromyxoid fibroma is an uncommon benign tumour of cartilaginous origin arising in the metaphysis of long bones. Most common locations are upper end of tibia and lower end of femur i.e. around the knee joint. Majority of tumours appear in 2nd to 3rd decades of life with male preponderance. Radiographically, the tumour appears as a sharply-outlined radiolucent area with foci of calcification and expansion of affected end of the bone.

G/A Chondromyxoid fibroma is sharply-demarcated, grey-white lobulated mass, not exceeding 5 cm in diameter, lying in the metaphysis. Cut surface of the tumour is soft to firm and lobulated but calcification within the tumour is not as common as with other cartilage-forming tumours.

M/E The tumour has essentially lobulated pattern. The lobules are separated by fibrous tissue and variable number of osteoclast-like giant cells. The lobules themselves are composed of immature cartilage consisting of spindle-shaped or stellate cells with abundant myxoid or chondroid intercellular matrix.

CHONDROSARCOMA

Chondrosarcoma is a malignant tumour of chondroblasts. In frequency, it is next in frequency to osteosarcoma but is relatively slow-growing and thus has a much better prognosis than that of osteosarcoma. Two types of chondrosarcoma are distinguished:

◈ **Central chondrosarcoma** is more common and arises within the medullary cavity of diaphysis or metaphysis. This type of chondrosarcoma is generally primary i.e. occurs *de novo.*

◈ **Peripheral chondrosarcoma** arises in the cortex or periosteum of metaphysis. It may be primary or secondary occurring on a pre-existing benign cartilaginous tumour such as osteocartilaginous exostoses (osteochondromas), multiple enchondromatosis, and rarely, chondroblastoma.

Both forms of chondrosarcoma usually occur in patients between 3rd and 6th decades of life with slight male preponderance. In contrast to benign cartilaginous tumours, majority of chondrosarcomas are found more often in the central skeleton (i.e. in the pelvis, ribs and shoulders); sometimes around the knee joint. Radiologic appearance is of hugely expansile and osteolytic growth with foci of calcification.

G/A Chondrosarcoma may vary in size from a few centimeters to extremely large and lobulated masses of firm consistency. Cut section of the tumour shows translucent, bluish-white, gelatinous or myxoid appearance with foci of ossification.

M/E The two hallmarks of chondrosarcoma are: invasive character and formation of lobules of anaplastic cartilage cells. These tumour cells show cellular features of malignancy such as hyperchromatism, pleomorphism, two or more cells in the lacunae and tumour giant cells.

GIANT CELL TUMOUR (OSTEOCLASTOMA)

The tumour arises in the epiphysis of long bones close to the articular cartilage. Most common sites of involvement are lower end of femur and upper end of tibia (i.e. about the knee), lower end of radius and upper end of fibula. Giant cell tumour occurs in patients between 20 and 40 years of age with no sex predilection. Radiologically, giant cell tumour appears as a large, lobulated and osteolytic lesion at the end of an expanded long bone with characteristic *'soap bubble'* appearance.

G/A Giant cell tumour is eccentrically located in the epiphyseal end of a long bone which is expanded. The tumour is well-circumscribed, dark-tan and covered by a thin shell of subperiosteal bone. Cut surface of the tumour is characteristically haemorrhagic, necrotic, and honey-combed due to focal areas of cystic degeneration.

M/E The hallmark features of giant cell tumour are the presence of large number of multinucleate osteoclast-like giant cells regularly scattered throughout the stromal mononuclear cells:

1. Giant cells often contain as many as 100 benign nuclei and have many similarities to normal osteoclasts. These cells have very high acid phosphatase activity.

2. Stromal cells are mononuclear cells and are the real tumour cells and their histologic appearance determines the biologic behaviour of the tumour. Typically, they are uniform, plump, spindle-shaped or round to oval cells with numerous mitotic figures.

3. Other features of the stroma include its scanty collagen content, rich vascularity, areas of haemorrhages and presence of macrophages.

Giant cell tumour of the bone has certain peculiarities which deserve further elaboration.

CELL OF ORIGIN Though designated as giant cell tumour or osteoclastoma, the actual tumour cells are round to spindled mononuclear cells while proliferated osteoclastic giant cells are seen as background cells.

OTHER GIANT CELL LESIONS Giant cells are present in several other benign tumours and tumour-like lesions from which the giant cell tumour is to be distinguished. These *benign giant cell lesions* are: chondroblastoma, brown tumour of hyperparathyroidism, reparative giant cell granuloma, aneurysmal bone cyst, simple bone cyst and metaphyseal fibrous defect (non-ossifying fibroma).

BIOLOGIC BEHAVIOUR Giant cell tumours are best described as aggressive and recurrent tumours. Approximately 4% cases result in distant metastases, mainly to lungs.

Ewing's sarcoma (ES) is a highly malignant small round cell tumour occurring in patients between the age of 5 and 20 years with predilection for occurrence in females. Currently it is settled for its origin from primitive neuroectodermal cells. Now, Ewing's sarcoma includes 3 variants:

i)   classic (skeletal) Ewing's sarcoma;
ii)   soft tissue Ewing's sarcoma; and
iii) primitive neuroectodermal tumour (PNET).

The three are linked together by a common neuroectodermal origin and by a common cytogenetic translocation abnormality t(11; 22) (q24; q12).

The skeletal Ewing's sarcoma arises in the medullary canal of diaphysis or metaphysis. The common sites are shafts and metaphysis of long bones, particularly femur, tibia, humerus and fibula.

Clinical features include pain, tenderness and swelling of the affected area accompanied by fever, leucocytosis and elevated ESR. X-ray examination reveals a predominantly osteolytic lesion with patchy subperiosteal reactive bone formation producing characteristic *'onion-skin'* radiographic appearance.

G/A Ewing's sarcoma is typically located in the medullary cavity and produces expansion of the affected diaphysis (shaft) or metaphysis, often extending into the adjacent soft tissues. The tumour tissue is characteristically grey-white, soft and friable.

M/E Ewing's tumour is a member of *small round cell tumours* which includes other tumours such as: PNET, neuroblastoma, embryonal rhabdomyosarcoma, lymphoma-leukaemias, and metastatic small cell carcinoma. Ewing's tumour shows the following histologic characteristics:

1.   **Pattern** The tumour is divided by fibrous septa into irregular lobules of closely-packed tumour cells. These tumour cells are characteristically arranged around capillaries forming *pseudorosettes*.

2.   **Tumour cells** The individual tumour cells comprising the lobules are small and uniform resembling lymphocytes and have ill-defined cytoplasmic outlines, scanty cytoplasm and round nuclei having 'salt and pepper' chromatin and frequent mitoses. Based on these cytological features the tumour is also called *round cell tumour* or *small blue cell tumour*. The cytoplasm contains glycogen that stains with periodic acid-Schiff (PAS) reaction.

3.   **Other features** The tumour is richly vascularised and lacks the intercellular network of reticulin fibres. There may be areas of necrosis and acute inflammatory cell infiltration.

Ewing's sarcoma metastasises early by haematogenous route to the lungs, liver, other bones and brain. Currently, use of combined regimen consisting of radiotherapy and systemic chemotherapy has improved the outcome greatly (5-year survival rate 40-80%).

CHORDOMA

Chordoma is a slow-growing malignant tumour arising from remnants of notochord. Notochord is the primitive axial skeleton which subsequently develops into the spine. Chordomas thus occur in the axial skeleton, particularly sacrum and coccyx (50%), spheno-occipital region (35%), and less often in the spine (15%). Chordoma is usually found in patients over the age of 40 years with no sex predilection. Radiographically, the tumour usually appears as an osteolytic lesion.

G/A The tumour is soft, lobulated, translucent and gelatinous with areas of haemorrhages.

ME Chordoma is composed of highly vacuolated physaliphorous cells surrounded by a sea of intercellular mucoid material.

METASTATIC BONE TUMOURS

Metastases to the skeleton are more frequent than the primary bone tumours. Metastatic bone tumours are exceeded in frequency by only 2 other organs—lungs and liver. Most skeletal metastases are derived from haematogenous spread.

Bony metastases of carcinomas predominate over the sarcomas. Some of the common *carcinomas* metastasising to the bones are from: breast, prostate, lung, kidney, stomach, thyroid, cervix, body of uterus, urinary bladder, testis, melanoma and neuroblastoma of adrenal gland. Examples of *sarcomas* which may metastasise to the bone are: embryonal and alveolar rhabdomyosarcoma, Ewing's sarcoma and osteosarcoma.

Skeletal metastases may be single or multiple. Most commonly involved bones are: the spine, pelvis, femur, skull, ribs and humerus. Usual radiographic appearance is of an *osteolytic* lesion. *Osteoblastic* bone metastases occur in cancer of the prostate, carcinoid tumour and small cell carcinoma of lung.

JOINTS (p. 841)

NORMAL STRUCTURE

The articular surfaces of bones are covered by hyaline cartilage which is thicker in weight-bearing areas than in nonweight-bearing areas. The joint space is lined by synovial membrane or synovium which forms synovial fluid that lubricates the joint during movements. The synovium may be smooth or thrown into numerous folds and villi. The synovial membrane is composed of inner layer of 1-4 cell thick synoviocytes and outer layer of loose vascular connective tissue.

DEGENERATIVE JOINT DISEASE (OSTEOARTHRITIS) (p. 842)

TYPES AND PATHOGENESIS OA occurs in 2 clinical forms:

◆ **Primary OA** occurs in the elderly, more commonly in women than in men. The process begins by the end of 4th decade and then progressively and steadily increases producing clinical symptoms. Probably, wear and tear with repeated minor trauma, heredity, obesity, ageing *per se*, all contribute to focal degenerative changes in the articular cartilage of the joints. Genetic factors favouring susceptibility to develop OA have been observed.

◆ **Secondary OA** may appear at any age and is the result of any previous wear and tear phenomena involving the joint such as previous injury, fracture, inflammation, loose bodies and congenital dislocation of the hip.

MORPHOLOGIC FEATURES As mentioned above, the weight-bearing joints such as hips, knee and vertebrae are most commonly involved but interphalangeal joints of fingers may also be affected.

1. Articular cartilages The regressive changes are most marked in the weight-bearing regions of articular cartilages. Initially, there is loss of cartilaginous matrix (proteoglycans). Further progression of the process causes loosening, flaking and fissuring of the articular cartilage resulting in breaking off of pieces of cartilage exposing subchondral bone.

2. Bone The denuded subchondral bone appears like polished ivory. There is death of superficial osteocytes and increased osteoclastic activity causing rarefaction, microcyst formation and occasionally microfractures of the subjacent bone. The margins of the joints respond to cartilage damage by *osteophyte* or *spur formation*. Loosened and fragmented osteophytes may form free 'joint mice' or loose bodies.

3. Synovium Initially, there are no pathologic changes in the synovium but in advanced cases there is low-grade chronic synovitis and villous hypertrophy.

The manifestations of OA are most conspicuous in large joints such as hips, knee and back. In symptomatic cases, clinical manifestations are joint stiffness, diminished mobility, discomfort and pain.

INFLAMMATORY JOINT DISEASES (p. 843)

RHEUMATOID ARTHRITIS

Rheumatoid arthritis (RA) is a chronic multisystem disease of unknown cause. Though the most prominent manifestation of RA is inflammatory arthritis of the peripheral joints, usually with a symmetrical distribution, its systemic manifestations include haematologic, pulmonary, neurological and cardiovascular abnormalities.

RA is a common disease having peak incidence in 3rd to 4th decades of life, with 3-5 times higher preponderance in females. The onset of disease is insidious, beginning with prodrome of fatigue, weakness, joint stiffness, vague arthralgias and myalgias. This is followed by pain and swelling of joints usually in symmetrical fashion, especially involving joints of hands, wrists and feet.

ETIOPATHOGENESIS Present concept on etiology and pathogenesis proposes that RA occurs in an *immunogenetically predisposed individual to the effect of microbial agents acting as trigger antigen.* The role of *superantigens* which are produced by several microorganisms with capacity to bind to HLA-DR molecules (MHC-II region) has also emerged.

The proposed events in **immunopathogenesis** of RA are as under:

i) In response to antigenic exposure (e.g. infectious agent) in a genetically predisposed individual (HLA-DR), *CD4+ T-cells* are activated.

ii) These cells elaborate *cytokines,* the important ones being tumour necrosis factor (TNF)-α, interferon (IF)-γ, interleukin (IL)-1 and IL-6.

iii) These cytokines *activate* endothelial cells, B lymphocytes and macrophages.

iv) Activation of B-cells releases IgM antibody against IgG (i.e. anti-IgG); this molecule is termed *rheumatoid factor (RF).*

v) IgG and IgM immune complexes trigger *inflammatory damage* to the synovium, small blood vessels and collagen.

vi) Activated endothelial cells express *adhesion molecules* which stimulate collection of inflammatory cells.

vii) Activation of macrophages releases more cytokines which cause damage to joint tissues and vascularisation of cartilage termed *pannus formation.*

viii) Eventually damage and destruction of bone and cartilage are followed by *fibrosis* and *ankylosis* producing joint deformities.

LABORATORY FINDINGS These include the following:

i) About 80% of cases are seropositive for *RA factor.*

ii) *HLA-DR4 and HLA-DR1* association in familial cases.

iii) *Anti-CCP antibodies* for evaluation of association of RA factor with HLA.

iv) Other laboratory findings include mild normocytic and normochromic anaemia, elevated ESR, mild leucocytosis and hypergammaglo-bulinaemia.

MORPHOLOGIC FEATURES Main findings are seen in the joints and tendons, and less often in the extra-articular tissues.

ARTICULAR LESIONS RA involves first the small joints of hands and feet and then symmetrically affects the joints of wrists, elbows, ankles and knees.

M/E Characteristic features are:

1. Numerous folds of large villi of synovium.

2. Marked thickening of the synovial membrane due to oedema, congestion and multilayering of synoviocytes.

3. Intense inflammatory cell infiltrate in the synovial membrane with predominance of lymphocytes, plasma cells and some macrophages, at places forming lymphoid follicles.

4. Foci of fibrinoid necrosis and fibrin deposition.

The pannus progressively destroys the underlying cartilage and subchondral bone.

EXTRA-ARTICULAR LESIONS Nonspecific inflammatory changes are seen in the blood vessels (acute vasculitis), lungs, pleura, pericardium, myocardium, lymph nodes, peripheral nerves and eyes. But one of the characteristic extra-articular manifestation of RA is occurrence of rheumatoid nodules in the skin.

1. **Juvenile RA** found in adolescent patients under 16 years of age is characterised by acute onset of fever and predominant involvement of knees and ankles.

2. **Felty's syndrome** consists of polyarticular RA associated with spleno-megaly and hypersplenism and consequent haematologic derangements.

3. **Ankylosing spondylitis or rheumatoid spondylitis** is rheumatoid involvement of the spine, particularly sacroiliac joints, in young male patients. The condition has a strong HLA-B27 association and may have associated inflammatory diseases such as inflammatory bowel disease, anterior uveitis and Reiter's syndrome.

SUPPURATIVE ARTHRITIS

Infectious or suppurative arthritis is invariably an acute inflammatory involvement of the joint. Bacteria usually reach the joint space from the bloodstream but other routes of infection by direct contamination of an open wound or lymphatic spread may also occur. Immunocompromised and debilitated patients are increasingly susceptible to suppurative arthritis.

MORPHOLOGIC FEATURES The haematogenous infectious joint involvement is more often monoarticular rather than polyarticular. The large joints of lower extremities such as the knee, hip and ankle, shoulder and sternoclavicular joints are particularly favoured sites. There may be formation of inflammatory granulation tissue and onset of fibrous adhesions between the opposing articular surfaces resulting in permanent ankylosis.

TUBERCULOUS ARTHRITIS

Tuberculous infection of the joints results most commonly from haemato-genous dissemination of the organisms from pulmonary or other focus of infection.

MORPHOLOGIC FEATURES Most commonly involved sites are the spine, hip joint and knees, and less often other joints are affected. Tuberculosis of the spine is termed *Pott's disease* or *tuberculous spondylitis*.

G/A The affected articular surface shows deposition of grey-yellow exudate and occasionally tubercles are present.

M/E The synovium is studded with solitary or confluent caseating tubercles. The underlying articular cartilage and bone may be involved by extension of tuberculous granulation tissue and cause necrosis *(caries)*.

GOUT AND GOUTY ARTHRITIS

Gout is a disorder of purine metabolism manifested by the following features, occurring singly or in combination:

1. Increased serum uric acid concentration *(hyperuricaemia)*.
2. Recurrent attacks of characteristic type of acute arthritis in which crystals of *monosodium urate monohydrate* may be demonstrable in the leucocytes present in the synovial fluid.
3. Aggregated deposits of monosodium urate monohydrate *(tophi)* in and around the joints of the extremities.
4. *Renal disease* involving interstitial tissue and blood vessels.
5. Uric acid *nephrolithiasis*.
    The disease usually begins in 3rd decade of life and affects men more often than women. A family history of gout is present in a fairly large proportion of cases indicating role of inheritance in hyperuricaemia.

TYPES AND PATHOGENESIS Hyperuricaemia and gout may be classified into 2 types: *metabolic* and *renal*, each of which may be *primary* or *secondary*. Primary refers to cases in which the underlying biochemical defect causing hyperuricaemia is not known, while secondary denotes cases with known causes of hyperuricaemia.

1. **Hyperuricaemia of metabolic origin** This group comprises about 10% cases of gout which are characterised by overproduction of uric acid. The causes of *primary metabolic gout* include a number of specific enzyme defects in purine metabolism which may be either of unknown cause or are inborn errors of metabolism. The *secondary metabolic gout* is due to either increased purine biosynthesis or a deficiency of glucose-6-phosphatase.

2. Hyperuricaemia of renal origin About 90% cases of gout are the result of reduced renal excretion of uric acid. Altered renal excretion could be due to reduced glomerular filtration of uric acid, enhanced tubular reabsorption or decreased secretion. The causes of gout of renal origin include diuretic therapy, drug-induced (e.g. aspirin, pyrazinamide, nicotinic acid, ethambutol and ethanol), adrenal insufficiency, starvation, diabetic ketosis, and disorders of parathyroid and thyroid.

MORPHOLOGIC FEATURES These are as under:

1. Acute gouty arthritis This stage is characterised by acute synovitis triggered by precipitation of sufficient amount of needle-shaped crystals of monosodium urate from serum or synovial fluid. There is joint effusion containing numerous polymorphs, macrophages and microcrystals of urates. Acute gouty arthritis is predominantly a disease of lower extremities, affecting most commonly *great toe*. Other joints affected, in order of decreasing frequency, are: the instep, ankles, heels, knees, wrists, fingers and elbows.

2. Chronic tophaceous arthritis Recurrent attacks of acute gouty arthritis lead to progressive evolution into chronic arthritis. The deposits of urate encrust the articular cartilage.

3. Tophi in soft tissue A *tophus* (meaning 'a porous stone') is a mass of urates measuring a few millimeters to a few centimeters in diameter. Tophi may be located in the periarticular tissues as well as subcutaneously such as on the hands and feet. Tophi are surrounded by inflammatory reaction consisting of macrophages, lymphocytes, fibroblasts and foreign body giant cells.

4. Renal lesions Chronic gouty arthritis frequently involves the kidneys. Three types of renal lesions are described in the kidneys:
i) Acute urate nephropathy
ii) Chronic urate nephropathy
iii) Uric acid nephrolithiasis

PSEUDOGOUT (PYROPHOSPHATE ARTHROPATHY)

Pseudogout refers to an inflammatory joint involvement due to deposition of calcium pyrophosphate in the joint space. The condition is seen in middle-aged and elderly individuals of either sex. The pain is usually less severe and involvement of big toe is rare.

PIGMENTED VILLONODULAR SYNOVITIS AND TENOSYNOVIAL GIANT CELL TUMOUR (NODULAR TENOSYNOVITIS)

The terms 'pigmented villonodular synovitis' and 'nodular tenosynovitis' represent diffuse and localised forms respectively of the same underlying process. The localised form of lesion is also termed *xanthofibroma* or *benign synovioma*. When the giant cells are numerous in localised tenosynovitis, the condition is called *giant cell tumour of tendon sheath*.

Clinically, they present with pain, swelling and limitation of movement of the affected joint and may be easily mistaken for rheumatoid or infective arthritis.

◈ **Giant cell tumour of tendon sheath (Nodular tenosynovitis)** The localised nodular tenosynovitis is seen most commonly in the tendons of fingers.

G/A It takes the form of a solitary, circumscribed, pedunculated, small and lobulated nodule, measuring less than 2 cm in diameter. It is closely attached to and sometimes grooved by the underlying tendon. On section, the lesion is yellowish-brown.

M/E It is well encapsulated and is composed of sheets of small oval to spindle-shaped cells, foamy xanthoma cells, scattered multinucleate giant cells and irregular bundles of collagen.

◈ **Pigmented villonodular tenosynovitis** This is a diffuse form of synovial overgrowth seen most commonly in the knee and hip.

G/A The synovium has characteristic sponge-like reddish-brown or tan appearance with intermingled elongated villous projections and solid nodules.

M/E The changes are modified by recurrent injury. The enlarged villi are covered by hyperplastic synovium and abundant subsynovial infiltrate of lymphocytes, plasma cells and macrophages, many of which are lipid-laden and haemosiderin-laden. Multinucleate giant cells are scattered in these areas.

CYST OF GANGLION

A ganglion is a small, round or ovoid, movable, subcutaneous cystic swelling of synovium. The most common location is dorsum of wrist but may be found on the dorsal surface of foot near the ankle. It may be the result of herniated synovium, embryologically displaced synovial tissue, or post-traumatic degeneration of connective tissue.

G/A A ganglion is a small cyst filled with clear mucinous fluid. It may or may not communicate with the joint cavity or tendon where it is located.

M/E The cyst has a wall composed of dense or oedematous connective tissue which is sometimes lined by synovial cells but more often has indistinct lining.

BURSITIS

Inflammation of bursa is termed bursitis. Bursae are synovial-lined sacs found over bony prominences. Bursitis occurs following mechanical trauma or inflammation.

G/A The bursal sac is thick-walled and may contain watery, mucoid or granular brown material.

M/E The bursal wall is composed of dense fibrous tissue lined by inflammatory granulation tissue. The wall is infiltrated by lymphocytes, plasma cells and macrophages and may show focal calcium deposits.

SKELETAL MUSCLES *(p. 848)*

NORMAL STRUCTURE

Individual muscle fibre is an elongated multinucleated syncytium-like cell about 100 µm in diameter and several centimeters in length. The muscle nuclei are spindle-shaped and lie at the periphery of fibre under the sarcolemma, the plasma membrane of muscle fibre. The cytoplasm of the muscle fibre contains myofilaments which are contractile elements. Myofilaments are of 2 types—*myosin* comprising thick filaments and *actin* constituting thin filaments.

The muscle, however, cannot function as a contractile organ without a nerve supply. For this purpose, there are **motor units,** each of which consists of the following:
1. Motor neuron cell body
2. The axon
3. The neuromuscular junction.

NEUROGENIC DISEASES *(p. 848)*

MYASTHENIA GRAVIS

Myasthenia gravis (MG) is a neuromuscular disorder of autoimmune origin in which the acetylcholine receptors (AChR) in the motor end-plates of the muscles are damaged. The term *'myasthenia'* means 'muscular weakness' and *'gravis'* implies 'serious'; thus both together denote the clinical characteristics of the disease. MG may be found at any age but adult women are affected more often than adult men in the ratio of 3:2. The condition presents clinically with muscular weakness and fatiguability, initially in the ocular musculature but later spreads to involve the trunk and limbs.

PATHOGENESIS It is best understood in the context of normal muscle metabolism.

◈ **Normally,** acetylcholine is synthesised in the motor nerve terminal and stored in vesicles that are released spontaneously when an action potential reaches the nerve terminal. Acetylcholine from released vesicles combines with AChRs, initiating an action potential which is propagated along the muscle fibre triggering muscle contraction.

◈ **In MG,** the basic defect is reduction in the number of available AChRs at the postsynaptic muscle membrane. In addition, the postsynaptic folds are flattened. The neuromuscular abnormalities in MG are mediated by autoimmune response.

DENERVATION ATROPHY

If the muscle or a part of muscle is deprived of its motor nerve supply, the affected muscle undergoes atrophy. In demyelination, on the other hand, there is conduction block in the nerve impulse but no denervation and hence muscle atrophy does not occur.

Denervating diseases are characterised by axonal degeneration and consequent muscle atrophy. These include *amyotrophic lateral sclerosis* as an example of anterior horn cell disease, and *peripheral neuropathy* causing injury to myelinated axon. The clinical manifestations of denervation atrophy are combination of muscular weakness and reduced muscle bulk. In amyotrophic lateral sclerosis, there are characteristic fasciculations of muscles of the shoulder and tongue.

MYOPATHIC DISEASES (MYOPATHIES) *(p. 850)*

Myopathies are primary skeletal muscle diseases resulting in chronic muscle weakness. These are divided into 5 broad groups: hereditary (muscular dystrophies), inflammatory, endocrine, metabolic and toxic myopathies.

MUSCULAR DYSTROPHIES

Muscular dystrophies are a group of genetically-inherited primary muscle diseases, having in common, progressive and unremitting muscular weakness. Six major forms of muscular dystrophies are described: *Duchenne's, Becker's, myotonic, facio-scapulohumeral, limb-girdle and oculopharyngeal type.* Each type of muscular dystrophy is a distinct entity having differences in inheritance pattern, age at onset, clinical features, other organ system involvements and clinical course. However, in general, muscular dystrophies manifest in childhood or in early adulthood.

M/E Common to all forms of muscular dystrophies are muscle fibre necrosis, regenerative activity, replacement by interstitial fibrosis and adipose tissue.

SELF ASSESSMENT

1. **The serum marker for increased osteoclastic activity is:**
   A. Total acid phosphatase level
   B. Bony acid phosphatase level
   C. Total alkaline phosphatase level
   D. Bony alkaline phosphatase level
2. **The serum marker for increased osteoblastic activity is:**
   A. Total acid phosphatase level
   B. Bony acid phosphatase level
   C. Total alkaline phosphatase level
   D. Bony alkaline phosphatase level
3. **Mineralisation of uncalcified osteoid matrix takes about:**
   A. 3-5 days   B. 5-8 days
   C. 8-12 days   D. 12-15 days

4. **Cartilage matrix largely consists of:**
   A. Chondroitin sulfate
   B. Keratan sulfate
   C. Heparan sulfate
   D. Dermatan sulfate

5. **Long-term complications of chronic osteomyelitis are as follows except:**
   A. Secondary amyloidosis
   B. Draining sinus tracts
   C. Development of Ewing's sarcoma
   D. Squamous carcinoma in sinus tract

6. **Osteopetrosis is characterised by the following features except:**
   A. Overgrowth of calcified dense bone
   B. Hereditary defect in osteoclast function
   C. There is hypercalcaemia
   D. Skeleton is susceptible to fractures

7. **Osteoporosis is characterised by the following laboratory investigations except:**
   A. Normal inorganic phosphate
   B. Raised serum calcium
   C. Normal alkaline phosphatase
   D. Normal acid phosphatase

8. **Renal osteodystrophy has the following biochemical parameters except:**
   A. Raised parathormone level
   B. Hyperphosphataemia
   C. Hypercalcaemia
   D. Calcium phosphorus product >70

9. **Paget's disease of the bone has following features except:**
   A. Affects older age past 50 years
   B. Elevation of serum alkaline phosphatase
   C. There is generally hypocalcaemia
   D. Role of virus in its etiology

10. **Albright's syndrome has the following features except:**
    A. There is monostotic bony lesion
    B. Skin pigmentation
    C. Sexual precocity
    D. More common in females

11. **Osteoblastoma differs from osteoid osteoma by the following features except:**
    A. It is larger than osteoid osteoma
    B. It is generally painful
    C. It is commonly located in the medulla of vertebrae, ribs, etc.
    D. There is absence of reactive bone formation

12. **Classic osteosarcoma has the following features except:**
    A. It occurs in age range of 10-20 years
    B. There is role of mutation in Rb gene in its etiology
    C. It is a highly malignant tumour
    D. Serum alkaline phosphatase levels are generally lowered

13. **Parosteal osteosarcoma has the following features except:**
    A. It occurs at extracortical location
    B. It occurs in older age group
    C. Worse prognosis than classic osteosarcoma
    D. It has no sex predilection

14. **There is a higher possibility of development of chondrosarcoma in the following benign cartilage-forming tumour:**
    A. Solitary enchondroma
    B. Multiple enchondroma
    C. Chondroblastoma
    D. Chondromyxoid fibroma

15. **In giant cell tumour of bone, the tumour cells are:**
    A. Osteoclastic giant cells
    B. Mononuclear stromal cells
    C. Fibroblastic cells
    D. Sinusoidal lining cells

16. **The cell of origin of Ewing's sarcoma is:**
    A. Endothelial cell
    B. Marrow cell
    C. Osteoblast
    D. Primitive neuroectodermal cell

17. Chordoma is a:
    A. Benign tumour
    B. Locally recurrent tumour
    C. Intermediate grade tumour
    D. Malignant tumour
18. Osteoblastic skeletal metastasis are characteristically seen in:
    A. Thyroid cancer
    B. Breast cancer
    C. Prostatic cancer
    D. Malignant melanoma
19. Osteoarthritis has the following pathologic changes except:
    A. Progressive loss of cartilaginous matrix
    B. Increased osteoclastic activity
    C. Osteophyte formation at the joint margin
    D. Atrophy of synovium
20. Most frequently and severely involved joints in rheumatoid arthritis are:
    A. Knees
    B. Elbows
    C. Interphalangeal
    D. Sacroiliac
21. Most frequently affected joint in acute gouty arthritis in the beginning is:
    A. Knee
    B. Elbow
    C. Shoulder
    D. Great toe
22. The origin of villonodular tenosynovitis and giant cell tumour of tendon sheath is:
    A. Inflammatory
    B. Neoplastic
    C. Traumatic
    D. Autoimmune
23. Patients of myasthenia gravis have the following features except:
    A. There is reduction in AChRs
    B. Majority of patients have anti-AChR antibodies in their serum
    C. Thymic hypoplasia has a risk in its etiology
    D. The disease has other autoimmune associations
24. All the following tumours are benign except:
    A. Osteoma
    B. Chondroma
    C. Chordoma
    D. Osteoblastoma
25. Most common etiologic agent implicated in chronic osteomyelitis is:
    A. *Staphylococcus aureus*
    B. *Escherichia coli*
    C. *Pseudomonas*
    D. *Klebsiella*
26. All are causes of avascular necrosis except:
    A. Long-term steroid therapy
    B. Chronic alcoholism
    C. Radiation therapy
    D. Fungal infection
27. All are types of skeletal dysplasia except:
    A. Achondroplasia
    B. Osteogenesis imperfecta
    C. Osteoporosis
    D. Osteopetrosis
28. All are benign bone forming tumours except:
    A. Osteoma
    B. Osteochondroma
    C. Osteoid osteoma
    D. Osteoblastoma
29. All of the following infectious agents are implicated in rheumatoid arthritis except:
    A. CMV
    B. Rubella
    C. Mycoplasma
    D. *Mycobacterium*

KEY

1 = B	2 = D	3 = D	4 = A	5 = C
6 = C	7 = B	8 = C	9 = C	10 = A
11 = B	12 = D	13 = C	14 = B	15 = B
16 = D	17 = D	18 = C	19 = D	20 = C
21 = D	22 = B	23 = C	24 = C	25 = A
26 = D	27 = C	28 = B	29 = D	

GENERAL FEATURES (p. 851)

INTRODUCTION

The WHO has defined soft tissues as all "non-epithelial extra-skeletal tissues of the body except the reticuloendothelial system, the glia and the supporting tissues of specific organs and viscera". Thus, soft tissues included for the purpose of categorisation of these tumours are: fibrous tissue, adipose tissue, muscle tissue, synovial tissue, blood vessels and neuroectodermal tissues of the peripheral and autonomic nervous system. The lesions of these tissues are embryologically derived from mesoderm, except those of peripheral nerve which are derived from ectoderm.

Benign soft tissue tumours are about 100 times more common than sarcomas. Sarcomas originate from the primitive mesenchymal cells having the capacity to differentiate along different cell pathways. Soft tissue sarcomas metastasise most frequently by the haematogenous route and disseminate commonly to the lungs, liver, bone and brain. Lymph node metastases are often late and are associated with widespread dissemination of the tumour. Histologic differentiation and grading of soft tissue sarcomas are important because of varying clinical behaviour, prognosis and response to therapy.

Majority of soft tissue tumours have following important general features:

1. Superficially-located tumours tend to be benign while *deep-seated* lesions are more likely to be malignant.
2. *Large-sized tumours* are generally more malignant than small ones.
3. *Rapidly-growing tumours* often behave as malignant tumours than those that develop slowly.
4. Malignant tumours have frequently *increased vascularity* while benign tumours are selectively avascular.
5. Although soft tissue tumours may arise anywhere in the body but in general *more common locations* are lower extremity (40%), upper extremity (20%), trunk and retroperitoneum (30%) and head and neck (10%).
6. Generally, *males* are affected more commonly than females.
7. Approximately 15% of soft tissue tumours occur in *children* and include some specific examples of soft tissue sarcomas e.g. rhabdomyosarcoma, synovial sarcoma.

ETIOLOGY AND PATHOGENESIS

1. Frequently there is history of antecedent *trauma* which may bring the tumour to attention of the patient.
2. Molecular and cytogenetic studies in many soft tissue tumours reveal *chromosomal abnormalities and mutations* in genes e.g. translocations, various fusion genes etc.
3. Most of the soft tissue tumours occur *sporadically;* however, there are a few examples which are components of *genetic syndromes* e.g. neurofibromatosis type 1, Li-Fraumeni syndrome, Osler-Weber-Rendu syndrome etc.

CLASSIFICATION

Currently, the WHO classification divides all soft tissue tumours into following 4 categories:

Benign These soft tissue tumours generally do not recur and are cured by complete excision. Common example is lipoma.

Intermediate, locally aggressive These tumours are locally destructive, infiltrative and often recur but do not metastasise. Such tumours are generally treated by wide excision; e.g. desmoid tumour.

Intermediate, rarely metastasising This category of tumours is also locally destructive, infiltrative and recurrent but in addition about 2% cases may have clinical metastasis e.g. dermatofibrosarcoma protuberans.

Malignant Tumours in this category are clearly malignant—they are locally destructive, infiltrative and they metastasise in a high percent of cases.

DIAGNOSTIC CRITERIA

1. CELL PATTERNS Several morphological patterns in which tumour cells are arranged are peculiar in different tumours e.g.

i) Smooth muscle tumours: interlacing fascicles.

ii) Fibrohistiocytic tumours: storiform pattern in which spindle tumour cells radiate from the centre in a spoke-wheel manner.

iii) Herringbone pattern: is seen in fibrosarcoma in which the tumour cells are arranged like the vertebral column of seafish.

iv) Palisaded arrangement: is characteristically seen in schwannomas in which the nuclei of tumour cells are piled upon each other.

v) Biphasic pattern: is the term used for a combination arrangement of two types—fascicles and epithelial-like e.g. in synovial sarcoma.

2. CELL TYPES Preliminary categorisation of soft tissue tumours is done on the basis of cell types comprising the soft tissue tumour:

i) Spindle cells: These are the most common cell types in most sarcomas e.g.

a) Fibrogenic tumours have spindle cells with light pink cytoplasm and tapering-ended nuclei.

b) Neurogenic (Schwann cell) tumours have tumour cells similar to fibrogenic cells but have curved nuclei.

c) Leiomyomatous tumours have spindle cells with blunt-ended (cigar-shaped) nuclei and more intense eosinophilic cytoplasm.

d) Skeletal muscle tumours have spindle cells similar to leiomyomatous cells but in addition have cytoplasmic striations.

ii) Small round cells: Some soft tissue sarcomas are characterised by dominant presence of small round cells or blue cells and are termed by various names such as malignant small round cell tumours, round cell sarcomas, or blue cell tumours e.g.

a) Rhabdomyosarcoma (embryonal and alveolar types)
b) Primitive neuroectodermal tumour (PNET)
c) Ewing's sarcoma
d) Neuroblastoma
e) Malignant lymphomas.

A few examples of epithelial tumours such as small cell carcinoma and malignant carcinoid tumours enter in the differential diagnosis of small round cell tumours.

iii) Epithelioid cells: Some soft tissue tumours have either epithelioid cells as the main cells (e.g. epithelioid sarcoma) or have epithelial-like cells as a part of biphasic pattern of the tumour (e.g. synovial sarcoma).

3. IMMUNOHISTOCHEMISTRY Soft tissue tumours are distinguished by application of immunohistochemical stains e.g.

i) *Smooth muscle actin (SMA):* for smooth muscle tumours.

ii) *Vimentin:* as common marker to distinguish mesenchymal cells from epithelium.

iii) *Desmin:* for skeletal muscle cells.

iv) *S-100:* for nerve fibres.

v) *Factor VIII:* antigen for vascular endothelium.

vi) *LCA (leucocyte common antigen):* common marker for lymphoid cells.

4. ELECTRON MICROSCOPY EM as such does not have much diagnostic value in soft tissue tumours but can be applied sometimes to look for tonofilaments or cell organelles.

5. CYTOGENETICS Many soft tissue tumours have specific genetic and chromosomal changes which can be done for determining histogenesis, or for diagnosis and prognosis.

GRADING

The number of pathological grades of soft tissue tumours may vary according to different grading systems: 2 grade system (grade I-II as low and high grade), 3-grade system (grade I, II, III as low, intermediate and high grade), and 4 grade system (grade I-IV). Pathological grading is based on following 3 features:
i)   Tumour differentiation or degree of cytologic atypia
ii) Mitotic count
iii) Tumour necrosis

STAGING

Enneking's staging: This staging system is accepted by most oncologists and is based on grade and location of tumour as under:
◈   *According to tumour location*: T1 (intracompartmental) and T2 (extracompartmental) tumours.
◈   *According to tumour grade*: G1 (low grade) and G2 (high grade) tumours.

Accordingly, the stages of soft tissue tumours vary from stage I to stage III as under:
Stage I: G1 and T1-T2 tumours, but no metastases.
Stage II: G2 and T1 -T2 tumours, but without metastases.
Stage III: G1 or G2 , T1 or T2 tumours, but with metastases.

AJC staging: This AJC system of staging is similar to staging for other tumours. It is based on TNM system in which the primary tumor (T), the status of lymph nodes (N) and presence or absence of metastases (M) are taken into consideration for staging, besides the histologic grade of the tumour.

SOFT TISSUE TUMOURS *(p. 853)*

TUMOURS AND TUMOUR-LIKE LESIONS OF FIBROUS TISSUE

FIBROMAS

True fibromas are uncommon tumours in soft tissues. Many fibromas are actually examples of hyperplastic fibrous tissue rather than true neoplasms. On the other hand, combinations of fibrous growth with other mesenchymal tissue elements are more frequent e.g. neurofibroma, fibromyoma etc.

Three types of fibromas are distinguished:

1. Fibroma durum is a benign, often pedunculated and well-circumscribed tumour occurring on the body surfaces and mucous membranes. It is composed of fully matured and richly collagenous fibrous connective tissue.

2. Fibroma molle or fibrolipoma, also termed **soft fibroma,** is similar type of benign growth composed of mixture of mature fibrous connective tissue and adult-type fat.

3. Elastofibroma is a rare benign fibrous tumour located in the subscapular region. It is characterised by association of collagen bundles and branching elastic fibres.

REACTIVE TUMOUR-LIKE PROLIFERATIONS

KELOID A keloid is a progressive fibrous overgrowth in response to cutaneous injury such as burns, incisions, insect bites, vaccinations and

G/A The keloid is a firm, smooth, pink, raised patch from which extend claw-like processes (keloid-claw).

M/E It is composed of thick, homogeneous, eosinophilic hyalinised bands of collagen admixed with thin collagenous fibres and large active fibroblasts. The adnexal structures are atrophic or destroyed.

NODULAR FASCIITIS Nodular fasciitis, also called pseudosarcomatous fibromatosis, is a form of benign and reactive fibroblastic growth extending from superficial fascia into the subcutaneous fat, and sometimes into the subjacent muscle. The most common locations are the upper extremity, trunk and neck region of young adults.

G/A The lesion appears as a solitary well-circumscribed nodule (true to its name) in the superficial fascia.

M/E Various morphologic patterns may be seen but most common is a whorled or S-shaped pattern of fibroblasts present in oedematous background. The individual cells are spindle-shaped, plump fibroblasts showing mild nuclear atypia. Typical mitoses are frequent but atypical mitoses are not present.

MYOSITIS OSSIFICANS Myositis ossificans is a benign, tumour-like lesion characterised by osteoid and heterotopic bone formation in the soft tissues.

Myositis ossificans is generally preceded by history of antecedent trauma to a skeletal muscle or its tendon. The trauma may be minor and repetitive e.g. to the adductor muscles of the thigh of a horseman, or may be single injury followed by haemorrhage into the muscle.

G/A The lesion appears as unencapsulated, gritty mass replacing the muscle.

M/E The central region of the mass shows loosely-arranged fibroblasts having high mitotic activity. Towards the periphery, there is presence of osteoid matrix and formation of woven mineralised bone with trapped skeletal muscle fibres and regenerating muscle (myogenic) giant cells. The appearance is sufficiently atypical to suggest osteosarcoma but osteosarcoma lacks maturation phenomena seen in myositis ossificans.

FIBROMATOSIS

'Fibromatosis' is the term used for tumour-like lesions of fibrous tissue which continue to proliferate actively and may be difficult to differentiate from sarcomas. These lesions may, therefore, be regarded as non-metastasising fibroblastic tumours which tend to invade locally and recur after surgical excision. Depending upon the anatomic locations and the age group affected, fibromatoses are broadly grouped as under:

A. Infantile or juvenile fibromatoses These include: fibrous hamartoma of infancy, fibromatosis colli, diffuse infantile fibromatosis, juvenile aponeurotic fibroma, juvenile nasopharyngeal angiofibroma and congenital (generalised and solitary) fibromatosis.

B. Adult type of fibromatoses These are: palmar and plantar fibromatosis, nodular fasciitis, cicatricial fibromatosis, keloid, irradiation fibromatosis, penile fibromatosis (Peyronie's disease), abdominal and extra-abdominal desmoid fibromatosis, and retroperitoneal fibromatosis. These are further categorised into *superficial or deep-seated*.

PALMAR AND PLANTAR (SUPERFICIAL) FIBROMATOSES These fibromatoses, also called Dupuytren-like contractures are the most common form of fibromatoses occurring superficially.

◈ **Palmar fibromatosis** is more common in the elderly males occurring in the palmar fascia and leading to flexion contractures of the fingers (Dupuytren's contracture). It appears as a painless, nodular or irregular, infiltrating, benign fibrous subcutaneous lesion.

◈ **Plantar fibromatosis** is a similar lesion occurring on the medial aspect of plantar arch. However, plantar lesions are less common than palmar type and do not cause contractures as frequently as palmar lesions. They are seen more often in adults and are infrequently multiple and bilateral. Essentially similar lesions occur in the shaft of the penis *(penile fibromatosis* or *Peyronie's disease)* and in the soft tissues of the knuckles *(knuckle pads).*

M/E Palmar and plantar fibromatoses have similar appearance. The nodules are composed of fibrovascular tissue having plump, tightly-packed fibroblasts which have high mitotic rate. The palmar lesions frequently extend into soft tissues causing contractures. Recurrence rate after surgical excision in both forms is as high as 50-60%.

DESMOID (DEEP-SEATED) FIBROMATOSES Desmoid fibromatoses or musculo-aponeurotic fibromatoses, commonly referred to as desmoid tumours, are of 2 types: abdominal and extra-abdominal. Clinically, both types behave in an aggressive manner and have to be distinguished from sarcomas. Recurrences are frequent and multiple. The pathogenesis of these lesions is not known but among the factors implicated are the role of antecedent trauma, genetic influences and relationship to oestrogen.

◈ **Abdominal desmoids** are locally aggressive infiltrating tumour-like fibroblastic growths, often found in the musculo-aponeurotic structures of the rectus muscle in the anterior abdominal wall in women during or after pregnancy.

◈ **Extra-abdominal desmoids,** on the other hand, are more common in men and are widely distributed such as in the upper and lower extremities, chest wall, back, buttocks, and head and neck region.

◈ **Intra-abdominal desmoids** present at the root of the small bowel mesentery are associated with Gardner's syndrome.

G/A Desmoids are solitary, large, grey-white, firm and unencapsulated tumours infiltrating the muscle locally. Cut surface is whorled and trabeculated.

M/E Their appearance is rather misleadingly bland in contrast with aggressive local behaviour. They are composed of uniform-looking fibroblasts arranged in bands and fascicles. Pleomorphism and mitoses are infrequent.

FIBROSARCOMA

Fibrosarcoma is a slow-growing tumour, affecting adults between 4th and 7th decades of life. Most common locations are the lower extremity (especially thigh and around the knee), upper extremity, trunk, head and neck, and retroperitoneum. The tumour is capable of metastasis, chiefly via the blood stream.

G/A Fibrosarcoma is a grey-white, firm, lobulated and characteristically circumscribed mass. Cut surface of the tumour is soft, fishflesh-like, with foci of necrosis and haemorrhages.

M/E The tumour is composed of uniform, spindle-shaped fibroblasts arranged in intersecting fascicles. In well-differentiated tumours, such areas produce *'herring-bone pattern'* (herring-bone is a sea fish). Poorly-differentiated fibrosarcoma, however, has highly pleomorphic appearance with frequent mitoses and bizarre cells.

FIBROHISTIOCYTIC TUMOURS *(p. 855)*

The group of fibrohistiocytic tumours is characterised by distinctive light microscopic features that include presence of cells with fibroblastic and histiocytic features in varying proportion and identification of characteristic *cart-wheel or storiform pattern* in which the spindle cells radiate outward from the central focus. The histogenesis of these cells is uncertain but possibly they arise from primitive mesenchymal cells or facultative fibroblasts which are capable of differentiating along different cell lines. The group includes full spectrum of lesions varying from *benign* (benign fibrous histiocytoma) malignant (malignant fibrous histiocytoma), with dermatofibrosarcoma protuberans occupying the *intermediate* (low-grade malignancy) position.

BENIGN FIBROUS HISTIOCYTOMA

Depending upon the location and predominant pattern, benign fibrous histiocytomas include a number of diverse entities such as dermatofibroma, sclerosing haemangioma, fibroxanthoma, xanthogranuloma, giant cell tumour of tendon sheath and pigmented villonodular synovitis.

DERMATOFIBROSARCOMA PROTUBERANS

Dermatofibrosarcoma protuberans is a low-grade malignant cutaneous tumour of fibrohistiocytic origin. The tumour recurs locally, and in rare instances gives rise to distant metastases.

G/A The tumour forms a firm, solitary or multiple, satellite nodules extending into the subcutaneous fat and having thin and ulcerated skin surface.

M/E The tumour is highly cellular and is composed of fibroblasts arranged in a cart-wheel or storiform pattern.

MALIGNANT FIBROUS HISTIOCYTOMA (PLEOMORPHIC SARCOMA)

Malignant fibrous histiocytomas (MFH), also called pleomorphic sarcoma now, represent approximately 20-30% of all soft tissue sarcomas. It is the most common soft tissue sarcoma and is the most frequent sarcoma associated with radiotherapy. The tumour occurs more commonly in males and more frequently in the age group of 5th to 7th decades. Most common locations are the lower and upper extremities and retroperitoneum.

G/A MFH is a multilobulated, well-circumscribed, firm or fleshy mass, 5-10 cm in diameter. Cut surface is grey-white, soft and myxoid.

M/E There is marked variation in appearance from area to area within the same tumour. In general, there is admixture of spindle-shaped *fibroblast-like cells* and mononuclear round to oval *histiocyte-like cells* which may show phagocytic function. There is tendency for the spindle shaped cells to be arranged in characteristic cart-wheel or storiform pattern. The tumour cells show varying degree of pleomorphism, hyperchromatism, mitotic activity and presence of multinucleate bizarre tumour giant cells. Important immunohistochemical markers for MFH include vimentin, α-chymotrypsin, CD68 and factor VIII-a.

As per current concept, corresponding WHO categories of MFH as pleomorphic sarcoma are as under:

1. Storiform-pleomorphic MFH as the prototype of *undifferentiated high-grade pleomorphic sarcoma*.

2. Inflammatory MFH is an undifferentiated high-grade MFH having prominent neutrophilic infiltrate besides the presence of eosinophils, histiocytes and xanthoma cells.

3. Giant cell MFH having prominent presence of tumour giant cells called as *undifferentiated pleomorphic sarcoma with giant cells*.

4. Myxoid MFH which shows areas of loose myxoid stroma in the cellular areas and has an overall better prognosis, is now categorised as a specific entity called *myxofibrosarcoma*.

Prognosis of MFH is determined by 2 parameters: depth of location and size of the tumour. Deep-seated and large MFH such as of the retroperitoneum have poorer prognosis than those small in size and located superficially which come to attention earlier. Metastases are frequent, most often to the lungs and regional lymph nodes. Five-year survival rate is approximately 30-50%.

TUMOURS OF ADIPOSE TISSUE *(p. 857)*

LIPOMA

Lipoma is the commonest soft tissue tumour. It appears as a solitary, soft, movable and painless mass which may remain stationary or grow slowly. Lipomas occur most often in 4th to 5th decades of life and are frequent in females. They may be found at different locations in the body but most common sites are the subcutaneous tissues in the neck, back and shoulder A lipoma rarely ever transforms into liposarcoma.

G/A A subcutaneous lipoma is usually small, round to oval and encapsulated mass. The cut surface is soft, lobulated, yellowish-orange and greasy.

M/E The tumour is composed of lobules of mature adipose cells separated by delicate fibrous septa. A thin fibrous capsule surrounds the tumour.

A variety of admixture of lipoma with other tissue components may be seen. These include: fibrolipoma (admixture with fibrous tissue), angiolipoma (combination with proliferating blood vessels) and myelolipoma (admixture with bone marrow elements as seen in adrenals). Infrequently, benign lipoma may infiltrate the striated muscle (infiltrating or intramuscular lipoma). Spindle cell lipoma and pleomorphic (atypical) lipoma are the other unusual variants of lipoma. The latter type may be particularly difficult to distinguish from well-differentiated liposarcoma.

LIPOSARCOMA

Liposarcoma is one of the most common soft tissue sarcomas in adults, perhaps next in frequency only to malignant fibrous histiocytoma. The peak incidence is in 5th to 7th decades of life. In contrast to lipomas which are more frequently subcutaneous in location, liposarcomas often occur in the deep tissues. Most frequent sites are intermuscular regions in the thigh, buttocks and retroperitoneum.

G/A Liposarcoma appears as a nodular mass, 5 cm or more in diameter. The tumour is generally circumscribed but infiltrative. Cut surface is grey-white to yellow, myxoid and gelatinous. Retroperitoneal masses are generally much larger.

M/E The hallmark of diagnosis of liposarcoma is the identification of variable number of *lipoblasts* which may be univacuolated or multivacuolated. The vacuoles represent fat in the cytoplasm. Four major histologic varieties of liposarcomas are distinguished: well-differentiated, myxoid, round cell, and pleomorphic.

The *prognosis* of liposarcoma depends upon the location and histologic type. In general, well-differentiated and myxoid varieties have excellent prognosis, while pleomorphic liposarcoma has significantly poorer prognosis. Round cell and pleomorphic variants metastasise frequently to the lungs, other visceral organs and serosal surfaces.

SKELETAL MUSCLE TUMOURS *(p. 859)*

RHABDOMYOMA

Rhabdomyoma is a rare benign soft tissue tumour. It should not be confused with glycogen-containing lesion of the heart designated as cardiac rhabdomyoma which is probably a hamartomatous lesion and not a true tumour. Soft tissue rhabdomyomas are predominantly located in the head and neck, most often in the upper neck, tongue, larynx and pharynx.

M/E The tumour is composed of large, round to oval cells, having abundant, granular, eosinophilic cytoplasm which is frequently vacuolated and contains glycogen. Cross-striations are generally demonstrable in some cells with phosphotungstic acid-haematoxylin (PTAH) stain.

RHABDOMYOSARCOMA

Rhabdomyosarcoma is a much more common soft tissue tumour than rhabdomyoma, and is the commonest soft tissue sarcoma in children and young adults. It is a highly malignant tumour arising from rhabdomyoblasts in varying stages of differentiation with or without demonstrable cross-striations. Depending upon the growth pattern and histology, 4 types are distinguished.

1. EMBRYONAL RHABDOMYOSARCOMA The embryonal form is the most common of the rhabdomyosarcomas. It occurs predominantly children under 12 years of age. The common locations are in the head and neck region, most frequently in the orbit, urogenital tract and the retroperitoneum.

G/A The tumour forms a gelatinous mass growing between muscles or in the deep subcutaneous tissues but generally has no direct relationship to the skeletal muscle.

M/E The tumour cells have resemblance to embryonal stage of development of muscle fibres. There is considerable variation in cell types. Generally, the tumour consists of a mixture of small, round to oval cells and spindle-shaped strap cells having tapering bipolar cytoplasmic processes in which cross-striations may be evident.

2. BOTRYOID RHABDOMYOSARCOMA Botryoid variety is regarded as a variant of embryonal rhabdomyosarcoma occurring in children under 10 years of age. It is seen most frequently in the vagina, urinary bladder and nose.

G/A The tumour forms a distinctive grape-like gelatinous mass protruding into the hollow cavity.

M/E The tumour grows underneath the mucosal layer, forming the characteristic *cambium layer* of tumour cells. The tumour is hypocellular and myxoid with predominance of small, round to oval tumour cells.

3. ALVEOLAR RHABDOMYOSARCOMA Alveolar type of rhabdomyosarcoma is more common in older children and young adults under the age of 20 years. The most common locations, unlike the embryonal variety, are the extremities.

G/A The tumour differs from embryonal type in arising directly from skeletal muscle and grows rapidly as soft and gelatinous mass.

M/E The tumour shows characteristic alveolar pattern resembling pulmonary alveolar spaces. These spaces are formed by fine fibrocollagenous septa. The tumour cells lying in these spaces and lining the fibrous trabeculae are generally small, lymphocyte-like with frequent mitoses and some multinucleate tumour giant cells. Cross-striation can be demonstrated in about a quarter of cases.

4. PLEOMORPHIC RHABDOMYOSARCOMA This less frequent variety of rhabdomyosarcoma occurs predominantly in older adults above the age of 40 years. They are most common in the extremities, most frequently in the lower limbs.

G/A The tumour forms a well-circumscribed, soft, whitish mass with areas of haemorrhages and necrosis.

M/E The tumour cells show considerable variation in size and shape. The tumour is generally composed of highly anaplastic cells having bizarre appearance and numerous multinucleate giant cells. Various shapes include racquet shape, tadpole appearance, large strap cells, and ribbon shapes containing several nuclei in a row.

Conventionally, the cross-striations can be demonstrated with PTAH stain in a few rhabdomyosarcomas. Immunohistochemical stains include: myogenin, Myo-D1, desmin, actin, myosin, myoglobin, and vimentin.

TUMOURS OF UNCERTAIN HISTOGENESIS (p. 861)

Some soft tissue tumours have a distinctive morphology but their exact histogenesis is unclear.

SYNOVIAL SARCOMA (MALIGNANT SYNOVIOMA)

Whether true benign tumours of synovial tissue exist is controversial. Pigmented villonodular synovitis and giant cell tumours of tendon sheaths. Synovial sarcoma or malignant synovioma, on the other hand, is a distinctive soft tissue sarcoma arising from synovial tissues close to the large joints, tendon sheaths, bursae and joint capsule but almost never arising within joint cavities. Most common locations are the extremities, frequently the lower extremity. The tumour principally occurs in young adults, usually under 40 years of age. The tumour grows slowly as a painful mass but ma~ metastasise via blood stream, chiefly to the lungs.

The *histogenesis* of tumour is, believed to be from multipoten~ mesenchymal cells which may differentiate along different cell lines.

G/A The tumour is of variable size and is grey-white, round to multilobulatec and encapsulated. Cut surface shows fishflesh-like sarcomatous appear~ ance with foci of calcification, cystic spaces and areas of haemorrhages anc necrosis.

M/E *Classic synovial sarcoma* shows a characteristic *biphasic cellula~ pattern* composed of clefts or gland-like structures lined by cuboidal tc columnar epithelial-like cells and plump to oval spindle cells. Reticulin fibres are present around spindle cells but absent within the epithelia foci. The spindle cell areas form interlacing bands similar to those seen in fibrosarcoma. Myxoid matrix, calcification and hyalinisation are frequently present in the stroma. Mitoses and multinucleate giant cells are infrequent.

An uncommon variant of synovial sarcoma is *monophasic pattern* in which the epithelial component is exceedingly rare and thus the tumour may be difficult to distinguish from fibrosarcoma.

ALVEOLAR SOFT PART SARCOMA

Alveolar soft part sarcoma is a histologically distinct, slow-growing malignant tumour of uncertain histogenesis. The tumour may occur a~ any age but affects children and young adults more often. Most alveola~ soft part sarcomas occur in the deep tissues of the extremities, along the musculofascial planes, or within the skeletal muscles.

G/A The tumour is well-demarcated, yellowish and firm.

M/E The tumour shows characteristic alveolar pattern. Organoid masses of tumour cells are separated by fibrovascular septa. The tumour cells are large and regular and contain abundant, eosinophilic, granular cytoplasm which contains diastase-resistant PAS-positive material. This feature distinguishes the tumour from paraganglioma, with which it closely resembles.

GRANULAR CELL TUMOUR

Granular cell tumour is a benign tumour of unknown histogenesis. It may occur at any age but most often affected are young to middle-aged adults. The most frequent locations are the tongue and subcutaneous tissue of the trunk and extremities.

G/A The tumour is generally small, firm, grey-white to yellow-tan nodular mass.

M/E The tumour consists of nests or ribbons of large, round or polygonal, uniform cells having finely granular, acidophilic cytoplasm and small dense nuclei. The tumours located in the skin are frequently associated with pseudoepitheliomatous hyperplasia of the overlying skin.

EPITHELIOID SARCOMA

This soft tissue sarcoma occurring in young adults is peculiar in that it presents as an ulcer with sinuses, often located on the skin and subcutaneous tissues as a small swelling. The tumour is slow growing but metastasising.

G/A The tumour is somewhat circumscribed and has nodular appearance with central necrosis.

M/E The tumour cells comprising the nodules have epithelioid appearance by having abundant pink cytoplasm and the centres of nodules show necrosis and thus can be mistaken for a granuloma.

CLEAR CELL SARCOMA

Clear cell sarcoma, first described by Enginzer, is seen in skin and subcutaneous tissues, especially of hands and feet.

M/E It closely resembles malignant melanoma, and is therefore also called melanoma of the soft tissues.

DESMOPLASTIC SMALL ROUND CELL TUMOUR

Desmoplastic small round cell tumour (DSRCT) is a rare and highly malignant tumour occurring more commonly in male children and juveniles under 2nd decade of life. The cell of origin is not clear. Some of the common locations are the abdomen, paratesticular region, ovaries, parotid, brain and thorax.

G/A The tumour appears as multiple soft to firm masses.

M/E Characteristic small and round tumour cells having epithelial, mesenchymal and neural differentiation.

SELF ASSESSMENT

1. **The term soft tissue tumours includes:**
   A. Mesodermal tissue
   B. Epithelial tissues
   C. Reticuloendothelial tissues
   D. Glial tissue

2. **Nodular fasciitis has the following features <u>except</u>:**
   A. It is an inflammatory condition
   B. Local excision is curative
   C. There are whorls of fibroblasts
   D. There is mild nuclear atypia and mitosis

3. **Desmoid tumour has the following characteristics <u>except</u>:**
   A. It has an aggressive behaviour
   B. The lesion is generally solitary and unencapsulated
   C. It has pleomorphic fibroblasts having moderate mitotic activity
   D. It may be abdominal or extra-abdominal

4. **The following lesions generally do not metastasise <u>except</u>:**
   A. Dermatofibrosarcoma protuberans
   B. Fibrosarcoma
   C. Granular cell myoblastoma
   D. Fibromatosis

5. **The most common soft tissue sarcoma is:**
   A. Fibrosarcoma
   B. Rhabdomyosarcoma
   C. Liposarcoma
   D. Malignant fibrous histiocytoma

6. **The commonest soft tissue sarcoma in children is:**
   A. Liposarcoma
   B. Rhabdomyosarcoma
   C. Malignant fibrous histiocytoma
   D. Synovial sarcoma

7. **Synovial sarcoma has the following characteristics <u>except</u>:**
   A. It generally arises from synovial tissues
   B. It has a biphasic growth pattern
   C. It always grows within joint cavities
   D. Most common locations are extremities

8. **Granular cell myoblastoma is seen most frequently in:**
   A. Extremities   B. Trunk
   C. Tongue   D. Visceral organs

9. **The term pseudomalignant osseous tumour is used for the following condition:**
   A. Myositis ossificans   B. Osteochondroma
   C. Osteoid osteoma   D. Osteoblastoma

10. **The following tumour is characterised by biphasic pattern of growth:**
   A. Osteosarcoma
   B. Osteochondroma
   C. Synovial sarcoma
   D. Malignant fibrous histiocytoma

11. **All of the following sarcomas are composed of small round cells <u>except</u>:**
    A. PNET
    B. Neuroblastoma
    C. Embryonal rhabdomyosarcoma
    D. Synovial sarcoma

12. **Pick the odd one out:**
    A. SMA – Smooth muscle tumours
    B. S-100 – Skeletal muscle tumours
    C. Factor VIII – Vascular tumours
    D. LCA – lymphoid cells

13. **Which of the following is associated with Gardner's syndrome?**
    A. Abdominal desmoids
    B. Extra-abdominal desmoids
    C. Intra-abdominal desmoids
    D. Plantar fibromatosis

14. **All are histologic variants of liposarcoma <u>except</u>:**
    A. Myxoid liposarcoma
    B. Round cell liposarcoma
    C. Pleomorphic liposarcoma
    D. Dedifferentiated liposarcoma

15. **Which one of the following variants of rhabdomyosarcoma is seen in adulthood?**
    A. Embryonal
    B. Botryoid
    C. Alveolar
    D. Pleomorphic

KEY

1 = A	2 = A	3 = C	4 = B	5 = D
6 = B	7 = C	8 = C	9 = A	10 = C
11 = D	12 = B	13 = C	14 = D	15 = D

NORMAL STRUCTURE

The skull and the vertebrae form a rigid compartment encasing the delicate brain and spinal cord. The average weight of the brain is about 1400 gm in men and 1250 gm in women. The two main divisions of the brain—the cerebrum and the cerebellum, are quite distinct in structure. The brain does not have lymphatic drainage. There are 2 types of tissues in the nervous system:

1. *Neuroectodermal tissues* which include neurons (nerve cells) and neuroglia, and together form the predominant constituent of the CNS.
2. *Mesodermal tissues* are microglia, dura mater, the leptomeninges (pia-arachnoid), blood vessels and their accompanying mesenchymal cells.

1. NEURONS The neurons are highly specialised cells of the body which are incapable of dividing after the first few weeks of birth.

Neuropil is the term used for the fibrillar network formed by processess of all the neuronal cells.

2. NEUROGLIA The neuroglia provides supportive matrix and maintenance to the neurons. It includes 3 types of cells: astrocytes, oligodendrocytes and ependymal cells. Neuroglia is generally referred to as *glia;* the tumours originating from it are termed *gliomas,* while reactive proliferation of the astrocytes is called *gliosis.*

i) Astrocytes The astrocytes are stellate cells with numerous fine branching processes. Depending upon the type of processes, two types of astrocytes are distinguished:
a) *Protoplasmic astrocytes*
b) *Fibrous astrocytes*

◈ *Gemistocytic astrocytes* are early reactive astrocytes having prominent pink cytoplasm. Long-standing progressive gliosis results in the development of *Rosenthal fibres* which are eosinophilic, elongated or globular bodies present on the astrocytic processes.

◈ *Corpora amylacea* are basophilic, rounded, sometimes laminated, bodies present in elderly people in the white matter and result from accumulation of starch-like material in the degenerating astrocytes.

ii) Oligodendrocytes Oligodendrocytes are so named because of their short and fewer processes when examined by light microscopy with special stains.

The major *function* of oligodendrocytes is formation and maintenance of myelin.

iii) Ependymal cells The ependymal cells are epithelium-like and form a single layer of cells lining the ventricular system, aqueduct, central canal of the spinal cord and cover the choroid plexus. They are cuboidal to columnar cells and have ciliated luminal surface.

The ependymal cells influence the formation and composition of the cerebrospinal fluid (CSF) by processes of active secretion, diffusion, absorption and exchange.

3. MICROGLIA Microglia is the nervous system counterpart of the monocyte-macrophage system.

4. DURA MATER The dura mater is a tough fibrous covering of the brain which is closely attached to the skull on its inner layer of endocranial periosteum. In the region of spinal canal, it encloses a potential space, the *epidural space,* between the bone and the dura. The dura is composed of dense collagen, fused with periosteum of the skull.

5. PIA-ARACHNOID (LEPTOMENINGES) The leptomeninges (*lepto*=thin, slender) consisting of the pia and arachnoid mater form the delicate vascular membranous covering of the central nervous system. The pia mater is closely applied to the brain and its convolutions, while the arachnoid mater lies between the pia mater and the dura mater without dipping into sulci. Thus, a space is left between the two layers of lepto-meninges, known as *subarachnoid space,* which contains the CSF. Extension of the subarachnoid space between the wall of blood vessels entering the brain and their pial sheaths form a circumvascular space called *Virchow-Robin space.* Another important potential space is enclosed between the dura and the arachnoid membrane known as *subdural space.*

DEVELOPMENTAL ANOMALIES AND HYDROCEPHALUS *(p. 865)*

SPINAL CORD DEFECTS

Spina bifida is the term applied to the malformations of the vertebral column involving incomplete embryologic closure of one or more of the vertebral arches (rachischisis), most frequently in the lumbosacral region. The vertebral defect is frequently associated with defect in the neural tube structures and their coverings. The bony defect may be of varying degree. The least serious form is **spina bifida occulta** in which there is only verte-bral defect but no abnormality of the spinal cord and its meninges. The site of bony defect is marked by a small dimple, or a hairy pigment mole in the overlying skin. The larger bony defect, however, appears as a distinct cystic swelling over the affected site called **spina bifida cystica.** This is associated with herniation of the meninges or the spinal cord, or both.

1. Herniation of the meninges alone through the bony defect is called **meningocele.** The herniated sac in meningocele consists of dura and arachnoid.

2. The commonest and more serious form is, however, **meningomyelocele** in which the spinal cord or its roots also herniate through the defect and are attached to the posterior wall of the sac. In this defect, the dura and the skin are in the sac are deficient.

3. A rare form of the defect is **myelocele** or **syringomyelocele** in which there is defective closure of the spinal canal so that the sac consists of an open flat neural tissue plate without skin covering and the CSF leaking through it.

5. The existence of defect in bony closure in the region of occipital bone or fronto-ethmoid junction may result in **cranial meningocele** and **encephalocele.**

ARNOLD-CHIARI MALFORMATIONS

Arnold-Chiari malformation is the term used for a group of malformations of the brain involving the brainstem and cerebellum. Approximately 50% of children with hydrocephalus have Arnold-Chiari malformation. Most patients of Arnold-Chiari malformation have, in addition, meningomyelocele. The major components of type II Arnold-Chiari malformation are as follows:

i) Elongation of the medulla with part of fourth ventricle in the cervical canal.

ii) Distortion of the medulla forming a characteristic S-shaped bend at the junction with the cervical spinal cord.

iii) Lengthening and herniation of the cerebellar vermis and cerebellar tonsils through the foramen magnum resulting in formation of a mass over the upper cervical cord.

HYDROCEPHALUS

Hydrocephalus is the term used for increased volume of CSF within the skull, accompanied by dilatation of the ventricles. In majority of cases of hydrocephalus, there is increased intracranial pressure. This type of hydrocephalus involving ventricular dilatation is termed *internal hydrocephalus*. A localised collection of CSF in the subarachnoid space is called *external hydrocephalus*.

SOURCE AND CIRCULATION OF CSF

CSF is mainly produced by choroid plexus in the lateral, third and fourth ventricle, and a small part is formed on the surface of the brain and spinal cord. The total volume of CSF is about 120-150 ml. CSF formed in the lateral ventricles flows through the foramina of Munro to the third ventricle and from there by the aqueduct of Sylvius to the fourth ventricle. It then spreads through the subarachnoid space over the surface of the spinal cord.

TYPES AND ETIOPATHOGENESIS

Hydrocephalus is classified into primary and secondary types, the former being much more common.

PRIMARY HYDROCEPHALUS Primary hydrocephalus is defined as actual increase in the volume of CSF within the skull along with elevated intracranial pressure. There are 3 possible mechanisms of primary hydrocephalus:
1. Obstruction to the flow of CSF.
2. Overproduction of CSF.
3. Deficient reabsorption of CSF.
   However, obstruction to the flow of CSF is by far the commonest cause and is termed *obstructive hydrocephalus*. The terms *non-communicating* and *communicating hydrocephalus* are used to denote the site of obstruction:

Non-communicating hydrocephalus When the site of obstruction of CSF pathway is in the third ventricle or at the exit foramina in the fourth ventricle, the ventricular system enlarges and CSF cannot pass into the subarachnoid space. Among the common causes are the following:
i) *Congenital non-communicating hydrocephalus* e.g. stenosis of the aqueduct, Arnold-Chiari malformation, progressive gliosis of the aqueduct and intra-uterine meningitis.
ii) *Acquired non-communicating hydrocephalus* may occur from expanding lesion within the skull. These conditions are as under:
◈ Tumours adjacent to the ventricular system e.g. ependymoma, choroid plexus papilloma, medulloblastoma and others.
◈ Inflammatory lesions e.g. cerebral abscess, meningitis.
◈ Haemorrhage e.g. parenchymal haemorrhage, intraventricular haemorrhage, and epidural and subdural haematoma.

Communicating hydrocephalus When obstruction to the flow of CSF is in the subarachnoid space at the base of the brain, it results in enlargement of the ventricular system but CSF flows freely between dilated ventricles and the spinal canal. The causes of communicating hydrocephalus are non-obstructive as follows:
i) *Overproduction of CSF* e.g. choroid plexus papilloma.
ii) *Deficient reabsorption of CSF* e.g. following meningitis, subarachnoid haemorrhage and dural sinus thrombosis.

SECONDARY HYDROCEPHALUS Secondary hydrocephalus is much less common and is defined as compensatory increase of CSF due to loss of neural tissue without associated rise in intracranial pressure (normal pressure hydrocephalus) e.g. from cerebral atrophy and infarction.

G/A There is dilatation of the ventricles depending upon the site of obstruction. There is thinning and stretching of the brain. The scalp veins overlying the enlarged head are engorged and the fontanelle remain open.

M/E Severe hydrocephalus may be associated with damage to ependymal lining of the ventricles and cause periventricular interstitial oedema.

A large number of pathogens comprising various kinds of bacteria, fungi, viruses, rickettsiae and parasites can cause infections of the nervous system. The micro-organisms may gain entry into the nervous system by one of the following routes:

1. Via blood stream
2. Direct implantation
3. Local extension
4. Along nerve

MENINGITIS

Meningitis is inflammatory involvement of the meninges. Meningitis may involve the dura called *pachymeningitis,* or the leptomeninges (pia-arachnoid) termed *leptomeningitis.*

◈ Pachymeningitis is invariably an extension of the inflammation from chronic suppurative otitis media or from fracture of the skull. An *extradural abscess* may form by suppuration between the bone and dura. Further spread of infection may penetrate the dura and form a *subdural abscess.* Other effects of pachymeningitis are localised or generalised leptomeningitis and *cerebral abscess.*

◈ Leptomeningitis, commonly called meningitis, is usually the result of infection but infrequently chemical meningitis and carcinomatous meningitis by infiltration of the subarachnoid space by cancer cells may occur. Infectious meningitis is broadly classified into 3 types:

ACUTE PYOGENIC MENINGITIS

Acute pyogenic or acute purulent meningitis is acute infection of the pia-arachnoid and of the CSF enclosed in the subarachnoid space. Since the subarachnoid space is continuous around the brain, spinal cord and the optic nerves, infection spreads immediately to whole of the cerebrospinal meninges as well as to the ventricles.

ETIOPATHOGENESIS The causative organisms vary with age of the patient:

1. *Escherichia coli* infection is common in neonates with neural tube defects.
2. *Haemophilus influenzae* is commonly responsible for infection in infants and children.
3. *Neisseria meningitidis* causes meningitis in adolescent and young adults and is causative for epidemic meningitis.
4. *Streptococcus pneumoniae* is causative for infection at extremes of age and following trauma.

G/A Pus accumulates in the subarachnoid space so that normally clear CSF becomes turbid or frankly purulent. The turbid fluid is particularly seen in the sulci and at the base of the brain where the space is wide.

M/E There is presence of numerous polymorphonuclear neutrophils in the subarachnoid space as well as in the meninges, particularly around the blood vessels. Gram-staining reveals varying number of causative bacteria.

CLINICAL FEATURES AND DIAGNOSIS Acute bacterial meningitis is a medical emergency. The immediate clinical manifestations are fever, severe headache, vomiting, drowsiness, stupor, coma, and occasionally, convulsions. The most important clinical sign is stiffness of the neck on forward bending.

The *diagnosis* is confirmed by examining CSF as soon as possible. The diagnostic alterations in the CSF in acute pyogenic meningitis are as under:

1. Naked eye appearance of cloudy or frankly purulent CSF.
2. Elevated CSF pressure (above 180 mm water).
3. Polymorphonuclear neutrophilic leucocytosis in CSF (between 10-10,000/µl).
4. Raised CSF protein level (higher than 50 mg/dl).

5. Decreased CSF sugar concentration (lower than 40 mg/dl).
6. Bacteriologic examination by Gram's stain or by CSF culture reveals causative organism.

ACUTE LYMPHOCYTIC (VIRAL, ASEPTIC) MENINGITIS

Acute lymphocytic meningitis is a viral or aseptic meningitis, especially common in children and young adults. Among the etiologic agents are numerous viruses such as enteroviruses, mumps, ECHO viruses, coxsackie virus, Epstein-Barr virus, herpes simplex virus-2, arthropode-borne viruses and HIV. However, evidence of viral infection may not be demonstrable in about a third of cases.

G/A Some cases show swelling of the brain while others show no distinctive change.

M/E There is mild lymphocytic infiltrate in the leptomeninges.

CLINICAL FEATURES AND DIAGNOSIS The clinical manifestations of viral meningitis are much the same as in bacterial meningitis with features of acute onset meningeal symptoms and fever. However, viral meningitis has a benign and self-limiting clinical course of short duration and is invariably followed by complete recovery.

The *CSF findings* in viral meningitis are as under:
1. Naked eye appearance of clear or slightly turbid CSF.
2. CSF pressure increased (above 250 mm water).
3. Lymphocytosis in CSF (10-100 cells/μl).
4. CSF protein usually normal or mildly raised.
5. CSF sugar concentration usually normal.
6. CSF bacteriologically sterile.

CHRONIC (TUBERCULOUS AND CRYPTOCOCCAL) MENINGITIS

There are two principal types of chronic meningitis.
◆ *Tuberculous meningitis* occurs in children and adults through haematogenous spread of infection from tuberculosis elsewhere in the body, or it may simply be a manifestation of miliary tuberculosis. Less commonly, the spread may occur directly from tuberculosis of a vertebral body.
◆ *Cryptococcal meningitis* develops particularly in debilitated or immunocompromised persons, usually as a result of haematogenous dissemination from a pulmonary lesion. Cryptococcal meningitis is especially an important cause of meningitis in patients with AIDS.

G/A In tuberculous meningitis, the subarachnoid space contains thick exudate, particularly abundant in the sulci and the base of the brain. Tubercles, 1-2 mm in diameter, may be visible, especially adjacent to the blood vessels. The exudate in cryptococcal meningitis is scanty, translucent and gelatinous.

M/E Tuberculous meningitis shows exudate of acute and chronic inflammatory cells, and granulomas with or without caseation necrosis and giant cells. Acid-fast bacilli may be demonstrated. Late cases show dense fibrous adhesions in the subarachnoid space and consequent hydrocephalus. Cryptococcal meningitis is characterised by infiltration by lymphocytes, plasma cells, an occasional granuloma and abundant characteristic capsulated cryptococci.

CLINICAL FEATURES AND DIAGNOSIS Tuberculous meningitis manifests clinically as headache, confusion, malaise and vomiting. The clinical course in cryptococcal meningitis may, however, be fulminant and fatal in a few weeks, or be indolent for months to years.

The *CSF findings* in chronic meningitis are as under:
1. Naked eye appearance of a clear or slightly turbid CSF which may form fibrin web on standing.
2. Raised CSF pressure (above 300 mm water).
3. Mononuclear leucocytosis consisting mostly of lymphocytes and some macrophages (100-1000 cells/μl).

4. Raised protein content.

5. Lowered glucose concentration.

6. Tubercle bacilli may be found on microscopy of centrifuged deposits by ZN staining in tuberculous meningitis. Pathognomonic capsulated cryptococci with a halo are appreciated in India ink preparation of CSF in cases of cryptococcal meningitis, while the capsule is better demonstrated by mucicarmine stain.

ENCEPHALITIS

Parenchymal infection of the brain is termed encephalitis. Encephalitis may be the result of bacterial, viral, fungal and protozoal infections.

BACTERIAL ENCEPHALITIS

Bacterial infection of the brain substance is usually secondary to involvement of the meninges rather than a primary bacterial parenchymal infection. This results in bacterial cerebritis that progresses to form *brain abscess*.

BRAIN ABSCESS Brain abscesses may arise by one of the following routes:

1. By direct implantation of organisms e.g. following compound fractures of the skull.

2. By local extension of infection e.g. chronic suppurative otitis media, mastoiditis and sinusitis.

3. By haematogenous spread e.g. from primary infection in the heart such as acute bacterial endocarditis, and from lungs such as in bronchiectasis.

Clinically, there is usually evidence of reactivation of infection at the primary site preceding the onset of cerebral symptoms.

G/A It appears as a localised area of inflammatory necrosis and oedema surrounded by fibrous capsule.

M/E The changes consist of liquefactive necrosis in the centre of the abscess containing pus. It is surrounded by acute and chronic inflammatory cells, neovascularisation, oedema, septic thrombosis of vessels, fibrous encapsulation and zone of gliosis. The CSF and overlying meninges also show evidence of acute and chronic inflammation.

TUBERCULOMA Tuberculoma is an intracranial mass occurring secondary to dissemination of tuberculosis elsewhere in the body.

G/A It has a central area of caseation necrosis surrounded by fibrous capsule.

M/E There is typical tuberculous granulomatous reaction around the central caseation necrosis. A zone of gliosis generally surrounds the tuberculoma. Advanced cases may show areas of calcification.

NEUROSYPHILIS Syphilitic lesions of the CNS used to be common and serious, but more recently there is evidence of atypical neurosyphilis in cases of HIV/AIDS. The lesions in syphilis may be in the form of *syphilitic meningitis* found in secondary syphilis, and *neurosyphilis* consisting of tabes dorsalis and generalised paralysis of the insane occurring in tertiary stage.

VIRAL ENCEPHALITIS

A number of viruses can infect the CNS and produce either aseptic meningitis or viral encephalitis, but sometimes combination of both termed meningo-encephalitis, is present. Most viral infections of the CNS are the end-result of preceding infection in other tissues and organs.

Most of the viruses reach the nervous system via blood stream before which they enter the body by various routes e.g. infection of the skin and mucous membrane (in herpes simplex and herpes zoster-varicella), by the alimentary tract (in enteroviruses including polio virus), by arthropod bite (in arbovirus), by transplacental infection (in cytomegalovirus), and through body fluids in AIDS (in HIV infection). Rabies virus travels along the peripheral nerves to reach the CNS. Herpes zoster-varicella is a distinct primary disease (chickenpox) but the virus remains latent for a long time

infections in which the agents have not only a long latent period but the
disease also develops slowly and may produce subacute sclerosing
panencephalitis, progressive multifocal leucoencephalopathy, progressive
rubella panencephalopathy and subacute spongiform encephalopathy.

HIV ENCEPHALOPATHY (AIDS-DEMENTIA COMPLEX)

Next to knocking off of the immune system, HIV has profound neurovirulence
but unlike tropism for CD4+ T cells of the immune system, HIV does not
have neurotropism. HIV has not been identified to infect the neuronal cells
but instead infects the cells of monocyte-macrophage cell line including
microglial cells.

Late in the course of AIDS, a group of signs and symptoms of CNS
disease appear termed HIV encephalopathy or *AIDS-dementia complex*.
One major clinical feature of this entity is the occurrence of *dementia* i.e. fall
in the cognitive ability of the individual compared to previous level.

PROGRESSIVE MULTIFOCAL LEUCOENCEPHALOPATHY

Progressive multifocal leucoencephalopathy (PML) is a slow viral infection of
the CNS caused by a papovavirus called *JC virus*. PML develops in immunocompromised individual like CMV and *Toxoplasma* encephalitis does, and
is, therefore, an important form of encephalitis due to increasing number of
cases of AIDS.

PML infects oligodendrocytes and causes progressive demyelination at
multifocal areas scattered throughout the CNS.

M/E The features are as under:
i) Focal areas of demyelination.
ii) Many lipid-laden macrophages in the centre of foci.

SPONGIFORM ENCEPHALOPATHY (CREUTZFELDT-JAKOB DISEASE)

Spongiform encephalopathy, also called Creutzfeldt-Jakob disease (CJD) or
mad-cow disease, though included under the group of viral encephalitis but
is caused by accumulation of prion proteins. *Prion proteins* are a modified
form of normal structural proteins present in the mammalian CNS and are
peculiar in two respects: they lack nucleic acid (DNA or RNA), and they can
be transmitted as an infectious proteinaceous particles.

Majority of cases occur sporadically though familial predisposition with
autosomal dominant inheritance has also been reported in 5-15% cases.
Other methods of transmission are by iatrogenic route (e.g. by tissue transplantation from an infected individual) and by human consumption of BSE
(bovine spongiform encephalopathy)-infected beef, hence called as mad-
cow disease.

Clinically, CJD is characterised by rapidly progressive dementia with
prominent association of myoclonus. CJD is invariably fatal with mean
survival of about 7 months after diagnosis.

M/E The hallmark is spongiform change i.e. there are small round vacuoles
in the neuronal cells. These changes are predominantly seen in the cortex
and other grey matter areas.

FUNGAL AND PROTOZOAL ENCEPHALITIS

Mycotic diseases of the CNS usually develop by blood stream from systemic
deep mycoses elsewhere in the body. They are particularly more common
in immunosuppressed individuals such as in AIDS, patients of lymphomas
and other cancers. Some of the fungi which may disseminate to the CNS are
*Candida albicans, Mucor, Aspergillus fumigatus, Cryptococcus neoformans,
Histoplasma capsulatum* and *Blastomyces dermatitidis*. These fungal
infections may produce one of the three patterns: fungal chronic meningitis,
vasculitis and encephalitis.

Besides fungal infections, CNS may be involved in protozoal diseases
such as in malaria, toxoplasmosis, amoebiasis, trypanosomiasis and
cysticerosis.

Cerebrovascular diseases are all those diseases in which one or more of the blood vessels of the brain are involved in the pathologic processes. Various pathologic processes commonly implicated in cerebrovascular diseases are: thrombosis, embolism, rupture of a vessel, hypoxia, hypertensive arteriolosclerosis, atherosclerosis, arteritis, trauma, aneurysm and developmental malformations. These processes can result in the following main types of parenchymal diseases of the brain:

A. Ischaemic brain damage:
a)   Generalised reduction in blood flow resulting in *global hypoxic-ischaemic encephalopathy*
b)   Local vascular obstruction causing *infarcts*.

B. Intracranial spontaneous (non-traumatic) haemorrhage:
a)   Haemorrhage in the brain parenchyma *(intracerebral haemorrhage)*
b)   Haemorrhage in the subarachnoid space *(subarachnoid haemorrhage)*.

C. Traumatic brain haemorrhage:
a)   Epidural haematoma
b)   Subdural haematoma
c)   Parenchymal brain damage.

The *stroke syndrome* is the cardinal feature of cerebrovascular disease. The term stroke is used for sudden and dramatic development of focal neurologic deficit, varying from trivial neurologic disorder to hemiplegia and coma. Other less common effects of vascular disease include: transient ischaemic attacks (TIA), vascular headache (e.g. in migraine, hypertension and arteritis), local pressure of an aneurysm and increased intracranial pressure (e.g. in hypertensive encephalopathy and venous thrombosis).

A. ISCHAEMIC BRAIN DAMAGE

Ischaemic necrosis in the brain results from ischaemia caused by considerable reduction or complete interruption of blood supply to neural tissue which is insufficient to meet its metabolic needs. The brain requires sufficient quantities of oxygen and glucose so as to sustain its aerobic metabolism, mainly by citric acid (Krebs') cycle which requires oxygen. Moreover, neural tissue has limited stores of energy reserves so that cessation of continuous supply of oxygen and glucose for more than 3-4 minutes results in permanent damage to neurons and neuroglial cells.

GLOBAL HYPOXIC-ISCHAEMIC ENCEPHALOPATHY

Depending upon the proneness of different cells of the brain to the effects of ischaemia-hypoxia, three types of lesion may occur:
1.   Selective neuronal damage
2.   Laminar necrosis
3.   Watershed infarcts

MORPHOLOGIC FEATURES The pathologic appearance of the brain in hypoxic encephalopathy varies depending upon the duration and severity of hypoxic episode and the length of survival.

◈   **Survival for a few hours:** No pathologic changes are visible.

◈   **Survival 12-24 hours:** No macroscopic change is discernible but microscopic examination reveals early neuronal damage in the form of eosinophilic cytoplasm and pyknotic nuclei, so called *red neurons*.

◈   **After 2-7 days:** There is focal softening. The area supplied by distal branches of the cerebral arteries suffers from the most severe ischaemic damage and may develop *border zone* or *watershed infarcts* in the junctional zones between the territories supplied by major arteries.

◈   *Longer duration:* Use of modern ventilators has led to maintenance of cardiorespiratory function in the presence of total brain necrosis unassociated with vital reaction.

Cerebral infarction is a localised area of tissue necrosis caused by local vascular occlusion—arterial or venous. Occasionally, it may be the result of non-occlusive causes such as compression on the cerebral arteries from outside and from hypoxic encephalopathy. Clinically, the signs and symptoms associated with cerebral infarction depend upon the region infarcted. In general, the focal neurologic deficit termed stroke, is present. However, significant atherosclerotic cerebrovascular disease may produce transient ischaemic attacks (TIA).

1. Arterial occlusion Occlusion of the cerebral arteries by either thrombi or emboli is the most common cause of cerebral infarction.

◈ Circle of Willis provides a complete collateral flow for internal carotid and vertebral arteries.

◈ Middle and anterior cerebral arteries have partial anastomosis of their distal branches. Their complete occlusion may cause infarcts.

◈ Small terminal cerebral arteries, on the contrary, are end-arteries and have no anastomosis. Hence, occlusion of these branches will invariably lead to an infarct.

2. Venous occlusion Venous infarction in the brain is an infrequent phenomenon due to good communications of the cerebral venous drainage.

3. Non-occlusive causes Compression of the cerebral arteries from outside such as occurs during herniation may cause cerebral infarction.

In any case, the extent of damage produced by any of the above causes depends upon:
i)   rate of reduction of blood flow;
ii)   type of blood vessel involved; and
iii) extent of collateral circulation.

G/A Cerebral infarcts may be anaemic or haemorrhagic. An *anaemic infarct* becomes evident 6-12 hours after its occurrence. The affected area is soft and swollen and there is blurring of junction between grey and white matter. Within 2-3 days, the infarct undergoes softening and disintegration. Eventually, there is central liquefaction with peripheral firm glial reaction and thickened leptomeninges, forming a cystic infarct. A *haemorrhagic infarct* is red and superficially resembles a haematoma. It is usually the result of fragmentation of occlusive arterial emboli or venous thrombosis.

M/E The sequential changes are as under:
1.   Initially, there is eosinophilic neuronal necrosis and lipid vacuolisation produced by breakdown of myelin. Simultaneously, the infarcted area is infiltrated by neutrophils.
2.   After the first 2-3 days, there is progressive invasion by macrophages and there is astrocytic and vascular proliferation.
3.   In the following weeks to months, the macrophages clear away the necrotic debris by phagocytosis followed by reactive astrocytosis, often with little fine fibrosis.
4.   Ultimately, after 3-4 months an old cystic infarct is formed which shows a cyst traversed by small blood vessels and has peripheral fibrillary gliosis. Small cavitary infarcts are called *lacunar infarcts* and are commonly found as a complication of systemic hypertension.

B. NON-TRAUMATIC INTRACRANIAL HAEMORRHAGE

Haemorrhage into the brain may be traumatic or non-traumatic, (or spontaneous). There are two main types of spontaneous intracranial haemorrhage:
1.   Intracerebral haemorrhage, which is usually of hypertensive origin.
2.   Subarachnoid haemorrhage, which is commonly aneurysmal in origin.

INTRACEREBRAL HAEMORRHAGE

Spontaneous intracerebral haemorrhage occurs mostly in patients of hypertension. Most hypertensives over middle age have microaneurysms in very small cerebral arteries in the brain tissue. Rupture of one of the numerous microaneurysms is believed to be the cause of intracerebral haemorrhage. Unlike subarachnoid haemorrhage, it is not common to have recurrent intracerebral haemorrhages.

The common sites of hypertensive intracerebral haemorrhage are the region of the basal ganglia (particularly the putamen and the internal capsule), pons and the cerebellar cortex.

G/A & M/E The haemorrhage consists of dark mass of clotted blood replacing brain parenchyma. The borders of the lesion are sharply-defined and have a narrow rim of partially necrotic parenchyma. Small ring haemorrhages in the Virchow-Robin space in the border zone are commonly present. After a few weeks to months, the haematoma undergoes resolution with formation of a slit-like space called *apoplectic cyst* which contains yellowish fluid.

SUBARACHNOID HAEMORRHAGE

Haemorrhage into the subarachnoid space is most commonly caused by rupture of an aneurysm, and rarely, rupture of a vascular malformation.

Berry aneurysms are saccular in appearance with rounded or lobulated bulge arising at the bifurcation of intracranial arteries and varying in size from 2 mm to 2 cm or more. They account for 95% of aneurysms which are liable to rupture. Berry aneurysms are rare in childhood but increase in frequency in young adults and middle life.

In more than 85% cases of subarachnoid haemorrhage, the cause is massive and sudden bleeding from a berry aneurysm on or near the circle of Willis. The four most common sites of such aneurysms are as under:

1. In relation to anterior communicating artery.
2. At the origin of the posterior communicating artery from the stem of the internal carotid artery.
3. At the first major bifurcation of the middle cerebral artery.
4. At the bifurcation of the internal carotid into the middle and anterior cerebral arteries.

The remaining 15% cases of subarachnoid haemorrhage are the result of rupture in the posterior circulation, vascular malformations and rupture of mycotic aneurysms that occurs in the setting of bacterial endocarditis.

MORPHOLOGIC FEATURES Rupture of a berry aneurysm frequently spreads haemorrhage throughout the subarachnoid space with rise in intracranial pressure and characteristic blood-stained CSF. An intracerebral haematoma may develop if the blood tracks into the brain parenchyma.

C. TRAUMA TO THE CNS

Trauma to the brain constitutes an important cause of death and permanent disability in the modern world. Important causes of head injuries are: motor vehicle accidents, accidental falls and violence. Traumatic injuries to the CNS may result in three consequences which may occur in isolation or in combination:

EPIDURAL HAEMATOMA

Epidural haematoma is accumulation of blood between the dura and the skull following fracture of the skull, most commonly from rupture of middle meningeal artery. The haematoma expands rapidly since accumulating blood is arterial in origin and causes compression of the dura and flattening of underlying gyri.

SUBDURAL HAEMATOMA

Subdural haematoma is accumulation of blood between the dura and subarachnoid and develops most often from rupture of veins which cross the surface convexities of the cerebral hemispheres. Subdural haematoma may be acute or chronic.

◈ **Acute subdural haematoma** develops following trauma and consists of clotted blood, often in the frontoparietal region. There is no significant compression of gyri. Since the accumulated blood is of venous origin, symptoms appear slowly and may become chronic with passage of time if not fatal.

◈ **Chronic subdural haematoma** occurs often with brain atrophy and less commonly following trauma. Chronic subdural haematoma is composed of liquid blood.

PARENCHYMAL BRAIN DAMAGE

Trauma to the CNS may result in damage to brain parenchyma and includes the following forms:

1. Concussion Concussion is caused by closed head injury and is characterised by transient neurologic dysfunction and loss of consciousness. Invariably, there is complete neurologic recovery after some hours to days.

2. Diffuse axonal injury Diffuse axonal injury is the most common cause of persistent coma or vegetative state following head injury. The underlying cause is sudden angular acceleration or deceleration resulting in widespread axonal shearing in the deep white matter of both the hemispheres.

3. Contusions and lacerations Contusions and lacerations are the result of direct damage to the brain parenchyma, particularly cerebral hemispheres, as occurs in the soft tissues.

4. Traumatic intracerebral haemorrhage On trauma to the CNS, the parenchymal vessels of the hemispheres may get torn and cause multiple intracerebral haemorrhages.

5. Brain swelling Head injury may be accompanied by localised or diffuse brain swelling.

MISCELLANEOUS DISEASES (p. 875)

DEMYELINATING DISEASES

Demyelinating diseases are an important group of neurological disorders which have, in common, the pathologic features of focal or patchy destruction of myelin sheaths in the CNS accompanied by an inflammatory response. Demyelination may affect peripheral nervous system as well. Some degree of axonal damage may also occur but demyelination is the predominant feature. The exact cause for demyelination is not known but currently viral infection and autoimmunity are implicated in its pathogenesis.

Loss of myelin may occur in certain other conditions as well, but without an inflammatory response. These conditions have known etiologies such as: genetically-determined defects in the myelin metabolism (leucodys-trophies), slow virus diseases of oligodendrocytes (progressive multifocal leucoencephalopathy), and exposure to toxins (central pontine myelinolysis). All these entities are currently not classified as demyelinating diseases. Only those conditions in which the myelin sheath or the myelin-forming cells (i.e. oligodendrocytes and Schwann cells) are primarily injured and are associated with considerable inflammatory exudate are included under the term 'demyelinating diseases'. Pathologically and clinically, two demyelinating diseases are distinguished:
1. Multiple or disseminated sclerosis
2. Perivenous encephalomyelitis.

DEGENERATIVE DISEASES

Degenerative diseases are disorders of unknown etiology and pathogenesis, characterised pathologically by progressive loss of CNS neurons and their processes accompanied by fibrillary astrocytosis.

Classification of degenerative diseases into individual syndromes is based on clinical aspects and anatomic distribution of the lesions.

ALZHEIMER'S DISEASE Alzheimer's disease is the most common cause of dementia in the elderly. The condition occurs after 5th decade of life and its incidence progressively increases with advancing age. The exact cause is not known but a few factors are implicated in its etiology which includes positive family history and deposition of Aβ amyloid derived from amyloid precursor protein (APP) forming *neuritic 'senile' plaques* and *neurofibrillary tangles*. Its pathogenesis is discussed in Chapter 3.

G/A The brain is often reduced in weight and bilaterally atrophic.

M/E The main features are as under:

i) *Senile neuritic plaque* is the most conspicuous lesion and consists of focal area which has a central core containing Aβ amyloid.

ii) *Neurofibrillary tangle* is a filamentous collection of neurofilaments and neurotubules within the cytoplasm of neurons.

iii) *Amyloid angiopathy* is deposition of the same amyloid in the vessel wall which is deposited in the amyloid core of the plaque.

iv) *Granulovacuolar degeneration* is presence of multiple, small intraneuronal cytoplasmic vacuoles, some of which contain one or more dark granules called *Hirano bodies*.

PARKINSONISM Parkinsonism is a syndrome of chronic progressive disorder of motor function and is clinically characterised by tremors which are most conspicuous at rest and worsen with emotional stress; other features are rigidity and disordered gait and posture. Parkinsonism is caused by several degenerative diseases, the most important being Parkinson's disease; other causes of parkinsonism are trauma, toxic agents, and drugs (dopamine antagonists).

G/A The brain is atrophic or may be normal externally.

M/E The hallmark is depigmentation of substantia nigra and locus ceruleus due to loss of neuromelanin pigment from neurons and accumulation of neuromelanin pigment in the glial cells. Some of the residual neurons in these areas contain intracytoplasmic, eosinophilic, elongated inclusions called *Lewy bodies*.

METABOLIC DISEASES

Metabolic diseases of the CNS result from neurochemical disturbances which are either inherited or acquired. *Hereditary metabolic disorders* predominantly manifest in infancy or childhood and include genetically-determined disorders of carbohydrate, lipid, amino acid and mineral metabolism. *Acquired or secondary metabolic diseases* are the disturbances of cerebral function due to disease in some other organ system such as the heart and circulation, lungs and respiratory function, kidneys, liver, endocrine glands and pancreas.

A. HEREDITARY METABOLIC DISEASES

1. Neuronal storage diseases These are characterised by storage of a metabolic product in the neurons due to specific enzyme deficiency. Common examples are: gangliosidoses (e.g. Tay-Sachs disease or GM2 gangliosidosis), mucopolysaccharidoses, Gaucher's disease and Niemann-Pick disease.

2. Leucodystrophies These are diseases of white matter characterised by diffuse demyelination and gliosis. They are caused by deficiency of one of the enzymes required for formation and maintenance of myelin. That is why these conditions are also called *dysmyelinating diseases*.

3. Other inborn errors of metabolism e.g. Wilson's disease (hepato-lenticular degeneration), glycogen-storage diseases, phenylketonuria and galactosaemia.

B. ACQUIRED METABOLIC DISEASES

1. Anoxic-ischaemic encephalopathy
2. Hypoglycaemic encephalopathy
3. Hyperglycaemic coma
4. Acute hepatic encephalopathy (Reye's syndrome)

5. Chronic hepatic encephalopathy
6. Kernicterus
7. Uraemic encephalopathy
8. Encephalopathy due to electrolyte and endocrine disturbances.

NUTRITIONAL DISEASES

Neurologic disorders may be caused by malnutrition from lack of adequate diet such as in many developing countries and many poor socio-economic groups.

Some of the common neurologic diseases included in the category of deficiency diseases are as under:

1. Wernicke's encephalopathy and Korsakoff's psychosis (vitamin B_1 or thiamine deficiency).
2. Subacute combined degeneration of the spinal cord (vitamin B_{12} deficiency).
3. Folic acid deficiency.
4. Spinocerebellar syndrome (vitamin E deficiency).
5. Pellagra (niacin deficiency).
6. Alcoholic cerebellar degeneration.

TUMOURS OF THE CNS (p. 878)

Tumours of the CNS may originate from the constituent cells in the brain or spinal cord (primary tumours), or may spread to the brain from another primary site of cancer (metastatic tumours). More than one-quarter of the CNS tumours are secondary metastases arising in patients undergoing treatment for systemic cancer. Primary CNS tumours are the second commonest form of cancer in infants and children under the age of 15 years, exceeded in frequency only by leukaemia. Childhood brain tumours arise from more primitive cells (e.g. neuroblastoma, medulloblastoma).

Among the primary brain tumours, gliomas constitute 50-60%, meningiomas 25%, schwannomas 10%, while other primary tumours comprise the remainder.

GLIOMAS

The term glioma is used for all tumours arising from neuroglia, or more precisely, from neuroectodermal epithelial tissue. Gliomas are the most common of the primary CNS tumours and collectively account for 40% of all intracranial tumours. They include tumours arising:

i) *from astrocytes* (astrocytomas and glioblastoma multiforme);
ii) *from oligodendrocytes* (oligodendroglioma);
iii) *from ependyma* (ependymoma); and
iv) *from choroid plexus* (choroid plexus papilloma).

ASTROCYTOMAS (INCLUDING GLIOBLASTOMA MULTIFORME)

Astrocytomas are the most common type of gliomas. In general, they are found in the late middle life with a peak in 6th decade of life. They occur predominantly in the cerebral hemispheres, and occasionally in the spinal cord. In children and young adults, pilocytic astrocytomas arise in the optic nerves, cerebellum and brainstem. Astrocytomas have tendency to progress from low grade to higher grades of anaplasia.

MORPHOLOGIC FEATURES Currently WHO classification of astrocytomas is widely used which divides them into 4 grades from grade I (low grade) to grade IV (glioblastoma multiforme) as under.

WHO GRADE I ASTROCYTOMA Also called as diffuse astrocytoma, it is a low-grade tumour having good prognosis and includes special histologic entities which mainly occur in children as under:

i) **Juvenile pilocytic astrocytoma** It occur in children and young adults in the cerebellum, third ventricle and optic nerve pathway.

G/A It is usually cystic or solid and circumscribed.

M/E It is predominantly composed of fusiform pilocytic astrocytes having unusually long, wavy fibrillary processes.

ii) Pleomorphic xanthoastrocytoma It looks histologically pleomorphic and alarming but has favourable prognosis.

WHO GRADE II (WELL-DIFFERENTIATED) ASTROCYTOMA It is also called as fibrillary astrocytoma and is the most common form of glioma occurring in 3rd to 4th decades of life.

G/A It is a poorly defined, grey-white tumour of variable size. The tumour distorts the underlying brain tissue and merges with the surrounding tissue.

M/E It is composed of well-differentiated astrocytes separated by variable amount of fibrillary background of astrocytic processes. Based on the type of astrocytes, three subtypes are distinguished: *fibrillary, protoplastic* and *gemistocytic astrocytoma.*

WHO GRADE III (ANAPLASTIC) ASTROCYTOMA It generally evolves from lower grade of astrocytoma.

G/A It may not be distinguishable from the low-grade astrocytoma.

M/E It contains features of anaplasia such as hypercellularity, pleomorphism, nuclear hyperchromatism and mitoses. Another characteristic feature of anaplastic variety of astrocytoma is the proliferation of vascular endothelium.

WHO GRADE IV ASTROCYTOMA (GLIOBLASTOMA MULTIFORME) Although its nomenclature means its origin from embryonal cells but now it is known that this tumour arises by neoplastic transformation of mature astrocytes. It is the most aggressive of astrocytomas.

G/A It shows variegated appearance, with some areas showing grey-white appearance while others are yellow and soft with foci of haemorrhages and necrosis. The surrounding normal brain tissue is distorted and infiltrated by yellow tumour tissue.

M/E The main features are as under:
i) It has highly anaplastic and cellular appearance. The cell types show marked variation consisting of fusiform cells, small poorly-differentiated round cells, pleomorphic cells and giant cells. Mitoses are quite frequent and glial fibrils are scanty.
ii) It shows areas of tumour necrosis around which tumour cells may form pseudopalisading.
iii) Microvascular endothelial proliferation is marked.

OLIGODENDROGLIOMA

Oligodendroglioma is an uncommon glioma of oligodendroglial origin and may develop in isolation or may be mixed with other glial cells. The tumour commonly presents in 3rd to 4th decades of life. It occurs in the cerebral hemispheres, most commonly in the frontal lobes or within the ventricles.

G/A Oligodendroglioma is well-circumscribed, grey-white and gelatinous mass having cystic areas, foci of haemorrhages and calcification.

M/E The tumour is characterised by uniform cells with round to oval nuclei surrounded by a clear halo of cytoplasm and well-defined cell membranes. Tumour cells tend to cluster around the native neurons forming *satellitosis.* Typically, there are varying degree of endothelial cell hyperplasia and foci of calcification.

EPENDYMOMA

Ependymoma is not an uncommon tumour, derived from the layer of epithelium that lines the ventricles and the central canal of the spinal cord. It occurs chiefly in children and young adults (below 20 years of age). Typically, it is encountered in the fourth ventricle (posterior fossa tumour). Other locations are the lateral ventricles, the third ventricle, and in the case of adults, the spinal cord in the region of lumbar spine. The usual biologic behaviour is of a slow-growing tumour over a period of years. Spinal ependymomas are associated with mutation of NF1 and NF2 genes.

G/A Ependymoma is a well-demarcated tumour but complete surgical removal may not be possible due to close proximity to vital structures in the medulla and pons.

M/E The tumour is composed of uniform epithelial (ependymal) cells forming rosettes, canals and perivascular pseudorosettes. By light microscopy under high magnification, PTAH-positive structures, blepharoplasts, representing basal bodies of cilia may be demonstrated in the cytoplasm of tumour cells. Most tumours are well-differentiated but anaplastic variants are also recognised.

Two variants of ependymoma deserve special mention:

Myxopapillary ependymoma It is a special variant of ependymoma which is common and occurs in adults. Characteristically, it occurs in the region of cauda equina and originates from the filum terminale. True to its name, it contains myxoid and papillary structures interspersed in the typical ependymal cells. It is a slow-growing tumour having a better prognosis.

Subependymoma It occurs as a small, asymptomatic, incidental solid nodule in the fourth and lateral ventricle of middle-aged or elderly patients. Areas of microcysts and calcification may be encountered.

CHOROID PLEXUS PAPILLOMA

Tumours derived from choroid plexus epithelium are uncommon intracranial tumours. They are found in the distribution of the choroid plexus. In children, they occur most frequently in the lateral ventricles, whereas in adults fourth ventricle is the most common site.

G/A The tumour projects as rounded, papillary mass into one of the ventricles.

M/E Choroid plexus papilloma is a papillary tumour resembling normal choroid plexus with a vascular connective tissue core covered by a single layer of cuboidal epithelium which lies upon a basement membrane.

POORLY-DIFFERENTIATED AND EMBRYONAL TUMOURS

MEDULLOBLASTOMA

Medulloblastoma is the most common variety of primitive neuroectodermal tumour. It comprises 25% of all childhood brain tumours but a quarter of cases occur in patients over the age of 20 years. The most common location is the cerebellum in the region of root of fourth ventricle, in the midline of cerebellum, in the vermis, and in the cerebellar hemispheres.

Medulloblastoma is a highly malignant tumour and spreads to local as well as to distant sites.

G/A The tumour typically protrudes into the fourth ventricle as a soft, grey-white mass or invades the surface of the cerebellum.

M/E Medulloblastoma is composed of small, poorly-differentiated cells with ill-defined cytoplasmic processes and has a tendency to be arranged around blood vessels and occasionally forms pseudorosettes (Homer-Wright rosettes). Another characteristic of the tumour is differentiation into glial or neuronal elements.

OTHER PRIMARY INTRAPARENCHYMAL TUMOURS

HAEMANGIOBLASTOMA

Haemangioblastoma is a tumour of uncertain origin and constitutes about 2% of all intracranial tumours. It is seen more commonly in young adults and is commoner in males. It may occur sporadically or be a part of von Hippel-Lindau syndrome (along with cysts in the liver, kidney, and benign/malignant renal tumour). *VHL* gene located on chromosome 3p25-p26 has an important function of regulating hypoxia induced factor-1 (HIF-1) which is responsible for the release of erythropoietin. Thus, about a quarter haemangioblastomas secrete erythropoietin and cause polycythaemia.

G/A The tumour is usually a circumscribed cystic mass with a mural nodule. The cyst contains haemorrhagic fluid.

M/E The features are as under:
i) Large number of thin-walled blood vessels lined by plump endothelium.
ii) Vascular spaces are separated by groups of polygonal lipid-laden foamy stromal cells.

PRIMARY CNS LYMPHOMA

Lymphomas in the brain may occur as a part of disseminated non-Hodgkin's lymphoma or may be a primary CNS lymphoma. The incidence of the primary CNS lymphoma has shown a rising trend in patients of AIDS and other immunosuppressed conditions.

G/A The tumour is frequently periventricular in location and may appear nodular or diffuse.

M/E The features are as under:
i) Characteristically, the tumour grows around blood vessels i.e. has an angiocentric growth pattern. Reticulin stain highlights this feature well.
ii) Typically, CNS lymphomas are diffuse, large cell type with high mitotic activity.
iii) They are generally B-cell type.

GERM CELL TUMOURS

Rarely, germ cell tumours may occur in the brain, especially in children. Common locations are suprasellar region and pineal area. Some common examples of such tumours are germinoma (seminoma/dysgerminoma), teratoma and embryonal carcinoma. Morphologically, they are similar to their counterparts elsewhere.

TUMOURS OF MENINGES

MENINGIOMA

Meningiomas arise from the cap cell layer of the arachnoid. Their most common sites are in the front half of the head and include: lateral cerebral convexities, midline along the falx cerebri adjacent to the major venous sinuses parasagittally, and olfactory groove. Less frequent sites are: within the cerebral ventricles, foramen magnum, cerebellopontine angle and the spinal cord. Meningiomas are generally solitary. They have an increased frequency in patients with neurofibromatosis 2 and are often multiple in these cases. They are usually found in 2nd to 6th decades of life, with slight female preponderance.

G/A Meningioma is well-circumscribed, solid, spherical or hemispherical mass of varying size (1-10 cm in diameter). The tumour is generally firmly attached to the dura and indents the surface of the brain but rarely ever invades it. The overlying bone usually shows hyperostosis. Cut surface of the tumour is firm and fibrous, sometimes with foci of calcification.

M/E Meningiomas are divided into 5 subtypes:

1. Meningotheliomatous (syncytial) meningioma This pattern of meningioma resembles the normal arachnoid cap cells. The tumour consists of solid masses of polygonal cells with poorly-defined cell membranes (i.e. syncytial appearance). The cells have round to oval, central nuclei with abundant, finely granular cytoplasm.

2. Fibrous (fibroblastic) meningioma A less frequent pattern is of a spindle-shaped fibroblastic tumour in which the tumour cells form parallel or interlacing bundles. Whorled pattern and psammoma bodies are less common features of this type.

3. Transitional (mixed) meningioma This pattern is characterised by a combination of cells with syncytial and fibroblastic features with conspicuous whorled pattern of tumour cells, often around central capillary-sized blood vessels. Some of the whorls contain psammoma bodies due to calcification of the central core of whorls.

4. Angioblastic meningioma An angioblastic meningioma includes 2 patterns: *haemangioblastic pattern* resembling haemangioblastoma of the cerebellum, and *haemangiopericytic pattern* which is indistinguishable from haemangiopericytoma elsewhere in the body. Both types of angioblastic meningiomas have high rate of recurrences.

5. Anaplastic (malignant) meningioma Rarely, a meningioma may display features of anaplasia and invade the underlying brain or spinal cord. This pattern of meningioma is associated with extraneural metastases, mainly to the lungs.

METASTATIC TUMOURS

Approximately a quarter of intracranial tumours are metastatic tumours. The clinical features are like those of a primary brain tumour. Most common primary tumours metastasising to the brain are: carcinomas of the lung, breast, skin (malignant melanoma), kidney and the gastrointestinal tract and choriocarcinoma. Infiltration from lymphoma and leukaemias may also occur.

G/A The metastatic deposits in the brain are usually multiple, sharply-defined masses at the junction of grey and white matter. A less frequent pattern is carcinomatous meningitis or meningeal carcinomatosis in which there is presence of carcinomatous nodules on the surface of the brain and spinal cord, particularly encountered in carcinomas of the lung and breast.

M/E Metastatic tumours in the brain recapitulate the appearance of the primary tumour of origin with sharp line of demarcation from adjoining brain tissue. It is usually surrounded by a zone of oedema.

PERIPHERAL NERVOUS SYSTEM (p. 884)

NORMAL STRUCTURE

The peripheral nervous system (PNS) consists of cranial and spinal nerves, sympathetic and parasympathetic autonomic nervous system and the peripheral ganglia. The PNS is involved in electric transmission of sensory and motor impulses to and from the CNS. A peripheral nerve is surrounded by an outer layer of fibrous tissue, the *epineurium*. Each nerve is made of several fascicles enclosed in multilayered membrane of flattened cells, the *perineurium*. *Myelinated axons* are thicker (diameter greater than 2 µm) and are surrounded by a chain of Schwann cells which produce myelin sheath. *Non-myelinated axons* have diameter of 0.2-3 µm and about ten non-myelinated fibres may be enclosed by a Schwann cell. *Nodes of Ranvier* on myelinated fibres are the boundaries between each Schwann cell surrounding the fibre.

PATHOLOGIC REACTIONS TO INJURY (p. 884)

The pathologic reactions of the PNS in response to injury may be in the form of one of the types of degenerations causing *peripheral neuropathy* or formation of a *traumatic neuroma*. There are 3 main types of degenerative processes in the PNS.

WALLERIAN DEGENERATION Wallerian degeneration occurs after transection of the axon which may be as a result of knife wounds, compression, traction and ischaemia. Following transection, initially there is accumulation of organelles in the proximal and distal ends of the transection sites. Subsequently, the axon and myelin sheath distal to the transection site undergo disintegration upto the next node of Ranvier, followed by phagocytosis.

AXONAL DEGENERATION In axonal degeneration, degeneration of the axon begins at the peripheral terminal and proceeds backward towards the nerve cell body. The cell body often undergoes chromatolysis. There is Schwann cell proliferation in the region of axonal degeneration.

SEGMENTAL DEMYELINATION Segmental demyelination is similar to demyelination within the brain. Segmental demyelination is loss of myelin of the segment between two consecutive nodes of Ranvier, leaving a denuded axon segment. The axon, however, remains intact.

TRAUMATIC NEUROMA Normally, the injured axon of a peripheral nerve regenerates at the rate of approximately 1 mm per day. However, if the process of regeneration is hampered due to an interposed haematoma or fibrous scar, the axonal sprouts together with Schwann cells and fibroblasts form a peripheral mass called as traumatic or stump neuroma.

PERIPHERAL NEUROPATHY (p. 884)

Peripheral neuropathy is the term used for disorders of the peripheral nerves of any cause.

POLYNEUROPATHY It is characteristically symmetrical with noticeable sensory features such as tingling, pricking, burning sensation or dysaesthesia in feet and toes. Motor features in the form of muscle weakness and loss of tendon reflexes may be present.

M/E Polyneuropathy may be the result of axonal degeneration (axonopathy) or segmental demyelination (demyelinating polyneuropathy).

MONONEUROPATHY MULTIPLEX (MULTIFOCAL NEUROPATHY) It is defined as simultaneous or sequential multifocal involvement of nerve trunks which are not in continuity. Multifocal neuropathy represents part of spectrum of chronic acquired demyelinating neuropathy.

MONONEUROPATHY Mononeuropathy on the other hand, is focal involvement of a single nerve. It is generally the result of local causes such as direct trauma, compression and entrapment.

NERVE SHEATH TUMOURS (p. 885)

SCHWANNOMAS (NEURILEMMOMAS)

Schwannomas or neurilemmomas arise from cranial and spinal nerve roots. An *acoustic schwannoma* or *acoustic neuroma* is an intracranial schwannoma located within the internal auditory canal originating from vestibular portion of the acoustic nerve. *Intraspinal schwannomas* are found as intradural tumours in the thoracic region. In the peripheral nerves, they occur as solitary nodule on any sheathed sensory, motor, or autonomic nerve.

G/A A schwannoma is an encapsulated, solid, sometimes cystic, tumour that produces eccentric enlargement of the nerve root from where it arises.

M/E The tumour is composed of fibrocellular bundles forming whorled pattern. There are areas of dense and compact cellularity (*Antoni A pattern*) alternating with loose acellular areas (*Antoni B pattern*). Areas of Antoni A pattern show palisaded nuclei called *Verocay bodies*. Nerve fibres are usually found stretched over the capsule but not within the tumour. Areas of degeneration contain haemosiderin and lipid-laden macrophages.

NEUROFIBROMAS AND VON RECKLINGHAUSEN'S DISEASE

Neurofibromas may occur as solitary, fusiform cutaneous tumour of a single nerve, but more often are multiple associated with von Recklinghausen's disease. Solitary neurofibroma is a tumour of adults but multiple neurofibromas or neurofibromatosis is a hereditary disorder with autosomal dominant inheritance. Solitary neurofibroma is generally asymptomatic but patients with von Recklinghausen's disease have a triad of features:

1. Multiple cutaneous neurofibromas.
2. Numerous pigmented skin lesions (*'café au lait'* spots).
3. Pigmented iris hamartomas.

Neurofibromatosis type 1 is a genetic disorder having mutation in chromosome 17 while type 2 has mutation in chromosome 22.

G/A Neurofibroma is an unencapsulated tumour producing fusiform enlargement of the affected nerve. Neurofibromatosis in von Recklinghausen's disease is characterised by numerous nodules of varying size, seen along the small cutaneous nerves but may also be found in visceral branches of sympathetic nerves. Neurofibromatosis may involve a group of nerves or may occur as multiple, oval and irregular swellings along the length of a nerve (plexiform neurofibroma).

M/E A neurofibroma is composed of bundles and interlacing fascicles of delicate and elongated spindle-shaped cells having wavy nuclei. The cellular area is separated by loose collagen and mucoid material. Residual nerve fibres (neurites) may be demonstrable. Histologic appearance of Antoni B pattern of schwannoma may be seen in neurofibroma and cause diagnostic difficulty. Immunohistochemically, neurofibroma is positive for epithelial membrane antigen (EMA) and some tumours express S-100 protein as schwannomas do.

Neurofibromas have tendency for local recurrences after excision. Neurilemmoma virtually never turns malignant, while sarcomatous transformation in neurofibroma, particularly in neurofibromatosis, is not unusual. It is estimated that about 3% of patients with von Recklinghausen's neurofibromatosis develop malignant transformation of one of the nodules.

MALIGNANT PERIPHERAL NERVE SHEATH TUMOUR

Malignant peripheral nerve sheath tumour (MPNST) is a poorly differentiated spindle cell sarcoma of the peripheral nerves occurring most often in adults. The tumour may arise *de novo* or from malignant transformation of a pre-existing neurofibroma than a schwannoma, generally at an early age (20-40 years).

G/A The tumour appears as an unencapsulated fusiform enlargement of a nerve.

M/E The tumour has the general appearance of tumour cells resembling a fibrosarcoma. The tumour has frequent mitosis and areas of necrosis. *Triton tumour* is the name used for MPNST which has areas of poorly-differentiated rhabdomyosarcoma, cartilage and bone.

Epithelioid MPNST has plump cells resembling epithelioid cells and is positive for HMB-45 immunostain. Most of the recurrent forms of MPNST are of epithelioid type.

Although relatively slow-growing, MPNST has local recurrences and haematogenous metastasis occur commonly; histology thus appears to have little correlation with clinical behaviour of the tumour.

SELF ASSESSMENT

1. **Astrocytic processes can be demonstrated by:**
   A. Reticulin stain
   B. Phosphotungstic acid haematoxylin (PTAH)
   C. Periodic acid Schiff (PAS)
   D. van Gieson
2. **Normally, the most numerous of the cells in the central nervous system are:**
   A. Astrocytes   B. Neurons
   C. Oligodendrocytes   D. Microglia
3. **Arnold-Chiari malformation consists of the following <u>except</u>:**
   A. Elongation of the medulla with part of 4th ventricle
   B. S-shaped bend in the medulla
   C. Encephalocele
   D. Lengthening and herniation of cerebellar vermix
4. **Secondary hydrocephalus has the following features <u>except</u>:**
   A. There is compensatory increase of CSF
   B. It occurs due to loss of neural tissue
   C. There is increased intracranial pressure
   D. Common causes are cerebral atrophy and infarction

5. **The most common route of spread of infection to the brain is:**
   A. Via venous route
   B. Via arterial route
   C. Via lymphatics
   D. Along nerves

6. **Glucose content of CSF is unaltered in the following type of meningitis:**
   A. Acute pyogenic meningitis
   B. Acute viral meningitis
   C. Cryptococcal meningitis
   D. Tuberculous meningitis

7. **The following viral infection of the brain produces intra-cytoplasmic inclusions:**
   A. Herpes simplex virus
   B. Cytomegalovirus
   C. Rabies virus
   D. Enteroviruses

8. **The etiologic agent for Creutzfeldt-Jakob disease (CJD) is as under:**
   A. HIV
   B. JC virus
   C. Prions
   D. Zoster-varicella virus

9. **The lowest limit of critical level of systolic pressure upto which the brain continues to be perfused is:**
   A. 70 mmHg
   B. 60 mmHg
   C. 50 mmHg
   D. 40 mmHg

10. **Subarachnoid haemorrhage results most often from the following:**
    A. Hypertension
    B. Aneurysm
    C. Vascular malformation
    D. Bleeding diathesis

11. **Acute subdural haematoma has the following features except:**
    A. Blood is of venous origin
    B. Accumulated blood is in liquid form
    C. No significant compression of gyri
    D. Symptoms develop slowly

12. **Neuritic plaques are seen in the brain in:**
    A. Multiple sclerosis
    B. Alzheimer's disease
    C. Parkinsonism
    D. Perivenous encephalomyelitis

13. **Primary CNS tumours may arise from the following constituent cells except:**
    A. Neuroglia
    B. Microglia
    C. Neurons
    D. Meninges

14. **Out of the following, the most common tumour in children is:**
    A. Ewing's sarcoma
    B. Neuroblastoma
    C. Glioma
    D. Embryonal rhabdomyosarcoma

15. **Astrocytoma occurring in children is commonly:**
    A. Fibrillary
    B. Pilocytic
    C. Anaplastic
    D. Glioblastoma multiforme

16. **Small foci of calcification are frequently seen on X-ray of the following glioma:**
    A. Ependymoma
    B. Oligodendroglioma
    C. Astrocytoma
    D. Choroid plexus papilloma

17. **Myxopapillary ependymoma characteristically occurs at the following location:**
    A. Lateral ventricles
    B. Fourth ventricle
    C. Third ventricle
    D. Filum terminale

18. **The following brain tumour has a tendency to metastasise by haematogenous route:**
    A. Anaplastic astrocytoma
    B. Glioblstoma multiforme
    C. Medulloblastoma
    D. Ependymoma

19. **The cell of origin of meningioma is:**
    A. Dura mater
    B. Arachnoid cap cell layer
    C. Pia mater
    D. Choroid plexus

20. **Transection of axon is followed by:**
    A. Wallerian degeneration
    B. Axonal degeneration

C. Segmental degeneration
D. Hypertrophy of Schwann cells

21. **Angiocentric growth pattern is typical of following CNS tumour:**
    A. Glioblastoma multiforme
    B. Haemangioblastoma
    C. Primary CNS lymphoma
    D. Medulloblastoma

22. **The most common cause of dementia is:**
    A. Parkinsonism
    B. Alzheimer's disease
    C. Multiple sclerosis
    D. Perivenous encephalomyelitis

23. **Common cause of meningitis in neonates with neural tube defects is:**
    A. *Escherichia coli*
    B. *Neisseria meningitides*
    C. *Streptococcus pneumoniae*
    D. *Staphylococcus aureus*

24. **Progressive multifocal leucoencephalopathy is caused by:**
    A. HIV
    B. CMV
    C. JC virus
    D. Prions

25. **Characteristic inclusions seen in parkinsonism are:**
    A. Hirano bodies
    B. Neurofibrillary tangle
    C. Negri bodies
    D. Lewy bodies

26. **Type of meningioma associated with extraneural metastasis:**
    A. Syncytial meningioma
    B. Fibrous meningioma
    C. Anaplastic meningioma
    D. Angioblastic meningioma

27. **Which of the following is not true about a schwannoma:**
    A. Unencapsulated
    B. Antoni A pattern
    C. Antoni B pattern
    D. Verocay bodies

28. **An 84 years old man, after an evening walk in the garden, is seen wandering in the street in search of his way back home and is helped by a passerby to find his way to home. The patient's family gives history of his deteriorating congnitive function progressively for the last 2 years. There is no history of any head injury, diabetes, hypertension or cardiovascular disease. What is the most likely cause of this patient's symptoms?**
    A. Parkinsonism
    B. Alzheimer's disease
    C. Cerebrovascular accident (CVA)
    D. Hypoxic-ischaemic encephalopathy

29. **A 10-year-old girl develops ataxia and hydrocephalus. CT scan shows a midline cerebellar mass. Which of the following is the most likely diagnosis?**
    A. Astrocytoma
    B. Meningioma
    C. Neurofibroma
    D. Medulloblastoma

30. **A one year old female child presented with an enlarging abdominal mass. Her 24-hour unrinary levels of metanephrine are elevated. Histopathology of the resected mass shows the tumour composed of numerous proliferating small round blue cells with occasional Homer-Wright rosettes. Which of the following is the most likely diagnosis?**
    A. Hepatoblastoma
    B. Nephroblastoma
    C. Neuroblastoma
    D. Embryonal rhabdosarcoma

KEY

1 = B	2 = C	3 = C	4 = C	5 = B
6 = B	7 = C	8 = C	9 = C	10 = B
11 = B	12 = B	13 = B	14 = B	15 = B
16 = B	17 = D	18 = C	19 = B	20 = A
21 = C	22 = B	23 = A	24 = C	25 = D
26 = C	27 = A	28 = B	29 = D	30 = C

Basic Diagnostic Cytology

Biopsy pathology has been the mainstay of diagnostic pathology at cellular level for over a century. This generated interest of workers towards obtaining cellular material by non-biopsy techniques to arrive at the diagnosis. As a result, diagnosis by cytopathologic technique was initially introduced in the 1920s by Dr. George N. Papanicolaou on cells naturally shed off (exfoliated) into cervical and vaginal secretion; subsequently its use was extended to cells shed off into other body cavities. Later, success of *bone marrow aspiration* for diagnosis of haematopoietic diseases created a parallel diagnostic cytopathologic technique of *fine needle aspiration cytology (FNAC)* for diagnosis of solid lesions.

ROLE OF DIAGNOSTIC CYTOLOGY

Among the numerous applications of cytodiagnostic techniques, the following are more important:

1. Diagnosis and management of cancer e.g.
i)   Cytodiagnosis in its traditional role is a *valuable adjunct* to histopathology.
ii) Cytologic techniques provide a *preliminary diagnosis* of cancer.
iii) As the *primary method* of establishing a tissue diagnosis e.g. in breast cancer.
iv) In the detection and diagnosis of clinically silent *early cancer* e.g. carcinoma *in situ* of the uterine cervix.
v)   Help in assessing *response to therapy* e.g. cervical smears for response to radiotherapy in carcinoma cervix.
vi) In detecting dissemination (metastasis) or recurrence of tumour.
2. Identification of benign neoplasms
3. Intraoperative cytopathologic consultation
4. Diagnosis of non-neoplastic/inflammatory conditions
5. Diagnosis of specific infections
6. In cytogenetics
7. Assessment of hormonal status in women
8. Identification of cell of origin
    For cytomorphological recognition of cancer, nuclear characteristics are used to determine the presence or absence of malignancy. Cytoplasmic characteristics help in typing the malignancy e.g. keratinisation in squamous cell carcinoma, mucin droplets in adenocarcinoma, melanin pigment in melanomas.

BRANCHES OF DIAGNOSTIC CYTOLOGY

Broadly speaking, there are two branches of diagnostic cytology:

EXFOLIATIVE CYTOLOGY This is the older branch that essentially involves the study of cells spontaneously shed off (as a result of continuous growth of epithelial linings) from epithelial surfaces into body cavities or body fluids. In addition, cells for study may also be obtained by scraping, brushing, or washing various mucosal surfaces (abrasive cytology).

Aspiration (FNA) which is also known as Aspiration Biopsy Cytology (ABC). In FNAC, the cytopathologist often performs the clinical procedure and interacts with the patient.

EXFOLIATIVE CYTOLOGY (p. 889)

Type of samples that can be obtained from different organ systems for exfoliative cytodiagnosis (gynaecologic and non-gynaecologic) and are listed below:

I.   GYNAECOLOGIC EXFOLIATIVE CYTOLOGY

Female genital tract	i)	Lateral vaginal smears (LVS)
	ii)	Vaginal 'pool' smears
	iii)	Cervical smears
	iv)	Combined (fast) smears
	v)	Triple smears (CVE)
	vi)	Endocervical/Endometrial aspiration

II.   NON-GYNAECOLOGIC EXFOLIATIVE CYTOLOGY

1. Respiratory tract	i)	Sputum
	ii)	Bronchial washings/brushing/ bronchioalveolar lavage (BAL)
2. Gastrointestinal tract		Endoscopic lavage/brushing
3. Urinary tract	i)	Urinary sediment
	ii)	Bladder washings
	iii)	Retrograde catheterisation
	iv)	Prostatic massage (secretions)
4. Body fluids	i)	Effusions
	ii)	Fluids of small volume
		a. Cerebrospinal fluid (CSF)
		b. Synovial fluid
		c. Amniotic fluid
		d. Hydrocele fluid
		e. Seminal fluid (semen)
		f. Nipple discharge
5. Other samples	—	Buccal smears (for sex chromatin)

I. GYNAECOLOGIC EXFOLIATIVE CYTOLOGY (p. 889)

Smears from the female genital tract have traditionally been known as 'Pap smears'. These smears may be prepared by different methods depending upon the purpose for which they are intended.

CELLS IN NORMAL COMBINED SMEARS

Combined smears normally contain epithelial cells (normal and variants) and other cells:

Epithelial cells   There are 4 types of squamous epithelial cells in the cervical smear: *superficial, intermediate, parabasal and basal cells*. A few variants of morphological forms and other epithelial cells are as under:

1.   *Navicular cells* are boat-shaped intermediate cells with folded cell borders.
2.   *Lactation cells* are parabasal cells with strongly acidophilic cytoplasm.
3.   *Endocervical cells* appear either as single dispersed nuclei, or as clusters of columnar cells.
4.   *Endometrial cells* are seen up to 12th day of menstrual cycle.
5.   *Trophoblastic cells* are seen following abortion or after delivery.

Other cells   Besides epithelial cells, other cells in cervical smears are leucocytes and Döderlein bacilli.

It includes application of Pap smears for hormonal evaluation and for categorising their abnormalities into non-neoplastic, benign, and malignant types.

CYTOHORMONAL EVALUATION

Assessment of hormonal status is best carried out from lateral vaginal smears although vaginal 'pool' or fast smears may also be used. Ideally, at least 3 smears obtained on alternate days should be scrutinised and cytologic indices determined for each smear for accurate assessment.

Several indices are available for description of cytohormonal patterns. The most commonly used are as under:

i)   *Acidophilic index (AI):* The relative proportion of cells containing acidophilic (pink) and basophilic (blue) cytoplasm are determined by AI.

ii)   *Pyknotic index (PI):* The percentage of cells having small, dark, shrunken nuclei (less than 6 μm in size) is determined by PI.

iii)   *Maturation index (MI):* MI is the most widely used method. One hundred squamous cells are counted and grouped according to their type—parabasal, intermediate, or superficial.

ABNORMAL COMBINED SMEARS

In order to evolve a system acceptable to clinicians and cytopathologists, National Cancer Institute Workshop in 1988 developed *the Bethesda System (TBS)* for uniformity in evaluation as well as limitations of reporting in cervicovaginal cytopathology; this was subsequently modified in 1991 and further updated in 2001. Criteria followed in the Bethesda system has three basic components in recommendations:

1.   Specimen adequacy It is an important component of quality assurance and provides feedback regarding sampling technique. It implies properly labelled, adequately fixed smears having sufficient number of evenly spread, well preserved cells as evaluated microscopically.

2.   General categorisation It includes categorising the smear in one of the three broad categories: within normal limits, benign cellular changes, and epithelial cell abnormalities.

3.   Descriptive diagnosis Final aspect of the Bethesda system includes detailed description of the benign cellular changes or epithelial cell abnormalities in the smear.

Based on it, the cellular changes in cervical smears are described under 2 headings: non-neoplastic (or benign) and neoplastic epithelial cell abnormalities.

NON-NEOPLASTIC (BENIGN) CELLULAR CHANGES:

i)   NON-SPECIFIC INFLAMMATORY CHANGES
◈   *Acute inflammatory changes* are characterised by an increase in the number of parabasal cells, cytoplasmic acidophilia and vacuolisation, leucocytic migration into cytoplasm, and perinuclear halos with nuclear pyknosis or enlargement.
◈   *Chronic inflammatory changes (Reactive changes)* manifest in squamous cells as nuclear enlargement, hyperchromatism, and nucleolar prominence, with multinucleation in some instances.

ii)   SPECIFIC INFLAMMATORY CHANGES
a)   *Bacterial agents:*
◈   *N. gonorrhoeae*
◈   *Gardnerella vaginalis*
◈   *Mycobacterium tuberculosis*

b)   *Viral agents:*
◈   *Human papillomavirus (HPV)*
◈   *Herpes simplex virus (HSV)*

c)   *Fungal agents:*
◈   *Candida albicans*
◈   *Torulopsis glabrata.*

d) Parasitic agents:
❖ *Trichomonas vaginalis*
❖ *Entamoeba histolytica*

NEOPLASTIC EPITHELIAL CELL ABNORMALITIES:

Carcinoma of the uterine cervix still ranks high in the list as the most frequent cancer in developing countries of the world and is the leading cause of cancer morbidity and mortality. Vast majority of cervical cancers are of the squamous cell type, and the diagnosis of squamous cell carcinoma of the cervix and its precursor lesions is considered as the most important application of exfoliative cytology.

Neoplastic epithelial changes are described below under 2 headings:

1. SQUAMOUS CELL ABNORMALITIES The fully-developed invasive squamous cell carcinoma of the uterine cervix is preceded by a pre-invasive intraepithelial neoplastic process that is recognisable on histologic and cytologic examination.

Morphogenesis and nomenclature The earliest recognisable change is *hyperplasia* of basal or reserve cells which normally constitute a single layer at the deepest part of the epithelium. The proliferating reserve cells next develop certain atypical features and progressive involvement of more and more layers of the epithelium is known as *dysplasia* (disordered growth). When dysplasia involves the full thickness of the epithelium and the lesion morphologically resembles squamous cell carcinoma without invasion of underlying stroma, it is termed *carcinoma in situ (CIS)*. CIS further progresses through the stage of *microinvasive carcinoma* (with depth of stromal invasion not exceeding 3 mm) into full-blown *invasive squamous cell carcinoma*.

Previously, depending on the degree of epithelial involvement, three grades of dysplasia were recognised: mild, moderate and severe. As the stages of dysplasia and CIS represented a continuous spectrum of lesions seen in the precancerous state, they were collectively termed 'cervical intraepithelial neoplasia' (CIN) and categorised CIN I, II and III.

Presently, *the Bethesda system* divides squamous cell abnormalities into four categories:

i) *Atypical squamous cells of undetermined significance (ASCUS)* which represents cellular changes falling short of intraepithelial lesion.

ii) *Low-grade squamous intraepithelial lesion (L-SIL)* that includes CIN-I and cellular changes associated with HPV infection.

iii) *High-grade squamous intraepithelial lesion (H-SIL)* includes CIN grade II, III and CIS.

iv) *Squamous cell carcinoma.*

Cytomorphology In dysplastic epithelium, stratification and maturation of cytoplasm occurs above the layers of proliferating primitive cells while the nuclear abnormalities persist. The character and type of dyskaryotic cells observed in smears reflect the severity of dysplasia:

i) In mild dysplasia (CIN-I or L-SIL), maturation occurs in the upper two-thirds of the epithelium and exfoliated dyskaryotic cells are of the superficial type. These cells show cytoplasmic vacuolation as perinuclear halo (koilocytosis) and nuclear enlargement.

ii) With increasing dysplasia (CIN-II and CIN-III, or H-SIL), the proliferating primitive cells reach closer to the epithelial surface, less cytoplasmic maturation/differentiation occurs, and dyskaryotic intermediate and parabasal cells are observed in smears.

iii) Progression to CIS (CIN-III or H-SIL) manifests as subtle alterations in cell arrangement and morphology (with predominantly basal and parabasal cells in smears).

iv) Onset of invasive carcinoma is heralded by the appearance of macronucleoli, cytoplasmic orangeophilia and presence of tumour diathesis (dirty, necrotic background).

2. GLANDULAR CELL ABNORMALITIES The Bethesda system categorises glandular abnormalities as under:

i) *Atypical glandular cells of undetermined significance (AGUS)* which represent nuclear atypia of endocervical and endometrial cells exceeding reparative changes.

ii)   *Endocervical* and *endometrial adenocarcinoma*, both of which can be detected from Pap smears.

iii) Cells from *extrauterine cancers* may also be present in Pap smears, majority originating from the ovaries.

AUTOMATION IN CERVICAL CYTOLOGY

Introduction of automated devices like PapNet for primary screening is a major technologic achievement in recent times. Automation offers routine pre-screening of hundreds of Pap smears, decreasing the workload of cytopathologists and at the same time providing quality assurance. It can be applied to conventional Pap smears or to *Thin-Preps*.

II. NON-GYNAECOLOGIC EXFOLIATIVE CYTOLOGY (p. 894)

RESPIRATORY TRACT

Cellular material from the respiratory tract may be obtained as a result of spontaneous expectoration (sputum), aspiration or brushing during broncho-scopic procedures.

GASTROINTESTINAL TRACT

Lesions in the oral cavity may be sampled by scraping the surface with wooden and metal tongue-depressors. For the oesophagus, stomach and duodenum, cytologic samples are obtained under direct vision by brushing or lavage through fibreoptic endoscopes.

URINARY TRACT

1.   URINARY SEDIMENT CYTOLOGY Cytological evaluation of the urinary tract is most often carried out by examining the sediment of voided or catheterised specimens of urine.

2.   BLADDER IRRIGATION (WASHINGS) Washings of the urinary bladder obtained at cystoscopy are preferred in symptomatic patients when bladder tumours are suspected. .

3.   RETROGRADE CATHETERISATION   In some instances, retrograde catheterisation and brushing of the ureter and renal pelvis are utilised for localisation of lesions.

4.   PROSTATIC MASSAGE   Prostatic secretions are obtained by prosta-tic massage and the sample is collected directly onto a glass slide and smeared.

BODY FLUIDS

Body fluids may be divided into 2 types:

A.   EFFUSIONS

Effusion refers to the accumulation of fluid in any of the three body cavities (pleural, pericardial and peritoneal). An effusion in the peritoneal cavity is also known as ascites. Effusions have traditionally been classed as transudates or exudates. This distinction is important in diagnostic cytology as malignant effusions are invariably exudates with a protein content greater than 3 gm/dl.

Diagnostic cytology of effusions on samples obtained by paracentesis is mainly related to the identification of malignancy, and wherever possible, its classification. In benign effusions, cytological findings are mostly non-specific.

CELLULAR COMPONENTS IN EFFUSIONS

Two main primary component cells of effusions are mesothelial cells and macrophages or histiocytes. Effusion causes disruption of the mesothelial lining and these cells collect in the fluid individually or as small groups. Macrophages appear as mononuclear cells of the size of mesothelial cells distributed singly or as loose clusters. However, macrophages have ill-defined cell border compared to mesothelial and may have cytoplasmic vacuoles. Moreover, the nuclei in the macrophages are eccentric and kidney-shaped while those of mesothelial cells are central and round.

In addition, the effusion may have the following cellular components:

CELLS IN BENIGN EFFUSIONS These include reactive proliferations of mesothelial cells in inflammation, polymorphonuclear neutrophils in acute suppurative inflammation, and lymphocytes in chronic fluid collections.

CELLS IN MALIGNANT EFFUSIONS Malignant cells in effusion may of origin from primary tumour (e.g. mesothelioma) or from secondary/ metastatic tumour; the latter being more common.

1. **Mesothelioma** It is an uncommon tumour and the cell yield is more often epithelial type since fibrous mesothelioma does not exfoliate cells in the effusion.

2. **Adenocarcinomas** These are the most common malignant cellular component in the effusions. They mostly represent metastasis from primary adenocarcinomas such as from the stomach, lung, breast, colon, and ovary.

3. **Squamous cell carcinoma** Effusion may rarely have malignant squamous cells in it and represent metastasis from carcinoma lung, oesophagus or uterine cervix.

4. **Small cell carcinoma** Cytologic features of small cell carcinoma of the lung are quite characteristic—hyperchromatic moulded nuclei and scanty or no cytoplasm.

5. **Lymphomas-leukaemias** Effusions may sometimes have malignant cells of leukaemia and lymphoma in line with primary disease in the body.

B. BODY FLUIDS OF SMALL VOLUME

Of the miscellaneous fluids included in this category, the most common samples submitted for cytological evaluation are cerebrospinal fluid (CSF) and seminal fluid (semen).

CEREBROSPINAL FLUID (CSF)

CSF examination is an important part of complete neurologic evaluation, both in non-neoplastic and neoplastic diseases of the central nervous system. Samples are usually obtained by lumbar puncture. Factors that are critical to the successful cytological evaluation of CSF are as under:

i) Speed of delivery to the laboratory and immediate processing, as diagnostic material may disintegrate within an hour resulting in false-negative diagnosis.

ii) Correct cytological processing and technique, since the cell yield of CSF is generally low and faulty technique may result in loss of cellular material or poor morphology.

SEMINAL FLUID (SEMEN)

Examination of seminal fluid (semen analysis) is one of the tests for investigating infertile couples, and is also used to check the adequacy of vasectomy. Samples are obtained by masturbation or coitus interruptus after observing at least 4 days of sexual abstinence and assessed on the following lines:

1. **Volume** Normal volume is between 2.5 and 5 ml.

2. **Viscosity and pH** When ejaculated, semen is fairly viscid but liquefies in about 10 to 30 minutes. It is usually alkaline (pH about 8).

3. **Motility** Normally, within 2 hours of ejaculation, at least 60% of the spermatozoa are vigorously motile; in 6 to 8 hours 25 to 40% are still motile.

4. **Count** Counting is done in a Neubauer chamber after suitable dilution. Normally, 60 million or more spermatozoa are present per ml.

5. **Morphology** Stained smears are used to assess morphology. Normally, not more than 20% of spermatozoa are morphologically abnormal (e.g. double-head, pointed-head, or swollen).

6. Fructose   Seminal fructose estimation (normal levels 150-600 mg/dl) complements cytological analysis. Low levels of seminal fructose indicate obstruction at the level of ejaculatory ducts.

BUCCAL SMEARS FOR SEX CHROMATIN BODIES

Sex-specific chromatin bodies are observed in interphase nuclei and comprise the Barr body (X chromatin) and the fluorescent or F body (Y chromatin).

DEMONSTRATION OF BARR BODY (X CHROMATIN)   In buccal smears, the Barr body appears as a plano-convex mass about 1 µm in diameter applied to the inner surface of the nuclear membrane.

DEMONSTRATION OF F BODY (Y CHROMATIN)   Demonstration of the F body requires fluorescent staining in contrast to the Barr body which may be observed on routine Papanicolaou-stained smears.

COUNTING OF DRUMSTICK APPENDAGE   The presence and frequency of drumstick appendages attached to nuclei of polymorphonuclear leucocytes on a peripheral blood film may also be used for determining sex.

TECHNIQUES IN EXFOLIATIVE CYTOLOGY (p. 897)

A.   COLLECTION OF SAMPLES

1.   PREPARATION OF PAP SMEARS   The procedure is as under:

i)   Smears are obtained under *direct vision* after introducing a Cusco's speculum with the patient in lithotomy position.

ii)   Ideally, *lubricants* and medical jellies should not be used for introducing the speculum. If required, the speculum may be moistened with a few drops of normal saline.

iii)   The posterior fornix of the vagina is aspirated with a *blunt-ended glass pipette* fitted with a rubber bulb.

iv)   The ectocervix is sampled with the *Ayre's spatula*.

v)   Thin uniform smears should be prepared and the slide immediately *immersed in fixative* to avoid artefacts in cells caused by drying.

vi)   Smears should be *transported* to the laboratory in the fixative in a Coplin's jar.

2.   LIQUID-BASED CYTOLOGY (LBC) PREPARATIONS   LBC is a special technique for preparation of gynaecologic and non-gynaecologic samples which provides uniform monolayered dispersion of cells on smears, without overlapping or clump formation and does not contain background material or debris. It is a pre-requisite for quantitative analysis and automated devices. Two types of LBC systems are commercially available—ThinPrep and SurePath, each with its own advantages.

3.   PREPARATION OF LATERAL VAGINAL SMEARS (LVS)   The LVS is obtained by scraping the lateral walls of the upper third of the vagina (at the level of the cervical external os) with the flat surface of a wooden tongue depressor and smearing the material directly onto labelled slides.

4.   COLLECTION OF SPUTUM   Fresh, unfixed, early morning specimens resulting from overnight accumulation of secretions are best for diagnostic purposes. A minimum of at least three specimens collected on three successive days should be examined.

5.   BRONCHIAL MATERIALS   All aspirated bronchial secretions, lavage (BAL), washings (BW) and brushings (BB) must be dispatched to the laboratory without delay.

6.   BUCCAL SMEARS   The mouth is rinsed with water or normal saline and the buccal mucosa scraped vigorously with a wooden or metal tongue depressor.

7.   G.I. CYTOLOGY   In a case of suspected malignancy or specific infections of GI tract, or for screening for Barrett's oesophagus, cytologic examination is indicated. The cytology specimen is collected during fibreoptic endoscopy of the part being visualised.

8.   URINE   Fresh catheterised specimens are preferred in female patients while voided urine is satisfactory in males. The initial morning specimen is discarded as cells deteriorate extremely quickly in acidic urine, and the morphology of cells accumulating overnight in bladder urine is distorted to an extreme degree.

9.   EFFUSIONS   Pericardial, pleural and peritoneal fluids are obtained by paracentesis. As these fluids are often exudative in character, they may clot after removal from respective cavities. Anticoagulants may be used to prevent coagulation.

10.   CEREBROSPINAL FLUID (CSF)   CSF samples should be dispatched without delay to the laboratory for immediate processing as the cells contained are extremely fragile.

11. SEMEN   Samples of seminal fluid obtained by masturbation are best collected at the laboratory.

B.   FIXATION AND FIXATIVES

All material for cytological examination must be properly fixed to ensure preservation of cytomorphological details. Methods of fixation vary depending upon the type of staining employed:

◈   Material for exfoliative cytodiagnosis is usually *wet-fixed* i.e. smears are immersed in fixative without allowing them to dry. These smears are then stained with Papanicolaou (Pap) or haematoxylin and eosin (H & E) stains.

◈   Sometimes, exfoliative cytology smears are *air-dried* for use with the Romanowsky stains as are used in haematologic studies. In Romanowsky staining, fixation is effected during the staining procedure.

1.   ROUTINE FIXATIVES   The ideal fixative for routine use is Papanicolaou's fixative comprising a solution of equal parts of ether and 95% ethanol. Most laboratories use 95% ethanol alone with excellent results. Where ethanol is not available, 100% methanol, 95% denatured alcohol, or 85% isopropyl alcohol (isopropanolol) may be used. Smears prepared at the bedside as well as those prepared in the laboratory from fluid samples are immediately placed in 95% ethanol *without allowing them to dry prior to fixation.*

2.   COATING FIXATIVES   Coating fixatives are applied as aerosol-sprays or with a dropper to the surface of freshly prepared smears.

3.   SPECIAL PURPOSE FIXATIVES   Buffered neutral formalin, Bouin's fluid and picric acid are used for specific purposes when required.

4.   PRESERVATION OF FLUID SAMPLES   Samples of fluids are best submitted to the laboratory in a fresh state for immediate processing. The best *preservative for general use* is 50% ethanol in volumes equal to that of the fluid sample.

C.   PROCESSING OF SAMPLES IN THE LABORATORY

1.   **PREPARED SMEARS**   Smears prepared at the bedside and wet-fixed in ethanol need no further processing in the laboratory prior to staining.

2.   **SPUTUM**   The procedure is as follows:

i)   The sample is placed in a petridish and inspected against a dark background.

ii)   Bloody, discoloured or solid particles are removed with wooden applicator sticks and placed on glass slides. Strands of ropy mucus are also selected (exfoliated cells adhere to mucus strands).

iii)   Clean glass slides are used to crush the particles/mucus and spread the material evenly.

iv)   Four such smears are prepared and immediately placed in 95% ethanol for fixation.

3.   **FLUID SPECIMENS**   Large volumes of fluid received are allowed to stand in the refrigerator for half to one hour. After that, all except the bottom 200 ml is discarded. The retained fluid is then processed. Commonly employed techniques for processing of fluids are as under:

Appendices

Sediment smears The sample is poured into 50 ml centrifuge tubes and centrifuged at 600 g for 10 minutes. Following centrifugation, the supernatant is decanted and smears prepared from the sediment or cell button by recovering the material with a glass pipette or a platinum wire loop. Smear preparation from samples collected in a preservative require albuminised slides as cell adhesiveness is reduced by prefixation. Smears are wet-fixed in 95% ethanol (or air-dried in some instances).

Cytocentrifuge and membrane filter preparations These methods are most useful for small volume fluids of low cell content. The interested reader is referred to specialised texts for descriptions of these methods.

D.   STAINING OF SMEARS

Three staining procedures are commonly employed: Papanicolaou and H&E stains are used for *wet-fixed smears* while Romanowsky stains are used for *air-dried smears.*

1.   PAPANICOLAOU STAIN Papanicolaou staining is the best method for routine cytodiagnostic studies. Three solutions are used comprising a nuclear stain (Harris' haematoxylin) and two cytoplasmic counter-stains (Orange G or OG-6, and eosin-azure or EA-65 or EA-50). Nuclear stain gives basophilic colour to the nucleus while the two cytoplasmic stains impart the orange and cyanophilic tints to cytoplasm respectively.

2.   H & E STAIN The stain is essentially the same that is used for histological sections. Harris' haematoxylin is the nuclear stain, and eosin is the cytoplasmic counterstain.

3.   ROMANOWSKY STAINS Romanowsky stains used in haematological preparations may also be used for cytological smear preparations. Leishman's, May-Grünwald-Giemsa (MGG) and Wright's stains are most commonly used.

INTERVENTIONAL CYTOLOGY *(p. 899)*

In interventional cytology, samples are obtained by aspiration or surgical biopsy. This branch includes fine needle aspiration cytology, imprint cytology, crush smear cytology and biopsy sediment cytology.

I.   FINE NEEDLE ASPIRATION CYTOLOGY *(p. 899)*

Interventional cytology is virtually synonymous with Fine Needle Aspiration Cytology (FNAC). The technique has gained wide acceptance in the last four decades and is increasingly being used to sample a wide variety of body tissues.

A.   APPLICATIONS OF FNAC

In routine practice, FNAC is most often used for diagnosis of palpable mass lesions. Palpable lesions commonly sampled are: breast masses, enlarged lymph nodes, enlarged thyroid and superficial soft tissue masses. The salivary glands, palpable abdominal lesions and the testicles are also frequently sampled for FNAC. Other sites and lesions accessible to FNAC are the prostate, pelvic organs, bone and joint spaces, lungs, retroperitoneum and orbit.

B.   ADVANTAGES OF FNAC

i)   FNAC is an OPD procedure and requires *no hospitalisation.*
ii)   *No anaesthesia* is required.
iii) The procedure is *quick, safe and least painful.*
iv)   *Multiple attempts* are possible.
v)   Results are obtained *rapidly.*
vi)   It is a *cost-effective* procedure.
vii) *First-hand knowledge* of the clinical findings.

MATERIALS

For performing FNAC, a syringe with a well-fitting needle, syringe holder, some microscopic glass slides and a suitable fixative are the only material required in most instances:

NEEDLES Fine needles range from 25 to 20 gauge (0.6 mm to 0.9 mm outer diameter). The standard 21 gauge disposable needle of 38 mm length is suitable for routine transcutaneous FNAC of palpable masses.

SYRINGES Syringes of 10 to 20 ml capacity are suitable. Syringe holders such as the Franzen handle permit a single-hand grip during aspiration, employing disposable syringes.

GLASS SLIDES AND FIXATIVE Four or six standard microscopic glass slides and a Coplin jar containing 95% ethyl alcohol (as a fixative) are the only other material required for routine FNAC.

METHOD OF ASPIRATION

Transcutaneous FNAC of palpable masses is routinely performed without anaesthesia:

i)   The patient is asked to *lie down* in a position that best exposes the target area.

ii) The target area is thoroughly *palpated* and the firmest portion of the lesion or mass delineated.

iii) The skin is *cleaned* with an alcohol pad.

iv) The mass is *fixed* by the palpating hand of the operator or by an assistant.

v)   The needle is *inserted* into the target area. On reaching the lesion, the plunger of the syringe is retracted and at least 10 ml of suction applied while moving the needle back and forth within the lesion; the direction or angle of the needle may be changed to access different areas of the lesion.

vi) Aspiration is *terminated* when aspirated material or blood becomes visible at the base or hub of the needle.

vii) On completion of aspiration, suction is *released* and pressure within the syringe allowed to equalise before withdrawing the needle.

viii) *Pressure* is applied to the site of puncture by the assistant or patient himself for 2 to 3 minutes in order to arrest bleeding.

ix) Aspirated material is *recovered* by detaching the needle from the syringe and filling the syringe with air; the syringe and needle are then reconnected and the aspirate expressed onto one end of a glass slide.

PREPARATION OF SMEARS

Preparation of smears is crucial to the success of FNAC. Poorly-prepared smears with distorted cellular morphology will frustrate the best efforts of the most competent cytopathologist, and often result in errors of interpretation or in failure to arrive at any specific diagnosis.

i)   Aspirates deposited on the slide are *inspected* with the naked eye.

ii) Semisolid particulate aspirates are *crush-smeared* by flat pressure with a glass slide or a thick coverslip.

iii) Prepared smears are either *wet-fixed* or *air-dried*. Half the number of smears are immediately immersed in 95% ethanol, transported to the laboratory in the fixative (wet-fixed), and used for Papanicolaou or H&E staining. The remaining smears are air-dried, wrapped in tissue paper for transport to the laboratory, and stained by Romanowsky stains (e.g. Leishman's, May-Grünwald-Giemsa).

SPECIAL AND ANCILLARY STUDIES

1.   SPECIAL STAINS Wet-fixed smears are used for a variety of special stains such as Alcian blue, mucicarmine and PAS (for mucin and carbohydrates); methyl violet or congo red (for amyloid); and bacterial and fungal stains (for microbial agents).

2. MICROBIOLOGICAL STUDIES Aspirates may also be submitted for viral, fungal, mycobacterial and bacterial culture.

3. CELL BLOCK Aspirated material may be processed as surgical pathology material by preparing paraffin blocks from cell button of the centrifuged deposit.

4. IMMUNOCYTOCHEMICAL STUDIES The smears or cell block sections can be further evaluated by immunocytochemical stains by employing panel of antibodies.

5. IMAGE ANALYSIS AND MORPHOMETRY These techniques when applied to cytological smears bring quantitation and objectivity to cytodiagnosis.

6. FLOW CYTOMETRY Determination of ploidy status and S phase fraction of tumour cells using flow cytometry enhances the diagnostic and prognostic information available on routine cytology.

7. ULTRASTRUCTURAL STUDIES Aspirates obtained by FNAC are also suitable for electron microscopy (both TEM and SEM).

8. MOLECULAR BIOLOGIC TECHNIQUES These techniques are now being widely applied to cytopathology also. Detection of oncogenes like *ERBB-2* in breast cancer, *BCL-2* in lymphomas, DNA sequence analysis, gene expression profiling and fluorescence *in situ* hybridisation (FISH) can all be used for aspiration samples.

RADIOLOGICAL IMAGING AIDS FOR FNAC

Non-palpable lesions require some form of localisation by radiological aids for FNAC to be carried out. *Plain X-ray films* are usually adequate for lesions within bones and for some lesions within the chest. FNAC of the chest may also be attempted under *image amplified fluoroscopy* which allows visualisation of needle placement on the television monitor. *Computerised tomographic-(CT) guidance* is also used for lesions within the chest and abdomen. The most versatile radiological aid is *ultrasonographic (US)-guidance* which allows direct visualisation of needle placement in real time and is free from radiation hazards. It is an extremely valuable aid for FNAC of thyroid nodules, soft tissue masses, intra-abdominal lesions and for intrathoracic lesions which abut the chest wall.

D. COMPLICATIONS AND HAZARDS OF FNAC

1. Haematomas
2. Infection
3. Pneumothorax
4. Dissemination of tumour

E. PRECAUTIONS AND CONTRAINDICATIONS OF FNAC

While FNAC is generally a safe procedure, precautions have to be taken when aspiration is contemplated of some sites under certain circumstances:

1. **Bleeding disorders** Thrombocytopenia *per se* is not a contraindication to FNAC. In patients with coagulopathies such as haemophilia, aspiration of joint spaces, chest and abdominal viscera is contraindicated.

2. **Liver** Estimation of prothrombin time is an essential pre-requisite for aspiration of the liver.

3. **Lung** FNAC of the lung should not be undertaken in elderly patients with emphysema or pulmonary hypertension.

4. **Pancreas** FNAC is contraindicated in acute pancreatitis.

5. **Prostate** Transrectal aspiration in acute prostatitis may cause bacteraemia/septicaemia.

6. **Testis** Aspiration is extremely painful in acute epididymo-orchitis and should be deferred till such time the acute inflammatory process subsides.

7. **Adrenal** FNAC of a suspected pheochromocytoma is inadvisable as it may sometimes provoke extreme fluctuations in blood pressure.

F. CYTOLOGIC DIAGNOSIS

The cytopathologist can render a preliminary diagnosis within one hour after the FNAC procedure when urgently required. Basic cytologic features in FNAC are similar to those in histopathology but smear cytology depends upon the technique for smear and stains employed. Emphasis in FNA cytology is on pattern recognition or arrangement of cells, nuclear and cytoplasmic features of individual cells or groups of cells, and comment on the background morphology.

G. LIMITATIONS OF FNAC

The main limitation of FNAC lies in the fact that only a small population of cells is sampled by the procedure. The reliability of the test, thus, depends upon the adequacy of the sample and its representative character. An inadequate sample which is not representative of the true lesion results in a 'false-negative' diagnosis. If the FNAC report is 'negative' despite a strong clinical suspicion of malignancy, the patient should be investigated further. FNAC may be repeated or a surgical biopsy performed to obtain a tissue diagnosis in such instances.

II. IMPRINT CYTOLOGY (p. 905)

In imprint cytology, touch preparations from cut surfaces of fresh unfixed surgically excised mass lesions are examined. Imprints may also be obtained from draining sinuses or ulcerated areas. For surgically resected specimens (e.g. lymph nodes), smears are prepared by bisecting or slicing the specimen and lightly touching or pressing a glass slide onto the freshly exposed surface without smearing it. Smears cannot be prepared from fixed specimens. Imprint smears are wet-fixed or air-dried and stained as per routine.

III. CRUSH SMEAR CYTOLOGY (p. 905)

Crush smear preparations of tissue particles obtained by craniotomy have been used in the diagnosis of brain tumours. These smears are preferred by many workers as they allow recognition of tissue architecture to some degree, in addition to better cytological details.

IV. BIOPSY SEDIMENT CYTOLOGY (p. 905)

Biopsy sediment cytology entails the examination of sediment obtained by centrifugation of fixatives/fluids in which surgical biopsy specimens are dispatched to the laboratory. The method may be useful in the rapid diagnosis of bone tumours as histological sections are usually obtained after many days on account of the delay necessitated by decalcification.

SELF ASSESSMENT

1. For cytomorphological recognition of cancer, the following characteristics are used to determine the presence or absence of cancer <u>except</u>:
   A. Cytoplasmic content
   B. Nulcear size
   C. N:C ratio
   D. Mitoses
2. The following statements are true for Bethesda system <u>except</u>:
   A. It is employed for cytologic reporting of Pap smears
   B. It divides dysplasias into three grades: mild, moderate and severe
   C. All forms of dysplasias are graded into two grades: L-SIL and H-SIL
   D. Bethesda system is current modification of reporting over conventional system
3. The number of Barr bodies observed in interphase nuclei is:
   A. Equal to the number of X chromosomes
   B. One less than the number of X chromosomes

C. Equal to the number of Y chromosomes

D. One less than the number of Y chromosomes

4. **Drum-stick appendages seen in neutrophils in stained blood film in females are:**

A. > 20%   B. 10-20 %

C. 3-6%   D. < 0.3%

5. **CSF cytology is not useful for the diagnosis of:**

A. Leukaemia   B. Medulloblastoma

C. Ependymoma   D. Meningioma

6. **For pleural effusion, if a delay of more than 12 hours is anticipated for processing, it should be fixed in:**

A. 95% ethanol

B. Equal volume of 10% formalin

C. Bouin's fluid

D. Picric acid

7. **Haematoxylin and eosin staining is employed as cytologic stain for:**

A. Wet-fixed smears

B. Air-dried smears

C. All FNAC smears only

D. All cases of crush smear only

8. **The following features characterise wet-fixed smears over air-dried smears except:**

A. Pap and H & E stain are applied for the former

B. The nuclear details are better seen

C. Cytoplasmic details are better seen

D. Cell size is comparable to tissue section

9. **Liquid based cytology:**

A. provides uniform monolayered cell dispersion

B. is useful only for gynaecological samples

C. is useful only for non-gynaecological samples

D. causes cellular clumping

10. **Imprint cytology is most useful in the lesions of following organ:**

A. Bones   B. Breast

C. Lymph nodes   D. Brain tumours

11. **Navicular cells are:**

A. Superficial squamous cells   B. Intermediate squamous cells

C. Parabasal cells   D. Basal cells

12. **Maturation index denotes:**

A. Relative proportion of cells containing acidophilic cytoplasm

B. Relative proportion of cells containing basophilic cytoplasm

C. Percentage of cells having small shrunken nuclei

D. Relative proportion of various cell types in a smear

13. **Which of the following is automated cytological technique?**

A. Membrane filtration   B. PapNet

C. Cell block technique   D. Cytospin

14. **F body is:**

A. X chromatin   B. Y chromatin

C. Chromosome 1   D. Chromosome 21

15. **Abdominal fat aspiration is done for the diagnosis of:**

A. Obesity   B. Amyloidosis

C. Metastatic cancer   D. Multiple myeloma

KEY

1 = A	2 = B	3 = B	4 = C	5 = D
6 = B	7 = A	8 = C	9 = A	10 = C
11 = B	12 = D	13 = B	14 = B	15 = B

Clinical Cases

PREAMBLE

With introduction of clinical cases as a method of learning pathology in this edition, a newer dimension has been added to enliven the field of "basic pathology" by directing the learner towards "applied pathology" as applied to clinical problems. These clinical cases (case 1 to 30) given at the end of most chapters are structured clinical exercises to stimulate the students of pathology to apply their knowledge and skills gained from the study of particular disease/s covered in that chapter in pathology to clinical settings as encountered in real life.

 CLINICAL CASE 1 (Chapter 3, Page 77)

A 46 years old male is admitted to medical ward with history of shortness of breath, loss of weight and appetite, and low-grade fever, all for the last one month. He has been smoking *bidis* for 25 years, and gives history of having productive cough with foul smelling expectoration for 15 years, interspersed with haemoptysis off and on. During these years, he had two episodes of bronchopneumonia.

On examination, he is poorly built and poorly nourished. His pulse rate is 90 per minute, respiratory rate 45 per minute, and blood pressure 130/90 mmHg. He has pallor ++, icterus +, pedal oedema +, and grade II clubbing of fingers. On auscultation of chest, rhonchi and crepts are heard.

PROBABLE DIAGNOSIS Bronchiectasis with nephrotic syndrome, possibly due to secondary systemic amyloidosis

Case Discussion and Investigations on page 906

 CLINICAL CASE 2 (Chapter 4, Page 115)

A 35 years old female admitted with pain lower abdomen following abortion by village midwife 3 days back. She has been having high-grade fever and bleeding from gums for 2 days. Now, she has been unconsciousness for the last 3 hours.

On examination, she is moderately built and nourished and unconscious. Her blood pressure and pulse are not recordable; while respiration rate is 40/min. She has pallor +++, oral bleeding + but no jaundice, cyanosis or lymphadenopathy. Auscultation of chest showed bilateral crepts and wheezing.

PROBABLE DIAGNOSIS Septic shock and disseminated intravascular coagulation (DIC)

Case Discussion and Investigations on page 906.

 CLINICAL CASE 3 (Chapter 5, Page 164)

A 35 years old male truck driver reports to hospital emergency with high-grade fever, headache and productive cough and rapid breathing. He gives history of progressive fatigue and weight loss of about 20 kg during the last 6 months.

On examination, he has generalised lymphadenopathy and mild hepatosplenomegaly. The skin shows many warts on neck, hands and genitals. On auscultation, lung fields are clear and CVS examination is normal. CNS examination shows stiffness of neck, positive Kernig's sign. Fundus examination shows papilloedema.

PROBABLE DIAGNOSIS HIV infection with opportunistic infections, disseminated tuberculosis, with possibly tuberculous meningitis (TBM)

Case Discussion and Investigations on page 907.

 CLINICAL CASE 4 (Chapter 10, Page 303)

A 25 years old female daily wager presented with progressive pallor, malaise and dyspnoea for 4 weeks. She gives history of two abortions in the last 6 months and heavy and irregular menstrual bleeding for the same duration.

On examination, she has no significant lymphadenopathy or organomegaly.

PROBABLE DIAGNOSIS Nutritional anaemia due to blood loss, likely iron deficiency anaemia

Case Discussion and Investigations on page 907.

 CLINICAL CASE 5 (Chapter 10, Page 304)

A 3 years old female child is brought by the mother to the paediatrician with persisting pallor, stunted growth and protuberant abdomen. The mother herself is also mildly anaemic which, according to her, has remained like this ever since she remembers and it did not improve with any medication.

The facial appearance of the child shows prominence of forehead and cheeks and slightly protruding upper teeth. On examination, the child has pallor ++ but no apparent jaundice or cyanosis. On palpation of the abdomen, the spleen is enlarged by two fingers below the costal margin and the liver is just palpable. There is no lymphadenopathy. CVS and respiratory system are unremarkable.

PROBABLE DIAGNOSIS Congenital haemolytic anaemia, likely β-thalassaemia major

Case Discussion and Investigations on page 907.

 CLINICAL CASE 6 (Chapter 11, Page 320)

A 30 years old female reports to physician with complaints of appearance of petechial haemorrhages on the skin of her legs and arms for the last 2 days. She further gives history of four episodes of epistaxis in the last 6 months. She has also been having heavy periods for the last 6-7 cycles.

On examination, the petechiae are purpuric and blanch on pressing. No jaundice is seen. On abdominal examination, the spleen is just palpable but the liver is not enlarged. There is no lymphadenopathy.

PROBABLE DIAGNOSIS Chronic immune thrombocytopenic purpura (ITP)

Case Discussion and Investigations on page 908.

 CLINICAL CASE 7 (Chapter 12, Page 369)

A 4 years old male child is brought by the mother to the paediatrician with low-grade fever, headache and bleeding from nose.

On examination, the child is found to have mild hepatosplenomegaly but no lymphadenopathy. A routine complete blood count (CBC) reveals haemoglobin 6 g/dl, white blood cell count 80,000/μl and platelet count 40,000/μl.

Case Discussion and Investigations on page 908.

 CLINICAL CASE 8 (Chapter 12, Page 369)

A 70 years old man complains of pain lower back, fatigue and increasing pallor for one month.

On examination, he has tenderness over the lower vertebral region. An X-ray shows multiple lytic lesions in the pelvis and sacrum.

PROBABLE DIAGNOSIS Multiple myeloma

Case Discussion and Investigations on page 908.

 CLINICAL CASE 9 (Chapter 13, Page 396)

A 50 years old male bank officer feels sudden onset of severe constricting chest pain while attending a meeting in his office. He gives history of intermittent pain over the sternum earlier too almost once a week which would go away when he sits down. He has mild hypertension, for which he is on dietary therapy. He also gives family history of diabetes. His cholesterol level is elevated. He is not a smoker.

PROBABLE DIAGNOSIS Coronary artery disease (acute myocardial infarction)

Case Discussion and Investigations on page 908.

 CLINICAL CASE 10 (Chapter 14, Page 441)

An 18 years old male reports to medical outpatient department with complaints of palpitation and joint pains for one year. The palpitation does not show any improvement on rest. Joint pain is fleeting type involving multiple major joints, associated with redness and swelling. Lately, for one month he has been having low-grade fever, sometimes with chills, and dyspnoea on out-door activity. There is no history of IV drug abuse.

On examination, his blood pressure is 100/70 mmHg, pulse rate 88/min, respiration rate 16/min. Pedal oedema: +, no pallor, jaundice, cyanosis, lymphadenopathy, or clubbing of fingers. On CVS examination, pansystolic murmur is heard.

PROBABLE DIAGNOSIS Rheumatic heart disease and mitral stenosis with superimposed infective endocarditis

Case Discussion and Investigations on page 909.

 CLINICAL CASE 11 (Chapter 15, Page 487)

A 75 years old man living on his own brought by the neighbour to the emergency department of the hospital with fever, fatigue, malaise, and a productive cough for the last 15 days. He also gives history of chills and rigors.

On examination, he has crepts and rhonchi in both lungs.

PROBABLE DIAGNOSIS Lobar pneumonia

Case Discussion and Investigations on page 909.

 CLINICAL CASE 12 (Chapter 15, Page 487)

A 54 years old male complains of persistent productive cough for 2 years. Lately, for the last 2 months there is intermittent blood in the sputum. There is history of progressive loss of weight and appetite for 1 month and

occasional chest pain. He has been a chronic smoker, smoking about 20 cigarettes/day for the last 30 years and is an occasional alcoholic.

On examination, Pallor: ++, Icterus: -ve, clubbing of fingers-grade II. On inspection of chest, left half of chest is not moving equally with respiration. On auscultation, breath sounds absent on left side.

PROBABLE DIAGNOSIS Bronchogenic carcinoma

Case Discussion and Investigations on page 909.

 CLINICAL CASE 13 (Chapter 16, Page 503)

A 20 years old medical student presents to ENT outpatient with complaints of nasal obstruction and partial loss of smell for 2 weeks. There is a history of perennial sneezing, increased nasal discharge and frequent nagging headache for the last 2 years for which he has been taking intermittent antibiotics, painkillers and anti-allergic whenever the symptoms get worse.

On local examination, the septum of nose is normal but there is soft polypoid mass, 1.5 cm in diameter, projecting from ostium of maxillary sinus into the nasal cavity.

PROBABLE DIAGNOSIS Antrochoanal polyp, allergic type

Case Discussion and Investigations on page 910.

 CLINICAL CASE 14 (Chapter 17, Page 520)

A 50 years old roadside tailor reports to surgeon with right lateral cervical lymphadenopathy and progressive pallor for 2 months. He has a non-healing ulcer with intermittent bleeding in the vestibule on right side for the last 2 years. He further gives history of chewing and keeping a bolus of tobacco throughout the day when he is awake on the same side of cheek ever since early adulthood.

On examination, there is induration around the ulcer in the vestibule. Multiple matted lymph nodes are palpable on lateral cervical region.

PROBABLE DIAGNOSIS Carcinoma oral cavity

Case Discussion and Investigations on page 910.

 CLINICAL CASE 15 (Chapter 18, Page 576)

A 35 years old male executive in a multinational company complains of dull pain in the midepigastric region for the last one month. The pain gets worse at night and is somewhat better immediately after he eats his meals. There is no history of any fever, nausea, or vomiting. He has been frequently taking analgesic (about 1-2 tablets per week) for headache but there is no history of intake of any other medications.

He underwent upper GI endoscopy once earlier but no records are available with him.

PROBABLE DIAGNOSIS Chronic peptic ulcer, gastric

Case Discussion and Investigations on page 910.

 CLINICAL CASE 16 (Chapter 18, Page 576)

A 25 years old man returns home after playing cricket, and starts complaining of pain in the mid-abdomen without history of any injury. The pain remains unremitting for the next few hours; instead it becomes more severe and gets localised to the lower right quadrant. He also develops nausea and vomiting but no diarrhoea. Over the next 24 hours, he remains sick and keeps rolling in bed with severe pain and is brought to the hospital emergency.

On examination, his body temperature is 102°F and appears ill. His abdomen is mildly distended and diffusely tender on palpation, especially in the right lower quadrant.

PROBABLE DIAGNOSIS   Acute appendicitis

Case Discussion and Investigations on page 910.

 CLINICAL CASE 17 (Chapter 19, Page 634)

A 65 years old male complains of progressive abdominal distension, H/O loss of weight and appetite, progressive weakness and malaise, all for the last 6 months. He also had two episodes of haematemesis during this period. He gives history of having undergone coronary bypass surgery 15 years back when he received multiple blood transfusions. He denies use of alcohol since then, although prior to his surgery he used to occasionally drink. He also gives history of smoking about 20 cigarettes/day for about 20 years prior to bypass surgery but is now a non-smoker.

On examination, he has pallor, mild pedal oedema and jaundice. Abdomen is distended, the liver is palpable 4 cm below costal margin, tender and has a nodular feel. Spleen is palpable up to mid-umbilicus.

PROBABLE DIAGNOSIS   Post-necrotic cirrhosis with portal hypertension and superimposed hepatocellular carcinoma

Case Discussion and Investigations on page 910.

 CLINICAL CASE 18 (Chapter 19, Page 634)

A 48 years old obese woman complains of severe ache in the right upper quadrant of the abdomen with radiation to interscapular area and yellowish discoloration of sclera for 2 days. She has also been having nausea and vomiting. She gives history of intermittent dull pain in the upper abdomen and bloating for the last 6 months, lasting for 1-2 days and gets relieved after taking some home remedies but she did not consult any physician for this. She has also been having intermittent malabsorption and flatulence, especially after meal for the last 6 months.

On examination, she has pallor +, icterus++, pedal edema+, pulse 90/min, blood pressure 130/90 mmHg. On deep palpation of the abdomen, there is pain in right hypochondrium. However, there is no fever, or any hepatosplenomegaly.

PROBABLE DIAGNOSIS   Chronic cholecysitis with cholelithiasis and cholestatic jaundice

Case Discussion and Investigations on page 911.

 CLINICAL CASE 19 (Chapter 19, Page 635)

A 65 years old male patient is brought to the hospital emergency with deep jaundice, moderate fever and pain in right hyochondrium for the last 2 weeks. He is also passing high coloured urine and clay coloured stools for the same duration. He also complains of intense itching, especially after taking bath. On further inquiry, he is found to have lost 10 kg weight during the last 2 months. He also gives history of smoking about 20 cigarettes/day for 40 years. There is history of alcohol intake on social occasions, 2-3 pegs about once a week, for the last 40 years.

On physical examination, there is a hard nodular mass in the midepigastrium. The liver is just palpable below costal margin, tender with smooth lower border.

PROBABLE DIAGNOSIS   Carcinoma head of pancreas with obstructive jaundice

Case Discussion and Investigations on page 911.

CLINICAL CASE 20 (Chapter 20, Page 690)

A 5 years old male child is brought by the mother to Paediatric Outpatient with chief complaints of puffiness of face, particularly more marked in the morning, and pitting oedema on both legs for about one month. The child is passing smoky urine but no oliguria. There is history of appearance of multiple boils repeatedly on the skin of both legs which remained neglected and partly healed.

On examination, the blood pressure is 150/110 mmHg, pulse rate 90/min, respiration rate 22/min. pallor+, pedal oedema+. There is no cyanosis, lymphadenopathy or icterus. Systemic examination did not show any abnormality in respiratory system, abdomen, CVS and CNS.

PROBABLE DIAGNOSIS Nephritic syndrome due to acute post-streptococcal glomerulonephritis

Case Discussion and Investigations on page 911.

CLINICAL CASE 21 (Chapter 20, Page 690)

A 50 years old man presents to General Surgery Outpatient with complaints of gross painless haematuria and pain in right flank. There is also history of loss of 10 kg weight in the last 6 months.

On physical examination, a right-sided flank mass is palpable on bimanual examination.

PROBABLE DIAGNOSIS Renal cell carcinoma, right kidney

Case Discussion and Investigations on page 912.

CLINICAL CASE 22 (Chapter 21, Page 709)

A 25 years old man complains of enlargement of right testis for about one month without history of antecedent trauma. In personal history, he is a non-smoker and non-alcoholic.

On local examination, there is a 5 cm firm, single, non-tender, testicular mass inside the right scrotum. The swelling is negative for transillumination. Regional lymph nodes are not palpable.

PROBABLE DIAGNOSIS Germ cell tumour, right testis

Case Discussion and Investigations on page 912.

CLINICAL CASE 23 (Chapter 22, Page 744)

A 50 years old woman gives history of progressive vaginal discharge with a foul odour for 6 months. There is also history of post-coital spotting. She had menopause 5 years back. She also has right back pain and swelling in right leg.

On per vaginum and speculum examination, the cervix is ulcerated and bleeds on touch.

PROBABLE DIAGNOSIS Carcinoma cervix

Case Discussion and Investigations on page 912.

CLINICAL CASE 24 (Chapter 23, Page 758)

A 65 years old woman reports to surgeon for soreness and oozing from the nipple of her left breast. There is no history of trauma to the breast.

On physical examination, there is fissuring and ulceration of the areola and nipple. Deep palpation of the breast shows a hard lump 5 cm in diameter, with irregular margins underneath the nipple. One lymph node 3 cm size is palpable in the apex of right axilla.

PROBABLE DIAGNOSIS Carcinoma breast with Paget's disease and axillary nodal metastasis

Case Discussion and Investigations on page 913.

 CLINICAL CASE 25 (Chapter 24, Page 781)

A 60 years old male complains of a tiny persisting ulcer on his forehead for 6 months. There is a history of presence of small waxy nodule initially for about one year which slowly increased in size followed by its ulceration.

On examination, there is a single nodule with central ulceration, 4 mm in diameter, having pearly white rolled up margins. There is no regional lymphadenopathy.

PROBABLE DIAGNOSIS Basal cell carcinoma skin

Case Discussion and Investigations on page 913.

 CLINICAL CASE 26 (Chapter 25, Page 820)

A 25 years old female presents with gradually progressive painless swelling in the midline of her neck for 6 months. She also complains of irregular and heavy periods, weight loss, intermittent headache, nervousness, palpitation, excessive sweating and tremors in both hands. Of late, her both eyes have also become prominent.

On physical examination, the thyroid gland is diffusely enlarged, non-tender and prominent but there is no nodularity. Her blood pressure is 140/90 mmHg and pulse rate is 100 per minute.

PROBABLE DIAGNOSIS Graves' disease (diffuse toxic goitre)

Case Discussion and Investigations on page 913.

 CLINICAL CASE 27 (Chapter 25, Page 820)

A 57 years old male, reports to his physician with complaints of intermittent fever for 3-4 months and pain in both legs and darkening of right great toe. He is a known case of diabetes for 7 years and hypertension for the last 10 years and has been on irregular treatment and intermittent follow up. He gives history of myocardial infarction 4 years back. He is not alcoholic or smoker.

On examination, the blood pressure is 130/94 mmHg, pulse rate 86 per minute. On auscultation, pericardial rub and bilateral crepts are heard.

PROBABLE DIAGNOSIS Systemic hypertension and uncontrolled and complicated diabetes mellitus type 2 (gangrene toe, pulmonary tuberculosis, pleurisy)

Case Discussion and Investigations on page 913.

CLINICAL CASE 28 (Chapter 26, Page 850)

A 12 years old boy is brought to orthopaedic surgeon with complaints of pain and progressive swelling around his right knee for one month which does not improve with rest. There is no history of any trauma.

Local examination shows diffuse hard swelling around upper part of right knee. An X-ray of the right knee shows an expanded and osteolytic mass in the right lower femur in the region of metaphysis.

PROBABLE DIAGNOSIS Osteosarcoma lower end of femur

Case Discussion and Investigations on page 914.

CLINICAL CASE 29 (Chapter 27, Page 862)

A 55 years old male complains of a progressively increasing swelling on right upper arm for the last 2 months. It has been growing rapidly and lately he has noticed that he has started having tightness of shirt on this side due to increase in size of swelling.

On examination, the swelling is 6 x 4 cm size, firm to hard subcutaneous mass which is fixed to underlying soft tissues. It is not attached to the underlying bone, and has well-defined margins. The overlying skin is shining and stretched but not ulcerated. Multiple right axillary lymph nodes are palpable.

PROBABLE DIAGNOSIS   Soft tissue sarcoma

Case Discussion and Investigations on page 914.

CLINICAL CASE 30 (Chapter 28, Page 887)

A 62 years old man notices sudden onset of weakness and numbness of right side of his body and inability to walk or stand upright on his own. Earlier in the day, he had experienced severe headache.

He gives history of hypertension for 12 years, diabetes mellitus for 10 years and has been a smoker for 30 years before he quit smoking 10 years back. He has been well with treatment for hypertension and diabetes mellitus except for occasional episodes of angina which were relieved by rest.

PROBABLE DIAGNOSIS   Stroke (cerebrovascular accident or CVA)

Case Discussion and Investigations on page 914.

Appendix III

Normal Values

WEIGHTS AND MEASUREMENTS OF NORMAL ORGANS (p. 915)

Table A-III.1	Weights and measurements of normal organs.
ORGAN	IN ADULTS
Adrenal gland	
Weight	4–5 gm
Brain	
Weight (in males)	1400 gm
Weight (in females)	1250 gm
Volume of cerebrospinal fluid	120–150 ml
Heart	
Weight (in males)	300–350 gm
Weight (in females)	250–300 gm
Thickness of right ventricular wall	0.3–0.5 cm
Thickness of left ventricular wall	1.3–1.5 cm
Circumference of mitral valve	10 cm
Circumference of aortic valve	7.5 cm
Circumference of pulmonary valve	8.5 cm
Circumference of tricuspid valve	12 cm
Intestines	
Length of duodenum	30 cm
Total length of small intestine	550–650 cm
Length of large intestine	150–170 cm
Kidneys	
Weight each (in males)	150 gm
Weight each (in females)	135 gm
Liver	
Weight (in males)	1400–1600 (1500) gm
Weight (in females)	1200–1400 (1300) gm
Lungs	
Weight (right lung)	375–500 (450) gm
Weight (left lung)	325–450 (400) gm

Contd...

Table A-III.1	Weights and measurements of normal organs. (Contd...)
ORGAN	**IN ADULTS**
Oesophagus	
Length (cricoid cartilage to cardia)	25 cm
Distance from incisors to gastro-oesophageal junction	40 cm
Ovaries	
Weight (each)	4–8 (6) gm
Pancreas	
Total weight	60–100 (80) gm
Weight of endocrine pancreas	1–1.5 gm
Pituitary gland (Hypophysis)	
Weight	500 mg
Placenta	
Weight at term	400–600 gm
Prostate	
Weight	20 gm
Spleen	
Weight	125–175 (150) gm
Stomach	
Length	25–30 cm
Testis and epididymis	
Weight each (in adults)	20–27 gm
Thymus	
Weight	5–10 gm
Thyroid	
Weight	15–40 gm
Uterus	
Weight (in nonpregnant woman)	35–40 gm

LABORATORY VALUES OF CLINICAL SIGNIFICANCE *(p. 916)*

The concept of 'normal values' and 'normal ranges' has been replaced by 'reference values' and 'reference limits' in which the variables for establishing the values for the reference population in a particular test are well defined.

In SI system, whole-unit multiple of three as power of ten is used (i.e. 10^3, 10^6, 10^9, 10^{12}, 10^{15}, 10^{18}).

| Table A-III.2 | Prefixes and conversion factors in SI system. | | | | |

PREFIX	PREFIX SYMBOL	FAC-TOR	UNITS OF LENGTH	UNITS OF WEIGHT	UNITS OF VOLUME
kilo-	k	10^3	kilometre (km)	kilogram (kg)	kilolitre (kl)
		1	metre (m)	gram (g)	litre (l)
deci-	d	10^{-1}	decimetre (dm)	decigram (dg)	decilitre (dl)
centi-	c	10^{-2}	centimetre (cm)	centigram (cg)	centilitre (cl)
milli-	m	10^{-3}	millimetre (mm)	milligram (mg)	millilitre (ml)
micro-	µ	10^{-6}	micrometre (µm)	microgram (µg)	microlitre (µl)
nano-	n	10^{-9}	nanometre (nm)	nanogram (ng)	nanolitre (nl)
pico-	p	10^{-12}	picometre (pm)	picogram (pg)	picolitre (pl)
femto-	f	10^{-15}	femtometre (fm)	femtogram (fg)	femtolitre (fl)
alto-	a	10^{-18}	altometre (am)	altogram (ag)	altolitre (al)

| Table A-III.3 | Clinical chemistry of blood. | |

COMPONENT	SPECIMEN	CONVENTIONAL RANGE
Aminotransferases (transaminases)	Serum	12–38 U/L
aspartate (AST, SGOT)	Serum	7–41 U/L
alanine (ALT, SGPT)		
Amylase	Serum	20–96 U/L
Bilirubin		
total	Serum	0.3–1.3 mg/dl
direct (conjugated)	Serum	0.1–0.4 mg/dl
indirect (unconjugated)	Serum	0.2–0.9 mg/dl
Calcium, total	Serum	8.7–10.2 mg/dl
Calcium, ionised	Whole blood	4.5–5.3 mg/dl
Chloride (Cl⁻)	Serum	102–109 mEq/L
Cholesterol	Serum	
total desirable for adults		<200 mg/dl
borderline high		200–239 mg/dl
high undesirable		≥240 mg/dl

Contd...

Table A-III.3	Clinical chemistry of blood. *(Contd...)*	
COMPONENT	**SPECIMEN**	**CONVENTIONAL RANGE**
LDL-cholesterol,	Serum	
desirable range		100–130 mg/dl
borderline high		130–159 mg/dl
high undesirable		≥160 mg/dl
HDL-cholesterol,		
protective range		>60 mg/dl
low		<40 mg/dl
triglycerides		<160 mg/dl
CO_2 content	Plasma	22–30 mEq/L (arterial)
Creatine kinase (CK), total	Serum	
males		51–294 U/L
females		39–238 IU/L
Creatine kinase-MB (CK-MB)	Serum	0–5.5 ng/ml
Creatinine	Serum	0.6–1.2 mg/dl
Gamma-glutamyl transpeptidase (transferase) (γ-GT)	Serum	9–58 IU/L
Gases, arterial		
Bicarbonate (HCO_3^-)	Whole blood	22–30 mEq/L
pH	Whole blood	7.35–7.45
P_{CO_2}	Whole blood	22–45 mmHg
P_{O_2}	Whole blood	72–104 mmHg
Glucose (fasting)	Plasma	
normal		70–100 mg/dl
impaired fasting glucose (IFG)		101–125 mg/dl
diabetes mellitus		≥126 mg/dl
Glucose (2-hr post-prandial)	Plasma	
normal		<140 mg/dl
impaired glucose tolerance (IGT)		140–200 mg/dl
diabetes mellitus		>200 mg/dl
Haemoglobin A_{1C}	Whole blood	4–6%
Lactate dehydrogenase (LDH)	Serum	115–221 U/L
Lactate/pyruvate ratio		10/1
Lipase	Serum	3–43 U/L
Lipoproteins	Serum	0–30 mg/dl
pH	Blood	7.35–7.45
Phosphatases		
acid phosphatase	Serum	0–5.5 U/L
alkaline phosphatase	Serum	33–96 U/L
Phosphorus, inorganic	Serum	2.5–4.3 mg/dl
Potassium	Serum	3.5–5.0 mEq/L
Prostate specific antigen (PSA)	Serum	0–4.0 ng/ml

Contd...

Table A-III.3   Clinical chemistry of blood. *(Contd...)*

COMPONENT	SPECIMEN	CONVENTIONAL RANGE
Proteins	Serum	
total		6.7–8.6 g/dl
albumin		3.5–5.5 g/dl (50–60%)
globulins		2.0–3.5 g/dl (40–50%)
A/G ratio		1.5–3 : 1
Sodium	Serum	136–146 mEq/L
Thyroid function tests		
radioactive iodine uptake (RAIU) 24-hr		5–30%
thyroxine (T_4) total	Serum	5.4–11.7 µg/dl
triiodothyronine (T_3) total	Serum	77–135 ng/dl
thyroid stimulating hormone (TSH)	Serum	0.4–5.0 µU/ml
Troponins, cardiac (cTn)		
troponin I (cTnI)	Serum	0–0.08 ng/ml
troponin T (cTnT)	Serum	0–0.01 ng/ml
Urea	Blood	20–40 mg/dl
Uric acid	Serum	
males		3.1–7.0 mg/dl
females		2.5–5.6 mg/dl

Table A-III.4   Other body fluids.

COMPONENT	SPECIMEN	CONVENTIONAL RANGE
Cerebrospinal fluid (CSF)	CSF	
CSF volume		120–150 ml
CSF pressure		60–150 mm water
leucocytes		0–5 lymphocytes/µl
pH		7.31–7.34
glucose		40–70 mg/dl
proteins		20–50 mg/dl
Glomerular filtration rate (GFR)	Urine	180 L/day (about 125 ml/min)
Microalbumin	24-hr urinary excretion	0–30 mg/24 hr
Seminal fluid	Semen	
liquefaction		Within 20 min
sperm morphology		>70% normal, mature spermatozoa
sperm motility		>60%
pH		>7.0 (average 7.7)
sperm count		60–150 million/ml
volume		1.5–5.0 ml

Contd...

Table A-III.4   Other body fluids. *(Contd...)*

COMPONENT	SPECIMEN	CONVENTIONAL RANGE
Urine examination	24-hr volume	600–1800 ml (variable)
pH	Urine	5.0–9.0
specific gravity, quantitative	Urine (random)	1.002–1.028 (mean 1.008)
protein excretion	24-hr urine	<150 mg/day
protein, qualitative	Urine (random)	Negative
glucose excretion, quantitative	24-hr urine	50–300 mg/day
glucose, qualitative	Urine (random)	Negative
porphobilinogen	Urine (random)	Negative
urobilinogen	24-hr urine	1.0–3.5 mg/day
microalbuminuria (24 hour)		0–30 mg/24 hr (0–30 μg/mg creatinine)
Urobilinogen	Urine (random)	Present in 1: 20 dilution

Table A-III.5   Normal haematologic values.

COMPONENT	SPECIMEN	CONVENTIONAL RANGE
Erythrocytes and Haemoglobin		
Erythrocyte count	Blood	
males		4.5–6.5×10^{12}/L (mean 5.5×10^{12}/L)
females		3.8–5.8×10^{12}/L (mean 4.8×10^{12}/L)
Erythrocyte diameter		6.7–7.7 μm (mean 7.2 μm)
Erythrocyte thickness		
peripheral		2.4 μm
central		1.0 μm
Erythrocyte indices (Absolute values)	Blood	
mean corpuscular haemoglobin (MCH)		27–32 pg
mean corpuscular volume (MCV)		77–93 fl
mean corpuscular haemoglobin concentration (MCHC)		30–35 g/dl
Erythrocyte life-span	Blood	120±30 days
Erythrocyte sedimentation rate (ESR)	Blood	
Westergren 1st hr,		
males		0–15 mm 1st hour
females		0–20 mm 1st hour
Wintrobe, 1st hr,		
males		0–9 mm 1st hour
females		0–20 mm 1st hour

Contd...

| Table A-III.5 | Normal haematologic values. *(Contd...)* |

COMPONENT	SPECIMEN	CONVENTIONAL RANGE
Ferritin	Serum	
males		30–250 ng/ml
females		10–150 ng/ml
Folate		
body stores		2–3 mg
daily requirement		100–200 µg
red cell level	Red cells	150–450 ng/ml
serum level	Serum	6–18 ng/ml
Haematocrit (PCV)	Blood	
males		40–54%
females		37–47%
Haemoglobin (Hb)		
adult haemoglobin (HbA)	Whole blood	95–98%
males		13.0–18.0 g/dl
females		11.5–16.5 g/dl
plasma Hb (quantitative)		0.5–5 mg/dl
haemoglobin A_2 (HbA$_2$)		1.5–3.5%
haemoglobin, foetal (HbF)		
in adults		<0–2%
HbF, children under 6 months		<5%
Iron, total	Serum	40–140 µg/dl
total iron binding capacity (TIBC)	Serum	250–406 µg/dl
iron saturation	Serum	20–45% (mean 33%)
Iron, storage form (ferritin and haemosiderin)		30% of body iron
Osmotic fragility	Blood	
slight haemolysis		at 0.45 to 0.39 g/dl NaCl
complete haemolysis		at 0.33 to 0.36 g/dl NaCl
mean corpuscular fragility		0.4–0.45 g/dl NaCl
Reticulocytes	Blood	
adults		0.5–2.5%
infants		2–6%
Transferrin	Serum	200–400 mg/dl
Vitamine B$_{12}$		
body stores		10–12 mg
daily requirement		2–4 µg
serum level	Serum	280–1000 pg/ml
Leucocytes		
Differential leucocyte count (DLC)	Blood film/CBC counter	
P (polymorphs or neutrophils)		40–75% (2,000–7,500/µl)
L (lymphocytes)		20–50% (1,500–4,000/µl)
M (monocytes)		2–10% (200–800/µl)
E (eosinophils)		1–6% (40–400/µl)
B (basophils)		< 1% (10–100/µl)

Contd...

Table A-III.5   Normal haematologic values. *(Contd...)*

COMPONENT	SPECIMEN	CONVENTIONAL RANGE

Total leucocyte count (TLC)
  adults
  infants (full term, at birth)
  infants (1 year)
	Blood	4,000–11,000/µl
		10,000–25,000/µl
		6,000–16,000/µl

Platelets and Coagulation		

Bleeding time (BT)
  Ivy's method
  template method
	Prick blood	2–7 min
		2.5–9.5 min

Clot retraction time
Clotted blood
  qualitative
 	
  quantitative
		Visible in 60 min
		(complete in <24–hr)
		48–64% (55%)

Clotting time (CT) Lee and White method	Whole blood	4–9 min at 37°C

Partial thromboplastin time
  with kaolin (PTTK) or
  activated partial thrombo-
  plastin time (APTT)
	Plasma	30–40 sec

Platelet count	Blood	150,000–400,000/µl
Prothrombin time (PT) (Quick's one-stage method)	Plasma	10–14 sec

Index

The page numbers given below indicate the first page at the beginning of the topic only.